Respiratory Medicine

Series Editors

Sharon I. S. Rounds
Alpert Medical School of Brown University
Providence, RI, USA

Anne Dixon
University of Vermont, College of Medical
Burlington, VT, USA

Lynn M. Schnapp
Medical University of South Carolina
Charleston, SC, USA

More information about this series at http://www.springer.com/series/7665

Jose L. Gomez • Blanca E. Himes
Naftali Kaminski
Editors

Precision in Pulmonary, Critical Care, and Sleep Medicine

A Clinical and Research Guide

We help the world breathe®
PULMONARY · CRITICAL CARE · SLEEP

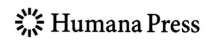

Editors
Jose L. Gomez, MD, MS, ATSF
Assistant Professor Pulmonary, Critical
Care and Sleep Medicine Section
Department of Medicine
Yale University School of Medicine
New Haven, CT
USA

Blanca E. Himes, PhD
Assistant Professor of Informatics
Department of Biostatistics,
Epidemiology and Informatics
University of Pennsylvania
Philadelphia, PA
USA

Naftali Kaminski, MD, FERS, ATSF
Boehringer-Ingelheim Endowed
Professor of Internal Medicine
Chief of Pulmonary, Critical Care
and Sleep Medicine
Yale University School of Medicine
New Haven, CT
USA

ISSN 2197-7372   ISSN 2197-7380   (electronic)
Respiratory Medicine
ISBN 978-3-030-31506-1   ISBN 978-3-030-31507-8   (eBook)
https://doi.org/10.1007/978-3-030-31507-8

This Humana imprint is published by the registered company Springer Nature Switzerland AG
The registered company address is: Gewerbestrasse 11, 6330 Cham, Switzerland

Preface

Precision medicine is rooted in the principle of individual variability and the design of diagnostic, preventive and therapeutic strategies to address the needs of each person. The commoditization of high-throughput assays for many types of biological data coupled with advances in imaging, sensors, data science and computing has enabled studies that seek to better understand the molecular basis underlying diseases. Most notably, such approaches are helping to redefine diseases based on the identification of groups of patients with similarities in molecular pathways that lead to common symptoms and presentations of what are increasingly recognized as heterogeneous conditions, including asthma, chronic obstructive pulmonary disease (COPD), interstitial lung disease (ILD) and lung cancer. As molecular similarities in groups of patients are identified, tailored preventive and therapeutic approaches can be designed. Inspired by the recent progress and transformative potential of precision medicine, this textbook presents its current state in pulmonary, critical care and sleep medicine.

Leading clinicians and researchers with expertise in precision medicine contributed valuable insights on various related topics, including genetics, molecular biomarkers, imaging, sensors, mobile health, phenotyping and therapeutics. With Springer's help, we assembled contributions on these key themes as applied to pulmonary, critical care and sleep medicine, and we edited this book to summarize related advances and knowledge gaps. The intended audience is healthcare providers and researchers who specialize in one or more pulmonary, critical care or sleep-related discipline(s). Both trainees and established clinicians and investigators will gain insights, as the topics presented are current.

Precision medicine will have an increasing impact on the practice and science of medicine, and we hope that this book will serve as a central resource for the implementation of precision medicine in pulmonary, critical care and sleep disorders for years to come. We are also hopeful that progress in precision medicine will become more symmetric and inclusive of *all* to decrease health disparities.

New Haven, CT, USA   Jose L. Gomez, MD
Philadelphia, PA, USA   Blanca E. Himes, PhD
New Haven, CT, USA   Naftali Kaminski, MD

Contents

Contributors

Samuel Y. Ash, MD, MPH Pulmonary and Critical Care Medicine, Brigham and Women's Hospital, Boston, MA, USA

Brett C. Bade, MD Section of Pulmonary, Critical Care, and Sleep Medicine, Department of Internal Medicine, Yale School of Medicine, New Haven, CT, USA

Stephen R. Baldassarri, MD, MHS Department of Internal Medicine, Section of Pulmonary, Critical Care, and Sleep Medicine, Yale School of Medicine, New Haven, CT, USA

Fabio Balli, MAS, GradD Breathing Games, Geneva, Switzerland
Concordia University, Montreal, QC, Canada

Hanne Beeckmans, MD KU Leuven and University Hospitals Leuven, Department of Chronic Diseases, Metabolism and Ageing (CHROMETA), Division of Respiratory Diseases, Lung Transplant Unit, Leuven, Belgium

Jessica Bon, MD, MS Division of Pulmonary, Allergy and Critical Care Medicine, Department of Medicine, University of Pittsburgh, Pittsburgh, PA, USA

Yohan Bossé, PhD Institut universitaire de cardiologie et de pneumologie de Québec, Québec, Canada
Department of Molecular Medicine, Laval University, Québec, Canada

Clemente J. Britto, MD Adult Cystic Fibrosis Program, Center for Pulmonary Infection Research and Treatment (CPIRT), Section of Pulmonary, Critical Care & Sleep Medicine, Department of Internal Medicine, Yale University, New Haven, CT, USA

Joshua D. Campbell, PhD Division of Computational Biomedicine, Department of Medicine, Boston University Medical Center, Bioinformatics Program, Boston University, Boston, MA, USA

Juan C. Celedón, MD, DrPH, ATSF Medicine, Epidemiology and Human Genetics, University of Pittsburgh, Pittsburgh, PA, USA
Pediatric Pulmonary Medicine, Children's Hospital of Pittsburgh of UPMC, Pittsburgh, PA, USA

Michael H. Cho, MD, MPH Channing Division of Network Medicine, Division of Pulmonary and Critical Care Medicine, Brigham and Women's Hospital, Harvard Medical School, Boston, MA, USA

Charles S. Dela Cruz, MD, PhD Yale School of Medicine, Department of Internal Medicine, Section of Pulmonary, Critical Care, and Sleep Medicine and Department of Microbial Pathogenesis, New Haven, CT, USA

Karen C. Dugan, MD Kaiser Permanente, Pulmonary and Critical Care, Portland, OR, USA

Oliver Eickelberg, MD Division of Pulmonary Sciences and Critical Care Medicine, Department of Medicine, University of Colorado, Aurora, CO, USA

Raúl San José Estépar, PhD Radiology, Brigham and Women's Hospital, Boston, MA, USA

Isis E. Fernandez, MD, PhD Comprehensive Pneumology Center, Ludwig-Maximilians-University and Helmholtz Zentrum München, Member of the German Center for Lung Research, Munich, Germany

Finbar T. Foley, MD Section of Pulmonary, Critical Care, and Sleep Medicine, Department of Internal Medicine, Yale School of Medicine, New Haven, CT, USA

Anna E. Frick, MD KU Leuven and University Hospitals Leuven, Department of Chronic Diseases, Metabolism and Ageing (CHROMETA), Division of Respiratory Diseases, Lung Transplant Unit, Leuven, Belgium

Catherine A. Gao, MD Yale School of Medicine, Department of Internal Medicine, New Haven, CT, USA

Samir Gautam, MD, PhD Yale School of Medicine, Department of Internal Medicine, Section of Pulmonary, Critical Care, and Sleep Medicine, New Haven, CT, USA

Jose L. Gomez, MD, MS, ATSF Pulmonary, Critical Care and Sleep Medicine Section, Department of Medicine, Yale University School of Medicine, New Haven, CT, USA

Tobias Heigl, MSc KU Leuven and University Hospitals Leuven, Department of Chronic Diseases, Metabolism and Ageing (CHROMETA), Division of Respiratory Diseases, Lung Transplant Unit, Leuven, Belgium

Erica L. Herzog, MD, PhD Section of Pulmonary, Critical Care and Sleep Medicine, Department of Internal Medicine, Yale School of Medicine, New Haven, CT, USA

Blanca E. Himes, PhD Department of Biostatistics, Epidemiology and Informatics, University of Pennsylvania, Philadelphia, PA, USA

Shyoko Honiden, MSc, MD Yale School of Medicine, New Haven, CT, USA

John C. Huston, MD Yale School of Medicine, Department of Internal Medicine, New Haven, CT, USA

Janne Kaes, MSc KU Leuven and University Hospitals Leuven, Department of Chronic Diseases, Metabolism and Ageing (CHROMETA), Division of Respiratory Diseases, Lung Transplant Unit, Leuven, Belgium

Naftali Kaminski, MD Pulmonary, Critical Care and Sleep Medicine, Department of Medicine, Yale University School of Medicine, New Haven, CT, USA

Mengyuan Kan, PhD Department of Biostatistics, Epidemiology and Informatics, University of Pennsylvania, Philadelphia, PA, USA

Rachel S. Kelly, BSc(Hons), MPH, PhD Systems Genetics and Genomics Unit, Channing Division of Network Medicine, Brigham and Women's Hospital, Harvard Medical School, Boston, MA, USA

Jonathan A. Kropski, MD Division of Allergy, Pulmonary and Critical Care Medicine, Department of Medicine, Vanderbilt University Medical Center, Nashville, TN, USA

Department of Cell and Developmental Biology, Vanderbilt University, Nashville, TN, USA

Department of Veterans Affairs Medical Center, Nashville, TN, USA

Yukiko Kunitomo, MD Yale University School of Medicine, Department of Internal Medicine, New Haven, CT, USA

Simon P. F. Lambden, MBBS, PhD NIHR Clinical Lecturer in Intensive Care Medicine, Department of Medicine, University of Cambridge School of Clinical Medicine, Cambridge, UK

Peter S. Marshall, MD, MPH Yale School of Medicine, Section of Pulmonary, Critical Care & Sleep Medicine, New Haven, CT, USA

Susan K. Mathai, MD Interstitial Lung Disease Program, Center for Advanced Heart & Lung Disease, Baylor University Medical Center at Dallas, Dallas, TX, USA

Department of Internal Medicine, Texas A&M University College of Medicine, Dallas, TX, USA

Nuala J. Meyer, MD, MS Pulmonary, Allergy, and Critical Care Division, University of Pennsylvania Perelman School of Medicine, Hospital of the University of Pennsylvania, Philadelphia, PA, USA

Emmet O'Brien, MD, PhD Department of Medicine, Beaumont Hospital, Dublin, Ireland

William M. Oldham, MD, PhD Division of Pulmonary and Critical Care Medicine, Brigham and Women's Hospital, Boston, MA, USA

Sofie Ordies, MD KU Leuven and University Hospitals Leuven, Department of Chronic Diseases, Metabolism and Ageing (CHROMETA), Division of Respiratory Diseases, Lung Transplant Unit, Leuven, Belgium

Victor E. Ortega, MD, PhD Department of Internal Medicine, Center for Precision Medicine, Wake Forest School of Medicine, Medical Center Boulevard, Winston-Salem, NC, USA

Allan I. Pack, MBChB, PhD Division of Sleep Medicine/Department of Medicine, University of Pennsylvania Perelman School of Medicine, Translational Research Laboratories, Philadelphia, PA, USA

Bhakti K. Patel, MD University of Chicago, Department of Medicine, Section of Pulmonary and Critical Care, Chicago, IL, USA

Margaret Ann Pisani, MD, MPH Yale School of Medicine, New Haven, CT, USA

Farbod Nick Rahaghi, MD, PhD Division of Pulmonary and Critical Care Medicine, Brigham and Women's Hospital, Boston, MA, USA

Angela J. Rogers, MD Department of Medicine, Stanford University, Palo Alto, CA, USA

Annelore Sacreas, MSc KU Leuven and University Hospitals Leuven, Department of Chronic Diseases, Metabolism and Ageing (CHROMETA), Division of Respiratory Diseases, Lung Transplant Unit, Leuven, Belgium

Berta Saez, MD, PhD KU Leuven and University Hospitals Leuven, Department of Chronic Diseases, Metabolism and Ageing (CHROMETA), Division of Respiratory Diseases, Lung Transplant Unit, Leuven, Belgium

David A. Schwartz, MD Department of Medicine, University of Colorado School of Medicine, Aurora, CO, USA

Frank C. Sciurba, MD Department of Medicine, Beaumont Hospital, Dublin, Ireland

Don D. Sin, MD, MPH University of British Columbia Centre for Heart Lung Innovation (HLI), Department of Medicine, St. Paul's Hospital, Vancouver, BC, Canada

Inderjit Singh, MD Division of Pulmonary, Critical Care and Sleep Medicine, Division of Applied Hemodynamics, Yale New Haven Hospital, New Haven, CT, USA

Katrina Steiling, MD, MSc Division of Computational Biomedicine, Department of Medicine, Boston University Medical Center, Bioinformatics Program, Boston University, The Pulmonary Center, Boston University Medical Center, Boston, MA, USA

Kathleen A. Stringer, PharmD Department of Clinical Pharmacy, College of Pharmacy and Division of Pulmonary and Critical Care Medicine, Department of Medicine, School of Medicine, University of Michigan, Ann Arbor, MI, USA

Charlotte Summers, BM, PhD University Lecturer in Intensive Care Medicine, Department of Medicine, University of Cambridge School of Clinical Medicine, Cambridge, UK

Lynn T. Tanoue, MD Section of Pulmonary, Critical Care, and Sleep Medicine, Department of Internal Medicine, Yale School of Medicine, New Haven, CT, USA

Patricia Valda Toro, MSc Yale School of Medicine, New Haven, CT, USA

Sze Man Tse, MDCM, MPH Department of Pediatrics, Sainte-Justine University Hospital Center, Montreal, QC, Canada

University of Montreal, Montreal, QC, Canada

Anke Van Herck, MD KU Leuven and University Hospitals Leuven, Department of Chronic Diseases, Metabolism and Ageing (CHROMETA), Division of Respiratory Diseases, Lung Transplant Unit, Leuven, Belgium

Bart M. Vanaudenaerde, MSc, PhD Department of Chronic Diseases, Metabolism and Ageing (CHROMETA), Lab of Respiratory Diseases, Lung Transplantation Unit, KU Leuven and UZ Leuven, Leuven, Belgium

Arno Vanstapel, MD KU Leuven and University Hospitals Leuven, Department of Chronic Diseases, Metabolism and Ageing (CHROMETA), Division of Respiratory Diseases, Lung Transplant Unit, Leuven, Belgium

Geert M. Verleden, MD, PhD KU Leuven and University Hospitals Leuven, Department of Chronic Diseases, Metabolism and Ageing (CHROMETA), Division of Respiratory Diseases, Lung Transplant Unit, Leuven, Belgium

Stijn E. Verleden, MSc, PhD KU Leuven and University Hospitals Leuven, Department of Chronic Diseases, Metabolism and Ageing (CHROMETA), Division of Respiratory Diseases, Lung Transplant Unit, Leuven, Belgium

Robin Vos, MD, PhD KU Leuven and University Hospitals Leuven, Department of Chronic Diseases, Metabolism and Ageing (CHROMETA), Division of Respiratory Diseases, Lung Transplant Unit, Leuven, Belgium

George R. Washko, MD, MS Pulmonary and Critical Care Medicine, Brigham and Women's Hospital, Boston, MA, USA

Chris H. Wendt, MD Pulmonary, Critical Care and Sleep Medicine, University of Minnesota, Minneapolis VAMC, Minneapolis, MN, USA

Julia Winkler, BS Section of Pulmonary, Critical Care and Sleep Medicine, Department of Internal Medicine, Yale School of Medicine, New Haven, CT, USA

Ann Chen Wu, MD, MPH PRecisiOn Medicine Translational Research (PROMoTeR) Center, Department of Population Medicine, Harvard Medical School, Boston, MA, USA

Sherrie Xie, BS Department of Biostatistics, Epidemiology and Informatics, University of Pennsylvania, Philadelphia, PA, USA

Part I

Introduction

Introduction

Jose L. Gomez, Naftali Kaminski,
and Blanca E. Himes

The goal of precision has been at the center of medicine for centuries. Hippocrates', and more broadly Greek medicine's, contribution to the practice of medicine ca 460–370 BC was the realization that diseases arise from natural causes rather than via divine curse [1]. Based on this principle, diseases were subject to scientific study and observations made via physical examination became a centerpiece in the practice of medicine [1]. Centuries later, Vesalius's anatomical studies summarized in the publication *De Humanis Corporis Fabrica* (*On the Structure of the Human Body*, Fig. 1.1) transformed medical knowledge by propagating insights obtained through human dissection [1]. These two early examples, first, of how a conceptual shift can lead to changes in practice and second, how new methods and dissemination of knowledge can transform a field, are foundational concepts that apply to *precision medicine*.

Thomas Sydenham (1624–1689) brought additional conceptual changes to the medical sciences through his foundational work in nosology, a term derived from the Greek roots *nosos*, meaning 'disease' and *logia*, meaning 'study of'. Nosology is the branch of medical science that deals with the concept, definition, classification and nomenclature of diseases [1], and one of Sydenham's principles remains at the center of modern medicine: 'the manifestations that are constant in each patient with a particular disease should be distinguished from other phenomena that could be due to the age, constitution, or treatment of the patient'. Thanks to incremental conceptual and technical advances in the modern period of Western civilization, including the development of the stethoscope by Laennec and growth of medical schools with subsequent global dissemination of knowledge, medicine transitioned from a descriptive, observational practice into a discipline centered on the investigation of causes of disease using experimental approaches [1]. This conceptual shift that experimental methods should be used to study disease and health established the scientific foundation of medicine of the past 150 years.

The first half of the twentieth century saw important diagnostic developments that arose from research in the physical sciences, such as X-rays [2], and therapeutic developments that

J. L. Gomez (✉)
Pulmonary, Critical Care and Sleep Medicine Section, Department of Medicine, Yale University School of Medicine, New Haven, CT, USA
e-mail: jose.gomez-villalobos@yale.edu

N. Kaminski
Pulmonary, Critical Care and Sleep Medicine, Department of Medicine, Yale University School of Medicine, New Haven, CT, USA
e-mail: naftali.kaminski@yale.edu

B. E. Himes
Department of Biostatistics, Epidemiology and Informatics, University of Pennsylvania, Philadelphia, PA, USA
e-mail: bhimes@pennmedicine.upenn.edu

© Springer Nature Switzerland AG 2020
J. L. Gomez et al. (eds.), *Precision in Pulmonary, Critical Care, and Sleep Medicine*, Respiratory Medicine, https://doi.org/10.1007/978-3-030-31507-8_1

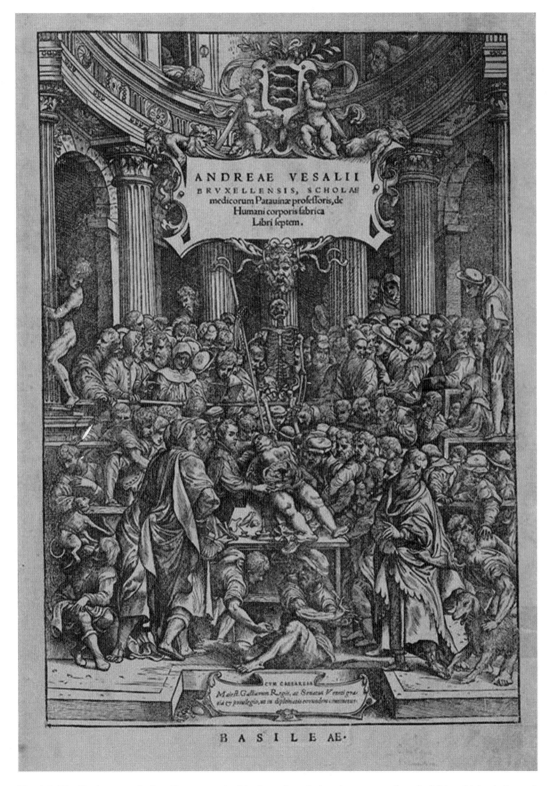

Fig. 1.1 Vesalius's anatomical studies summarized in the publication *De Humanis Corporis Fabrica* (*On the Structure of the Human Body*) transformed medical knowledge by propagating insights obtained through human dissection. (Courtesy of Yale University, Harvey Cushing/John Hay Whitney Medical Library)

arose from research in microbiology, such as anti-biotics [3]. These transformative advances led to the recognition that the medical sciences could not grow in isolation, but rather, medicine could benefit from advances in other scientific disciplines. Under this principle, the medical sciences in the second half of the twentieth century borrowed heavily from rapid advances in genetics, including the use of recombinant DNA for the synthesis of insulin [4] and the identification of genetic variation leading to diseases such as cystic fibrosis [5]. The integration of medicine and genetics has grown even stronger during the past two decades, following the completion of the Human Genome Project [6, 7]. More broadly, medicine has increasingly become interdisciplinary in nature and technology has more rapidly been developed for, and integrated into, the practice of medicine.

Advances in high-throughput biotechnologies have enabled the collection of an unprecedentedly large number of so-called *omics* datasets by biomedical researchers. Starting with DNA microarrays in the 1990s and expanding to next-generation sequencing (NGS) in the 2000s, omics approaches capture a wide variety of biological measurements, including DNA variation and modifications, expression of transcripts and levels of proteins and metabolites [8–10]. As the repertoire of available omics approaches continues to expand to include single-cell technologies and measures of 3D configuration of DNA, the full characterization of biological systems at ever-increasing resolutions is possible [11–13]. Early successes in the use of omics technologies to understand disease and enable drug development [14, 15] have resulted in optimism that many more effective diagnostic tests and treatments tailored to a person's genetic, environmental and lifestyle factors will be developed. Concurrently, there is increased recognition that the molecular mechanisms driving complex diseases differ among patients as does response to therapy and predisposition to adverse effects. *Precision medicine*, also referred to as *personalized medicine*, is a vision of medicine that incorporates person-specific genetic and molecular information to guide the prevention of disease and therapeutic strategies [15, 16].

In addition to benefiting from advances in genetics and other omics technologies that enable the collection of large datasets representing layers of biological data, precision medicine is made possible by developments in computing [17] and the creation of sophisticated algorithms to analyze single modality data as well as integrate heterogeneous datasets [18–20]. The exponential growth in computational processing power predicted by Moore's law [21] has led to changes across many aspects of modern life, including medicine (Fig. 1.2). Some specialties, such as radiology, stand out as having benefited from the early integration of computing in their practice [22]. The consulting firm Frost & Sullivan estimated that by 2016 medical imaging alone had generated 1 exabyte (i.e., 1 billion gigabytes) of data [23]. Omics data also requires advanced computing resources for its storage and analysis to enable the generation of insights that impact our knowledge of biology and disease [24–26]. The increasing salience of this need is evidenced by the exponential growth of human genomic data that has followed the decreasing costs of DNA sequencing (Fig. 1.3) [27].

Important ethical and social challenges arise in precision medicine [28]. For medicine to be precise, the preferences, health behavior and social determinants of each person must be taken into account [29]. Although clinicians and researchers are often aware of this well-established aspect of medicine [30], careful consideration for how it applies to precision medicine is warranted. For example, the development of precision medicine must include input and participation of diverse populations to ensure precision medicine will work for *all*, including those who are at peak risk for various diseases. Another concern regarding the proliferation of precision diagnostics and therapies is that individuals of the lowest socioeconomic groups will not be able to afford them, rendering them unable to advance health for all.

The impact of precision medicine is recognized across all medical specialties, including pulmonary, critical care and sleep medicine [31–39]. Using Collins and Varmus's definition of precision medicine as 'prevention and treatment

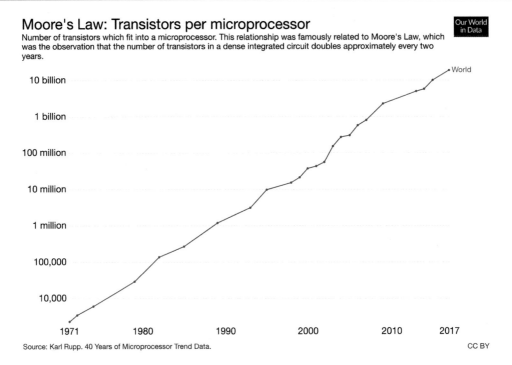

Fig. 1.2 The exponential growth in computational processing power predicted by Moore's law has led to changes across many aspects of modern life, including medicine. (Reproduced under Creative Commons License CC-BY4.0: https://creativecommons.org/licenses/by/4.0/deed.en_US)

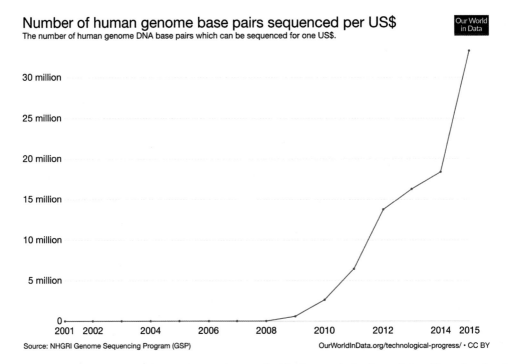

Fig. 1.3 The cost of DNA sequencing has decreased dramatically over the last decade, enabling the generation of large amounts of data in a cost-efficient manner to power the big data revolution in medicine. (Reproduced under Creative Commons License CC-BY4.0: https://creativecommons.org/licenses/by/4.0/deed.en_US)

strategies that take individual variability into account' [15], we can build a framework that includes use of technology, science and the humanities to guide our understanding, development and implementation of precision medicine. We have adhered to this framework across the book, and each chapter provides specific details on how to integrate different strategies to solve clinical problems in pulmonary, critical care and sleep medicine. The chapters also provide an overview of how to account for individual variability through improved phenotyping, molecular and imaging characterization as well as clinical practice to improve disease outcomes. As ongoing research efforts provide insights by integrating multi-omics datasets, and these insights enable the discovery of novel drug targets and preventive strategies, a major shift in pulmonary precision medicine that benefits all people will occur.

References

1. Walker HK. The origins of the history and physical examination. In: Walker HK, Hall WD, Hurst JW, editors. Clinical methods: the history, physical, and laboratory examinations. Boston: Butterworths; 2011.
2. Assmus A. Early history of X rays. Beam Line. 1995;25(2):10–24.
3. Aminov RI. A brief history of the antibiotic era: lessons learned and challenges for the future. Front Microbiol. 2010;1:134.
4. Institute of medicine (US) committee on technological innovation in medicine. In: Rosenberg N, Gelijns AC, Dawkins H, editors. Incentives and focus in university and industrial research: the case of synthetic insulin. USA: National Academies Press; 1995.
5. Kerem B, Rommens JM, Buchanan JA, et al. Identification of the cystic fibrosis gene: genetic analysis. Science. 1989;245(4922):1073–80.
6. Lander ES, Linton LM, Birren B, et al. Initial sequencing and analysis of the human genome. Nature. 2001;409(6822):860–921.
7. Venter JC, Adams MD, Myers EW, et al. The sequence of the human genome. Science. 2001;291(5507):1304–51.
8. Duggan DJ, Bittner M, Chen Y, Meltzer P, Trent JM. Expression profiling using cDNA microarrays. Nat Genet. 1999;21(1 Suppl):10–4.
9. Mardis ER. Next-generation DNA sequencing methods. Annu Rev Genomics Hum Genet. 2008;9:387–402.
10. Altelaar AFM, Munoz J, Heck AJR. Next-generation proteomics: towards an integrative view of proteome dynamics. Nat Rev Genet. 2013;14(1):35–48.
11. Ramani V, Shendure J, Duan Z. Understanding spatial genome organization: methods and insights. Genomics Proteomics Bioinf. 2016;14(1):7–20.
12. Saliba A-E, Westermann AJ, Gorski SA, Vogel J. Single-cell RNA-seq: advances and future challenges. Nucleic Acids Res. 2014;42(14):8845–60.
13. Yardımcı GG, Noble WS. Software tools for visualizing Hi-C data. Genome Biol. 2017;18(1):26.
14. Plenge RM, Scolnick EM, Altshuler D. Validating therapeutic targets through human genetics. Nat Rev Drug Discov. 2013;12(8):581–94.
15. Collins FS, Varmus H. A new initiative on precision medicine. N Engl J Med. 2015;372(9):793–5.
16. Nimmesgern E, Benediktsson I, Norstedt I. Personalized medicine in Europe [Internet]. Clin Transl Sci. 2017;10(2):61–3. https://doi.org/10.1111/cts.12446.
17. Hansen J, Iyengar R. Computation as the mechanistic bridge between precision medicine and systems therapeutics. Clin Pharmacol Ther. 2013;93(1):117–28.
18. Ritchie MD, Holzinger ER, Li R, Pendergrass SA, Kim D. Methods of integrating data to uncover genotype-phenotype interactions. Nat Rev Genet. 2015;16(2):85–97.
19. Brookes AJ, Robinson PN. Human genotype–phenotype databases: aims, challenges and opportunities. Nat Rev Genet. 2015;16:702.
20. Moore JH, Boland MR, Camara PG, et al. Preparing next-generation scientists for biomedical big data: artificial intelligence approaches. Per Med. 2019;16(3):247–57.
21. Moore GE, Others. Cramming more components onto integrated circuits [Internet]. 1965. Available from: https://www.funkschau.de/uploads/media_uploads/documents/1429521922-13-gordonmoore1965article.pdf.
22. Bradley WG. History of medical imaging. Proc Am Philos Soc. 2008;152(3):349–61.
23. Frost.com|Medical imaging & informatics [Internet]. 2019. Available from: http://www.frost.com/c/10280/home.do.
24. Alyass A, Turcotte M, Meyre D. From big data analysis to personalized medicine for all: challenges and opportunities. BMC Med Genet. 2015;8:33.
25. Rajkomar A, Dean J, Kohane I. Machine learning in medicine. N Engl J Med. 2019;380(14):1347–58.
26. Schmidt B, Hildebrandt A. Next-generation sequencing: big data meets high performance computing. Drug Discov Today. 2017;22(4):712–7.
27. Goodwin S, McPherson JD, McCombie WR. Coming of age: ten years of next-generation sequencing technologies. Nat Rev Genet. 2016;17(6):333–51.
28. Juengst ET, Settersten RA Jr, Fishman JR, McGowan ML. After the revolution? Ethical and social challenges in "personalized genomic medicine". Per Med. 2012;9(4):429–39.

29. Glasgow RE, Kwan BM, Matlock DD. Realizing the full potential of precision health: the need to include patient-reported health behavior, mental health, social determinants, and patient preferences data. J Clin Transl Sci. 2018;2(3):183–5.

30. Seeman MV, Becker RE. Osler and the way we were taught. Med Sci Educ. 2017;27(3):555–7.

31. Steiling K, Christenson SA. Targeting 'types: precision medicine in pulmonary disease. Am J Respir Crit Care Med. 2015;191(10):1093–4.

32. Politi K, Herbst RS. Lung cancer in the era of precision medicine. Clin Cancer Res. 2015;21(10):2213–20.

33. Maher TM. Precision medicine in idiopathic pulmonary fibrosis. QJM. 2016;109(9):585–7.

34. Khalyfa A, Gileles-Hillel A, Gozal D. The challenges of precision medicine in obstructive sleep Apnea. Sleep Med Clin. 2016;11(2):213–26.

35. Gomez JL, Kaminski N. Toward precision medicine of symptom control in asthma. Am J Respir Crit Care Med. 2017;195(2):147–8.

36. Wu AC, Kiley JP, Noel PJ, et al. Current status and future opportunities in lung precision medicine research with a focus on biomarkers. An American Thoracic Society/National Heart, Lung, and Blood Institute Research Statement. Am J Respir Crit Care Med. 2018;198(12):e116–36.

37. Savale L, Guignabert C, Weatherald J, Humbert M. Precision medicine and personalising therapy in pulmonary hypertension: seeing the light from the dawn of a new era. Eur Respir Rev [Internet]. 2018;27(148):180004. Available from: https://doi.org/10.1183/16000617.0004-2018.

38. Zhang H, Li Y, Slutsky AS. Precision medicine for cell therapy in acute respiratory distress syndrome. Lancet Respir Med. 2019;7(4):e13.

39. Hersh CP, Adcock IM, Celedón JC, et al. High-throughput sequencing in respiratory, critical care, and sleep medicine research. An official American Thoracic Society workshop report. Ann Am Thorac Soc. 2019;16(1):1–16.

Part II

Genetics

Differential Diagnosis of Diffuse Pulmonary Disorders Using Genetics

2

Jonathan A. Kropski

Key Point Summary

- In multiple clinical scenarios, establishing a genetic diagnosis of a pulmonary disease can impact clinical care of affected patients and their relatives.
- Genetic evaluation of patients with pulmonary diseases should be performed in coordination with genetic counselors with disease-specific experience.
- Interpretation of genetic information in a clinical context remains challenging, particularly because of the frequent identification of ultra-rare, novel variants of uncertain significance.
- Genotype-driven precision therapies are available or under study for patients with cystic fibrosis, pulmonary alveolar proteinosis, pulmonary Langerhans cell histiocytosis, and alpha-1 antitrypsin disease.

Introduction

Through the past several decades, there has been dramatic progress in defining genetic risk for a wide variety of lung diseases. These advances have led to remarkable insights into disease pathobiology, facilitated biomarker development, provided prognostic information to clinicians, and are now rapidly being translated into precision therapies.

While a decade ago the role of genetics in the evaluation of pulmonary disease was largely restricted to the research realm, the development of massively parallel next-generation sequencing technologies [1–3] has led to a rapid increase of recognized genetic causes of a variety of pulmonary diseases: mutations in more than 50 different genes have been linked to lung diseases. These studies have also revealed the complexity of genetic risk mechanisms; in particular, this work has demonstrated that mutations in a given gene may lead to multiple distinct phenotypes of pulmonary disease.

With growing understanding of discreet genetic risk mechanisms, there has been a rapid proliferation of commercially available pulmonary gene panels and other genetic tests. Below, we review the current state of genetic testing and evaluation in lung diseases and summarize how established genotype-phenotype relationships can inform the use of genetic information in the evaluation of patients with select diffuse pulmonary disorders.

J. A. Kropski (✉)
Division of Allergy, Pulmonary and Critical Care Medicine, Department of Medicine, Vanderbilt University Medical Center, Nashville, TN, USA

Department of Cell and Developmental Biology, Vanderbilt University, Nashville, TN, USA

Department of Veterans Affairs Medical Center, Nashville, TN, USA
e-mail: jon.kropski@vumc.org

© Springer Nature Switzerland AG 2020
J. L. Gomez et al. (eds.), *Precision in Pulmonary, Critical Care, and Sleep Medicine*, Respiratory Medicine, https://doi.org/10.1007/978-3-030-31507-8_2

Overview of Genetic Testing

"Genetic testing" is a broad term that refers to medical tests that evaluate for alterations in DNA sequence or structure that may be associated with risk for one or more diseases. Genetic testing can evaluate for mutations acquired in an individual (i.e., somatic mutations, most commonly tested for in the setting of cancer) or inherited (i.e., germline) mutations. In the context of evaluating for pulmonary diseases, testing for germline mutations is typically the relevant approach. The Genetics Home Reference (available at http://ghr.nlm.nih.gov) is an excellent resource that provides in-depth discussion of a variety of considerations related to genetic testing, including risks, benefits, costs, utility, and protections from genetic discrimination. Most authorities strongly recommend that patients undergo genetic counseling prior to performing any genetic test.

In the event that a genetic test is recommended, there are several different methods of genetic testing that can be performed: single gene sequencing/genotyping, targeted "panel" testing focused on relevant genes for a certain disease or phenotype, and whole-exome/whole-genome sequencing. Currently, panel-based testing is the most commonly used platform in most settings. A large number of laboratories currently offer different pulmonary-related gene panels, and their components change rapidly. In most cases, when a gene panel is requested, the DNA sample undergoes whole-exome sequencing, but only a targeted set of genes are analyzed to identify clinically relevant sequence variation. These gene panels generally have high sensitivity for detection of single-nucleotide variations (SNVs) and small insertions/deletions in the coding region of genes but, for technical reasons related to short-read sequencing methodology, have limited ability to detect structural variation (e.g., large insertions, deletions, or copy-number variations) and will not detect deep intronic or inter-genic variants. Thus, in general, a "positive" finding on a genetic test is informative, but a "negative" test does not exclude the possibility of genetic variants contributing to a given disease.

The American College of Medical Genetics has established a framework for reporting of results from genetic tests that assigns a likelihood of pathogenicity based on a variety of factors, including frequency of the variant in the general population, the effect of a variant on the protein sequence/structure, whether a given variant has been previously associated with the same phenotype, and, where available, functional studies of a given variant [4]. In general, variants that are novel or have very low frequency in the general population are more likely to be pathogenic. Variants that introduce frameshifts, premature termination codons, or alter splice donor/acceptor sites are generally considered pathogenic or likely pathogenic. Missense variations (i.e., those leading to a change in the amino acid sequence of the protein) are classified based on previous association with disease and/or functional studies and frequently are reported as "variants of uncertain significance." The interpretation and communication of findings for variants of uncertain significance remains one of the most challenging aspects of genetic testing today.

As the average individual carries approximately 200 monoallelic loss-of-function variants across the genome, and 2–3 de novo loss-of-function variants in the coding region of the genome (i.e., the exome) [1], in most cases, a Bayesian approach to genetic testing is advisable. By using clinical criteria to select cases in which a genetic cause is likely and specifically interrogating the genes most relevant for the given clinical scenario, the yield and positive predictive value of a genetic test can be maximized [5]. Next, we discuss genetics findings corresponding to diffuse pulmonary disorders that aid in the differential diagnosis of pediatric (Table 2.1) and adult (Table 2.2) patients.

Table 2.1 Genes with variants that are known to cause neonatal and pediatric diffuse pulmonary disorders

Gene symbol	Associated clinical features
SFTPB	Neonatal RDS, PAP
SFTPC	Neonatal RDS, PAP, adult ILD
ABCA3	Neonatal RDS, PAP
NKX2.1	Neonatal RDS, hypothyroidism, seizures, neuroendocrine hyperplasia of infancy
COPA	Autoantibodies, pulmonary hemorrhage, arthritis
TMEM173	Cutaneous vasculopathy, ILD, autoantibodies

RDS Respiratory distress syndrome, PAP Pulmonary alveolar proteinosis, ILD Interstitial lung disease

Table 2.2 Genes with variants that are associated with diffuse pulmonary disorders in adults

Disease	Gene symbols
PAP	CFSR2A, CFSR2B, MARS, GATA2
Cystic lung disease	
LAM	TSC1, TSC2
PLCH	BRAF (Somatic)
BHD	FCN
Bronchiectasis	
Cystic fibrosis	CFTR
PCD	Over 35 genes
A1AD	SERPINA1
ILD	TERT, TERC, RTEL1, PARN, TINF2, NAF1, HPS1, HPS2, HPS4, SFTPC, SFTPA2, ABCA3

PAP Pulmonary alveolar proteinosis, LAM Lymphangioleiomyomatosis, PLCH Pulmonary Langerhans cell histiocytosis, BHD Birt-Hogg-Dube, PCD Primary ciliary dyskinesia, A1AD Alpha-1 antitrypsin deficiency, ILD Interstitial lung disease

Neonatal Respiratory Distress Syndrome (RDS) and Diffuse Lung Disease in Childhood

Neonatal RDS is characterized by physical signs of impaired lung function (e.g., tachypnea, retractions) combined with a compatible chest radiograph demonstrating reticular infiltrates and/or air bronchograms [6]. Neonatal RDS is most frequently observed in preterm infants and in the era before surfactant replacement therapy had high morbidity and mortality. In premature neonates, risk for RDS is related largely to the stage of lung developmental maturation, and in term infants, RDS is uncommon [6]. The development of RDS in a term infant should prompt consideration of a potential genetic etiology. Mutations in a number of different genes have now been implicated in cases of neonatal RDS, including de novo mutations as well as those with autosomal dominant and recessive inheritance patterns.

Most of the mutations associated with neonatal RDS occur in genes related to surfactant biosynthesis, trafficking, or function [7]. The first locus linked to neonatal RDS was SFTPB [8], which encodes for surfactant protein B (SPB). SPB disease follows a recessive inheritance pattern, and biallelic mutations lead to low or absent levels of SPB protein. SFTPB mutations leading to SPB deficiency appear to be exceedingly rare (<1:100,000) and are associated with failure of trafficking of surfactant protein C (SPC) and functional surfactant deficiency [9]. SPB deficiency is almost uniformly fatal in the first year of life, although now a small number of cases, typically those in which one allele retains some SPB function, have been described as surviving beyond infancy [7].

Mutations in SFTPC, the gene encoding SPC, have also been identified in infants with RDS [10]. In contrast to SPB disease, SFTPC mutations are typically monoallelic and associated with a toxic gain-of-function mechanism [11–16]. The clinical presentation of SPC disease is substantially more variable than SPB disease; while neonatal RDS/childhood interstitial lung disease (ILD) is the typically presentation, there are reports of initial presentation in adults with pulmonary fibrosis [17, 18]. De novo and autosomal dominant inheritance patterns have been observed for SPC disease.

Mutations in the ATP binding cassette subfamily A member 3 (ABCA3) gene are the most prevalent genetic cause of RDS [7, 19–21]. Similar to SPB disease, RDS-associated *ABCA3* mutations are biallelic loss-of-function and contribute to disease by impairing surfactant processing and trafficking. Estimates based on population carrier rates suggest the prevalence of ABCA3 disease could be as high as 1 in 3000 live births [7]. There is good evidence that *ABCA3* genotypes influence biochemical and clinical phenotypes [22]. Studies using heterologous cell lines suggest there may be a critical threshold of ABCA3 function that is required for alveolar type II (AT2) cell homeostasis, and the disease phenotype may be related to retained ABCA3 activity [23]. For example, biallelic null mutations are almost uniformly fatal in the first few months of life, whereas survival into adolescence and beyond has been reported for genotypes with partially retained ABCA3 activity [7, 24].

Neonatal RDS has also been described in infants with "brain-thyroid-lung" syndrome, which results from mutations in *NKX2-1* [25, 26], the gene encoding thyroid transcription factor 1 (TTF-1), a homeobox transcription factor that is critical in lung development. *NKX2-1* mutations described to date have been monoallelic; it is not yet clear whether these mutations function primarily through a haploinsufficiency mechanism or gain-of-function. In contrast to SPB and ABCA3 disease, there is considerable heterogeneity of disease phenotype associated with *NKX2-1* mutations: neonatal RDS is common and often associated with hypothyroidism, but later onset disease has also been reported. *NKX2-1* mutations have also been described in families with a rare pulmonary disorder known as "neuroendocrine hyperplasia of infancy" [27], which is characterized by a dramatic increase in numbers of cells expressing neuroendocrine markers in distal airways. The mechanisms explaining these diverse presentations remain uncertain.

Mutations in several other genes have been linked to rarer pulmonary disorders of the neonatal period. Mutations in the transcription factor Forkhead Box F1 (*FOXF1*) have been reported in children with alveolar capillary dysplasia, a developmental disorder that may be associated with misalignment of the pulmonary veins [28]. The *FOXF1* locus appears subject to paternal imprinting [28, 29] and somatic mosaicism [30]; phenotypic variability within a given family carrying the same mutation has been reported [28]. Autoimmune arthritis, alveolar hemorrhage, and high-titer autoantibodies have been reported in children with mutations in the Coatomer Protein Complex Subunit Alpha (*COPA*) gene [31]. COPA syndrome is rare, but pulmonary involvement appears nearly ubiquitous and presents from the neonatal period to early childhood [32]. Mutations in *TMEM173*, encoding the stimulator of interferon genes protein (STING), have also been reported in children with a cutaneous vasculopathy and pulmonary involvement [33].

Together, these data suggest that an accurate genetic diagnosis may provide important prognostic information that can inform considerations around prolonged mechanical ventilation and lung transplantation. It is frequently most informative to perform sequencing of both an affected child and both parents to evaluate for *de novo* variants and enable phase determination when multiple variants are detected in a given gene. A key question for the field is when to integrate genetic evaluation in critically ill neonates, as despite advances in sequencing technology, cost remains considerable and results often take weeks to obtain.

Pulmonary Alveolar Proteinosis (PAP)

PAP is a syndrome characterized by progressive accumulation of surfactant within alveolar spaces, leading to gas exchange defects and characteristic "crazy-paving" patterns on chest computed tomography (CT) [34]. A breakthrough in understanding the biology of PAP occurred in the early 1990s when it was discovered that mice deficient for granulocyte-monocyte colony-stimulating factor (*Gm-csf*) developed a spontaneous pulmonary phenotype that closely resembled PAP [35]. Subsequent work demonstrated that there are multiple mechanisms converging on the GM-CSF pathway that can lead to the clinical phenotype of PAP. A diagnosis of PAP is made by bronchoscopy or bronchoalveolar lavage with lung biopsy in most cases [36]. After a diagnosis of PAP is established, it must be determined whether the patient has "primary" or "secondary" PAP [34]. In adults, an autoimmune mechanism is the most common cause of primary PAP wherein autoantibodies to GM-CSF lead to ineffective signaling. Secondary PAP can develop after a variety of pulmonary insults, including toxic inhalational exposures and bone marrow transplantation. In children and, occasionally, adults with primary PAP, biallelic (recessive) mutations in the genes encoding for the GM-CSF receptor (*CSF2RA* and *CSF2RB*) have been identified [37–39]. Much less commonly, mutations in the solute transporter *SLC7A7* [40], the tRNA synthetase *MARS* [41], and transcription factor *GATA2* [42, 43] have been associated with PAP phenotypes. In neonates, PAP can also be seen in the setting of *SFTPB*, *SFTPC*, and *ABCA3* mutations [7].

PAP treatment approaches are driven by understanding of the underlying mechanism of disease. Autoimmune PAP is typically treated with GM-CSF supplementation and immune suppression. In patients with a genetic form of PAP, immunosuppression and GM-CSF replacement are not effective, and supportive therapy in the form of whole-lung lavage remains the primary treatment. In many cases, supportive therapy is sufficient for long-term management, and spontaneous disease remission occurs in some patients. In severe or refractory cases of genetic PAP, hematopoetic stem-cell transplantation [44] has successfully repopulated the lung with functional alveolar macrophages.

Pulmonary Vascular Disease

Pulmonary hypertension is a syndrome defined by detection of elevated mean pulmonary artery pressure >25 mmHg. Pulmonary hypertension can occur in isolation, referred to as pulmonary arterial hypertension (PAH), and in the setting of an underlying chronic disease [45]. The current guidelines define five classes of pulmonary

hypertension. Group I pulmonary hypertension (i.e., PAH) is characterized by a primary pulmonary vasculopathy and elevated pulmonary vascular resistance. The clinical phenotype of PAH can be observed in patients with connective tissue disease, heritable pulmonary arterial hypertension (hPAH), congenital heart disease, and idiopathic PAH (iPAH) [45].

Heritable PAH typically has an autosomal dominant inheritance pattern with incomplete penetrance; thus, in evaluating patients with PAH, obtaining a thorough family history is crucial [46]. A family history of early-onset heart failure or unexplained sudden death in a young individual raises suspicion of previously unrecognized hPAH. In hPAH, heterozygous mutations in the gene encoding for bone morphogenic protein receptor 2 (*BMPR2*) are found in approximately 75% patients [47, 48]. Some reports suggest up to 20% of patients with "idiopathic" PAH also carry pathogenic *BMPR2* mutations, presumably due to de novo mutations or low-penetrance alleles [49].

While *BMPR2* mutations are the predominant cause of hPAH, mutations in a potassium channel (*KCNK3*) and caveolin 1 (*CAV1*) have also been reported in families with hPAH [48]. The prevalence of these mutations in hPAH and iPAH has not yet been reported from large cohorts. More recently, mutations in transcription factor *TBX4* have been reported in hPAH families and may be more common in pediatric pulmonary hypertension. *TBX4* mutations have also been associated with "small patella syndrome." The observation of patellar abnormalities in a patient with unexplained dyspnea or pulmonary hypertension should prompt consideration of *TBX4* mutations as an underlying diagnosis [50, 51].

PAH has also been observed in patients and families with hereditary hemorrhagic telangiectasia (HHT). A personal or family history of frequent epistaxis, unexplained anemia, or arteriovenous malformations should prompt more comprehensive evaluation for HHT. The etiology of pulmonary hypertension in HHT is complex and may be related to both high cardiac output and a primary pulmonary vasculopathy. PAH associated with HHT has been reported in patients with mutations in other TGF-β super-family receptors, including *ALK1*, *Endoglin*, and *SMAD9*. Within a given family, the manifestations of HHT can vary significantly [52].

Pulmonary venoocclusive disease (PVOD) and pulmonary capillary hemangiomatosis (PCH) are extremely rare pulmonary disorders that are often not correctly diagnosed until the time of lung transplantation or after death. Several groups have recently reported biallelic (recessive) mutations in *EIF2AK4* [53], a kinase related to initiation of protein translation, as leading to PVOD. In contrast to PAH, patients with PVOD and PCH typically have poor responses to pulmonary vasodilator therapy (i.e., phosphodiesterase inhibitors, endothelin antagonists, prostacyclin analogs), and, in some cases, clinical deterioration after initiation of pulmonary vasodilator therapy in a patient with suspected PAH has been observed in patients ultimately recognized to have PVOD [54].

To date, there are limited data with regard to genotype-phenotype relationships in terms of disease progression, outcomes, and treatment responses for patients with pulmonary vascular disease. While the evidence for a genetic etiology of many cases of PAH is considerable, the penetrance of mutations in a family varies substantially with estimates as low as 20%. Thus, while genetic testing and counseling can be performed in patients and families with PAH, the low penetrance of a disease-associated mutation limits the clinical value of a positive genetic test, and its value beyond a known family history has not been clearly established. As such, the primary role of genetic evaluation for hPAH is for unaffected family members to decide whether they should undergo testing and/or more frequent screening for PAH by echocardiography.

Cystic Lung Disease and Spontaneous Pneumothorax

Diffuse cystic lung diseases are a broad group of disorders that share the common characteristic of thin-walled, radiolucent cystic structures on chest imaging. The clinical features and manifestations include high prevalence of spontaneous pneumothorax and, in some cases, progressive lung parenchymal destruction and respiratory failure. Cystic lung diseases may be a feature of systemic disorders, and an accurate genetic diagnosis can aid in defining the scope of evaluation for extrapulmonary disease features.

The differential diagnosis of cystic lung disease is broad, including neoplastic, autoimmune, infectious, genetic, developmental, and other conditions [55, 56]. In patients with diffuse cystic lung disease, the primary genetic considerations center around patients with lymphangioleiomyomatosis (LAM) and Langerhans cell histiocytosis. LAM is believed to be a benign neoplastic process that occurs almost exclusively in women [57]. LAM can occur sporadically or in patients with tuberous sclerosis complex (TSC). The cystic structures found in chest imaging are typically round, <2 cm in size, and randomly distributed throughout both lungs [56]. Pathologic examination of explanted lung tissue from patients with LAM demonstrates expansion of HMB-45+ LAM cells. Patients with tuberous sclerosis carry germline mutations in *TSC1* or *TSC2*, two tumor suppressor genes. In patients with sporadic LAM, somatic mutations in TSC genes are found in the cystic lung lesions. Patients with TSC are at risk for the development of angiomyolipomas (AMLs), most commonly in the kidney, as well as brain tumors, seizures, and skin cancers [58]. Patients with sporadic LAM also appear to be at increased risk for renal AMLs but not other systemic manifestations of TSC. Germline genetic testing for TSC can inform both heritability risk and the risk of extrapulmonary disease.

Pulmonary Langerhans cell histiocystosis (PLCH) is a cystic lung disease that occurs almost exclusively in adults who are active or former tobacco users. In children, PLCH can occur more frequently in the setting of systemic histiocytosis (termed Erdheim-Chester disease). In contrast to LAM, PLCH occurs in men and women and is characterized by irregularly shaped cysts that are found more commonly in the lung apex and only rarely involve the lung base [56]. Histopathologically, PLCH is characterized by CD1a Langerhans cells. Up to 50% of

PLCH cases are found to have somatic mutations in B-Raf Proto-Oncogene, Serine/Threonine Kinase (*BRAF*) [59], which can be detected in circulating peripheral blood [60]. A potential role for targeted therapies for *BRAF*-mutant PLCH is an area of ongoing investigation; at present there are case reports and series of disease stabilization and/or improvement with BRAF and MEK inhibitors [61–64], but no large-scale studies have yet determined efficacy of these targeted therapies in patients with PLCH.

While LAM and PLCH can lead to progressive lung parenchymal destruction and respiratory failure, isolated cystic lung disease can also present with primary spontaneous pneumothorax. Several genetic disorders, including Birt-Hogg-Dube (BHD), as well as connective tissue disorders, including Ehlers-Danlos Syndrome, Marfan's Synrome, and Loeys-Dietz syndromes have been recognized as causes of primary spontaneous pneumothorax [65]. BHD is characterized by subpleural cysts, dermal fibrofolliculinomas, and risk of renal tumors, and is caused by autosomal dominant inheritance of mutations in Folliculin (*FLCN*), a tumor suppressor gene [66]. In contrast to LAM and PLCH, pulmonary cysts in patients with BHD resemble emphysematous cysts, and the mechanism of their development is not well understood [67]. Establishing a genetic diagnosis as cause of primary spontaneous pneumothorax has direct therapeutic implications for patients; as the recurrence risk is >75% among BHD patients with a first pneumothorax, pleurodesis is recommended in the initial management of these patients [68]. Patients with BHD are at increased risk of renal tumors, and periodic screening is recommended if a diagnosis of BHD is established [69].

Bronchiectasis and Obstructive Lung Disease

Bronchiectasis is a clinical syndrome characterized by clinical symptoms of a persistent productive cough and evidence of dilated, thickened airways on chest imaging. The differential diagnosis of bronchiectasis includes immunodeficiencies, postinfectious etiologies, autoimmune disease, and genetic disorders, including cystic fibrosis (CF), primary ciliary dyskinesia (PCD), and alpha-1 antitrypsin deficiency (A1AD).

CF is a systemic disease caused by biallelic loss-of-function mutations in a chloride ion transporter gene called Cystic Fibrosis Transmembrane Conductance Regulator (*CFTR*). In the lungs, loss of CFTR function leads to impaired mucociliary clearance, recurrent infections, mucous impaction, bronchiectasis, and progressive respiratory failure. CF-associated *CFTR* mutations are grouped into six classes based on the mechanism of dysfunction (e.g., null, mistrafficking, gating, reduced protein levels/impaired stability), and mutation-class driven precision therapies are available for many patients with CF [70, 71]. Consequently, *CFTR* genotyping is recommended for all patients with CF. It is becoming increasingly recognized that some CF phenotypes are relatively mild and may present in adulthood as isolated bronchiectasis. Sweat chloride test values may be near the upper limits of normal in these individuals; thus, an equivocal sweat chloride test with appropriate clinical suspicion should prompt *CFTR* genotyping.

PCD is a syndrome of impaired ciliary assembly and/or function that leads to abnormal mucociliary clearance and bronchiectasis [72]. Evaluation of ciliary ultrastructure by electron microscopy (EM) can aid in the diagnosis of PCD, but considerable experience is required for proper processing and evaluation of ciliary EM. Elevated nasal nitric oxide (NO) can be observed in many patients with PCD, although some genetic causes of PCD have been associated with normal nasal NO levels [73]. PCD typically follows an autosomal recessive inheritance pattern, and biallelic variants in >35 genes encoding for components of the inner dynein arm, outer dynein arm, and those related to axonemal disorganization have been reported; mutations in several PCD genes do not appear to affect ciliary ultrastructure [72]. PCD can be associated with Kartagener's syndrome and other malrotation disorders.

A1AD is a syndrome characterized by biallelic mutations in *SERPINA1*, the gene encoding for the antiprotease alpha-1 antitrypsin [74]. There are several different classes of *SERPINA1* mutations that lead to different A1AD phenotypes as detected by gel electrophoresis, including the M allele (normal), S allele (low protein), and Z allele (null) [74]. In the lung, loss of antiprotease activity in patients with ZZ genotypes is associated with early onset and severe emphysema, dramatically exacerbated by tobacco smoking. Individuals with SZ genotypes are also at increased risk for developed emphysema [75]. In total, it is estimated that 1–3% of all patients with COPD have A1AD, but this is likely significantly underrecognized in clinical practice. The Current Global Initiative for Chronic Obstructive Lung Disease (GOLD) guidelines recommend testing for A1AD in all patients newly diagnosed with COPD [75]. The clinical spectrum of A1AD includes both pulmonary and liver disease. Misfolding of mutant alpha-1 antitrypsin in the liver leads to a toxic gain-of-function and chronic hepatocyte injury, leading to chronic liver disease that progresses to cirrhosis in some patients [76]. In the lung, while emphysema is the primary clinical manifestation, isolated bronchiectasis can also be observed. As both the S and Z alleles have low frequency in the general population, despite need for biallelic mutations to develop disease, A1AD can run in families with complex inheritance patterns, including different primary disease manifestations in different individuals. Genetic testing for A1AD is widely available through the alpha-1 foundation (available at https://www.alpha1.org). For patients with low alpha-1 antitrypsin levels and disease-associated genotypes, alpha-1 antitrypsin replacement therapy is available and has been demonstrated to slow loss of lung function [77].

Adult Interstitial Lung Disease

There are more than 150 reported causes of diffuse parenchymal lung disease, also termed interstitial lung disease (ILD) in adults, including occupational, environmental and toxic exposures, autoimmune conditions, inherited/genetic syndromes, and idiopathic interstitial pneumonias (IIP) [78]. Among the IIPs, idiopathic pulmonary fibrosis (IPF) is the most common and most severe [78], and the role of genetic risk in IPF is most clearly defined [79]. More than 20 common genetic variants have been associated with risk of IPF [79–82], including a striking association with a promoter polymorphism in the gene encoding for the airway mucin *MUC5B,* which is associated with a four- to six-fold increased risk for IPF in patients of European ancestry [83]. More recent studies have suggested this locus confers disease risk in patients with rheumatoid arthritis-associated ILD with usual interstitial pneumonia (UIP) disease patterns [84] and also in patients with chronic hypersensitivity pneumonitis [85]. While the *MUC5B* promoter polymorphism is associated with an unusually large effect size on disease risk for a common genetic variant, among IPF patients, risk (T) allele carriers have better outcomes than patients homozygous for the major (G) allele [86]. Given the high background prevalence (18–20%) of the *MUC5B* promoter SNP in populations of European ancestry, and the recognition that this variant is associated with multiple forms of ILD, testing for this variant is not recommended in the evaluation of patients with ILD; in the future, it may be explored as a prognostic marker [5].

Upon careful ascertainment, studies from multiple groups indicate that approximately 20% of patients with IIP have a family history of IIP [87]; this syndrome is termed familial interstitial pneumonia (FIP). The inheritance pattern of FIP is autosomal dominant with incomplete penetrance [79]. Consistent with the phenotypic heterogeneity seen in other genetic pulmonary syndromes, within a single family, several different IIP radiologic/histopathologic patterns can be observed [88]. Among FIP kindreds, mutations in genes related to telomere biology, including *TERT* [89, 90], *TERC* [89, 90], *RTEL1* [91–93], *PARN* [93, 94], *TINF2* [95], *NAF1* [96], and *DKC1* [97, 98] have been implicated. Within these families, other features of short-telomere syndromes are frequently present, including bone marrow dyscrasias (e.g., macrocytosis, MDS, aplastic anemia), and chronic liver disease (e.g., cryptogenic cirrhosis). In patients with telomere pathway mutations, limited available data suggest that genetic risk, rather than radiologic/pathologic disease pattern, is the primary determinant of disease course [99]. Most FIP-associated telomere pathway mutations are ultra-rare or novel; thus, there are limited data on genotype-phenotype relationships and variant-specific disease penetrance. As described in brief above, in a small proportion of families with surfactant pathway mutations, delayed presentation into adulthood occurs in few individuals. Compared to other forms of adult ILD, the disease course of patients who present in adulthood with surfactant pathway mutations may have early onset but slower disease progression, although there are cases of adults with surfactant protein mutations progressing to lung transplantation in the fifth to sixth decades of life. To date, there are no formal guidelines for genetic testing in patients with FIP, although emerging evidence suggests that a specific genetic diagnosis may inform considerations around lung transplantation [100–104].

In addition to short telomere syndromes, pulmonary fibrosis is a prevalent feature of Hermansky-Pudlak syndrome (HPS), an autosomal recessive disorder characterized by oculocutaneous albinism, platelet dysfunction, and highly penetrant pulmonary fibrosis in some subtypes [105]. The current standard for diagnosis of HPS is demonstration of absent dense granules in platelets by EM. Once a diagnosis of HPS is established, genetic evaluation for HPS mutations is recommended. Ten HPS subtypes have been identified as associated with mutations in different components related to biogenesis of lysosome-derived organelles with mutations in *HPS1* (HPS subtype 1), *AP3B1* (HPS subtype 2), and *HPS4* (HPS subtype 4) having associations with pulmonary fibrosis [105]. As is the case in scenarios described above, a positive result of a genetic test is informative whereas a negative test does not exclude a diagnosis.

Challenges and Future Directions

As genetic testing and evaluation is more frequently performed, there will be an increasing opportunity to refine understanding of genotype-phenotype relationships across lung diseases. This will have implications for both patients with chronic lung disease and, in many situations, will inform disease risk for other family members. Currently, there are several major barriers to integration of genetic information into the clinical evaluation of patients with chronic lung disease, largely centered around cost of testing, limited or absent insurance coverage for testing, and access to genetic counseling. The implication of heterogeneous disease phenotypes associated with mutations in a single gene suggests understanding of fundamental disease mechanisms needs further refinement. Although much more work remains to be done, one can imagine a future scenario for pulmonary diseases analogous to what has occurred in the field of oncology where disease classification and corresponding therapeutic approaches are directed by the genetic drivers of disease.

References

1. Bamshad MJ, Ng SB, Bigham AW, Tabor HK, Emond MJ, Nickerson DA, et al. Exome sequencing as a tool for Mendelian disease gene discovery. Nat Rev Genet. 2011;12(11):745–55.
2. Rabbani B, Mahdieh N, Hosomichi K, Nakaoka H, Inoue I. Next-generation sequencing: impact of exome sequencing in characterizing Mendelian disorders. J Hum Genet. 2012;57(10):621–32.
3. Yang Y, Muzny DM, Reid JG, Bainbridge MN, Willis A, Ward PA, et al. Clinical whole-exome sequencing for the diagnosis of Mendelian disorders. N Engl J Med. 2013;369(16):1502–11.
4. Richards S, et al. Standards and guidelines for the interpretation of sequence variants: a joint consensus recommendation of the American College of Medical Genetics and Genomics and the Association for Molecular Pathology. Genet Med. 2015;17(5):405–24.
5. Kropski JA, Young LR, Cogan JD, Mitchell DB, Lancaster LH, Worrell JA, et al. Genetic evaluation and testing of patients and families with idiopathic pulmonary fibrosis. Am J Respir Crit Care Med. 2017;195(11):1423–8.

6. Sweet DG, Carnielli V, Greisen G, Hallman M, Ozek E, Plavka R, et al. European consensus guidelines on the management of neonatal respiratory distress syndrome in preterm infants–2013 update. Neonatology. 2013;103(4):353–68.

7. Nogee LM. Genetic causes of surfactant protein abnormalities. Curr Opin Pediatr. 2019;31:330.

8. Nogee LM, Garnier G, Dietz HC, Singer L, Murphy AM, deMello DE, et al. A mutation in the surfactant protein B gene responsible for fatal neonatal respiratory disease in multiple kindreds. J Clin Invest. 1994;93(4):1860–3.

9. Vorbroker DK, Profitt SA, Nogee LM, Whitsett JA. Aberrant processing of surfactant protein C in hereditary SP-B deficiency. Am J Phys. 1995;268(4 Pt 1):L647–56.

10. Nogee LM, Dunbar AE 3rd, Wert SE, Askin F, Hamvas A, Whitsett JA. A mutation in the surfactant protein C gene associated with familial interstitial lung disease. N Engl J Med. 2001;344(8):573–9.

11. Beers MF, Hawkins A, Maguire JA, Kotorashvili A, Zhao M, Newitt JL, et al. A nonaggregating surfactant protein C mutant is misdirected to early endosomes and disrupts phospholipid recycling. Traffic. 2011;12(9):1196–210.

12. Lawson WE, Cheng DS, Degryse AL, Tanjore H, Polosukhin VV, Xu XC, et al. Endoplasmic reticulum stress enhances fibrotic remodeling in the lungs. Proc Natl Acad Sci U S A. 2011;108(26):10562–7.

13. Maguire JA, Mulugeta S, Beers MF. Endoplasmic reticulum stress induced by surfactant protein C BRICHOS mutants promotes proinflammatory signaling by epithelial cells. Am J Respir Cell Mol Biol. 2011;44(3):404–14.

14. Mulugeta S, Maguire JA, Newitt JL, Russo SJ, Kotorashvili A, Beers MF. Misfolded BRICHOS SP-C mutant proteins induce apoptosis via caspase-4- and cytochrome c-related mechanisms. Am J Physiol Lung Cell Mol Physiol. 2007;293(3):L720–9.

15. Mulugeta S, Nguyen V, Russo SJ, Muniswamy M, Beers MF. A surfactant protein C precursor protein BRICHOS domain mutation causes endoplasmic reticulum stress, proteasome dysfunction, and caspase 3 activation. Am J Respir Cell Mol Biol. 2005;32(6):521–30.

16. Wang WJ, Mulugeta S, Russo SJ, Beers MF. Deletion of exon 4 from human surfactant protein C results in aggresome formation and generation of a dominant negative. J Cell Sci. 2003;116(Pt 4):683–92.

17. Thomas AQ, Lane K, Phillips J 3rd, Prince M, Markin C, Speer M, et al. Heterozygosity for a surfactant protein C gene mutation associated with usual interstitial pneumonitis and cellular nonspecific interstitial pneumonitis in one kindred. Am J Respir Crit Care Med. 2002;165(9):1322–8.

18. Crossno PF, Polosukhin VV, Blackwell TS, Johnson JE, Markin C, Moore PE, et al. Identification of early interstitial lung disease in an individual with genetic variations in ABCA3 and SFTPC. Chest. 2010;137(4):969–73.

19. Bullard JE, Wert SE, Nogee LM. ABCA3 deficiency: neonatal respiratory failure and interstitial lung disease. Semin Perinatol. 2006;30(6): 327–34.

20. Bullard JE, Wert SE, Whitsett JA, Dean M, Nogee LM. ABCA3 mutations associated with pediatric interstitial lung disease. Am J Respir Crit Care Med. 2005;172(8):1026–31.

21. Shulenin S, Nogee LM, Annilo T, Wert SE, Whitsett JA, Dean M. ABCA3 gene mutations in newborns with fatal surfactant deficiency. N Engl J Med. 2004;350(13):1296–303.

22. Wambach JA, Casey AM, Fishman MP, Wegner DJ, Wert SE, Cole FS, et al. Genotype-phenotype correlations for infants and children with ABCA3 deficiency. Am J Respir Crit Care Med. 2014;189(12):1538–43.

23. Wambach JA, Yang P, Wegner DJ, Heins HB, Kaliberova LN, Kaliberov SA, et al. Functional characterization of ATP-binding cassette transporter A3 mutations from infants with respiratory distress syndrome. Am J Respir Cell Mol Biol. 2016;55(5):716–21.

24. Young LR, Nogee LM, Barnett B, Panos RJ, Colby TV, Deutsch GH. Usual interstitial pneumonia in an adolescent with ABCA3 mutations. Chest. 2008;134(1):192–5.

25. Doyle DA, Gonzalez I, Thomas B, Scavina M. Autosomal dominant transmission of congenital hypothyroidism, neonatal respiratory distress, and ataxia caused by a mutation of NKX2-1. J Pediatr. 2004;145(2):190–3.

26. Guillot L, Carre A, Szinnai G, Castanet M, Tron E, Jaubert F, et al. NKX2-1 mutations leading to surfactant protein promoter dysregulation cause interstitial lung disease in "Brain-Lung-Thyroid Syndrome". Hum Mutat. 2010;31(2):E1146–62.

27. Young LR, Deutsch GH, Bokulic RE, Brody AS, Nogee LM. A mutation in TTF1/NKX2.1 is associated with familial neuroendocrine cell hyperplasia of infancy. Chest. 2013;144(4):1199–206.

28. Reiter J, Szafranski P, Breuer O, Perles Z, Dagan T, Stankiewicz P, et al. Variable phenotypic presentation of a novel FOXF1 missense mutation in a single family. Pediatr Pulmonol. 2016;51(9):921–7.

29. Sen P, Gerychova R, Janku P, Jezova M, Valaskova I, Navarro C, et al. A familial case of alveolar capillary dysplasia with misalignment of pulmonary veins supports paternal imprinting of FOXF1 in human. Eur J Hum Genet. 2013;21(4):474–7.

30. Luk HM, Tang T, Choy KW, Tong MF, Wong OK, Lo FM. Maternal somatic mosaicism of FOXF1 mutation causes recurrent alveolar capillary dysplasia with misalignment of pulmonary veins in siblings. Am J Med Genet A. 2016;170(7):1942–4.

31. Watkin LB, Jessen B, Wiszniewski W, Vece TJ, Jan M, Sha Y, et al. COPA mutations impair ER-Golgi transport and cause hereditary autoimmune-mediated lung disease and arthritis. Nat Genet. 2015;47:654–60.

32. Tsui JL, Estrada OA, Deng Z, Wang KM, Law CS, Elicker BM, et al. Analysis of pulmonary features and treatment approaches in the COPA syndrome. ERJ Open Res. 2018;4(2):00017–2018. https://doi.org/10.1183/23120541.00017-2018.

33. Liu Y, Jesus AA, Marrero B, Yang D, Ramsey SE, Sanchez GAM, et al. Activated STING in a vascular and pulmonary syndrome. N Engl J Med. 2014;371(6):507–18.

34. Trapnell BC, Nakata K, Bonella F, Campo I, Griese M, Hamilton J, et al. Pulmonary alveolar proteinosis. Nat Rev Dis Primers. 2019;5(1):16.

35. Dranoff G, Crawford AD, Sadelain M, Ream B, Rashid A, Bronson RT, et al. Involvement of granulocyte-macrophage colony-stimulating factor in pulmonary homeostasis. Science. 1994;264(5159):713–6.

36. McCarthy C, Avetisyan R, Carey BC, Chalk C, Trapnell BC. Prevalence and healthcare burden of pulmonary alveolar proteinosis. Orphanet J Rare Dis. 2018;13(1):129.

37. Dirksen U, Nishinakamura R, Groneck P, Hattenhorst U, Nogee L, Murray R, et al. Human pulmonary alveolar proteinosis associated with a defect in GM-CSF/IL-3/IL-5 receptor common beta chain expression. J Clin Invest. 1997;100(9):2211–7.

38. Suzuki T, Sakagami T, Rubin BK, Nogee LM, Wood RE, Zimmerman SL, et al. Familial pulmonary alveolar proteinosis caused by mutations in CSF2RA. J Exp Med. 2008;205(12):2703–10.

39. Trapnell BC, Whitsett JA, Nakata K. Pulmonary alveolar proteinosis. N Engl J Med. 2003;349(26):2527–39.

40. Borsani G, Bassi MT, Sperandeo MP, De Grandi A, Buoninconti A, Riboni M, et al. SLC7A7, encoding a putative permease-related protein, is mutated in patients with lysinuric protein intolerance. Nat Genet. 1999;21(3):297–301.

41. Hadchouel A, Wieland T, Griese M, Baruffini E, Lorenz-Depiereux B, Enaud L, et al. Biallelic mutations of methionyl-tRNA synthetase cause a specific type of pulmonary alveolar proteinosis prevalent on reunion island. Am J Hum Genet. 2015;96(5):826–31.

42. Griese M, Zarbock R, Costabel U, Hildebrandt J, Theegarten D, Albert M, et al. GATA2 deficiency in children and adults with severe pulmonary alveolar proteinosis and hematologic disorders. BMC Pulm Med. 2015;15:87.

43. Spinner MA, Sanchez LA, Hsu AP, Shaw PA, Zerbe CS, Calvo KR, et al. GATA2 deficiency: a protean disorder of hematopoiesis, lymphatics, and immunity. Blood. 2014;123(6):809–21.

44. Fremond ML, Hadchouel A, Schweitzer C, Berteloot L, Bruneau J, Bonnet C, et al. Successful haematopoietic stem cell transplantation in a case of pulmonary alveolar proteinosis due to GM-CSF receptor deficiency. Thorax. 2018;73(6):590–2.

45. Galie N, Humbert M, Vachiery JL, Gibbs S, Lang I, Torbicki A, et al. ESC/ERS Guidelines for the diagnosis and treatment of pulmonary hypertension: The Joint Task Force for the Diagnosis and Treatment of Pulmonary Hypertension of the European Society of Cardiology (ESC) and the European Respiratory Society (ERS): Endorsed by: Association for European Paediatric and Congenital Cardiology (AEPC), International Society for Heart and Lung Transplantation (ISHLT). Eur Heart J. 2016;37(1):67–119.

46. Chew JD, Loyd JE, Austin ED. Genetics of pulmonary arterial hypertension. Semin Respir Crit Care Med. 2017;38(5):585–95.

47. Evans JD, Girerd B, Montani D, Wang XJ, Galie N, Austin ED, et al. BMPR2 mutations and survival in pulmonary arterial hypertension: an individual participant data meta-analysis. Lancet Respir Med. 2016;4(2):129–37.

48. Machado RD, Southgate L, Eichstaedt CA, Aldred MA, Austin ED, Best DH, et al. Pulmonary arterial hypertension: a current perspective on established and emerging molecular genetic defects. Hum Mutat. 2015;36(12):1113–27.

49. Soubrier F, Chung WK, Machado R, Grunig E, Aldred M, Geraci M, et al. Genetics and genomics of pulmonary arterial hypertension. J Am Coll Cardiol. 2013;62(25 Suppl):D13–21.

50. Kerstjens-Frederikse WS, Bongers EM, Roofthooft MT, Leter EM, Douwes JM, Van Dijk A, et al. TBX4 mutations (small patella syndrome) are associated with childhood-onset pulmonary arterial hypertension. J Med Genet. 2013;50(8):500–6.

51. Nimmakayalu M, Major H, Sheffield V, Solomon DH, Smith RJ, Patil SR, et al. Microdeletion of 17q22q23.2 encompassing TBX2 and TBX4 in a patient with congenital microcephaly, thyroid duct cyst, sensorineural hearing loss, and pulmonary hypertension. Am J Med Genet A. 2011;155a(2):418–23.

52. McDonald J, Wooderchak-Donahue W, VanSant Webb C, Whitehead K, Stevenson DA, Bayrak-Toydemir P. Hereditary hemorrhagic telangiectasia: genetics and molecular diagnostics in a new era. Front Genet. 2015;6:1.

53. Eyries M, Montani D, Girerd B, Perret C, Leroy A, Lonjou C, et al. EIF2AK4 mutations cause pulmonary veno-occlusive disease, a recessive form of pulmonary hypertension. Nat Genet. 2014;46(1):65.

54. Montani D, Lau EM, Dorfmuller P, Girerd B, Jais X, Savale L, et al. Pulmonary veno-occlusive disease. Eur Respir J. 2016;47(5):1518–34.

55. Gupta N, Vassallo R, Wikenheiser-Brokamp KA, McCormack FX. Diffuse cystic lung disease. Part I. Am J Respir Crit Care Med. 2015;191(12):1354–66.

56. Gupta N, Vassallo R, Wikenheiser-Brokamp KA, McCormack FX. Diffuse cystic lung disease. Part II. Am J Respir Crit Care Med. 2015;192(1):17–29.

57. Moss J, Avila NA, Barnes PM, Litzenberger RA, Bechtle J, Brooks PG, et al. Prevalence and clinical characteristics of lymphangioleiomyomatosis

(LAM) in patients with tuberous sclerosis complex. Am J Respir Crit Care Med. 2001;164(4):669–71.

58. Gupta N, Henske EP. Pulmonary manifestations in tuberous sclerosis complex. Am J Med Genet C Semin Med Genet. 2018;178(3):326–37.

59. Badalian-Very G, Vergilio JA, Degar BA, MacConaill LE, Brandner B, Calicchio ML, et al. Recurrent BRAF mutations in Langerhans cell histiocytosis. Blood. 2010;116(11):1919–23.

60. Schwentner R, Kolenova A, Jug G, Schnoller T, Ahlmann M, Meister B, et al. Longitudinal assessment of peripheral blood BRAFV600E levels in patients with Langerhans cell histiocytosis. Pediatr Res. 2019;85(6):856–64.

61. Haroche J, Cohen-Aubart F, Emile JF, Arnaud L, Maksud P, Charlotte F, et al. Dramatic efficacy of vemurafenib in both multisystemic and refractory Erdheim-Chester disease and Langerhans cell histiocytosis harboring the BRAF V600E mutation. Blood. 2013;121(9):1495–500.

62. Haroche J, Cohen-Aubart F, Emile JF, Donadieu J, Amoura Z. Vemurafenib as first line therapy in BRAF-mutated Langerhans cell histiocytosis. J Am Acad Dermatol. 2015;73(1):e29–30.

63. Heritier S, Jehanne M, Leverger G, Emile JF, Alvarez JC, Haroche J, et al. Vemurafenib use in an infant for high-risk Langerhans cell histiocytosis. JAMA Oncol. 2015;1(6):836–8.

64. Hyman DM, Puzanov I, Subbiah V, Faris JE, Chau I, Blay JY, et al. Vemurafenib in multiple nonmelanoma cancers with BRAF V600 mutations. N Engl J Med. 2015;373(8):726–36.

65. Boone PM, Scott RM, Marciniak SJ, Henske EP, Raby BA. The genetics of pneumothorax. Am J Respir Crit Care Med. 2019;199:1344.

66. Gupta N, et al. Birt-Hogg-Dubé syndrome. Clin Chest Med. 2016;37(3):475–86.

67. Kennedy JC, et al. Mechanisms of pulmonary cyst pathogenesis in Birt-Hogg-Dube syndrome: the stretch HYPOTHESIS. Semin Cell Dev Biol. 2016;52:47–52.

68. Gupta N, et al. Spontaneous pneumothoraces in patients with Birt-Hogg-Dubé syndrome. Ann Am Thorac Soc. 2017;14(5):706–13.

69. Gupta N, Sunwoo BY, Kotloff RM. Birt-Hogg-Dube syndrome. Clin Chest Med. 2016;37(3):475–86.

70. Ramsey BW, Davies J, McElvaney NG, Tullis E, Bell SC, Drevinek P, et al. A CFTR potentiator in patients with cystic fibrosis and the G551D mutation. N Engl J Med. 2011;365(18):1663–72.

71. Wainwright CE, Elborn JS, Ramsey BW, Marigowda G, Huang X, Cipolli M, et al. Lumacaftor-Ivacaftor in patients with cystic fibrosis homozygous for Phe508del CFTR. N Engl J Med. 2015;373(3):220–31.

72. Horani A, Ferkol TW. Advances in the genetics of primary ciliary dyskinesia: clinical implications. Chest. 2018;154(3):645–52.

73. Shapiro AJ, Josephson M, Rosenfeld M, Yilmaz O, Davis SD, Polineni D, et al. Accuracy of nasal nitric oxide measurement as a diagnostic test for primary ciliary dyskinesia. A systematic review and meta-analysis. Ann Am Thorac Soc. 2017;14(7):1184–96.

74. American Thoracic Society, European Respiratory Society. American Thoracic Society/European Respiratory Society statement: standards for the diagnosis and management of individuals with alpha-1 antitrypsin deficiency. Am J Respir Crit Care Med. 2003;168(7):818–900.

75. Torres-Duran M, Lopez-Campos JL, Barrecheguren M, Miravitlles M, Martinez-Delgado B, Castillo S, et al. Alpha-1 antitrypsin deficiency: outstanding questions and future directions. Orphanet J Rare Dis. 2018;13(1):114.

76. Marciniak SJ, Ordonez A, Dickens JA, Chambers JE, Patel V, Dominicus CS, et al. New concepts in Alpha-1 antitrypsin deficiency disease mechanisms. Ann Am Thorac Soc. 2016;13(Suppl 4):S289–96.

77. Edgar RG, Patel M, Bayliss S, Crossley D, Sapey E, Turner AM. Treatment of lung disease in alpha-1 antitrypsin deficiency: a systematic review. Int J Chron Obstruct Pulmon Dis. 2017;12:1295–308.

78. Lederer DJ, Martinez FJ. Idiopathic pulmonary fibrosis. N Engl J Med. 2018;378(19):1811–23.

79. Kropski JA, Blackwell TS, Loyd JE. The genetic basis of idiopathic pulmonary fibrosis. Eur Respir J. 2015;45:1717.

80. Allen RJ, Porte J, Braybrooke R, Flores C, Fingerlin TE, Oldham JM, et al. Genetic variants associated with susceptibility to idiopathic pulmonary fibrosis in people of European ancestry: a genome-wide association study. Lancet Respir Med. 2017;5(11):869–80.

81. Fingerlin TE, Murphy E, Zhang W, Peljto AL, Brown KK, Steele MP, et al. Genome-wide association study identifies multiple susceptibility loci for pulmonary fibrosis. Nat Genet. 2013;45(6):613–20.

82. Noth I, Zhang Y, Ma SF, Flores C, Barber M, Huang Y, et al. Genetic variants associated with idiopathic pulmonary fibrosis susceptibility and mortality: a genome-wide association study. Lancet Respir Med. 2013;1(4):309–17.

83. Seibold MA, Wise AL, Speer MC, Steele MP, Brown KK, Loyd JE, et al. A common MUC5B promoter polymorphism and pulmonary fibrosis. N Engl J Med. 2011;364(16):1503–12.

84. Juge PA, Lee JS, Ebstein E, Furukawa H, Dobrinskikh E, Gazal S, et al. MUC5B promoter variant and rheumatoid arthritis with interstitial lung disease. N Engl J Med. 2018;379:2209.

85. Ley B, Newton CA, Arnould I, Elicker BM, Henry TS, Vittinghoff E, et al. The MUC5B promoter polymorphism and telomere length in patients with chronic hypersensitivity pneumonitis: an observational cohort-control study. Lancet Respir Med. 2017;5(8):639–47.

86. Peljto AL, Zhang Y, Fingerlin TE, Ma SF, Garcia JG, Richards TJ, et al. Association between the MUC5B promoter polymorphism and survival in patients with idiopathic pulmonary fibrosis. JAMA. 2013;309(21):2232–9.

87. Loyd JE. Pulmonary fibrosis in families. Am J Respir Cell Mol Biol. 2003;29(3 Suppl):S47–50.
88. Steele MP, Speer MC, Loyd JE, Brown KK, Herron A, Slifer SH, et al. Clinical and pathologic features of familial interstitial pneumonia. Am J Respir Crit Care Med. 2005;172(9):1146–52.
89. Armanios MY, Chen JJ, Cogan JD, Alder JK, Ingersoll RG, Markin C, et al. Telomerase mutations in families with idiopathic pulmonary fibrosis. N Engl J Med. 2007;356(13):1317–26.
90. Tsakiri KD, Cronkhite JT, Kuan PJ, Xing C, Raghu G, Weissler JC, et al. Adult-onset pulmonary fibrosis caused by mutations in telomerase. Proc Natl Acad Sci U S A. 2007;104(18):7552–7.
91. Cogan JD, Kropski JA, Zhao M, Mitchell DB, Rives L, Markin C, et al. Rare variants in RTEL1 are associated with familial interstitial pneumonia. Am J Respir Crit Care Med. 2015;191:646.
92. Kannengiesser C, Borie R, Menard C, Reocreux M, Nitschke P, Gazal S, et al. Heterozygous RTEL1 mutations are associated with familial pulmonary fibrosis. Eur Respir J. 2015;46(2):474–85.
93. Stuart BD, Choi J, Zaidi S, Xing C, Holohan B, Chen R, et al. Exome sequencing links mutations in PARN and RTEL1 with familial pulmonary fibrosis and telomere shortening. Nat Genet. 2015;47(5):512–7.
94. Kropski JA, Reiss S, Markin C, Brown KK, Schwartz DA, Schwarz MI, et al. Rare genetic variants in PARN are associated with pulmonary fibrosis in families. Am J Respir Crit Care Med. 2017;196(11):1481–4.
95. Alder JK, Stanley SE, Wagner CL, Hamilton M, Hanumanthu VS, Armanios M. Exome sequencing identifies mutant TINF2 in a family with pulmonary fibrosis. Chest. 2015;147(5):1361–8.
96. Stanley SE, Gable DL, Wagner CL, Carlile TM, Hanumanthu VS, Podlevsky JD, et al. Loss-of-function mutations in the RNA biogenesis factor NAF1 predispose to pulmonary fibrosis-emphysema. Sci Transl Med. 2016;8(351):351ra107.
97. Alder JK, Parry EM, Yegnasubramanian S, Wagner CL, Lieblich LM, Auerbach R, et al. Penetrant telomere phenotypes in females with heterozygous mutations in the dyskeratosis congenita 1 (DKC1) gene. Hum Mutat. 2013;34:1481.
98. Kropski JA, Mitchell DB, Markin C, Polosukhin VV, Choi L, Johnson JE, et al. A novel dyskerin (DKC1) mutation is associated with familial interstitial pneumonia. Chest. 2014;146(1):e1–7.
99. Newton CA, Batra K, Torrealba J, Kozlitina J, Glazer CS, Aravena C, et al. Telomere-related lung fibrosis is diagnostically heterogeneous but uniformly progressive. Eur Respir J. 2016;48(6):1710–20.
100. Newton CA, Kozlitina J, Lines JR, Kaza V, Torres F, Garcia CK. Telomere length in patients with pulmonary fibrosis associated with chronic lung allograft dysfunction and post-lung transplantation survival. J Heart Lung Transplant. 2017;36(8):845–53.
101. Faust HE, Golden JA, Rajalingam R, Wang AS, Green G, Hays SR, et al. Short lung transplant donor telomere length is associated with decreased CLAD-free survival. Thorax. 2017;72:1052–4. England: Published by the BMJ Publishing Group Limited. For permission to use (where not already granted under a licence) please go to http://www.bmj.com/company/products-services/rights-and-licensing/.
102. George G, Rosas IO, Cui Y, McKane C, Hunninghake GM, Camp PC, et al. Short telomeres, telomeropathy, and subclinical extrapulmonary organ damage in patients with interstitial lung disease. Chest. 2015;147(6):1549–57.
103. Silhan LL, Shah PD, Chambers DC, Snyder LD, Riise GC, Wagner CL, et al. Lung transplantation in telomerase mutation carriers with pulmonary fibrosis. Eur Respir J. 2014;44(1):178–87.
104. Tokman S, Singer JP, Devine MS, Westall GP, Aubert JD, Tamm M, et al. Clinical outcomes of lung transplant recipients with telomerase mutations. J Heart Lung Transplant. 2015;34(10):1318–24.
105. El-Chemaly S, Young LR. Hermansky-Pudlak syndrome. Clin Chest Med. 2016;37(3):505–11.

Genetics and Pharmacogenetics of Asthma

3

Mengyuan Kan and Blanca E. Himes

Key Point Summary
- Several genetic variants have been associated with asthma and asthma-related traits, including highly replicated loci. The most notable is at 17q21, spanning genes that include ORMDL sphingolipid biosynthesis regulator 3 (*ORMDL3*) and gasdermin B (*GSDMB*).
- Fewer asthma pharmacogenetic loci have been identified and widely replicated due in part to the limited number of large cohorts with appropriate and similarly captured drug response measures.
- Genetics may contribute to observed racial/ethnic and sex disparities in asthma prevalence and severity, and, thus, asthma genetics studies must include diverse groups to inform precision medicine efforts.
- Although the exact mechanisms via which asthma-related variants confer susceptibility to asthma are not yet understood, genetic discoveries are the subject of ongoing functional studies to understand the role of novel molecular pathways in disease pathogenesis, which may ultimately improve asthma precision medicine.

Introduction

Asthma, a chronic lung disease characterized by variable airflow limitation, affects 22 million Americans and costs $81.9 billion annually [1]. Episodes of worsening asthma symptoms requiring the use of systemic corticosteroids or other treatments to prevent serious outcomes, termed exacerbations, are a major cause of asthma morbidity and health care costs that in severe cases lead to death [1–4]. While there is no cure for asthma, providing treatment according to existing clinical guidelines successfully controls symptoms, prevents exacerbations, and improves lung function in most patients [5]. Bronchodilator and glucocorticoid medications are commonly used drugs in the treatment of asthma [4]: short-acting bronchodilators (β_2-agonists) are used to provide quick symptom relief; inhaled glucocorticoids that act directly in the lung are prescribed to individuals with persistent asthma to decrease

M. Kan · B. E. Himes (✉)
Department of Biostatistics, Epidemiology and Informatics, University of Pennsylvania, Philadelphia, PA, USA
e-mail: mengykan@pennmedicine.upenn.edu; bhimes@pennmedicine.upenn.edu

© Springer Nature Switzerland AG 2020
J. L. Gomez et al. (eds.), *Precision in Pulmonary, Critical Care, and Sleep Medicine*, Respiratory Medicine, https://doi.org/10.1007/978-3-030-31507-8_3

inflammation, and some individuals with severe disease require long-term use of oral glucocorticoids. Thus, the goal of asthma clinical therapy is to prevent lung damage and control symptoms so that these do not interfere with daily activities.

Asthma is one of the most common diseases of childhood, and some patients continue to manifest symptoms, or develop asthma, as adults. Disparities in asthma prevalence and severity by race/ethnicity and socioeconomic status are a well-known problem in the United States [6–9] where childhood asthma prevalence is highest among Puerto Ricans (36.5%), intermediate among African Americans (13.4%), and lowest among European Americans (7.6%) and Mexicans (7.5%) [10], while asthma mortality is four-fold higher in Puerto Ricans and African Americans compared to Mexican Americans and European Americans [11]. In addition, studies have found that African American and Puerto Rican children have lower drug response to the most commonly used asthma therapies, bronchodilators [12, 13] and glucocorticoids [14], consistent with trends observed for asthma morbidity and mortality. Similar disparities by race/ethnicity are observed among adults in the United States with additional disparities arising by sex: women have 1.7 times greater prevalence of asthma than men and have 30% greater asthma death rates [11, 15, 16].

Beyond increased airway responsiveness to specific exposures or exercise, characteristics exhibited by patients with asthma are variable, but they often include elevated serum total IgE levels, increased Th2 cells, eosinophils, mast cells and lymphocytes, and in the case of persistent and/or severe disease, airway remodeling (i.e., increased airway smooth muscle mass, epithelial goblet cell hyperplasia) [17]. Accordingly, asthma is recognized as being composed of several endotypes that have been, and continue to be, identified via linkage of precise phenotypes to molecular signatures [18, 19]. Further, specific characteristics of asthma are increasingly being used to identify biomarkers for specific disease subtypes and provide therapy tailored to them. For example, biologics like

mepolizumab (an anti-IL5 monoclonal antibody) are now indicated for patients with eosinophilic asthma [20].

Asthma has long been recognized as a heritable condition [21–26] for which genetic variation influences risk [27]. It is estimated that genetic factors explain 35–95% of asthma heritability, 35–84% of total serum IgE levels heritability, 24–41% of blood eosinophil count heritability, and 30–60% of bronchodilator response heritability [28–30]. For the past two decades, genetics studies of asthma and asthma-related traits, such as IgE levels and eosinophil count, have been pursued to identify genetic loci that may clarify the complex mechanisms that lead to what is currently broadly labeled as asthma [31].

Early asthma genetic studies took a candidate gene approach whereby investigators selected single-nucleotide polymorphisms (SNPs) within genes for which there was a biological rationale they be involved in asthma based on disease knowledge at the time, and subsequently, measured the association between these genotyped SNPs and asthma. Although several nominally significant associations were reported in candidate gene studies, very few were independently replicated [27]. Starting in 2005, as commercially available genome-wide genotyping microarrays became available, investigators sought to relate common SNPs (defined as those with minor allele frequency >1–5%) to diseases via genome-wide association studies (GWAS) [32]. Since then, over 3955 GWAS have been completed for a wide range of phenotypes [33, 34]. With the advent of next generation sequencing (NGS) in the late 2000s, attempts to relate DNA sequence variants to diseases have extended to whole-exome and whole-genome sequencing, expanding the genome-wide association approach to include rare and structural variants [35]. In this chapter, we review genetic loci that have been associated with asthma (Fig. 3.1) and asthma drug response (Fig. 3.2) using genome-level studies, and we summarize some of the pathobiological and treatment insights gained via functional studies of these loci (Table 3.1).

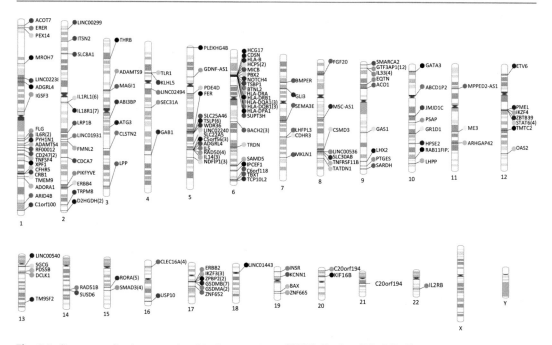

Fig. 3.1 Summary of asthma-associated loci across the human genome. Asthma-related GWAS association results with *p*-value <10⁻⁶ were downloaded from the GWAS Catalog [33, 34]. Figures were generated with PhenoGram (available at: http://visualization.ritchielab.org/phenograms/plot)

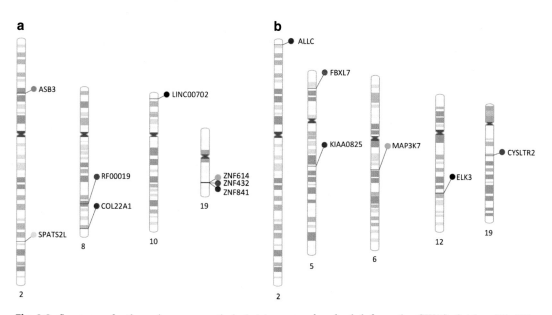

Fig. 3.2 Summary of asthma pharmacogenetic loci. (**a**) Bronchodilator response (BDR) and (**b**) glucocorticoid response GWAS association results with *p*-value <10⁻⁶ were downloaded from the GWAS Catalog [33, 34]. Figures were generated with PhenoGram (available at: http://visualization.ritchielab.org/phenograms/plot)

Table 3.1 Summary of main findings of asthma genetic and pharmacogenetic studies

Phenotype	Main findings
Asthma	Prominent asthma-associated loci are 17q21 locus (including *ORMDL3* and *GSDMB*), HLA region, *TSLP*, *IL33*, *IL13*, and *IL1RL1* [28, 37–39]
	Robust asthma loci identified in persons of African descent include 17q21, *IL33*, *RORA*, and *STAT6* [40]
	There are more significant loci for childhood-onset versus adult-onset asthma. Shared loci across age-of-onset include *IL1RL1*, *IL33* and the HLA region while 17q21 is specific to childhood-onset asthma [58, 59]
Asthma severity	Loci associated with early-childhood severe asthma include *CDHR3* and other asthma loci (17q21, *IL33*, *IL1RL1*, *RAD50*) [62]
	Loci associated with severe-to-moderate asthma include *GATA3*, *MUC5AC*, and *KIAA1109* and other asthma loci (17q21, *TSLP*, *IL1RL1*, *IL33*, *HLA-DQB1*) [64]
IgE levels	Loci associated with IgE levels include IgE level-specific ones (*FCER1A*) and some overlapping with asthma risk (*RAD50*, *STAT6*, and *HLA-DQB1*) in European populations [66, 68]
	Loci associated with IgE levels in non-European populations include *HLA-DQA1* (Latinos) and *HLA-C* (Japanese) [69, 70]
Eosinophil count	A rare loss-of-function variant in *IL33* was associated with lower blood eosinophil counts and reduced asthma risk [72]
Allergic diseases (asthma, allergic rhinitis, atopic dermatitis)	Loci associated with allergic diseases include known asthma loci (17q21, *IL1RL1*, *SMAD3*, *TSLP*), and a hay fever locus *CLEC16A* [74, 75]
Bronchodilator response	BDR-associated loci include *SPATS2L* [78], *COL22A1* [79], and *ASB3* [80]
	ZNF432 was associated with BDR via interaction with inhaled corticosteroid treatment [81]
	BDR-associated loci in minority children with asthma include genes related to lung capacity (*DNAH5*), immunity (*NFKB1* and *PLCB1*), and β-adrenergic signaling (*ADAMTS3* and *COX18*) [90]
Glucocorticoid response	A *GLCCI1* SNP that was nominally associated with glucocorticoid response in patients treated with inhaled glucocorticoids was in high linkage disequilibrium with a variant that was associated with decreased GLCCI1 expression in B cells [91]
	No genetic variants met pre-specified genome-wide significant statistical criteria in the largest published GWAS of glucocorticoid response to date [96]

Genetics of Asthma

Several asthma GWAS have been conducted over the past decade, providing researchers with a relatively solid understanding of which findings are generalizable, which require further verification to determine whether statistical associations truly represent a biologically significant process related to disease, and how GWAS are limited in explaining the heritability of asthma and its related traits [28, 31]. After initial GWAS were completed, investigators noticed that most complex trait associations had relatively small effect sizes, and, hence, cohorts of 100s or 1000s of subjects were inappropriately powered to detect associations [36]. Accordingly, the asthma GWAS that have provided the most consistent results are large meta-analyses of pooled cohorts gathered by different groups of investigators around the world. The first such efforts in asthma were the GABRIEL consortium [37], consisting of 10,365 European persons with physician-diagnosed asthma and 16,110 European controls, and the EVE consortium [38], consisting of 3246 cases with asthma, 3385 non-asthmatic controls, 1702 asthma case-parent trios, and 355 family-based cases and 468 family-based controls, comprising European American, African American and African Caribbean, and Latino subjects. Larger meta-analyses that followed include the Trans-National Asthma Genetic Consortium (TAGC), consisting of 23,948 asthma cases and 118,538 controls without asthma of diverse ancestries from 75 independent asthma GWAS, and the Consortium on Asthma Among African Ancestry Populations (CAAPA), consisting of 7645 asthma cases and 7009 controls without asthma of African ancestry [39–42].

The most well-known and highly replicated asthma association signal, which appears to be specific to childhood-onset asthma [43], is within the 17q21 locus [37, 38, 44]. Many functional studies have sought to understand which gene(s) and variant(s) in this region modify asthma susceptibility. Four genes, IKAROS family zinc finger 3 (*IKZF3*), gasdermin B (*GSDMB*), ORMDL sphingolipid biosynthesis regulator 3 (*ORMDL3*), and zona pellucida binding protein 2 (*ZPBP2*), were proposed as functional candidates in early studies based on their proximity to the association signal and results from expression quantitative trait loci (eQTL) studies, which found that the asthma-associated SNPs were also associated with these genes' mRNA expression levels in various tissues [45–48]. More detailed experimental studies lend support to *ORMDL3* and *GSDMB* as being the genes that are relevant to asthma: overexpression of either *ORMDL3* or *GSDMB* in bronchial epithelium in mice leads to increased airway remodeling and responsiveness [49–51]. A study by Panganiban and colleagues found that GSDMB protein induces pyroptosis of airway epithelia cells during inflammation and that a *GSDMB* splice variant abolishes its pyroptotic activity, thus hypothesizing that this variant contributes to the protective association signal observed in asthma [52]. The 17q21 locus associations have also been observed in Puerto Rican children [53] and admixed African populations in CAAPA [40], suggesting the signal is not limited to people of European ancestry, although the linkage disequilibrium patterns at this locus differ across populations and their relationship with asthma is not fully characterized. Further, there is inconsistent evidence of association in some studies of African American people with asthma [54–56], underscoring the need for a better understanding of how genetic ancestry influences this locus. In asthma GWAS conducted in adults, it is not always clear whether subjects had childhood-onset asthma; thus, some lack of replication may reflect type of asthma rather than racial/ethnic differences. For example, in GWAS among Asian and Hispanic adults [54, 55] where

the 17q21 locus was not associated with asthma, it is unclear whether this was due to differences in genetic ancestry or the fact that few cases had childhood-onset asthma. Ongoing GWAS and functional studies may shed further light on this association signal and one day lead to clinically useful insights.

Other robust asthma associations have been discovered in European cohorts within and near the genes coding for thymic stromal lymphopoietin (*TSLP*) (5q22), interleukin 33 (*IL33*) (9q24), and interleukin 1 receptor like 1 (*IL1RL1*) (2q12), and the human leukocyte antigen (HLA) regions (6p21) [37, 38]. These genes represent pathways in which epithelial cell-derived cytokines promote the differentiation and activation of T helper 2 (Th2) cells [28], and unlike the 17q21 association, they are consistent with what is known about asthma biology. However, the fact that SNPs in/near these specific genes arise via GWAS, while those of other cytokine-related genes do not, points to the ability of unbiased approaches to identify the most promising disease loci. Fewer consistent asthma GWAS results specific to non-European populations have been observed, partly because there are fewer non-European GWAS cohorts, and those that do exist are of limited sample size [57]. For example, the EVE study found that SNPs near pyrin and HIN domain family member 1 (*PYHIN1*) were associated with asthma in subjects of African descent [38], a finding that has not been definitively observed in subsequent GWAS of African Americans. GWAS of non-European persons, however, have served to validate trans-ethnic loci: the TAGC meta-analyses of multi-ancestry populations replicated GWAS findings at *IL33*, *IL1RL1*, RAR related orphan receptor A (*RORA*), SMAD family member 3 (*SMAD3*), and signal transducer and activator of transcription 6 (*STAT6*), which were initially discovered in European populations [39], while CAAPA found that asthma associations among individuals of African descent included variants at/near the 17q21 locus, *IL33*, *RORA*, and *STAT6* [40].

The majority of subjects in asthma GWAS have been children or persons with childhood-onset asthma, but more recent studies have been able to formally search for genetic factors specific to childhood- versus adult-onset asthma. UK Biobank studies have found that there are more loci associated with childhood- versus adult-onset asthma [58, 59]. Specifically, Ferreira and colleagues conducted GWAS of childhood-onset asthma (13,962 affected individuals; 300,671 controls) and adult-onset asthma (26,582 affected individuals; 300,671 controls) and identified 123 independent associations for childhood-onset asthma and 56 for adult-onset asthma with 37 overlapping [58]. Attempted replication of these findings in an independent study of 262,767 subjects found that 98 and 34 loci replicated for childhood- and adult-onset, respectively [58]. Pividori and colleagues, using data for 376,358 British white individuals (9433 adults with childhood onset asthma; 21,564 adults with adult-onset asthma), identified 23 childhood-onset specific loci, one adult-onset specific locus, and 37 shared loci [59]. Genes that were shared across age-of-onset in both of these UK Biobank studies included the known asthma-associated genes *IL1RL1*, *IL33*, and the HLA region while the 17q21 locus was specific to childhood-onset asthma, consistent with results of previous asthma GWAS. Overall, these studies suggest that genetic variation contributes more strongly to childhood-onset asthma while non-genetic risk factors (e.g., environmental factors) are more prominent in adult-onset asthma [58, 59].

Sex is a non-modifiable risk factor related to genetics, and, thus, considering sex in GWAS may help clarify the pathobiological mechanisms that lead to observed asthma sex disparities. A meta-analysis of sex-specific GWAS was conducted in 2653 male and 2566 female asthma cases versus 3830 pooled non-asthma controls from EVE found six loci with a p-value $<10^{-6}$. Two loci were male-specific: interferon regulatory factor 1 (*IRF1*) in European Americans and RAB11 family interacting protein 2 (*RAB11FIP2*) in African Americans, while four loci were female-specific: long intergenic non-protein coding RNA 1931 (*LINC01931*) in African Americans, and Erb-B2 receptor tyrosine kinase 4 (*ERBB4*), chromosome 6 open reading frame

118 (*C6orf118*) and RAB11 family interacting protein 2 (*RAB11FIP2*) in Latinos [60]. This sex-specific study was limited by the reduced power resulting from diminished sample size inherent when restricting analysis by sex, and no major sex-specific asthma GWAS have been published with genome-wide significant findings.

Rare variants do not appear to confer much risk for asthma based on studies published thus far, suggesting that rare variants are unlikely to account for a significant proportion of asthma heritability. An exome study by Igartua and colleagues based on some of the EVE cohorts reported evidence of population-specific low-frequency variants being associated with asthma in/near the general receptor for phosphoinositides 1 associated scaffold protein (*GRASP*) and *GSDMB* among Latinos, and methylenetetrahydrofolate reductase (*MTHFR*) among African Americans/African Caribbeans [61].

Genetics of Traits Related to Asthma

Genetic studies of people selected via a more specific asthma definition than "doctor's diagnosis" and of secondary quantitative phenotypes related to asthma have been performed in an attempt to increase power to detect associations and clarify the potential functional role of associated loci. This approach has been successful in some cases. A GWAS of early-childhood severe asthma, defined on the basis of repeated acute hospitalizations, consisting of 1173 cases and 2522 controls, identified several known asthma susceptibility loci such as the 17q21 locus, *IL33, IL1RL1*, and RAD50 double-strand break repair protein (*RAD50*), but additionally, it identified a locus that had not been observed using broader asthma definitions: cadherin-related family member 3 (*CDHR3*) [62]. A GWAS of childhood acute asthma exacerbations, defined on the basis of having a 5-day course of oral steroids, found promising variants in/near catenin alpha 3 (*CTNNA3*) and semaphorin 3D (*SEMA3D*), two genes with potential roles in immune response and airway remodeling, respectively [63]. The SNP near *CTNNA3* reached genome-wide significance while a SNP near *SEMA3D* was significant in a replication cohort; however, further support for these associations has not yet been published. A more recent GWAS of moderate-to-severe asthma from the UK Biobank, where patients were selected based on medications used and doctor diagnosis, identified novel asthma-associated loci at the GATA binding protein 3 (*GATA3*) gene, which encodes a transcription factor related to T-cell response in asthma and eosinophilia, mucin 5 AC, oligomeric mucus/gel-forming gene (*MUC5AC*), and uncharacterized protein KIAA1109 (*KIAA1109*) [64]. Additionally, this study replicated previously identified asthma GWAS loci such as 17q21, *TSLP*, *IL1RL1*, *IL33*, and *HLA-DQB1* [64].

GWAS of immunoglobulin E (IgE), an antibody that mediates allergic diseases and is elevated in some persons with asthma [65], have found robust genetic associations that are specific to IgE levels, such as variants in/near Fc fragment of IgE receptor Ia (*FCER1A*), as well as associations that are shared with asthma susceptibility (e.g., *STAT6*, *RAD50*, and *HLA-DQB1*) [66–68]. IgE GWAS of non-European populations have identified variants in/near the major histocompatibility complex, class II, DQ Alpha 1 (*HLA-DQA1*) as associated with IgE levels in Latinos [69] and the major histocompatibility complex, class I, C (*HLA-C*) in Japanese individuals [70]. Genetic studies of count of eosinophils, effector cells activated by Th2-type cytokines such as IL33 [71], include a whole-genome sequencing study that identified a rare loss-of-function variant in *IL33* as associated with lower blood eosinophil counts and reduced asthma risk [72].

Shared Genetics of Asthma and Allergic Diseases

Allergic asthma shares some of its genetic origin with other diseases, such as allergic rhinitis (hay fever) and atopic dermatitis (eczema) [73, 74]. GWAS in which cases include persons with at least one allergic disease have been pursued to detect associations that underlie shared biological pathways that lead to allergic diseases [74, 75]. Ferreira and colleagues conducted such a

GWAS with 180,129 cases with self-reported or doctor-diagnosed asthma and/or hay fever and/or eczema and 180,709 controls of European ancestry in which they identified 99 independent associations with allergic disease, most with similar effects in individual allergic diseases [75]. Zhu and colleagues performed a GWAS using 76,768 controls from the UK Biobank and restricting cases to 33,593 subjects with a doctor-diagnosed allergic disease, and they identified 38 genome-wide significant loci including seven novel shared loci [74]. Both of these studies identified prominent asthma GWAS loci (i.e.,17q21, *IL1RL1*, *SMAD3*, *TSLP*) as well as some novel loci with suggestive associations such as the C-type lectin domain containing 16A (*CLEC16A*) gene that was previously associated with hay fever among asthma patients [76]. Functional annotation of allergic-disease-associated loci revealed enrichment of immune/inflammatory pathways, suggesting that variants in/near several genes contribute to the co-existence of allergic diseases [74, 75].

Genetics of Bronchodilator Response

Bronchodilator response (BDR), measured as the percent change in forced expiratory volume in 1 second (FEV_1) following administration of a β_2-agonist (usually albuterol) according to recommended guidelines [77], has been used as a quantitative and dichotomous outcome for GWAS of β_2-agonist response. Early genome-wide efforts to study BDR include a study by Himes and colleagues in which the primary cohort consisted of 1644 white asthma subjects from six clinical trials, and replication was performed in two independent populations [78]. The top association signal was near the spermatogenesis-associated serine rich 2 like (*SPATS2L*) gene with a combined p-value $<10^{-6}$; further evidence that this gene of unknown function was involved in BDR was provided by experiments in which *SPATS2L* mRNA knockdown in airway smooth muscle, a target tissue of bronchodilators, resulted in increased levels of

β_2-adrenergic receptor, the receptor via which β_2-agonists exert their airway relaxation effect [78]. Duan and colleagues performed a BDR GWAS based on 403 white trios with asthma children from the Childhood Asthma Management Program (CAMP) and applied five different statistical approaches to determine that the most robust associations were within the collagen type XXII alpha 1 (COL22A1) gene [79]. A BDR GWAS study in 724 white subjects, including the CAMP cohort, used two distinct measures of BDR to screen SNPs for replication in an attempt to control for phenotypic variability in β_2-agonist response [80]. This study by Israel and colleagues found that a novel locus near the ankyrin repeat (ASB3) gene was associated with BDR. While the three BDR GWAS discussed thus far used subjects from clinical trials in which BDR was measured while no other medications had been taken (i.e., after a "wash-out" period), most people with persistent asthma are treated with both inhaled corticosteroids (ICS) and β_2-agonists, and the effects of these two drugs are synergistic. To account for this, a BDR GWAS that included interactions with ICS treatment in 581 white asthmatic children from CAMP was performed by Wu and colleagues [81]. After combining primary and replication cohort results, a genome-wide significant locus was found near the zinc finger protein 432 (ZNF432) gene [81]. BDR loci that had been identified via candidate gene studies, including the adrenoceptor beta 2 (ADRB2), adenylate cyclase 9 (ADCY9), corticotropin-releasing hormone receptor 2 (CRHR2), and arginase 1 (ARG1) genes [82–87], have not been identified in BDR GWAS, again demonstrating that most results from candidate gene studies are not generalizable. BDR GWAS, however, have been limited relative to asthma GWAS by smaller sample sizes and the lack of convenience cohorts: BDR tests are not readily available via Biobanks or studies that rely on self-reported outcomes.

Differences in response to albuterol have been observed between racial/ethnic groups: Puerto Rican and African American children with asthma are significantly less responsive to albuterol than Mexican children [12, 13], and, thus, studies of BDR in diverse populations have been performed as they may shed light on asthma disparities. Drake and colleagues performed a BDR GWAS in 1782 Latino children with asthma and identified rare variants in SLC22A15, SLC24A4, and IGF2R genes as associated with BDR [88]. More recently, BDR studies have been conducted as part of the Trans-Omics for Precision Medicine (TOPMed) Program of the National Heart, Lung, and Blood Institute [89]. Specifically, a whole-genome sequencing study performed in 1441 minority children (i.e., Puerto Ricans, Mexicans, and African Americans) with asthma used a dichotomous BDR outcome based on the tails of the continuous BDR distribution (i.e., high vs. low responder status) and found several promising loci near genes previously associated with lung capacity (dynein axonemal heavy chain 5 (DNAH5)), immunity (nuclear factor kappa B subunit 1 (NFKB1), phospholipase C beta 1 (PLCB1)), β-adrenergic signaling (ADAM metallopeptidase with thrombospondin type 1 motif 3 (ADAMTS3), cytochrome C oxidase assembly factor COX18 (COX18)) [90]. Functional evidence that a variant near NFKB1 influences transcription of this gene was provided, resulting in the strongest evidence for this locus. Due to the unavailability of additional cohorts for replication, however, these findings have not been further tested. As the TOPMed program grows, the identification of robust BDR-associated loci may increase.

Genetics of Glucocorticoid Response

Asthma glucocorticoid response studies have addressed the question of whether patients' symptoms improve with ICS use. Unlike BDR, which refers to a more clearly defined acute outcome measured in a laboratory setting, response to ICS is assessed over the course of weeks to months, and specific outcomes measured are variable although usually involving the number of asthma exacerbations and/or improved lung function (e.g., improved baseline FEV_1). Because glucocorticoid response outcomes are related to asthma severity and medication adherence, it is difficult to ensure that the same actual outcome is being assessed across patients. This is particularly the case when using cross-sectional data to assess glucocorticoid response, and it is thus not surprising that most glucocorticoid response GWAS are based on clinical trials cohorts. Tantisira and colleagues performed one of the first GWAS of glucocorticoid response using 181 white asthma-proband trios from CAMP and four independent clinical trial cohorts for attempted replication. In a discovery stage, the quantitative outcome selected was residuals of the difference between FEV_1 following months of budesonide treatment after adjustment for age, sex, and height. Of the 13 top variants from this stage that were selected for replication, SNP rs37972, near glucocorticoid induced 1 (*GLCCI1*), was nominally associated with glucocorticoid response ($p < 0.05$). Functional analysis showed that SNP rs37973, which was in high linkage disequilibrium with rs37972, was associated with decreased GLCCI1 expression in B cells, suggesting that rs37973 leads to decreased response to glucocorticoids in patient with asthma via changes in GLCCI1 expression [91]. The *GLCCI1* associations have not been replicated in some independent studies [92, 93]. A GWAS of glucocorticoid response defined as the change in percent FEV_1 after 4 weeks of treatment with ICS was performed in 189 Korean subjects with asthma found that the top SNPs (p-value $<10^{-6}$) mapped to allantoicase (*ALLC*) [94]. A GWAS of changes in asthma symptom scores after ICS treatment (i.e., average asthma symptom score from the last week of ICS treatment minus average asthma symptom score from the week before ICS treatment was initiated) was performed in 124 white children from CAMP. Three SNPs near rhabdomyosarcoma 2 associated transcript (*RMST*), long intergenic non-protein coding RNA 2140 (*LINC02140*), and F-box and leucine rich repeat protein 7 (*FBXL7*) were nominally replicated in children, but not adults, from independent clinical trial cohorts [95].

Most glucocorticoid response GWAS results published thus far have not been replicated in independent studies, partly because the GWAS studies have been based on small sample sizes. The largest published GWAS of glucocorticoid response to date was conducted using data from 2675 asthma subjects who were part of GSK clinical trials of fluticasone furoate and fluticasone propionate [96]. This study by Mosteller and colleagues found that no genetic variants met pre-specified genome-wide significant statistical criteria, and while *GLCCI1* variants were nominally associated with change in FEV_1, the authors concluded that common genetic variants are unlikely to serve as biomarkers of steroid responsiveness [96]. With the advent of inhaler-based sensors and health information technologies that permit convenient and remote tracking of ICS use in many individuals, larger pharmacogenetics studies of asthma may be possible in the near future [97].

Conclusion

Asthma genetics and pharmacogenetics studies have identified numerous genetic loci associated with asthma and asthma-related traits, including drug response. Associations at some loci, most notably the 17q21 region with asthma, have been replicated in several independent studies, leaving little doubt the associations reflect true disease pathways. Nonetheless, linking specific alleles to asthma pathobiology has been a slow process due, in part, to the difficulty in determining what experimental assays should be used to validate associations representing the complex trait that is asthma. Based on BDR and glucocorticoid response GWAS results thus far, it is unlikely that pharmacogenetic tests for commonly used asthma drugs will be useful at the point of care. Results of asthma pharmacogenetic studies are valuable, however, to identify novel loci involved in asthma drug response pathways. Ongoing efforts such as the TOPMed Program will provide insights via larger and more diverse whole-genome sequencing studies of asthma that link multi-omics data to genetics, leading to the discovery of novel drug targets and preventive strategies for improved asthma precision medicine.

References

1. Nurmagambetov T, Kuwahara R, Garbe P. The economic burden of asthma in the United States, 2008–2013. Ann Am Thorac Soc. 2018;15(3):348–56.
2. Mazurek J, Syamlal G. Prevalence of asthma, asthma attacks, and emergency department visits for asthma among working adults — National Health Interview Survey, 2011–2016. MMWR Morb Mortal Wkly Rep. 2018;67:377–86.
3. Zahran H, Bailey C, Damon S, Garbe P, Breysse P. Vital signs: asthma in children — United States, 2001–2016. MMWR Morb Mortal Wkly Rep. 2018;67:149–55.
4. Fanta CH. Asthma. N Engl J Med. 2009;360(10): 1002–14.
5. National Asthma Education Program. Expert panel report 3: guidelines for the diagnosis and management of asthma. National Institutes of Health. Bethesda: US Department of Health and Human Services; 2007.
6. Burchard EG. Medical research: missing patients. Nature. 2014;513(7518):301–2.
7. Forno E, Celedon JC. Health disparities in asthma. Am J Respir Crit Care Med. 2012;185(10):1033–5.
8. Celedon JC, Roman J, Schraufnagel DE, Thomas A, Samet J. Respiratory health equality in the United States. The American thoracic society perspective. Ann Am Thorac Soc. 2014;11(4):473–9.
9. Moorman JE, Akinbami LJ, Bailey CM, Zahran HS, King ME, Johnson CA, et al. National surveillance of asthma: United States, 2001–2010. National Center for Health Statistics. Vital Health Stat 3. 2012;2012(35):1–58.
10. Barr RG, Aviles-Santa L, Davis SM, Aldrich TK, Gonzalez F 2nd, Henderson AG, et al. Pulmonary disease and age at immigration among Hispanics. Results from the Hispanic community health study/study of Latinos. Am J Respir Crit Care Med. 2016;193(4):386–95.
11. Akinbami L, Moorman J, Bailey C, Zahran H, King M, Johnson C, et al. Trends in asthma prevalence, health care use, and mortality in the United States, 2001–2010. Hyattsville: National Center for Health Statistics; 2012.
12. Naqvi M, Thyne S, Choudhry S, Tsai HJ, Navarro D, Castro RA, et al. Ethnic-specific differences in bronchodilator responsiveness among African Americans, Puerto Ricans, and Mexicans with asthma. J Asthma. 2007;44(8):639–48.
13. Burchard EG, Avila PC, Nazario S, Casal J, Torres A, Rodriguez-Santana JR, et al. Lower bronchodilator responsiveness in Puerto Rican than in Mexican subjects with asthma. Am J Respir Crit Care Med. 2004;169(3):386–92.
14. Akinbami LJ, Moorman JE, Simon AE, Schoendorf KC. Trends in racial disparities for asthma outcomes among children 0 to 17 years, 2001–2010. J Allergy Clin Immunol. 2014;134(3):547–53 e5.
15. Greenblatt R, Mansour O, Zhao E, Ross M, Himes BE. Gender-specific determinants of asthma among U.S. adults. Asthma Res Pract. 2017;3:2.
16. Zein JG, Erzurum SC. Asthma is different in women. Curr Allergy Asthma Rep. 2015;15(6):28.
17. Davies DE, Wicks J, Powell RM, Puddicombe SM, Holgate ST. Airway remodeling in asthma: new insights. J Allergy Clin Immunol. 2003;111(2):215–25; quiz 26.
18. Wenzel SE. Asthma phenotypes: the evolution from clinical to molecular approaches. Nat Med. 2012;18(5):716–25.
19. Lotvall J, Akdis CA, Bacharier LB, Bjermer L, Casale TB, Custovic A, et al. Asthma endotypes: a new approach to classification of disease entities within the asthma syndrome. J Allergy Clin Immunol. 2011;127(2):355–60.
20. Ortega HG, Liu MC, Pavord ID, Brusselle GG, FitzGerald JM, Chetta A, et al. Mepolizumab treatment in patients with severe eosinophilic asthma. N Engl J Med. 2014;371(13):1198–207.
21. Nieminen MM, Kaprio J, Koskenvuo M. A population-based study of bronchial asthma in adult twin pairs. Chest. 1991;100(1):70–5.
22. Laitinen T, Rasanen M, Kaprio J, Koskenvuo M, Laitinen LA. Importance of genetic factors in adolescent asthma: a population-based twin-family study. Am J Respir Crit Care Med. 1998;157(4 Pt 1):1073–8.
23. Duffy DL, Martin NG, Battistutta D, Hopper JL, Mathews JD. Genetics of asthma and hay fever in Australian twins. Am Rev Respir Dis. 1990;142(6 Pt 1):1351–8.
24. Harris JR, Magnus P, Samuelsen SO, Tambs K. No evidence for effects of family environment on asthma. A retrospective study of Norwegian twins. Am J Respir Crit Care Med. 1997;156(1):43–9.
25. Koeppen-Schomerus G, Stevenson J, Plomin R. Genes and environment in asthma: a study of 4 year old twins. Arch Dis Child. 2001;85(5):398–400.
26. Skadhauge LR, Christensen K, Kyvik KO, Sigsgaard T. Genetic and environmental influence on asthma: a population-based study of 11,688 Danish twin pairs. Eur Respir J. 1999;13(1):8–14.
27. Ober C, Hoffjan S. Asthma genetics 2006: the long and winding road to gene discovery. Genes Immun. 2006;7(2):95–100.
28. Ober C, Yao TC. The genetics of asthma and allergic disease: a 21st century perspective. Immunol Rev. 2011;242(1):10–30.
29. McGeachie MJ, Stahl EA, Himes BE, Pendergrass SA, Lima JJ, Irvin CG, et al. Polygenic heritability estimates in pharmacogenetics: focus on asthma and related phenotypes. Pharmacogenet Genomics. 2013;23(6):324–8.
30. Thomsen SF, van der Sluis S, Kyvik KO, Skytthe A, Backer V. Estimates of asthma heritability in a large twin sample. Clin Exp Allergy. 2010;40(7):1054–61.
31. Kim KW, Ober C. Lessons learned from GWAS of asthma. Allergy Asthma Immunol Res. 2019;11(2):170–87.
32. Kan M, Shumyatcher M, Himes BE. Using omics approaches to understand pulmonary diseases. Respir Res. 2017;18(1):149.

33. Buniello A, MacArthur JAL, Cerezo M, Harris LW, Hayhurst J, Malangone C, et al. The NHGRI-EBI GWAS catalog of published genome-wide association studies, targeted arrays and summary statistics 2019. Nucleic Acids Res. 2019;47(D1):D1005–12.

34. MacArthur J, Bowler E, Cerezo M, Gil L, Hall P, Hastings E, et al. The new NHGRI-EBI catalog of published genome-wide association studies (GWAS catalog). Nucleic Acids Res. 2017;45(D1):D896–901.

35. Goodwin S, McPherson JD, McCombie WR. Coming of age: ten years of next-generation sequencing technologies. Nat Rev Genet. 2016;17(6):333–51.

36. Tam V, Patel N, Turcotte M, Bosse Y, Pare G, Meyre D. Benefits and limitations of genome-wide association studies. Nat Rev Genet. 2019;20:467.

37. Moffatt MF, Gut IG, Demenais F, Strachan DP, Bouzigon E, Heath S, et al. A large-scale, consortium-based genomewide association study of asthma. N Engl J Med. 2010;363(13):1211–21.

38. Torgerson DG, Ampleford EJ, Chiu GY, Gauderman WJ, Gignoux CR, Graves PE, et al. Meta-analysis of genome-wide association studies of asthma in ethnically diverse North American populations. Nat Genet. 2011;43(9):887–92.

39. Demenais F, Margaritte-Jeannin P, Barnes KC, Cookson WOC, Altmuller J, Ang W, et al. Multiancestry association study identifies new asthma risk loci that colocalize with immune-cell enhancer marks. Nat Genet. 2018;50(1):42–53.

40. Daya M, Rafaels N, Brunetti TM, Chavan S, Levin AM, Shetty A, et al. Association study in African-admixed populations across the Americas recapitulates asthma risk loci in non-African populations. Nat Commun. 2019;10(1):880.

41. Stein MM, Thompson EE, Schoettler N, Helling BA, Magnaye KM, Stanhope C, et al. A decade of research on the 17q12–21 asthma locus: piecing together the puzzle. J Allergy Clin Immunol. 2018;142(3):749–64 e3.

42. Mathias RA, Taub MA, Gignoux CR, Fu W, Musharoff S, O'Connor TD, et al. A continuum of admixture in the Western Hemisphere revealed by the African Diaspora genome. Nat Commun. 2016;7:12522.

43. Ono JG, Worgall TS, Worgall S. 17q21 locus and ORMDL3: an increased risk for childhood asthma. Pediatr Res. 2014;75(1–2):165–70.

44. Moffatt MF, Kabesch M, Liang L, Dixon AL, Strachan D, Heath S, et al. Genetic variants regulating ORMDL3 expression contribute to the risk of childhood asthma. Nature. 2007;448(7152):470–3.

45. Verlaan DJ, Berlivet S, Hunninghake GM, Madore AM, Lariviere M, Moussette S, et al. Allele-specific chromatin remodeling in the ZPBP2/GSDMB/ ORMDL3 locus associated with the risk of asthma and autoimmune disease. Am J Hum Genet. 2009;85:377–93.

46. Caliskan M, Bochkov YA, Kreiner-Moller E, Bonnelykke K, Stein MM, Du G, et al. Rhinovirus wheezing illness and genetic risk of childhood-onset asthma. N Engl J Med. 2013;368(15):1398–407.

47. Li X, Hastie AT, Hawkins GA, Moore WC, Ampleford EJ, Milosevic J, et al. eQTL of bronchial epithelial cells and bronchial alveolar lavage deciphers GWAS-identified asthma genes. Allergy. 2015;70(10):1309–18.

48. Schmiedel BJ, Seumois G, Samaniego-Castruita D, Cayford J, Schulten V, Chavez L, et al. 17q21 asthma-risk variants switch CTCF binding and regulate IL-2 production by T cells. Nat Commun. 2016;7:13426.

49. Miller M, Tam AB, Cho JY, Doherty TA, Pham A, Khorram N, et al. ORMDL3 is an inducible lung epithelial gene regulating metalloproteases, chemokines, OAS, and ATF6. Proc Natl Acad Sci. 2012;109:16648–53.

50. Miller M, Rosenthal P, Beppu A, Mueller JL, Hoffman HM, Tam AB, et al. ORMDL3 transgenic mice have increased airway remodeling and airway responsiveness characteristic of asthma. J Immunol. 2014;192:3475–87.

51. Das S, Miller M, Beppu AK, Mueller J, McGeough MD, Vuong C, et al. GSDMB induces an asthma phenotype characterized by increased airway responsiveness and remodeling without lung inflammation. Proc Natl Acad Sci U S A. 2016;113(46):13132–7.

52. Panganiban RA, Sun M, Dahlin A, Park HR, Kan M, Himes BE, et al. A functional splice variant associated with decreased asthma risk abolishes the ability of gasdermin B to induce epithelial cell pyroptosis. J Allergy Clin Immunol. 2018;142(5):1469–78 e2.

53. Yan Q, Brehm J, Pino-Yanes M, Forno E, Lin J, Oh SS, et al. A meta-analysis of genome-wide association studies of asthma in Puerto Ricans. Eur Respir J. 2017;49(5):1601505.

54. Almoguera B, Vazquez L, Mentch F, Connolly J, Pacheco JA, Sundaresan AS, et al. Identification of four novel loci in asthma in European American and African American populations. Am J Respir Crit Care Med. 2017;195(4):456–63.

55. Dahlin A, Sordillo JE, Ziniti J, Iribarren C, Lu M, Weiss ST, et al. Large-scale, multiethnic genome-wide association study identifies novel loci contributing to asthma susceptibility in adults. J Allergy Clin Immunol. 2019;143(4):1633–5.

56. Mathias RA, Grant AV, Rafaels N, Hand T, Gao L, Vergara C, et al. A genome-wide association study on African-ancestry populations for asthma. J Allergy Clin Immunol. 2010;125(2):336–46 e4.

57. Oh SS, Galanter J, Thakur N, Pino-Yanes M, Barcelo NE, White MJ, et al. Diversity in clinical and biomedical research: a promise yet to be fulfilled. PLoS Med. 2015;12(12):e1001918.

58. Ferreira MAR, Mathur R, Vonk JM, Szwajda A, Brumpton B, Granell R, et al. Genetic architectures of childhood- and adult-onset asthma are partly distinct. Am J Hum Genet. 2019;104(4):665–84.

59. Pividori M, Schoettler N, Nicolae DL, Ober C, Im HK. Shared and distinct genetic risk factors for childhood-onset and adult-onset asthma: genome-wide and transcriptome-wide studies. Lancet Respir Med. 2019;7:509.

60. Myers RA, Scott NM, Gauderman WJ, Qiu W, Mathias RA, Romieu I, et al. Genome-wide interaction studies reveal sex-specific asthma risk alleles. Hum Mol Genet. 2014;23(19):5251–9.

61. Igartua C, Myers RA, Mathias RA, Pino-Yanes M, Eng C, Graves PE, et al. Ethnic-specific associations of rare and low-frequency DNA sequence variants with asthma. Nat Commun. 2015;6:5965.

62. Bonnelykke K, Sleiman P, Nielsen K, Kreiner-Moller E, Mercader JM, Belgrave D, et al. A genome-wide association study identifies CDHR3 as a susceptibility locus for early childhood asthma with severe exacerbations. Nat Genet. 2014;46(1):51–5.

63. McGeachie MJ, Wu AC, Tse SM, Clemmer GL, Sordillo J, Himes BE, et al. CTNNA3 and SEMA3D: promising loci for asthma exacerbation identified through multiple genome-wide association studies. J Allergy Clin Immunol. 2015;136(6):1503–10.

64. Shrine N, Portelli MA, John C, Soler Artigas M, Bennett N, Hall R, et al. Moderate-to-severe asthma in individuals of European ancestry: a genome-wide association study. Lancet Respir Med. 2019;7(1):20–34.

65. Gould HJ, Sutton BJ. IgE in allergy and asthma today. Nat Rev Immunol. 2008;8(3):205–17.

66. Granada M, Wilk JB, Tuzova M, Strachan DP, Weidinger S, Albrecht E, et al. A genome-wide association study of plasma total IgE concentrations in the Framingham Heart Study. J Allergy Clin Immunol. 2012;129(3):840–5 e21.

67. Levin AM, Mathias RA, Huang L, Roth LA, Daley D, Myers RA, et al. A meta-analysis of genome-wide association studies for serum total IgE in diverse study populations. J Allergy Clin Immunol. 2013;131(4):1176–84.

68. Weidinger S, Gieger C, Rodriguez E, Baurecht H, Mempel M, Klopp N, et al. Genome-wide scan on total serum IgE levels identifies FCER1A as novel susceptibility locus. PLoS Genet. 2008;4(8):e1000166.

69. Pino-Yanes M, Gignoux CR, Galanter JM, Levin AM, Campbell CD, Eng C, et al. Genome-wide association study and admixture mapping reveal new loci associated with total IgE levels in Latinos. J Allergy Clin Immunol. 2015;135(6):1502–10.

70. Yatagai Y, Sakamoto T, Masuko H, Kaneko Y, Yamada H, Iijima H, et al. Genome-wide association study for levels of total serum IgE identifies HLA-C in a Japanese population. PLoS One. 2013;8(12):e80941.

71. Brusselle GG, Maes T, Bracke KR. Eosinophils in the spotlight: eosinophilic airway inflammation in nonallergic asthma. Nat Med. 2013;19(8):977–9.

72. Smith D, Helgason H, Sulem P, Bjornsdottir US, Lim AC, Sveinbjornsson G, et al. A rare IL33 loss-of-function mutation reduces blood eosinophil counts and protects from asthma. PLoS Genet. 2017;13(3):e1006659.

73. van Beijsterveldt CE, Boomsma DI. Genetics of parentally reported asthma, eczema and rhinitis in 5-yr-old twins. Eur Respir J. 2007;29(3):516–21.

74. Zhu Z, Lee PH, Chaffin MD, Chung W, Loh PR, Lu Q, et al. A genome-wide cross-trait analysis from UK biobank highlights the shared genetic architecture of asthma and allergic diseases. Nat Genet. 2018;50(6):857–64.

75. Ferreira MA, Vonk JM, Baurecht H, Marenholz I, Tian C, Hoffman JD, et al. Shared genetic origin of asthma, hay fever and eczema elucidates allergic disease biology. Nat Genet. 2017;49(12):1752–7.

76. Ferreira MA, Matheson MC, Tang CS, Granell R, Ang W, Hui J, et al. Genome-wide association analysis identifies 11 risk variants associated with the asthma with hay fever phenotype. J Allergy Clin Immunol. 2014;133(6):1564–71.

77. Miller MR, Hankinson J, Brusasco V, Burgos F, Casaburi R, Coates A, et al. Standardisation of spirometry. Eur Respir J. 2005;26(2):319–38.

78. Himes BE, Jiang X, Hu R, Wu AC, Lasky-Su JA, Klanderman BJ, et al. Genome-wide association analysis in asthma subjects identifies SPATS2L as a novel bronchodilator response gene. PLoS Genet. 2012;8(7):e1002824.

79. Duan QL, Lasky-Su J, Himes BE, Qiu W, Litonjua AA, Damask A, et al. A genome-wide association study of bronchodilator response in asthmatics. Pharmacogenomics J. 2014;14(1):41–7.

80. Israel E, Lasky-Su J, Markezich A, Damask A, Szefler SJ, Schuemann B, et al. Genome-wide association study of short-acting beta2-agonists. A novel genome-wide significant locus on chromosome 2 near ASB3. Am J Respir Crit Care Med. 2015;191(5):530–7.

81. Wu AC, Himes BE, Lasky-Su J, Litonjua A, Peters SP, Lima J, et al. Inhaled corticosteroid treatment modulates ZNF432 gene variant's effect on bronchodilator response in asthmatics. J Allergy Clin Immunol. 2014;133(3):723–8 e3.

82. Drysdale CM, McGraw DW, Stack CB, Stephens JC, Judson RS, Nandabalan K, et al. Complex promoter and coding region beta 2-adrenergic receptor haplotypes alter receptor expression and predict in vivo responsiveness. Proc Natl Acad Sci U S A. 2000;97(19):10483–8.

83. Litonjua AA, Lasky-Su J, Schneiter K, Tantisira KG, Lazarus R, Klanderman B, et al. ARG1 is a novel bronchodilator response gene: screening and replication in four asthma cohorts. Am J Respir Crit Care Med. 2008;178(7):688–94.

84. Poon AH, Tantisira KG, Litonjua AA, Lazarus R, Xu J, Lasky-Su J, et al. Association of corticotropin-releasing hormone receptor-2 genetic variants with acute bronchodilator response in asthma. Pharmacogenet Genomics. 2008;18(5):373–82.

85. Silverman EK, Kwiatkowski DJ, Sylvia JS, Lazarus R, Drazen JM, Lange C, et al. Family-based association analysis of beta2-adrenergic receptor polymorphisms in the childhood asthma management program. J Allergy Clin Immunol. 2003;112(5):870–6.

86. Tantisira KG, Small KM, Litonjua AA, Weiss ST, Liggett SB. Molecular properties and pharmacogenetics of a polymorphism of adenylyl cyclase

type 9 in asthma: interaction between beta-agonist and corticosteroid pathways. Hum Mol Genet. 2005;14(12):1671–7.

87. Vonk JM, Postma DS, Maarsingh H, Bruinenberg M, Koppelman GH, Meurs H. Arginase 1 and arginase 2 variations associate with asthma, asthma severity and beta2 agonist and steroid response. Pharmacogenet Genomics. 2010;20(3):179–86.

88. Drake KA, Torgerson DG, Gignoux CR, Galanter JM, Roth LA, Huntsman S, et al. A genome-wide association study of bronchodilator response in Latinos implicates rare variants. J Allergy Clin Immunol. 2014;133(2):370–8.

89. Wu AC, Kiley JP, Noel PJ, Amur S, Burchard EG, Clancy JP, et al. Current status and future opportunities in lung precision medicine research with a focus on biomarkers. An American Thoracic Society/National Heart, Lung, and Blood Institute research statement. Am J Respir Crit Care Med. 2018;198(12):e116–e36.

90. Mak ACY, White MJ, Eckalbar WL, Szpiech ZA, Oh SS, Pino-Yanes M, et al. Whole-genome sequencing of pharmacogenetic drug response in racially diverse children with asthma. Am J Respir Crit Care Med. 2018;197(12):1552–64.

91. Tantisira KG, Lasky-Su J, Harada M, Murphy A, Litonjua AA, Himes BE, et al. Genomewide association between GLCCI1 and response to glucocorticoid therapy in asthma. N Engl J Med. 2011;365(13):1173–83.

92. Hosking L, Bleecker E, Ghosh S, Yeo A, Jacques L, Mosteller M, et al. GLCCI1 rs37973 does not influence treatment response to inhaled corticosteroids in white subjects with asthma. J Allergy Clin Immunol. 2014;133(2):587–9.

93. Vijverberg SJ, Tavendale R, Leusink M, Koenderman L, Raaijmakers JA, Postma DS, et al. Pharmacogenetic analysis of GLCCI1 in three north European pediatric asthma populations with a reported use of inhaled corticosteroids. Pharmacogenomics. 2014;15(6):799–806.

94. Park TJ, Park JS, Cheong HS, Park BL, Kim LH, Heo JS, et al. Genome-wide association study identifies ALLC polymorphisms correlated with FEV(1) change by corticosteroid. Clin Chim Acta. 2014;436:20–6.

95. Park HW, Dahlin A, Tse S, Duan QL, Schuemann B, Martinez FD, et al. Genetic predictors associated with improvement of asthma symptoms in response to inhaled corticosteroids. J Allergy Clin Immunol. 2014;133(3):664–9 e5.

96. Mosteller M, Hosking L, Murphy K, Shen J, Song K, Nelson M, et al. No evidence of large genetic effects on steroid response in asthma patients. J Allergy Clin Immunol. 2017;139(3):797–803 e7.

97. Himes BE, Weitzman ER. Innovations in health information technologies for chronic pulmonary diseases. Respir Res. 2016;17:38.

Genetics and Pharmacogenetics of COPD

Yohan Bossé and Michael H. Cho

The Era of Precision Medicine Needs in COPD

Chronic obstructive pulmonary disease (COPD) is a non-curable disorder characterized by irreversible airway obstruction caused by airway and/or parenchymal abnormalities. It is associated with persistent respiratory symptoms and characterized by a heterogeneous clinical presentation. COPD is ranked among the top global causes of death, reaching a staggering figure of nearly 3 million deaths in 2016 [1]. Projections estimate that the total number of diagnosed COPD patients will increase by more than 150% from 2010 to 2030, giving rise to an escalating burden of COPD on the healthcare system [2].

Just in United States, medical costs attributable to COPD exceeded $32 billion in 2010 and were projected to reach $49 billion in 2020 [3]. In Canada, the average annual excess direct costs of COPD were estimated at nearly $5500 per patient compared to a matched cohort of subjects without COPD [4]. Novel prevention and treatments strategies must be rapidly developed and implemented to stem the progression of this disease.

Cigarette smoking is the main risk factor for COPD. However, only 20–25% of smokers develop clinically significant airflow obstruction [5]. In addition, COPD susceptibility and lung function decline vary considerably among individuals with similar smoking exposure. Interventions to prevent smoking initiation and use for all are of paramount importance to decrease the burden of COPD. The age-standardized COPD morbidity and mortality continue to rise despite declining rates of smoking in most high-income countries [6, 7] and never-smokers accounted for up to one-quarter of all COPD cases [8]. Thus, we must understand the determinants of COPD susceptibility beyond smoking.

Other than eliminating noxious particles or gases exposure (such as cigarette smoking), the current management of patients with COPD is based on therapeutics that alleviate the symptoms, improve lung function, or reduce exacerbations. However, there are no treatments available to stop or reverse the underlying disease

Y. Bossé (✉)
Institut universitaire de cardiologie et de pneumologie de Québec, Québec, Canada

Department of Molecular Medicine, Laval University, Québec, Canada
e-mail: yohan.bosse@criucpq.ulaval.ca

M. H. Cho
Channing Division of Network Medicine, Division of Pulmonary and Critical Care Medicine, Brigham and Women's Hospital, Harvard Medical School, Boston, MA, USA
e-mail: remhc@channing.harvard.edu

© Springer Nature Switzerland AG 2020
J. L. Gomez et al. (eds.), *Precision in Pulmonary, Critical Care, and Sleep Medicine*, Respiratory Medicine, https://doi.org/10.1007/978-3-030-31507-8_4

processes – no pharmacologic therapies have convincingly been shown to alter decline in lung function or reduce mortality [9], and several recent clinical trials in COPD enrolling large numbers of patients failed their therapeutic targets [10, 11]. In addition, there is substantial heterogeneity in patient response [12, 13].

A deeper understanding of the disease is essential to develop new therapeutics and achieve greater therapeutic precision. Genomic research holds promise to reveal host susceptibility to develop COPD, discover new therapeutic targets, and find new biomarkers to refine disease classification and guide therapies [14, 15]. In this chapter, we describe recent progress to elucidate the genetic factors underlying COPD susceptibility and response to pharmacotherapy. We also discuss the translation of this new knowledge into clinical applications highlighting successes, promises, challenges, and failures.

The Evolving Genetic Map of COPD

For more than half a century, we have known that alpha-1 antitrypsin deficiency (AATD) is a genetic determinant of COPD. AATD is caused by inherited variants in the *SERPINA1* gene located on chromosome 14q32.13, which encodes an antiprotease called alpha-1 antitrypsin. Previous studies suggested that AATD occurs only in 1–5% of COPD cases [16–19]. *SERPINA1* is thus the first and still the most well-proven genetic risk factor for COPD but only explains a minority of cases. Studies based on twins, families, and population-based studies, many excluding known AATD, have demonstrated a substantial contribution of genetic factors to COPD, with estimates of heritability – the proportion of susceptibility from genetic factors – ranging from 35 to above 50% [20–24]. Thus, AATD and *SERPINA1* do not account for the strong genetic component to COPD and lung function phenotypes predicted from genetic epidemiology studies [25], which implies there are additional genes to be discovered.

Elucidating COPD genes is key to understand the underlying pathobiological processes giving rise to this disease. During the pre-genome-wide association study (GWAS) era, investigators relied on candidate gene and genome-wide linkage studies to identify the genetic factors of COPD. A large number of candidate gene studies were performed focusing on genes governing molecular processes involved in the current understanding of COPD pathogenesis, namely protease-antiprotease balance, inflammation, xenobiotic metabolism, immune response, and oxidative stress. In 2009, the genetic map of COPD contained 57 susceptibility genes derived from candidate gene studies [26]. Three years later, this number grew to 144 genes associated with COPD or related-phenotypes [27]. Although we need to appreciate the worldwide and intense effort from the COPD research community to find the responsible genes, unfortunately, most candidate genes were not replicated. In 2012, seven genes were supported by at least 10 genetic association studies: *ADRB2*, *TGFB1*, *TNF*, *GSTM1*, *GSTP1*, *SERPINA1*, and *EPHX1*. However, many studies were flawed by poor phenotype definition, small sample size, publication bias, and low genetic coverage, among others. Subsequent studies found rather inconsistent results and the global outcome from candidate gene studies is largely negative, a phenomenon echoed in many other diseases [28]. As of today, excluding *SERPINA1*, none of the other genes reported by candidate gene studies are well-proven susceptibility gene for COPD. Compared to candidate gene studies, fewer genome-wide linkage studies were performed as they required recruitment of families. More thorough reviews on genome-wide linkage studies in COPD and related-phenotypes have been reported [26]. Briefly, these studies revealed the multilocus nature of COPD, i.e., many genetic loci potentially harboring susceptibility genes for COPD. However, linkage loci consist of very large intervals with several putative genes. Fine mapping studies identified several genes, but similar to candidate gene studies, many have not been subsequently replicated in larger studies [29].

In retrospect, earlier studies had failed to fully appreciate the complex and polygenic architecture of COPD. Advances in genotyping and sequencing technology and statistical methodology led to the era of GWAS. For COPD research, as for other fields of medicine, the pre-GWAS era will be known as the period where geneticists were learning how to find genes of complex diseases. To date, GWAS have been the most successful approach to identify the genetic determinants of COPD. During the last decade, GWAS have been progressively more successful by enlarging sample sizes and improving SNP coverage. Figure 4.1 shows landmark GWAS in COPD and depicts their sample sizes as well as the number of discovered genomic loci and their effect sizes. There is a clear correlation between the sample size and the number of discovered COPD loci. Early COPD GWAS identified, and consistently replicated, one to few associations and suggested many others that the studies were underpowered to demonstrate. It is well known that GWAS needs to reach a certain threshold sample size above which the rate of locus discovery accelerates [30], and this threshold has recently been achieved in COPD research (Fig. 4.1). The latest of these GWAS was performed combining resources from the International COPD Genetics Consortium and the UK Biobank [31]. The allele frequencies of

35,735 COPD cases defined by moderate to very severe airflow limitation were compared to 222,076 controls for more than 6 million genetic variants. Figure 4.2 summarizes the findings of this study. At genome-wide significance, 82 loci were identified, of which 60 were clearly replicated, and the remainder had varying levels of replication evidence. Conditional analyses then revealed secondary associations in 50 of these loci, indicating independent variants associated with COPD in the same loci. The nearest genes to all independent variants are illustrated in Fig. 4.2. Odds ratio of the 82 genome-wide significant variants vary from 1.06 to 1.21 and explained 7.0% of the COPD phenotypic variance. As is typical with other complex diseases, most important COPD loci have small effect sizes (OR < 1.3). As sample sizes of GWAS increase, more loci are detected at a corresponding lower effect sizes. It should also be emphasized that this large COPD GWAS did not identify the *SERPINA1* Z allele, even though this was identified in a previous, smaller GWAS of more specific phenotypes [32, 33]. Thus, the absence of identification by GWAS of some of the most robust candidate genes associated with COPD including *SERPINE2* [29], *MMP12* [34], *FGF7* [35], *TGFB1* [36], *GSTM1* [37], *XRCC5* [38], and *SOX5* [39] does not necessarily refute their involvement in COPD.

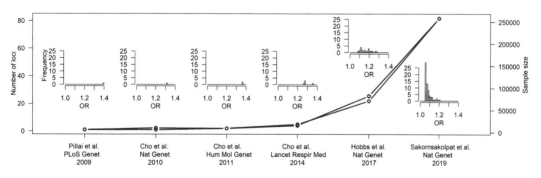

Fig. 4.1 Landmark GWAS on COPD. The x-axis denotes the name of the first author, journal, and year of publication of GWAS on COPD. The left y-axis shows the number of COPD loci identified and corresponds to the blue line. The right y-axis shows the sample size and corresponds to the red line. Only COPD loci reaching genome-wide significance were considered ($p < 5 \times 10^{-8}$). A histogram showing the distribution of odds ratios (OR) of COPD loci for each GWAS is illustrated. Note that ORs lower than 1 were converted into their reciprocal (1/OR) for illustration purpose

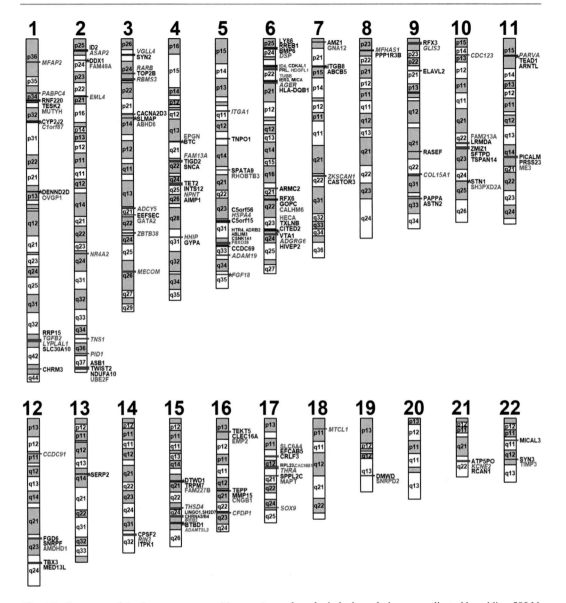

Fig. 4.2 Summary of the largest genome-wide association study on COPD including 35,735 cases and 222,076 controls [31]. Ideograms of the 22 autosomal chromosomes are illustrated. A total of 82 genome-wide significant loci were identified. These include 47 loci previously reported to be associated with COPD or lung function depicted in blue and 35 novel loci depicted in red. Thirteen out of 35 novel COPD risk loci were associated with lung function in the SpiroMeta cohort (79,055 individuals) and are highlighted by a red asterisk. The boundaries of each locus were defined by 500 kb up and downstream of the sentinel SNP. The nearest gene to the lead GWAS SNP is indicated on the right side of each locus. By conditional analysis, secondary signals were observed at 50 loci. For these loci, the boundaries were adjusted by adding 500 kb downstream of the most 5′ SNP and 500 kb upstream of the most 3′ SNP. The nearest genes to all independent SNPs at each locus are indicated. Candidate target genes revealed by integrative genomics are illustrated in magenta. Only the single gene with the most supportive evidences at each locus is illustrated. The candidate target genes that are also the nearest genes to the GWAS SNPs are in italics. The alternating grey and white colors on the chromosomes have been used to distinguish cytogenic bands from the adjacent ones and do not correspond to the band colors observed on giemsa-stained chromosomes. Information to construct the ideogram was obtained from the UCSC Genome Browser (hg19)

Overlapping Loci with Lung Function, COPD-Related Phenotypes, and Other Diseases

The most common respiratory phenotypes that have generated the largest GWAS in terms of sample size are derived from spirometry, which is the gold standard method for the diagnosis of COPD. The most common lung function measurements are the volume of air that can be maximally expired after a full inspiration or forced vital capacity (FVC) and the volume of air that can be expired in the first second of the same breathing maneuver or forced expiratory volume in the first second (FEV_1). Recommendations from guidelines defined COPD based on an FVC/FEV_1 lower than 0.7, which is an indication of airway obstruction [40]. FEV_1 grades disease severity as mild, moderate, severe, and very severe in patients with FEV_1 ≥80%, <80%, <50%, and <30% of predicted values, respectively. This relationship between the diagnosis of COPD and lung function, and the potentially greater statistical power that results from studying a quantitative trait, explains the relevance of studying the genetic determinants of lung function to study COPD and vice versa.

The latest GWAS on lung function measures was conducted in 400,102 individuals of European ancestry [41]. A total of 279 replicated distinct signals of association were identified with four lung function traits, namely, FVC, FEV_1, FEV_1/FVC, and peak expiratory flow (PEF). These include 139 new signals not reported in previous GWAS on lung function. Globally, these 279 signals explained 9.3%, 6.7%, 13.1%, 7.8% of the estimated heritability of FEV_1, FVC, FEV_1/FVC, and PEF, respectively, and a risk score constructed using these variants was strongly associated with COPD (see below). Among these signals, 107 putative causal genes were identified using integrative genomic approaches (see below).

Apart from COPD affection status and baseline lung function measurements, a range of respiratory phenotypes has been investigated to study the genetics of COPD. So far, GWAS have been performed on lung function decline [42–44],

airway responsiveness [45], chronic bronchitis [46], cachexia-related phenotypes [47], chronic mucus hypersecretion [48], circulating biomarkers (CC16, SP-D, and inflammatory markers) [49] as well as many phenotypes derived from computed tomography imaging including qualitative emphysema [50], percent emphysema [51], emphysema patterns [52], airway wall thickness [53], emphysema, and airway quantitative imaging phenotypes [33]. Table 4.1 summarizes the results of these studies. In all scenarios, investigators have tried to balance sample size and phenotype measurements to produce GWAS of the highest possible quality. In general, the more refined the phenotype, the smaller the sample size. Deep phenotyping is clearly a promising avenue to increase the yield of genetic studies. The main challenges are data harmonization across cohorts and to have studies of sufficient sample size.

One of the striking findings from genetic association studies is the identification of multiple phenotypes affected by genetic loci. In COPD, *FAM13A* was independently discovered as a locus for COPD and for pulmonary fibrosis [54, 55]. Subsequent papers identified four additional loci shared between COPD and pulmonary fibrosis [31, 54]. For all of these loci, the COPD risk variant appears to decrease risk of fibrosis. In addition, these papers first identified an overall genetic correlation between COPD and asthma and identified individual loci shared between COPD and asthma.

Integrative Genomic Approaches

GWAS identify a locus, not the causal variant, and the function of most variants in the human genome is unknown. Post-GWAS analyses using orthogonal data sources are now standard to leverage the outcomes and facilitate biological interpretation of genetic association results. Thus, one of the key issues in follow-up of genetic associations is identifying the causal variant, gene, and cell type. Most GWAS variants appear to be non-coding, i.e., they are not known to directly alter the structure or function of genes but instead are suspected to

Table 4.1 Susceptibility loci for COPD-related phenotypes identified by GWAS

Phenotype	Study	Loci (possible gene)
Lung function decline	Imboden et al. [42]	13q14 (*DLEU7*), 8p22 (*TUSC3*)
	Hansel et al. [43]	10q21.2 (*ANK3, CDK1, RHOBTB1, TMEM26*), 14q21.1 (*FOXA1*)
	Tang et al. [44]	15q25.1 (*IL16, STARD5, TMC3*), 11q14.2 (*ME3*)
Airway responsiveness	Hansel et al. [45]	9p21.2 (*LINGO2*), 6q21 (*PDSS2*), 5q33 (*SGCD*), 3q13.1 (*DZIP3, MYH15, RETNLB*)
Chronic bronchitis	Lee et al. [46]	4q22.1 (*FAM13A*), 11p15.5 (*EFCAB4A, CHID1, AP2A2*), 1q23.3 (*RPL31P11, ATF6*)
Cachexia-related phenotypes	Wan et al. [47]	16q12 (*FTO*)
Chronic mucus hypersecretion	Dijkstra et al. [48]	3p24.3 (*SATB1*)
Circulating biomarkers	Kim et al. [49]	
CC16		11q12.3 (*SCGB1A1, AHNAK, ASRGL1*), 11p13 (*APIP, EHF*)
SP-D		10q22.3 (*SFTPD, ANXA11*), 16q24.1 (*ATP2C2*), 6p21.33 (*CCHCR1, HLA-C FGFR3P, PSORS1C1*)
Qualitative emphysema	Kong et al. [50]	12p11 (*BICD1*)
Percent emphysema	Manichaikul et al. [51]	12q23.1 (*SNRPF, CCDC38*), 6p21.32 (*PPT2, AGER*)
Upper-lower lobe ratio in Hispanic		19p13.13 (*MAN2B1*)
Upper-lower lobe ratio in Chinese		4p15.2 (*DHX15*), 17q25.2 (*MGAT5B*)
Emphysema patterns	Castaldi et al. [52]	
Emphysema pattern – normal		15q25 (*CHRNA5*), 4q31 (*HHIP*), 1q41 (*TGFB2*), 11q22 (*MMP12*)
Emphysema pattern – moderate centrilobular		15q25 (*CHRNA3*), 19q13 (*CYP2A6*), 11q22 (*MMP12*), 1q41 (*TGFB2*)
Emphysema pattern – severe centrilobular		15q25 (*AGPHD1*), 17q11 (*MYO1D*)
Emphysema pattern – panlobular		15q25 (*AGPHD1*), 13q14 (*VWA8*)
Airway wall thickness	Dirkstra et al. [53]	10q26.2 (*C10orf90, DOCK1*), 7q21 (*MAGI2*), 17q21.2 (*NT5C3B*), 15q21.2 (*TNFAIP8L3*), 2q36.1 (*SCG2, AP1S3, WDFY1, MRPL44, SERPINE2*), 14q32.2 (*RPL3P4, BCL11B*), 10p13 (*FAM107B*)
Emphysema and airway quantitative imaging phenotypes	Cho et al. [33]	
Emphysema (% LAA-950)		4q31 (*HHIP*), 15q25 (*CHRNA3, CHRNA5, IREB2*), 6p21.32 (*AGER*), 8p22 (*DLC1*), 14q32.13 (*SERPINA10*)
Emphysema (Perc15)		8p22 (*DLC1*), 4q31 (*HHIP*)
Wall area percent		4q28.1 (*MIR2054*)
Gas trapping		6p21.32 (*AGER*), 21q22.11 (*LINC00310, KCNE2*)

% LAA-950: percentage low attenuation area, using a threshold of −950 Hounsfield units; Perc15: the 15th percentile of the density histogram

affect gene regulation. Mapping of expression quantitative trait loci (eQTL) has thus become a major method of post-GWAS analyses [56]. In a disease-relevant tissue, eQTL can enhance GWAS findings in two major ways: (1) identify the putative causal gene underlying the GWAS signals and (2) delineate the direction of effect, i.e., determine whether the risk allele increases or decreases the expression of the gene of interest in the relevant tissue. For COPD, these extensions of GWAS findings were attempted using lung eQTL [57–59]. In addition, the field has also progressed based on the development of new bioinformatics approaches that integrate GWAS and eQTL data [60, 61]. As a result, integrative genomic approaches are becoming more sophisticated owing to progressively larger GWAS and eQTL datasets as well as new and more powerful bioinformatics methods. Recently, the largest lung eQTL mapping study [62] and the GWAS results from the International COPD Genetics Consortium (ICGC) [54] were combined to map new candidate causal genes for COPD and gain biological insights about COPD risk loci derived from the GWAS literature [63]. First, the results of 36 published GWAS on COPD and related-phenotypes were summarized into 129 non-overlapping genetic risk loci. Three methods were then used to integrate the GWAS summary statistics from ICGC and the lung eQTL dataset using a transcriptome-wide association study (TWAS) [61], colocalization [60], and Mendelian randomization-based (SMR) approaches [64].

Applied at the genome-wide level, 12 new candidate causal genes residing outside of the literature-based COPD risk loci were identified and six of them were replicated using an independent lung eQTL dataset from the Genotype-Tissue Expression (GTEx) dataset [65], namely *CAMK2A*, *DMPK*, *MYO15A*, *TNFRSF10A*, *BTN3A2*, and *TRBV30*. For previously established COPD risk loci, putative causal genes were identified in 60 out of the 129 non-overlapping risk loci derived from the literature. Figure 4.3 provides an example of the contribution of the integrative genomic approach to refine the COPD risk locus on chromosome 6p24. For this locus, two genes were suspected from GWAS, namely *BMP6* [66, 67] and *DSP* [54]. Integrative analyses were able to determine that the SNPs most strongly associated with COPD in the ICGC GWAS were also those associated with the expression of *DSP* in lung tissues (with a posterior probability of shared GWAS and eQTL signals of 1.0). This example demonstrates how integrative genomics can

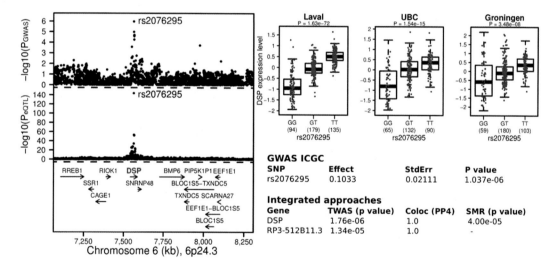

GWAS ICGC

SNP	Effect	StdErr	P value
rs2076295	0.1033	0.02111	1.037e-06

Integrated approaches

Gene	TWAS (p value)	Coloc (PP4)	SMR (p value)
DSP	1.76e-06	1.0	4.00e-05
RP3-512B11.3	1.34e-05	1.0	-

Fig. 4.3 *DSP* as the top candidate causal gene for COPD on chromosome 6p24. The upper left panel shows the genetic associations with COPD in ICGC. The bottom left panel shows the lung eQTL statistics for *DSP*. The location of genes at this locus is illustrated at the bottom. The upper right panel shows boxplots of *DSP* gene expression levels in lung tissues by genotyping groups for SNP rs2076295 (the lead GWAS SNP) in the eQTL datasets from three academic sites, Laval University, University of British Columbia (UBC), and University of Groningen. The number of individuals is indicated in parentheses.

The risk allele identified in the ICGC GWAS is shown in red. Box boundaries, whiskers, and center mark in box-plots represent the first and third quartiles, the most extreme data point which is no more than 1.5 times the interquartile range, and the median, respectively. The table shows the top GWAS SNP in ICGC and then the most likely causal gene(s) based on TWAS, colocalization, and SMR combining summary statistics at this locus from the ICGC GWAS and the lung eQTL study. (Reproduced from Lamontagne et al. [63], with permission from Oxford University Press)

narrow down the putative causal genes underneath GWAS loci. Similarly insightful, the COPD risk allele for the lead GWAS SNP in ICGC was associated with higher expression of *DSP* in the lung eQTL dataset, thus revealing the direction of effect. Together these results suggest that the SNPs associated with COPD on 6p24 confer susceptibility by increasing the mRNA expression levels of *DSP* in lung tissue. These insights represent major steps forward to understand the genetic basis of COPD and provide important information to prioritize follow-up functional studies.

A similar post-GWAS analysis using the summary statistics from the largest GWAS on lung function was also conducted using integrative genomic approaches [41]. In this case, the authors focused on the presence of QTL variants; eQTLs in lung, blood, and nine tissues known to contain smooth muscle; and protein QTLs in plasma, to identify a total of 107 putative causal genes. Pathway analyses revealed that these 107 genes are enriched in pathways governing elastic fiber, extracellular matrix organization, cilia development, and TGF-β superfamily signaling.

In the latest COPD GWAS described above [31], candidate target genes were investigated by combining the GWAS results with several data sources in addition to gene expression, including gene regulation (open chromatin and methylation data), chromatin interaction, co-regulation of gene expression with gene sets, and coding variant data. A total of 156 genes meeting criteria of statistical significance were identified. These target genes are located in 69 out of the 82 GWAS loci. The single gene with the most convincing functional evidence of being the putative causal gene underlying these 69 GWAS signals is illustrated in magenta in Fig. 4.2. Again, these analyses confirmed *DSP* as the target gene on chromosome 6p24. The different integrative genomic methods also converged consistently for *ADAM19* on 5q33.3, *ADAMTSL3* on 15q25.2, *EML4* on 2p21, and *RIN3* on 14q32.12. These studies and others highlight multiple integrative approaches used in dissecting genetic association signals.

Translating New COPD Genetics Knowledge into Clinical Applications

Finding genetic factors robustly associated with COPD provides valuable etiological insights with the hope that this will lead to new medical treatment. It is already clear that genetic discoveries have transformed the research activities of many laboratories in the world. Genes identified are prioritized for functional studies and are crucial to generate relevant cell and animal models based on human genetic etiology. However, actionable outcomes are yet to be experienced by COPD patients. Promises include new biomarkers for early detection of susceptible individuals, prediction and stratification of disease risk, drug target identification, and custom-tailored future medical treatments. Recent progress suggests that we may soon have the ability to turn some of these promises into reality.

One key insight from genetic studies is the role of early life factors and lung development in COPD pathogenesis [68]. This conclusion is based on the strong correlation between genetic risk of COPD with lung function in the general population, a lack of association of COPD loci with lung function decline, and overlap of COPD-associated loci with regulatory regions in fetal lung [54, 66, 69]. This genetic evidence is supported by epidemiologic observations, including a recent study showing that approximately half of older adults with COPD exhibit low lung function in early adulthood [70], suggesting that reduced maximal attained lung function caused by abnormal lung growth and development may be the etiology of half of COPD cases while the other half develop the disease owing to an accelerated decline of lung function.

The most near-term clinical application is likely in assisting with risk prediction. A genetic risk score based on the combination of 279 genetic variants associated with lung function was recently shown to predict the risk of COPD [41]. Figure 4.4 shows the gradation in susceptibility to moderate-to-severe COPD across deciles of the genetic risk score. The risk of COPD was nearly five times higher in the top decile than it

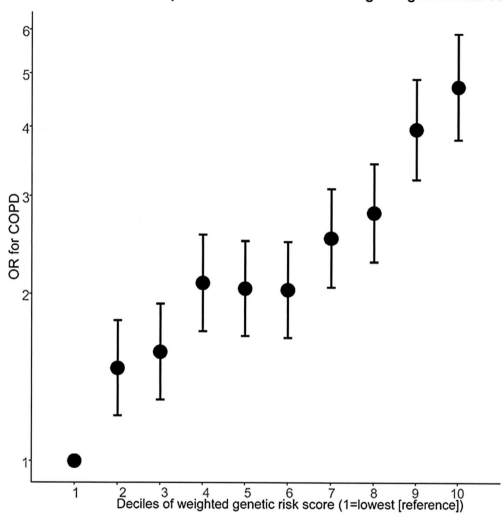

Fig. 4.4 Odds ratios (OR) for COPD according to membership of deciles 2–10 of the weighted genetic risk score, with decile 1 as the reference group (the 10% of individuals with the lowest genetic risk score). Each point represents a meta-analysis of results for a given comparison (i.e., decile 2 vs reference, decile 3 vs reference … decile 10 versus reference) in five external European-ancestry study groups (COPDGene, ECLIPSE, GenKOLS, SPIROMICS, NETT-NAS). Deciles were calculated and models were run in each group separately. Points represent odds ratios, and error bars correspond to 95% confidence intervals. (Reproduced from Shrine et al. [41])

was in the bottom decile (OR = 4.73). Interestingly, this genetic risk score derived from European ancestry individuals alone was also associated with COPD across other ancestry groups including African, South Asian, and Chinese. In contrast to most COPD risk factors, genetic markers can be obtained from birth and thus have great potential to facilitate early diagnosis. How useful would this genetic risk score be for a largely preventable disease like COPD? Obviously more studies are needed to answer this question, but new concrete options for the management of COPD patients are now emerging from the outcomes of genetic research. It should also be noted that further improvement is expected. The strength of association of this genetic risk score to predict COPD risk (OR = 4.73) is remarkable considering that the total heritability explained by the 279 signals vary from 6.7% to 13.1% depending on the lung function trait. A more comprehensive understanding of the genetic factors of COPD and lung function as well as disease heterogeneity is, thus, likely to generate more powerful predictors.

Ensuring translation all the way to point-of-care implementation is likely to be very challenging. This is demonstrated in the field of COPD by the case of AATD. AATD is still the only non-syndromic single gene disorder causing emphysema. This discovery made in the 1960s has transformed our molecular understanding of human emphysema, setting the protease/antiprotease imbalance hypothesis as a pathobiological hallmark of COPD. In addition, this discovery has led to prevention strategies as well as the development of new therapies (e.g., augmentation therapy) that are now available to prevent, or at least alleviate, serious lung and liver diseases associated with this condition. Clear guidelines about appropriate patients suitable for targeted testing for AATD have been published [18, 71]. Unfortunately, most patients with AATD are undiagnosed, and under-recognition of the disorder is a persistent problem [72]. The diagnosis is also potentially complex, consisting of multiple steps including the measurement of serum or plasma levels of alpha-1 antitrypsin, targeted genotyping, protease inhibitor phenotyping, and direct DNA sequencing. The results of these diagnostic algorithms are now apparent. In Canada, for example, there is a marked regional variation in the rate of diagnosis and the number of patients receiving augmentation therapy [73]. Accordingly, patient diagnosis and care vary by province. Recent technical advances have reduced the cost and improved availability of DNA diagnostics. There are now examples that demonstrated that DNA sequencing of *SERPINA1* to detect AATD is more precise (provide a definitive diagnosis), faster, and cheaper than existing diagnostic algorithms [74]. However, progress in genetic technologies has not always been appropriately translated into the clinical setting. The AATD case serves as an example that clinically valuable COPD genetic findings are not readily adopted in clinical practice and raises an important consideration for implementation of the other aforementioned genetic findings. Education and advances in regulatory processes are critical if we want to witness the full promise of precision medicine in COPD and other diseases.

COPD Pharmacogenetics

One area where recent developments in genetics have the potential to quickly improve patient care is pharmacogenetics. Wide interindividual variability is observed in response to COPD drugs. This is true for all phenotypes examined as outcomes in pharmacogenetics studies including bronchodilator responsiveness, lung function, exacerbation, extent and distribution of emphysema, adverse effects, and others. While the fraction of variability in drug response that is attributable to genetic factors is difficult to assess and remains largely unknown, the effect of individual genetic variants for drug response may be higher than those for disease risk [75]. The ultimate goal of pharmacogenetics-based tailoring of therapy is to maximize therapeutic benefits, define optimal drug dosage, and minimize adverse effects. The most common COPD medications are inhaled bronchodilators and inhaled corticosteroids (ICS). Different classes of bronchodilators include short- and long-acting β-agonists (SABA and LABA) and short- and long-acting muscarinic antagonists (SAMA and LAMA) as well as methylxanthines. Other anti-inflammatory agents include oral glucocorticoids, phosphodiesterase-4 inhibitors, antibiotics, and mucolytics/antioxidants. Many compounds within each class of medication exist. Combination therapies (e.g. SABA/SAMA, LABA/LAMA, ICS/LABA) are also frequently used and triple therapy (LABA/LAMA/ICS) is also an option.

Table 4.2 shows a summary of COPD pharmacogenetic studies. There are many limitations associated with these studies that parallel those described for COPD susceptibility, e.g., limited sample size, poor genetic coverage, and lack of consistent replication. In most cases, the genetic influence on drug response was evaluated using

Table 4.2 Summary of pharmacogenetic studies in COPD

Medication		Genes							
Class	Drug	*ADRB2*	*HCK*	*EPHX1*	*CYP1A2*	*PDGFD*	*CRHR1*	*GWAS*	
SABA	salbutamol	(76, 98-101)							
	isoproterenol	(102)	(80)						
	albuterol	(103)		(103)					
LABA	formoterol	(77)							
	indacaterol	(78)							
	salmeterol	(104, 105)							
ultra-LABA	vilanterol	(84)						(84)	
SAMA	oxitropium bromide	(99)							
LAMA	tiotropium	(104, 106)							
	umeclidinium	(84)						(84)	
Methylxanthines	theophylline				(82)				
ICS	fluticasone					(85)			
	budesonide	(77)							
Antioxidant agents	N-acetylcysteine			(81)					
	budesonide	(77)							
Antioxidant agents	N-acetylcysteine			(81)					
Combinations	salmeterol/fluticasone	(98)					(83)		
	formoterol/budesonide	(77)							
	vilanterol/umeclidinium	(84)						(84)	

Reference numbers are indicated in cells. The color of the background illustrates whether the genetic association is negative (white), conflicting (grey), or positive (black)
ICS inhaled corticosteroid, *LABA* long-acting β-agonist, *LAMA* long-acting muscarinic antagonist, *SABA* short-acting β-agonist, *SAMA* short-acting muscarinic antagonist

only specific polymorphisms in candidate genes, and the overall results are conflicting. This point is illustrated from the outcomes of studies that evaluated the impact of functional polymorphisms (Gly16Arg and Gln27Glu) in the *ADRB2* gene, which is the target for β-agonists and by far the gene most studied in COPD pharmacogenetics. Earlier studies demonstrated that these polymorphisms are associated with bronchodilator response to inhaled β-agonists in patients with COPD [76]. However, larger studies have not replicated these results [77, 78]. A recent systematic review and meta-analysis concludes

no consistent associations between *ADRB2* genotype and treatment response [79].

Other genes previously associated with genotype by response effects to COPD therapies include an insertion/deletion polymorphism in the *HCK* gene associated with bronchodilator response [80], a genotype affecting the enzyme activity of EPHX1 associated with change in FEV$_1$ and symptom scores after a 1-year intervention with antioxidant N-acetylcysteine [81], a polymorphism in *CYP1A2* associated with plasma theophylline levels [82], and an intronic variant in *CRHR1* associated with change in

FEV$_1$ following 12-week treatment with ICS combined with a LABA [83]. These studies have the merit of hypothesis-driven research focusing on functional polymorphisms in relevant candidate genes, but all these findings at this point require further replication. Similar to the *ADRB2* example, these studies only investigated a tiny portion of possible genetic effect. More comprehensive genetic studies are needed, i.e., we need to move from pharmacogenetics to pharmacogenomics. In this regard, a recent study showed that no variants were associated with treatment response to umeclidinium (LAMA) and vilanterol (LABA) in monotherapies or in combination at genome-wide significance [84]. Although negative, this study exemplified the minimum genetic coverage required to discover pharmacogenetic effects. More studies of this type are needed to identify robust genetic variants associated with treatment response. Genome-wide approaches may also be used to identify adverse drug effects. A recent GWAS identified an intronic SNP within the *PDGFD* gene associated with the risk of adrenal suppression in asthma and COPD patients using ICS [85]. Progress made and lessons learned in genetics of complex diseases are thus likely to be transferred into the field of pharmacogenomics and generate more of these promising results.

To date, these early pharmacogenetic studies have failed to deliver medically actionable results. In comparison to complex disease genetics, pharmacogenomics faces extra challenges [26, 86]. Drug development is a dynamic process where new or modified preparations are being produced continuously and with various modes of deliveries (inhaler, nebulizer, oral, injection). It may be important to study the inherited basis of therapeutic response to novel preparations and combinations that undergo full assessment as part of COPD clinical trials. This would identify pharmacogenetic effects during the clinical development stage and generate data to justify genotype-guided clinical trials. Clearly, future studies are needed to determine the pharmacogenetic determinants of COPD therapies. This also applies to other treatment modalities available to COPD patients including smoking cessation therapies, influenza and pneumococcal vaccinations, exercise and education programs, pulmonary rehabilitation, ventilator support, and oxygen therapy as well as surgical and bronchoscopic interventions. Given this large investigational space, identifying COPD patients most likely to respond to pharmacotherapy and nonpharmacologic interventions will require major and well-orchestrated research efforts by the COPD research community.

Future Directions

While the majority of discoveries in COPD genetics have been in common variants, rare variants are also likely important contributors. Rare, coding variants of large effect have the potential to directly implicate genes important for treatment [87]. Connective tissue pathway genes [88] are part of Mendelian syndromes which include emphysema, and, more recently, evidence has emerged implicating telomerase genes [89, 90]. Genome-wide approaches to rare variants – either through whole exome or whole genome sequencing – show promise but likely will require larger sample sizes or more specific phenotypes [91, 92]. In addition to rare variants, the relative importance of other types of variation, such as structural or somatic variants [93], in COPD remains to be seen.

The vast majority of COPD genetic studies has also been performed in subjects of European ancestry. While it is likely that a substantial portion of COPD genetic risk loci is shared between ancestries, studies of other ancestries may identify new loci, improve risk prediction, and allow refinement of association signals through fine mapping. Studies to date have demonstrated the potential promise of multiethnic approaches [51, 94], and larger studies with diverse people are clearly needed.

While larger studies will likely continue to increase the number of COPD-associated loci, COPD is a highly heterogeneous disease, and different genetic risks may underlie different phenotypes [95]. While some phenotype-specific investigations discussed above have made some progress, identifying specific subsets of disease processes ('endophenotypes') will be important for identifying new genetic loci or elucidating the impact of existing variants [96].

Finally, translating associations to disease understanding remains a major challenge as the number of loci outpaces the ability of functional studies to identify mechanism. Efforts to identify cell types using single-cell methods (such as the Human Cell Atlas), identifying not only expression and protein but other molecular QTLs (e.g. splicing, histone modification) across various conditions and performing high-throughput assays to annotate variant effect [97], will greatly facilitate the understanding of genetic associations.

Conclusions

Projections of COPD prevalence and associated mortality and morbidities as well as costs for management and treatment are alarming. Recent progress made in genetics of COPD provides some hope to counteract its large and underestimated socio-economic burden. We are currently living in a time period where the genetic basis of COPD is being unlocked. We now know dozens of risk loci, have an improved understanding of how genetics contributes to disease susceptibility, can identify subjects at highest genetic risk, and have many genes that give new insight into disease. However, "*Knowing is not enough; we must apply* – Goethe." Major challenges remain to apply new COPD genomic knowledge in a clinical setting. The difficulties of implementing DNA sequencing of a single gene to definitively detect AATD exemplify real-life resource and expertise barriers. Education is key to train the next-generation of clinicians, but all health-care providers must be willing and active in educating themselves about genomic medicine. Scientists must also find solutions to incorporate genomics in clinical practice without further stressing a health care system that is already out of breath. In terms of COPD pharmacogenetics, only a limited number of studies have been conducted, and so far, these have failed to reach results that are ready for clinical applications. The investigational space is particularly wide in

this area considering all treatment modalities (pharmacologic or not), the dynamic process of drug development (continuous development of new drugs and preparations), and the spectrum of possible phenotypes to monitor benefits and adverse effects. An orchestrated international effort is warranted.

References

1. GBD 2016 Causes of Death Collaborators. Global, regional, and national age-sex specific mortality for 264 causes of death, 1980–2016: a systematic analysis for the Global Burden of Disease Study 2016. Lancet. 2017;390(10100):1151–210.
2. Khakban A, Sin DD, FitzGerald JM, McManus BM, Ng R, Hollander Z, et al. The projected epidemic of chronic obstructive pulmonary disease hospitalizations over the next 15 years. A population-based perspective. Am J Respir Crit Care Med. 2017;195(3):287–91.
3. Ford ES, Murphy LB, Khavjou O, Giles WH, Holt JB, Croft JB. Total and state-specific medical and absenteeism costs of COPD among adults aged >/= 18 years in the United States for 2010 and projections through 2020. Chest. 2015;147(1):31–45.
4. Khakban A, Sin DD, FitzGerald JM, Ng R, Zafari Z, McManus B, et al. Ten-year trends in direct costs of COPD: a population-based study. Chest. 2015;148(3):640–6.
5. Lokke A, Lange P, Scharling H, Fabricius P, Vestbo J. Developing COPD: a 25 year follow up study of the general population. Thorax. 2006;61(11):935–9.
6. Doucet M, Rochette L, Hamel D. Incidence, prevalence, and mortality trends in chronic obstructive pulmonary disease over 2001 to 2011: a public health point of view of the burden. Can Respir J. 2016;2016:7518287.
7. Leone FT, Carlsen KH, Folan P, Latzka K, Munzer A, Neptune E, et al. An official American Thoracic Society Research statement: current understanding and future research needs in tobacco control and treatment. Am J Respir Crit Care Med. 2015;192(3):e22–41.
8. Tan WC, Sin DD, Bourbeau J, Hernandez P, Chapman KR, Cowie R, et al. Characteristics of COPD in never-smokers and ever-smokers in the general population: results from the CanCOLD study. Thorax. 2015;70(9):822–9.
9. Sliwka A, Jankowski M, Gross-Sondej I, Storman M, Nowobilski R, Bala MM. Once-daily long-acting beta(2)-agonists/inhaled corticosteroids combined inhalers versus inhaled long-acting muscarinic antagonists for people with chronic obstructive pulmonary disease. Cochrane Database Syst Rev. 2018;8:CD012355.

10. Criner GJ, Connett JE, Aaron SD, Albert RK, Bailey WC, Casaburi R, et al. Simvastatin for the prevention of exacerbations in moderate-to-severe COPD. N Engl J Med. 2014;370(23):2201–10.
11. The Long-Term Oxygen Treatment Trial Research Group, Albert RK, Au DH, Blackford AL, Casaburi R, Cooper JA Jr, et al. A randomized trial of long-term oxygen for COPD with moderate desaturation. N Engl J Med. 2016;375(17):1617–27.
12. Pavord ID, Chanez P, Criner GJ, Kerstjens HAM, Korn S, Lugogo N, et al. Mepolizumab for eosinophilic chronic obstructive pulmonary disease. N Engl J Med. 2017;377(17):1613–29.
13. Vestbo J, Leather D, Diar Bakerly N, New J, Gibson JM, McCorkindale S, et al. Effectiveness of fluticasone furoate-vilanterol for COPD in clinical practice. N Engl J Med. 2016;375(13):1253–60.
14. Visscher PM, Wray NR, Zhang Q, Sklar P, McCarthy MI, Brown MA, et al. 10 years of GWAS discovery: biology, function, and translation. Am J Hum Genet. 2017;101(1):5–22.
15. Nelson MR, Tipney H, Painter JL, Shen J, Nicoletti P, Shen Y, et al. The support of human genetic evidence for approved drug indications. Nat Genet. 2015;47(8):856–60.
16. Lieberman J, Winter B, Sastre A. Alpha 1-antitrypsin Pi-types in 965 COPD patients. Chest. 1986;89(3):370–3.
17. Abboud RT, Ford GT, Chapman KR. Alpha1-antitrypsin deficiency: a position statement of the Canadian Thoracic Society. Can Respir J. 2001;8(2):81–8.
18. American Thoracic Society; European Respiratory Society. American Thoracic Society/European Respiratory Society statement: standards for the diagnosis and management of individuals with alpha-1 antitrypsin deficiency. Am J Respir Crit Care Med. 2003;168(7):818–900.
19. de la Roza C, Rodriguez-Frias F, Lara B, Vidal R, Jardi R, Miravitlles M. Results of a case-detection programme for alpha1-antitrypsin deficiency in COPD patients. Eur Respir J. 2005;26(4):616–22.
20. Eriksson S. Pulmonary emphysema and alpha1-antitrypsin deficiency. Acta Med Scand. 1964;175:197–205.
21. McCloskey SC, Patel BD, Hinchliffe SJ, Reid ED, Wareham NJ, Lomas DA. Siblings of patients with severe chronic obstructive pulmonary disease have a significant risk of airflow obstruction. Am J Respir Crit Care Med. 2001;164(8 Pt 1):1419–24.
22. Silverman EK, Chapman HA, Drazen JM, Weiss ST, Rosner B, Campbell EJ, et al. Genetic epidemiology of severe, early-onset chronic obstructive pulmonary disease. Risk to relatives for airflow obstruction and chronic bronchitis. Am J Respir Crit Care Med. 1998;157(6 Pt 1):1770–8.
23. Zhou JJ, Cho MH, Castaldi PJ, Hersh CP, Silverman EK, Laird NM. Heritability of chronic obstructive pulmonary disease and related phenotypes in smokers. Am J Respir Crit Care Med. 2013;188(8):941–7.
24. Ingebrigtsen T, Thomsen SF, Vestbo J, van der Sluis S, Kyvik KO, Silverman EK, et al. Genetic influences on chronic obstructive pulmonary disease – a twin study. Respir Med. 2010;104(12):1890–5.
25. Sandford AJ, Weir TD, Pare PD. Genetic risk factors for chronic obstructive pulmonary disease. Eur Respir J. 1997;10(6):1380–91.
26. Bossé Y. Genetics of chronic obstructive pulmonary disease: a succinct review, future avenues and prospective clinical applications. Pharmacogenomics. 2009;10(4):655–67.
27. Bossé Y. Updates on the COPD gene list. Int J Chron Obstruct Pulmon Dis. 2012;7:607–31.
28. Siontis KC, Patsopoulos NA, Ioannidis JP. Replication of past candidate loci for common diseases and phenotypes in 100 genome-wide association studies. Eur J Hum Genet. 2010;18(7):832–7.
29. Demeo DL, Mariani TJ, Lange C, Srisuma S, Litonjua AA, Celedon JC, et al. The SERPINE2 gene is associated with chronic obstructive pulmonary disease. Am J Hum Genet. 2006;78(2):253–64.
30. Ahlqvist E, van Zuydam NR, Groop LC, McCarthy MI. The genetics of diabetic complications. Nat Rev Nephrol. 2015;11(5):277–87.
31. Sakornsakolpat P, Prokopenko D, Lamontagne M, Reeve NF, Guyatt AL, Jackson VE, et al. Genetic landscape of chronic obstructive pulmonary disease identifies heterogeneous cell-type and phenotype associations. Nat Genet. 2019;51(3):494–505.
32. Busch R, Hobbs BD, Zhou J, Castaldi PJ, McGeachie MJ, Hardin ME, et al. Genetic association and risk scores in a chronic obstructive pulmonary disease meta-analysis of 16,707 subjects. Am J Respir Cell Mol Biol. 2017;57(1):35–46.
33. Cho MH, Castaldi PJ, Hersh CP, Hobbs BD, Barr RG, Tal-Singer R, et al. A genome-wide association study of emphysema and airway quantitative imaging phenotypes. Am J Respir Crit Care Med. 2015;192(5):559–69.
34. Hunninghake GM, Cho MH, Tesfaigzi Y, Soto-Quiros ME, Avila L, Lasky-Su J, et al. MMP12, lung function, and COPD in high-risk populations. N Engl J Med. 2009;361(27):2599–608.
35. Brehm JM, Hagiwara K, Tesfaigzi Y, Bruse S, Mariani TJ, Bhattacharya S, et al. Identification of FGF7 as a novel susceptibility locus for chronic obstructive pulmonary disease. Thorax. 2011;66(12):1085–90.
36. Smolonska J, Wijmenga C, Postma DS, Boezen HM. Meta-analyses on suspected chronic obstructive pulmonary disease genes: a summary of 20 years' research. Am J Respir Crit Care Med. 2009;180(7):618–31.
37. Castaldi PJ, Cho MH, Cohn M, Langerman F, Moran S, Tarragona N, et al. The COPD genetic association compendium: a comprehensive online database of COPD genetic associations. Hum Mol Genet. 2010;19(3):526–34.
38. Hersh CP, Pillai SG, Zhu G, Lomas DA, Bakke P, Gulsvik A, et al. Multistudy fine mapping of chromosome 2q identifies XRCC5 as a chronic obstructive

pulmonary disease susceptibility gene. Am J Respir Crit Care Med. 2010;182(5):605–13.

39. Hersh CP, Silverman EK, Gascon J, Bhattacharya S, Klanderman BJ, Litonjua AA, et al. SOX5 is a candidate gene for chronic obstructive pulmonary disease susceptibility and is necessary for lung development. Am J Respir Crit Care Med. 2011;183(11):1482–9.

40. Vogelmeier CF, Criner GJ, Martinez FJ, Anzueto A, Barnes PJ, Bourbeau J, et al. Global strategy for the diagnosis, management, and prevention of chronic obstructive lung disease 2017 report. GOLD executive summary. Am J Respir Crit Care Med. 2017;195(5):557–82.

41. Shrine N, Guyatt AL, Erzurumluoglu AM, Jackson VE, Hobbs BD, Melbourne CA, et al. New genetic signals for lung function highlight pathways and chronic obstructive pulmonary disease associations across multiple ancestries. Nat Genet. 2019;51(3):481–93.

42. Imboden M, Bouzigon E, Curjuric I, Ramasamy A, Kumar A, Hancock DB, et al. Genome-wide association study of lung function decline in adults with and without asthma. J Allergy Clin Immunol. 2012;129(5):1218–28.

43. Hansel NN, Ruczinski I, Rafaels N, Sin DD, Daley D, Malinina A, et al. Genome-wide study identifies two loci associated with lung function decline in mild to moderate COPD. Hum Genet. 2013;132(1):79–90.

44. Tang W, Kowgier M, Loth DW, Soler Artigas M, Joubert BR, Hodge E, et al. Large-scale genome-wide association studies and meta-analyses of longitudinal change in adult lung function. PLoS One. 2014;9(7):e100776.

45. Hansel NN, Pare PD, Rafaels N, Sin DD, Sandford A, Daley D, et al. Genome-wide association study identification of novel loci associated with airway responsiveness in chronic obstructive pulmonary disease. Am J Respir Cell Mol Biol. 2015;53(2):226–34.

46. Lee JH, Cho MH, Hersh CP, McDonald ML, Crapo JD, Bakke PS, et al. Genetic susceptibility for chronic bronchitis in chronic obstructive pulmonary disease. Respir Res. 2014;15:113.

47. Wan ES, Cho MH, Boutaoui N, Klanderman BJ, Sylvia JS, Ziniti JP, et al. Genome-wide association analysis of body mass in chronic obstructive pulmonary disease. Am J Respir Cell Mol Biol. 2011;45(2):304–10.

48. Dijkstra AE, Smolonska J, van den Berge M, Wijmenga C, Zanen P, Luinge MA, et al. Susceptibility to chronic mucus hypersecretion, a genome wide association study. PLoS One. 2014;9(4):e91621.

49. Kim DK, Cho MH, Hersh CP, Lomas DA, Miller BE, Kong X, et al. Genome-wide association analysis of blood biomarkers in chronic obstructive pulmonary disease. Am J Respir Crit Care Med. 2012;186(12):1238–47.

50. Kong X, Cho MH, Anderson W, Coxson HO, Muller N, Washko G, et al. Genome-wide association study identifies BICD1 as a susceptibility gene for emphysema. Am J Respir Crit Care Med. 2011;183(1):43–9.

51. Manichaikul A, Hoffman EA, Smolonska J, Gao W, Cho MH, Baumhauer H, et al. Genome-wide study of percent emphysema on computed tomography in the general population. The multi-ethnic study of atherosclerosis lung/SNP health association resource study. Am J Respir Crit Care Med. 2014;189(4):408–18.

52. Castaldi PJ, Cho MH, San Jose Estepar R, McDonald ML, Laird N, Beaty TH, et al. Genome-wide association identifies regulatory loci associated with distinct local histogram emphysema patterns. Am J Respir Crit Care Med. 2014;190(4):399–409.

53. Dijkstra AE, Postma DS, van Ginneken B, Wielputz MO, Schmidt M, Becker N, et al. Novel genes for airway wall thickness identified with combined genome-wide association and expression analyses. Am J Respir Crit Care Med. 2015;191(5):547–56.

54. Hobbs BD, de Jong K, Lamontagne M, Bossé Y, Shrine N, Artigas MS, et al. Genetic loci associated with chronic obstructive pulmonary disease overlap with loci for lung function and pulmonary fibrosis. Nat Genet. 2017;49(3):426–32.

55. Fingerlin TE, Murphy E, Zhang W, Peljto AL, Brown KK, Steele MP, et al. Genome-wide association study identifies multiple susceptibility loci for pulmonary fibrosis. Nat Genet. 2013;45(6):613–20.

56. Bossé Y. Genome-wide expression quantitative trait loci analysis in asthma. Curr Opin Allergy Clin Immunol. 2013;13(5):487–94.

57. Lamontagne M, Couture C, Postma DS, Timens W, Sin DD, Paré PD, et al. Refining susceptibility loci of chronic obstructive pulmonary disease with lung eQTLs. PLoS One. 2013;8(7):e70220.

58. Lamontagne M, Joubert P, Timens W, Postma DS, Hao K, Nickle D, et al. Susceptibility genes for lung diseases in the major histocompatibility complex revealed by lung expression quantitative trait loci analysis. Eur Respir J. 2016;48(2):573–6.

59. Lamontagne M, Timens W, Hao K, Bossé Y, Laviolette M, Steiling K, et al. Genetic regulation of gene expression in the lung identifies CST3 and CD22 as potential causal genes for airflow obstruction. Thorax. 2014;69(11):997–1004.

60. Giambartolomei C, Vukcevic D, Schadt EE, Franke L, Hingorani AD, Wallace C, et al. Bayesian test for colocalisation between pairs of genetic association studies using summary statistics. PLoS Genet. 2014;10(5):e1004383.

61. Gusev A, Ko A, Shi H, Bhatia G, Chung W, Penninx BW, et al. Integrative approaches for large-scale transcriptome-wide association studies. Nat Genet. 2016;48(3):245–52.

62. Hao K, Bossé Y, Nickle DC, Pare PD, Postma DS, Laviolette M, et al. Lung eQTLs to help reveal the molecular underpinnings of asthma. PLoS Genet. 2012;8(11):e1003029.

63. Lamontagne M, Berube JC, Obeidat M, Cho MH, Hobbs BD, Sakornsakolpat P, et al. Leveraging lung

tissue transcriptome to uncover candidate causal genes in COPD genetic associations. Hum Mol Genet. 2018;27(10):1819–29.

64. Zhu Z, Zhang F, Hu H, Bakshi A, Robinson MR, Powell JE, et al. Integration of summary data from GWAS and eQTL studies predicts complex trait gene targets. Nat Genet. 2016;48(5):481–7.

65. GTEx Consortium. Genetic effects on gene expression across human tissues. Nature. 2017;550(7675): 204–13.

66. Wain LV, Shrine N, Artigas MS, Erzurumluoglu AM, Noyvert B, Bossini-Castillo L, et al. Genome-wide association analyses for lung function and chronic obstructive pulmonary disease identify new loci and potential druggable targets. Nat Genet. 2017;49(3):416–25.

67. Loth DW, Soler Artigas M, Gharib SA, Wain LV, Franceschini N, Koch B, et al. Genome-wide association analysis identifies six new loci associated with forced vital capacity. Nat Genet. 2014;46(7):669–77.

68. Smith BM, Traboulsi H, Austin JHM, Manichaikul A, Hoffman EA, Bleecker ER, et al. Human airway branch variation and chronic obstructive pulmonary disease. Proc Natl Acad Sci U S A. 2018;115(5):E974–E81.

69. John C, Soler Artigas M, Hui J, Nielsen SF, Rafaels N, Pare PD, et al. Genetic variants affecting cross-sectional lung function in adults show little or no effect on longitudinal lung function decline. Thorax. 2017;72(5):400–8.

70. Lange P, Celli B, Agusti A, Boje Jensen G, Divo M, Faner R, et al. Lung-function trajectories leading to chronic obstructive pulmonary disease. N Engl J Med. 2015;373(2):111–22.

71. Marciniuk DD, Hernandez P, Balter M, Bourbeau J, Chapman KR, Ford GT, et al. Alpha-1 antitrypsin deficiency targeted testing and augmentation therapy: a Canadian Thoracic Society clinical practice guideline. Can Respir J. 2012;19(2):109–16.

72. Stoller JK, Brantly M. The challenge of detecting alpha-1 antitrypsin deficiency. COPD. 2013;10(Suppl 1):26–34.

73. Bradi AC, Audisho N, Casey DK, Chapman KR. Alpha-1 antitrypsin deficiency in Canada: regional disparities in diagnosis and management. COPD. 2015;12(Suppl 1):15–21.

74. Maltais F, Gaudreault N, Racine C, Theriault S, Bosse Y. Clinical experience with SERPINA1 DNA sequencing to detect Alpha-1 antitrypsin deficiency. Ann Am Thorac Soc. 2018;15(2):266–8.

75. Maranville JC, Cox NJ. Pharmacogenomic variants have larger effect sizes than genetic variants associated with other dichotomous complex traits. Pharmacogenomics J. 2016;16(4):388–92.

76. Hizawa N, Makita H, Nasuhara Y, Betsuyaku T, Itoh Y, Nagai K, et al. Beta2-adrenergic receptor genetic polymorphisms and short-term bronchodilator responses in patients with COPD. Chest. 2007;132(5):1485–92.

77. Bleecker ER, Meyers DA, Bailey WC, Sims AM, Bujac SR, Goldman M, et al. ADRB2 polymor-

phisms and budesonide/formoterol responses in COPD. Chest. 2012;142(2):320–8.

78. Yelensky R, Li Y, Lewitzky S, Leroy E, Hurwitz C, Rodman D, et al. A pharmacogenetic study of ADRB2 polymorphisms and indacaterol response in COPD patients. Pharmacogenomics J. 2012;12(6):484–8.

79. Nielsen AO, Jensen CS, Arredouani MS, Dahl R, Dahl M. Variants of the ADRB2 gene in COPD: systematic review and meta-analyses of disease risk and treatment response. COPD. 2017;14(4):451–60.

80. Zhang X, Mahmudi-Azer S, Connett JE, Anthonisen NR, He JQ, Pare PD, et al. Association of Hck genetic polymorphisms with gene expression and COPD. Hum Genet. 2007;120(5):681–90.

81. Zhang JQ, Zhang JQ, Liu H, Zhao ZH, Fang LZ, Liu L, et al. Effect of N-acetylcysteine in COPD patients with different microsomal epoxide hydrolase genotypes. Int J Chron Obstruct Pulmon Dis. 2015;10:917–23.

82. Uslu A, Ogus C, Ozdemir T, Bilgen T, Tosun O, Keser I. The effect of CYP1A2 gene polymorphisms on Theophylline metabolism and chronic obstructive pulmonary disease in Turkish patients. BMB Rep. 2010;43(8):530–4.

83. Kim WJ, Sheen SS, Kim TH, Huh JW, Lee JH, Kim EK, et al. Association between CRHR1 polymorphism and improved lung function in response to inhaled corticosteroid in patients with COPD. Respirology. 2009;14(2):260–3.

84. Condreay L, Huang L, Harris E, Brooks J, Riley JH, Church A, et al. Genetic effects on treatment response of umeclidinium/vilanterol in chronic obstructive pulmonary disease. Respir Med. 2016;114:123–6.

85. Hawcutt DB, Francis B, Carr DF, Jorgensen AL, Yin P, Wallin N, et al. Susceptibility to corticosteroid-induced adrenal suppression: a genome-wide association study. Lancet Respir Med. 2018;6(6):442–50.

86. Hersh CP. Pharmacogenetics of chronic obstructive pulmonary disease: challenges and opportunities. Pharmacogenomics. 2010;11(2):237–47.

87. Cohen JC, Boerwinkle E, Mosley TH Jr, Hobbs HH. Sequence variations in PCSK9, low LDL, and protection against coronary heart disease. N Engl J Med. 2006;354(12):1264–72.

88. Callewaert B, Renard M, Hucthagowder V, Albrecht B, Hausser I, Blair E, et al. New insights into the pathogenesis of autosomal-dominant cutis laxa with report of five ELN mutations. Hum Mutat. 2011;32(4):445–55.

89. Nunes H, Monnet I, Kannengiesser C, Uzunhan Y, Valeyre D, Kambouchner M, et al. Is telomeropathy the explanation for combined pulmonary fibrosis and emphysema syndrome?: report of a family with TERT mutation. Am J Respir Crit Care Med. 2014;189(6):753–4.

90. Stanley SE, Chen JJ, Podlevsky JD, Alder JK, Hansel NN, Mathias RA, et al. Telomerase mutations in smokers with severe emphysema. J Clin Invest. 2015;125(2):563–70.

91. Wain LV, Sayers I, Soler Artigas M, Portelli MA, Zeggini E, Obeidat M, et al. Whole exome re-

sequencing implicates CCDC38 and cilia structure and function in resistance to smoking related airflow obstruction. PLoS Genet. 2014;10(5):e1004314.

92. Qiao D, Ameli A, Prokopenko D, Chen H, Kho AT, Parker MM, et al. Whole exome sequencing analysis in severe chronic obstructive pulmonary disease. Hum Mol Genet. 2018;27(21):3801–12.

93. Buscarlet M, Provost S, Zada YF, Barhdadi A, Bourgoin V, Lepine G, et al. DNMT3A and TET2 dominate clonal hematopoiesis and demonstrate benign phenotypes and different genetic predispositions. Blood. 2017;130(6):753–62.

94. Wyss AB, Sofer T, Lee MK, Terzikhan N, Nguyen JN, Lahousse L, et al. Multiethnic meta-analysis identifies ancestry-specific and cross-ancestry loci for pulmonary function. Nat Commun. 2018;9(1):2976.

95. Pillai SG, Kong X, Edwards LD, Cho MH, Anderson WH, Coxson HO, et al. Loci identified by genome-wide association studies influence different disease-related phenotypes in chronic obstructive pulmonary disease. Am J Respir Crit Care Med. 2010;182(12):1498–505.

96. Udler MS, Kim J, von Grotthuss M, Bonas-Guarch S, Cole JB, Chiou J, et al. Type 2 diabetes genetic loci informed by multi-trait associations point to disease mechanisms and subtypes: a soft clustering analysis. PLoS Med. 2018;15(9):e1002654.

97. Starita LM, Ahituv N, Dunham MJ, Kitzman JO, Roth FP, Seelig G, et al. Variant interpretation: functional assays to the rescue. Am J Hum Genet. 2017;101(3):315–25.

98. Kim WJ, Oh YM, Sung J, Kim TH, Huh JW, Jung H, et al. Lung function response to 12-week treatment with combined inhalation of long-acting beta2 agonist and glucocorticoid according to ADRB2 polymorphism in patients with chronic obstructive pulmonary disease. Lung. 2008;186(6):381–6.

99. Konno S, Makita H, Hasegawa M, Nasuhara Y, Nagai K, Betsuyaku T, et al. Beta2-adrenergic receptor polymorphisms as a determinant of preferential bronchodilator responses to beta2-agonist and anticholinergic agents in Japanese patients with chronic obstructive pulmonary disease. Pharmacogenet Genomics. 2011;21(11):687–93.

100. Hussein MH, Sobhy KE, Sabry IM, El Serafi AT, Toraih EA. Beta2-adrenergic receptor gene haplotypes and bronchodilator response in Egyptian patients with chronic obstructive pulmonary disease. Adv Med Sci. 2017;62(1):193–201.

101. Mokry M, Joppa P, Slaba E, Zidzik J, Habalova V, Kluchova Z, et al. Beta2-adrenergic receptor haplotype and bronchodilator response to salbutamol in patients with acute exacerbations of COPD. Med Sci Monit. 2008;14(8):CR392–8.

102. Joos L, Weir TD, Connett JE, Anthonisen NR, Woods R, Pare PD, et al. Polymorphisms in the beta2 adrenergic receptor and bronchodilator response, bronchial hyperresponsiveness, and rate of decline in lung function in smokers. Thorax. 2003;58(8):703–7.

103. Kim WJ, Hersh CP, DeMeo DL, Reilly JJ, Silverman EK. Genetic association analysis of COPD candidate genes with bronchodilator responsiveness. Respir Med. 2009;103(4):552–7.

104. Rabe KF, Fabbri LM, Israel E, Kogler H, Riemann K, Schmidt H, et al. Effect of ADRB2 polymorphisms on the efficacy of salmeterol and tiotropium in preventing COPD exacerbations: a prespecified substudy of the POET-COPD trial. Lancet Respir Med. 2014;2(1):44–53.

105. Mochizuki H, Nanjo Y, Kawate E, Yamazaki M, Tsuda Y, Takahashi H. β2-adrenergic receptor haplotype may be associated with susceptibility to desensitization to long-acting beta2-agonists in COPD patients. Lung. 2012;190(4):411–7.

106. Umeda N, Yoshikawa T, Kanazawa H, Hirata K, Fujimoto S. Association of beta2-adrenoreceptor genotypes with bronchodilatory effect of tiotropium in COPD. Respirology. 2008;13(3):346–52.

The Evolution of Precision Medicine in Cystic Fibrosis

5

Yukiko Kunitomo and Clemente J. Britto

Cystic Fibrosis (CF) is a life-shortening, multi-organ autosomal recessive disease that affects approximately 75,000 patients world-wide. CF is the most common fatal genetic disease in the US, affecting over 33,000 patients [1, 2]. CF is caused by a mutation in the cystic fibrosis transmembrane conductance regulator (*CFTR*) gene leading to abnormal chloride and bicarbonate transport on epithelial surfaces of the respiratory and gastrointestinal tracts. The disease was first described in 1938, when affected children were clinically characterized as having high mortality due to nutritional failure and pancreatic insufficiency [3–6]. The introduction of pancreatic enzyme replacement therapy changed the natural history of CF, making way for lung disease as a defining characteristic that eventually became its major cause of morbidity and mortality [7–9].

Improvements in CF diagnosis have helped uncover previously unidentified populations with milder presentations of CF later in life, while developments in the treatment of CF manifestations improved life expectancy. As a result, the adult CF population has exceeded the pediatric CF population since 2015 [2, 9]. There has been considerable improvement in CF survival since its original description, with a median predicted survival of 46.2 years in 2017 [2]. These remarkable gains can be largely attributed to effective disease management strategies ranging from early diagnosis to standardized clinical care guidelines. Despite the broad spectrum of clinical presentations of CF and a multitude of disease-causing *CFTR* mutations, CF has been historically treated as a single clinical entity, using a common approach to improve mucociliary clearance, nutritional management, antimicrobial therapy, and addressing multi-organ manifestations. Thanks to the introduction of novel diagnostic technologies and *CFTR*-specific therapies, personalized approaches that integrate genetic differences and clinical manifestations are becoming increasingly available in CF care.

From Clinical Phenotyping to Personalized Molecular Diagnosis

Standardized Approach to CF Diagnosis

A key breakthrough in CF diagnosis was the discovery of the disease-causing genetic defects on chromosome 7q31.2 in the mid-1980s [10, 11]. The entire *CFTR* gene was sequenced in 1989

Y. Kunitomo
Yale University School of Medicine, Department of Internal Medicine, New Haven, CT, USA
e-mail: Yukiko.kunitomo@yale.edu

C. J. Britto (✉)
Adult Cystic Fibrosis Program, Center for Pulmonary Infection Research and Treatment (CPIRT), Section of Pulmonary, Critical Care & Sleep Medicine, Department of Internal Medicine, Yale University, New Haven, CT, USA
e-mail: clemente.britto@yale.edu

© Springer Nature Switzerland AG 2020
J. L. Gomez et al. (eds.), *Precision in Pulmonary, Critical Care, and Sleep Medicine*, Respiratory Medicine, https://doi.org/10.1007/978-3-030-31507-8_5

[12, 13] and since then over 2000 disease-causing mutations have been identified. This information has allowed clinicians to stratify disease by CF-causing mutation severity, anticipate outcomes, and take steps beyond symptom management to target the basic molecular defects caused by specific *CFTR* mutations [14]. In this way, CF was perhaps one of the first lung diseases to adopt a personalized medicine approach to diagnosis and treatment.

Since the 1980s newborn screening has been the preferred approach to diagnose CF in the United States. This is typically a two-tier test. First, immunoreactive trypsinogen (IRT), a pancreatic enzyme precursor normally present at very low concentrations, is measured in the infant's blood. If IRT is increased, follow-up testing for *CFTR* mutations is ordered with a panel of 25 mutations accounting for >80% of CF alleles in the pan-ethnic US population with CF [15, 16]. The screening is considered positive if the IRT remains increased 7–14 days after the initial testing, or if two *CFTR* mutations are confirmed [17, 18]. However, it is predicted that more than one-third of all US CF diagnoses in 2014 were not a result of newborn screening, and rather included patients with residual-function *CFTR* mutations that manifested later in life, or as a milder phenotype [19].

In older children and adults, a diagnosis of CF requires a clinical phenotype consistent with CF and the presence of two disease-causing *CFTR* mutations on separate alleles. The diagnosis is often confirmed by high chloride sweat test concentrations or evidence of *CFTR* dysfunction on nasal potential difference measurements [20]. The pilocarpine iontophoresis sweat test measures sweat chloride concentrations, usually elevated in CF, and the range of increase can give insight into the degree of ion transport dysfunction [21–23].

The genotypic criteria for CF diagnosis require identifying two disease-causing mutations on the *CFTR* gene in distinct chromosomes with each mutation meeting one of the following conditions: *CFTR* sequence alteration that affects protein structure and/or function, introduction of a premature stop codon, intron splice site alteration, or the existence of a novel amino acid sequence that does not occur in normal *CFTR* genes of an individual's ethnic group [24, 25]. Since commercial laboratories initially only test for the most prevalent *CFTR* gene mutations, this may delay diagnosis and appropriate treatment in patients with rare mutations. This is particularly relevant in non-Caucasian ethnic groups whom, while less frequently affected by CF, often carry uncommon *CFTR* gene mutations that drive their disease [26]. For these rare mutations, whole exome sequencing of the *CFTR* gene is necessary to establish the diagnosis of CF.

Diagnostic Approaches to *CFTR* Mutations

Identification of the *CFTR* gene and its associated mutation classes improved disease stratification and prognostication at the time of diagnosis. Mutations in the *CFTR* gene can be categorized based on the primary abnormality resulting from the mutation: *Class I*) no functional *CFTR* protein production, *Class II*) *CFTR* trafficking defect, *Class III*) Defective *CFTR* channel regulation, *Class IV*) Decreased channel conductance, *Class V*) Reduced synthesis of *CFTR* protein, and *Class VI*) Decreased *CFTR* stability. Class I, II, and III are associated with profoundly impaired *CFTR* function and generally have a more severe clinical phenotype compared to Class IV, V, and VI mutations, where residual *CFTR* function is retained [9, 27, 28].

There are some challenges to the clinical application of specific *CFTR* mutations as tools for personalized medicine. First, of over 2000 *CFTR* mutations identified to date, only about 250 have well-documented disease-causing effects. Further, only a much smaller fraction of these mutations occurs at a worldwide frequency greater than 0.1%, making the rest of the known mutations extremely rare and difficult to characterize clinically [24]. The Clinical and Functional Translation of *CFTR* (*CFTR*2) Project is a global endeavor to tackle this challenge by creating a database of functional and clinical data associated with each *CFTR* mutation to better understand mutation–phenotype relationships. For each identified *CFTR* mutation, this publicly available database contains information including sweat chloride measurements, lung function scores, pancreatic function, and microbiology, as reported in clinical cases associated with each mutation [29].

Another challenge in the clinical application of *CFTR* mutations as tools for personalized medicine is the functional overlap of *CFTR* mutations in different mutation classes. Many *CFTR* variants have properties of more than one mutation Class. For example, the most common mutation of the *CFTR* gene is *F508del*, an in-frame deletion leading to loss of a phenylalanine residue. *F508del* occurs in 86.4% of US patients, of which 46.5% are homozygous and over 40% carry the mutation in at least one allele [2]. This Class II mutation causes improper processing of protein, which leads to *CFTR* misfolding, and subsequent degradation of the protein by proteasomes, preventing proper *CFTR* expression on the apical membrane [30, 31]. However, this mutation also results in characteristics of Class III mutations, as it results in impaired *CFTR* regulation with higher inactivation rates even when the channel is present in the apical membrane [32, 33]. On one hand, having multiple mechanisms of channel dysfunction due to a single mutation poses a challenge for prognostication and makes recovery of channel function complex. On the other hand, a treatment that can correct the effects of one mutation class may also treat many more mutations than originally expected based on mutation type, because of this overlap. The application of this concept in the selection of *CFTR* modulator drugs is discussed below. A third caveat to consider when applying CF mutation knowledge to clinical management is the presence of environmental exposures, comorbidities, ongoing therapy, and adherence to therapeutic interventions, as these factors may significantly change the overall clinical phenotype of individuals sharing similar genotypes.

From Disease Management to the Rise of Precision Medicine Therapies in CF

The current management of CF lung disease focuses on slowing disease progression by treating clinical manifestations and preventing pulmonary exacerbations [34]. Treatment regimens can be intensive, sometimes taking hours daily in order to maintain lung health in those with severe clinical presentations. The main components of treatment include daily airway clearance therapy, mucolytics and airway hydrators to improve mucus clearance, antibiotics, and anti-inflammatory drugs [9]. Airway clearance techniques include manual chest percussion, use of hand-held devices that provide oscillatory positive expiratory pressure, and high-frequency chest compression vests [35]. The recombinant human DNAse dornase alfa (mucolytic) and hypertonic saline improve mucus clearance and reduce the incidence of pulmonary exacerbations [36–42]. Anti-inflammatories can limit the chronic airway inflammation present in CF that contributes to the progressive lung parenchymal injury [8]. Antibiotics are an essential part of the regimen to treat acute and chronic airway infections. For example, colonization with *Pseudomonas aeruginosa* is associated with an accelerated decline in pulmonary function [43, 44], which has led to development of inhaled antibiotic formulations targeting this pathogen [45–49]. Although treatment choices may have been influenced by an individual's genotype, they have been traditionally guided by the severity of disease manifestations. The incorporation of personalized medicine adds another layer of complexity that is rapidly changing our approach to clinical decision-making in CF.

Precision Medicine Approaches to CF Therapy

Over the past decade, there have been at least two approaches to implement precision medicine in CF therapy: (1) Direct targeting of the

CFTR gene mutation and dysfunctional *CFTR* protein and (2) Seeking alternative targets in non-*CFTR* genetic variations or non-*CFTR* channels that modify the CF phenotype. The fundamental defect in *CFTR* can be addressed by gene therapy approaches to repair the *CFTR* gene or pharmacotherapy to correct abnormal *CFTR* protein function. While there have been breakthroughs with these strategies, twin/sibling studies of CF patients have demonstrated that less than 50% of variation in CF lung disease severity is reflected by *CFTR* gene variation. There is now growing interest in identifying non-*CFTR* genetic variations and environmental factors that influence CF lung disease phenotypes [50]. Examples of these genetic variations include small nucleotide polymorphisms (SNPs) identified through large-scale genome-wide association studies (GWAS), and associated gene variants such as T-polymorphisms within the *CFTR* gene. Further, other ion channels on the lung epithelium (e.g. the epithelial sodium channel ENaC) work in conjunction with *CFTR* to regulate ion transport and fluid balance across epithelial surfaces, providing potential therapeutic targets for addressing these non-*CFTR* contributions to clinical phenotypes [51].

Gene Therapy

After the *CFTR* gene was sequenced, developing gene therapy to repair the abnormal *CFTR* gene or mRNA through delivery of normal DNA became a goal of CF therapy research. However, throughout the 1990s there was limited progress in this field due to several setbacks [52–55]. Early clinical trials attempted oligonucleotide delivery with adenovirus or adeno-associated virus vectors which that were complicated by interactions with the innate immune defense mechanisms of the lung [56]. It was also found to be extremely difficult to deliver repair oligonucleotides into the lung epithelium of a patient with CF through thick mucus secretions and extensive lung parenchymal damage [57].

A novel approach to gene therapy developed in the early 2000s is the use of peptide nucleic acids (PNAs), synthetic DNA analogs which can bind to DNA or RNA, for targeted gene editing [58]. Genome modification is performed by using PNAs and a donor DNA containing the correct base pairs for the target mutation. The PNAs bind to target mutation sequences and induce recombination and repair of the mutation by endogenous DNA repair factors using the donor DNA [59]. Delivery of the PNAs and donor DNAs to target cells is accomplished using bio-degradable nanoparticles [60, 61]. Thus, because PNAs do not have any inherent nuclease activity, PNAs have emerged as a safe method of gene editing with very low off-target mutation frequencies [62]. In recent years progress has been made in cystic fibrosis with attempts to correct the *F508del* mutation using PNAs. In vitro experiments resulted in approximately 10% correction of *CFTR* function, and in vivo experiments using intranasal treatment in mice yielded approximately 6% *CFTR* mutation correction in the nasal epithelium without evidence of an inflammatory response [63]. A similar method using microRNAs instead of PNAs has also been used for targeted gene therapy in CF [64]. While this gene editing method has yet to make it to clinical trials in CF patients, it will likely play an important role in gene therapy for CF [65].

In addition to PNAs, there are several other methods for gene editing including zinc-finger nucleases (ZFNs) [66] and clustered regularly interspaced short palindromic repeats (CRISPR)/CRISPR-associated (Cas) systems [67]. Both are now common methods used in bench research for gene modification in vitro with the hopes of developing these techniques into clinical treatments. Efforts have also been made in the realm of CF with attempts to correct the *F508del* mutation with ZFNs and CRISPR/Cas [68–70], and while there has been success at the cellular level, they have not yet been translated into clinical trials due to higher rates of off-target effects seen in animal models [68]. While the gene therapy approach did not yield the expected results early on, recent developments in gene editing technologies may hold promise for a resurgence in years to come.

CFTR Modulators

CFTR modulators are small molecules that can correct functional abnormalities of *CFTR* protein and partially restore *CFTR* activity. While this does not eliminate the existing gene mutation or reverse the disease, it can greatly alter the trajectory and overall health of the patient. There are two main types of modulators: potentiators and correctors. Potentiators target gating mutations (Class III) by increasing the channel opening probability, allowing increased chloride secretion [71]. Correctors modify target protein misfolding and defective trafficking to increase cell surface expression of *CFTR* [72, 73].

Ivacaftor, a potentiator approved by the FDA in 2012, was the first medication developed as a personalized treatment based on a specific *CFTR* mutation. This molecule was identified by high-throughput screening as an agent to restore *CFTR* function in the mutation *G551D*, a Class III mutation characterized by aberrant ATP-dependent gating which reduces the open probability by nearly 100-fold compared to wild-type *CFTR* [74, 75]. In clinical trials there was a drastic improvement in lung function, weight, quality of life, and reduction in pulmonary exacerbation frequency [76–78]. It was later revealed that Ivacaftor potentiates other *CFTR* gating mutations, Class IV mutations such as *R117H*, as well as *F508del* to a minor degree [72, 79]. The KONNECTION trial demonstrated that ivacaftor is effective in a variety of other Class III gating mutations leading to FDA approval for eight additional gating mutations [80]. At this time there are close to 40 approved mutations in the target group for Ivacaftor [73]. Although the efficacy of Ivacaftor varies by patient and mutation, Ivacaftor can help attain up to 35–40% of normal *CFTR* activity, enough to have comparable function level to wild-type *CFTR* [81, 82]. Ivacaftor is well tolerated in children as young as 2 years of age with at least one Class III mutation [83]. It is now approved in the US, the EU, and Canada for patients with CF aged 2 years and older. While these are still new medications, studies thus far show a sustained effect with a good safety profile [72]. The use of Ivacaftor based on *CFTR*

mutation data in asymptomatic children is a prime example of how personalized medicine could change the natural history of a disease before clinical manifestations develop.

Lumacaftor was the first *CFTR* corrector approved for use in patients with at least one *F508del* mutation. By targeting *F508del*, this medication could treat almost the entire CF population. In initial in vitro studies, lumacaftor restored chloride transport close to 15% of wild-type *CFTR* levels, and phase 2 studies revealed no significant effect on lung function at 28 days [84]. Overall the improvement at the molecular and clinical level was much less robust compared to the effect of Ivacaftor on its target gating mutations [85]. Ivacaftor on its own was also studied in subjects homozygous for *F508del*, showing limited clinical effects on FEV_1 and sweat chloride [86]. Subsequently Ivacaftor was combined with Lumacaftor as a first combination regimen [57]. Together, they increased *CFTR* function in *F508del* to nearly 30% [71]. The Lumacaftor/Ivacaftor combination therapy in patients with two *F508del* mutations was studied in TRAFFIC and TRANSPORT, two large phase III trials, [87]. In these 24-week, randomized, placebo-controlled trials of patients over 12 years of age, the drug combination led to significant improvements in FEV_1, decreased pulmonary exacerbations, and was associated with significant weight gain. The Ivacaftor/Lumacaftor combination is now approved for patients with two *F508del* mutations in the *CFTR* gene [24].

In addition to the Lumacaftor/Ivacaftor combination therapy, there are numerous ongoing clinical trials for triple therapy combinations especially targeting *F508del* homozygous or heterozygous patients [88]. Due to the complexity of the *F508del* mutation, further correction of misfolding of the *CFTR* protein with an additional corrector can increase stability of the protein and enhance function [89]. There are several phase II and III trials for triple combination therapy consisting of Ivacaftor, Tezacaftor (a corrector already approved for use in combination with Ivacaftor), and new *CFTR* corrector molecules that have shown improvement in FEV_1 at 30 days compared to Ivacaftor/Tezacaftor alone [90–92].

These triple therapy combinations now have the potential to treat up to 90% of CF patients [88].

With the influx of new modulators, mounting evidence for combination therapy, and increasingly sophisticated screening methods for predicting drug efficacy, there is a great opportunity to develop individualized treatment regimens informed by a subject's biological data. A novel approach in this field is the use of nasal epithelial culture specimens from a single individual to test the effects of *CFTR* modulators on ion transport in vitro (e.g. electrophysiological measurements of *CFTR* activity, evaluation of ion transport). This personalized approach can predict a patient's response to these drugs regardless of their actual mutation Class [93, 94]. Bronchial epithelial cultures and rectal tissues from individual patients are also being tested in a similar manner [95, 96]. This technique will be crucial not only to screen candidates for existing medications but also in the development and approval of future modulators, many of which are already being tested in Phase II and III clinical trials [88]. This, along with the development on novel modulators and triple-drug combinations will continue to expand the reach of personalized medicine from a candidate group of individuals based on their mutation type, to further benefit individuals that may not have an identifiable *CFTR* mutation but do have a chloride transport defect susceptible of correction or modulation.

Evolving Concepts in CF Precision Medicine: Going Deeper and Beyond the *CFTR* Gene

Advances in human genomics have driven the development of precision medicine for numerous diseases, including CF. We are now able to look beyond the primary genetic mutation in the *CFTR* gene and find non-*CFTR* genetic variations that contribute to its clinical phenotype. With the advent of high-throughput genotyping, this field shifted focus from family-based studies of genotype–phenotype relationships to large studies of unrelated individuals, namely Genome-Wide Association Studies GWAS [97]. GWAS is a general term for a study design or statistical method which identifies genetic variants associated with a disease phenotype on a genome-wide scale [98]. In a case–control study, the allele frequency of the genetic variant of interest is compared with that in the target group (e.g. CF patients) compared with a control group. Before GWAS, research progressed from candidate SNP studies to gene studies of single-gene variants, and then to the study of multiple genes in a common biologic pathway [97]. Thus, in the case of CF we are now able to identify target genes that affect CF lung disease through mechanisms that do not involve a *CFTR* mutation.

Large-scale GWAS have made it possible to explore millions of polymorphisms as potential genetic determinants of phenotypic variation in CF. Earlier studies had been limited by the relatively small sample sizes and lack of consistency on phenotyping CF lung disease. However there have now been several large-scale GWAS in CF that have successfully overcome these challenges [99–102]. One example is the International CF Gene Modifier Consortium, a meta-analysis of GWAS [103]. By creating a standardized lung disease phenotype definition to use as an outcome phenotype, a large database was generated across international cohorts. Five loci were found to be associated with severity of lung disease, although ultimately GWAS only accounts for a small percentage of expected genetic influence [104]. These associated loci contain genes expressed in the lung, known to affect lung disease manifestations in CF [105, 106]. Examples include mucins that play a role in host defense and airway clearance, a crucial part of current airway management techniques [107], and ion channels like the cation proton antiporter 3 (NHE 3) that regulates pH via epithelial ion transport [108]. These studies also detected variation in HLA Class II region on chromosome 6 in CF individuals. This variation has been previously associated with asthma severity [109], lung function decline, and susceptibility to allergic bronchopulmonary aspergillosis in non-CF populations [110]. In CF, these pathways have been recently associated with CF lung disease and age of onset of persistent *Pseudomonas aeruginosa* colonization [111]. Functional analysis of associated SNPs and genes at each modifier locus could identify novel targets for treating CF [99].

Deep sequencing of the *CFTR* gene has revealed other associated gene variants such as T-polymorphisms that can provide insight into likely clinical phenotypes or response to treatment. An example is the *R117H-CFTR* mutation, a unique mutation in that phenotypic expression differs depending on the number of thymidine repeats within the introns of the *CFTR* gene [112, 113]. 5 T genotype (five repeats) correlate with a more severe disease phenotype, whereas 7 T and 9 T genotypes have a milder phenotype (aberrant gene splicing in 5 T). Investigation of Ivacaftor in this mutation has shown increased efficacy in *R117H* patients with the 5 T modifier despite being a non-Class II mutation [112].

In lung epithelial cells of CF patients, deficient *CFTR*-mediated chloride secretion leads to abnormal activity in other channels involved in electrolyte and pH balance, including the epithelial sodium channel ENaC [114, 115]. ENaC plays an essential part in the regulation of sodium and water transport across epithelial surfaces. Increased ENaC activity as a result of *CFTR* dysfunction causes airway dehydration and impaired mucociliary clearance. ENaC inhibitors have been pursued to improve airway surface, but this has yet to come into clinical practice [73]. Amiloride, a classic ENaC blocker was one of the first drugs trialed for this purpose; however, it failed to improve lung function due to its short half-life, low potency, and poor side effect profile [116]. New small-molecule ENaC inhibitors are being developed to overcome these problems and are now in early-phase clinical testing [51, 117].

Future Directions

Although the initial trials of gene therapy for CF in the 1990s were not successful, research in this area has been revived in recent years. The greatest advantage of gene therapy over *CFTR* modulating therapies is that it should be effective independently of mutation Class. A recent phase II trial by the UK Cystic Fibrosis Gene Therapy Consortium used a novel lipid-based, non-viral vector complexed with plasmid *CFTR* cDNA. Results stratified by lung function indicate improvement in those with severe respiratory disease and stabilization of lung disease (no progression of disease) in patients with less severe clinical presentations [56, 118]. There are also ongoing efforts to create novel viral vectors without the immunogenic components that can trigger lung inflammation as seen in the earlier trials with adenovirus [119, 120]. As mentioned above, PNAs and CRISPR technologies are being optimized to become viable treatments for humans that can be tested in clinical trials. If successful, gene therapy would limit the need for *CFTR* modulating therapy. More practically, this may be the solution for patients with rare mutations associated with a severe disease phenotype for whom targeted therapies are not available or in development. In regards to *CFTR* modulator therapies, in addition to next generation correctors and potentiators that may be used in triple combination therapies, there are drugs with new mechanisms under development to enhance the effects of modulators, including 'amplifiers' that increase the total amount of *CFTR* protein made in the cell [89, 121]. Finally, other treatment modalities using oligonucleotides to repair *CFTR*-encoded mRNA in phase 1 proof-of-concept studies are also underway [122].

As CF becomes a disease of adulthood with increased survival, the ultimate treatment for CF would be correction of the *CFTR* mutations before birth to prevent CF as a disease altogether. Research in the use of gene therapy in utero to correct gene mutations is currently being investigated for many hereditary diseases including CF [123]. Nanoparticle-based delivery of PNAs and the newer, safer viral vectors have been used to test this concept of in-utero gene mutation correction for CF [124, 125].

Summary

Since the first description of CF in 1938, the progression of CF research studies involving the clinical, molecular, and functional characterization of CF has reshaped our understanding of disease pathogenesis and informed our approach to diagnosis and treatment. Recent advances in personalized medicine and the establishment of international collaborations for the CF population have enabled the generation and sharing of information on a large scale, defining the disease truly at an individual level. The new technologies for individualized drug efficacy screening and combination therapies have opened treatment opportunities for those with the most prevalent CF-causing mutations, but importantly also for others with rare mutations that have functional responses these drugs. As we progress toward increasingly early applications of these technologies in a patient's life, we look forward to the prospect of treating individuals before clinical manifestations develop, to yet once more change the natural history of cystic fibrosis.

References

1. Farrell PM. The prevalence of cystic fibrosis in the European Union. J Cyst Fibros. 2008;7:450–3.
2. Foundation CF. Cystic fibrosis foundation patient registry 2017 annual data report; 2018.
3. Andersen DH. Cystic fibrosis of the pancreas and its relation to celiac disease: a clinical and pathologic study. Am J Dis Child. 1938;56:344–99.
4. Andersen DH. The present diagnosis and therapy of cystic fibrosis of the pancreas. Proc R Soc Med. 1949;42:25–32.
5. Andersen DH. Cystic fibrosis of the pancreas. J Chronic Dis. 1958;7:58–90.
6. Kopelman H, Corey M, Gaskin K, Durie P, Weizman Z, Forstner G. Impaired chloride secretion, as well as bicarbonate secretion, underlies the fluid secretory defect in the cystic fibrosis pancreas. Gastroenterology. 1988;95:349–55.
7. Castellani C, Conway S, Smyth AR, Stern M, Elborn JS. Standards of Care for Cystic Fibrosis ten years later. J Cyst Fibros. 2014;13(Suppl 1):S1–2.
8. Flume PA, O'Sullivan BP, Robinson KA, Goss CH, Mogayzel PJ Jr, Willey-Courand DB, Bujan J, Finder J, Lester M, Quittell L, Rosenblatt R, Vender RL, Hazle L, Sabadosa K, Marshall B. Cystic fibrosis pulmonary guidelines: chronic medications for maintenance of lung health. Am J Respir Crit Care Med. 2007;176:957–69.
9. Rowe SM, Miller S, Sorscher EJ. Cystic fibrosis. N Engl J Med. 2005;352:1992–2001.
10. Rommens JM, Zengerling S, Burns J, Melmer G, Kerem BS, Plavsic N, Zsiga M, Kennedy D, Markiewicz D, Rozmahel R, et al. Identification and regional localization of DNA markers on chromosome 7 for the cloning of the cystic fibrosis gene. Am J Hum Genet. 1988;43:645–63.
11. Tsui LC, Rommens JM, Burns J, Zengerling S, Riordan JR, Carlock LR, Grzeschik KH, Buchwald M. Progress towards cloning the cystic fibrosis gene. Philos Trans R Soc Lond Ser B Biol Sci. 1988;319:263–73.
12. Kerem B, Rommens JM, Buchanan JA, Markiewicz D, Cox TK, Chakravarti A, Buchwald M, Tsui LC. Identification of the cystic fibrosis gene: genetic analysis. Science (New York, NY). 1989;245:1073–80.
13. Riordan JR, Rommens JM, Kerem B, Alon N, Rozmahel R, Grzelczak Z, Zielenski J, Lok S, Plavsic N, Chou JL, et al. Identification of the cystic fibrosis gene: cloning and characterization of complementary DNA. Science. 1989;245:1066–73.
14. Spielberg DR, Clancy JP. Cystic fibrosis and its management through established and emerging therapies. Annu Rev Genomics Hum Genet. 2016;17:155–75.
15. Grody WW, Cutting GR, Klinger KW, Richards CS, Watson MS, Desnick RJ. Laboratory standards and guidelines for population-based cystic fibrosis carrier screening. Genet Med. 2001;3:149–54.
16. Ross LF. Newborn screening for cystic fibrosis: a lesson in public health disparities. J Pediatr. 2008;153:308–13.
17. Farrell PM, White TB, Derichs N, Castellani C, Rosenstein BJ. Cystic fibrosis diagnostic challenges over 4 decades: historical perspectives and lessons learned. J Pediatr. 2017;181S:S16–26.
18. Crossley JR, Smith PA, Edgar BW, Gluckman PD, Elliott RB. Neonatal screening for cystic fibrosis, using immunoreactive trypsin assay in dried blood spots. Clin Chim Acta. 1981;113:111–21.
19. Sosnay PR, White TB, Farrell PM, Ren CL, Derichs N, Howenstine MS, Nick JA, De Boeck K. Diagnosis of cystic fibrosis in nonscreened populations. J Pediatr. 2017;181s:S52–S57.e2.
20. Farrell PM, White TB, Ren CL, Hempstead SE, Accurso F, Derichs N, Howenstine M, McColley SA, Rock M, Rosenfeld M, Sermet-Gaudelus I, Southern KW, Marshall BC, Sosnay PR. Diagnosis of cystic fibrosis: consensus guidelines from the Cystic Fibrosis Foundation. J Pediatr. 2017;181s:S4–S15.e11.
21. Collaco JM, Blackman SM, Raraigh KS, Corvol H, Rommens JM, Pace RG, Boelle PY, McGready J, Sosnay PR, Strug LJ, Knowles MR, Cutting GR. Sources of variation in sweat chloride measurements in cystic fibrosis. Am J Respir Crit Care Med. 2016;194:1375–82.
22. Gibson LE, Cooke RE. A test for concentration of electrolytes in sweat in cystic fibrosis of the pancreas utilizing pilocarpine by iontophoresis. Pediatrics. 1959;23:545–9.
23. Gibson LE, Gottlieb R, Di Sant'Agnese PA, Huang NN. Reliability of sweat tests in diagnosis of cystic fibrosis. J Pediatr. 1972;81:193–7.

24. Paranjape SM, Mogayzel PJ Jr. Cystic fibrosis in the era of precision medicine. Paediatr Respir Rev. 2018;25:64–72.

25. Rosenstein BJ, Cutting GR. The diagnosis of cystic fibrosis: a consensus statement. J Pediatr. 1998;132:589–95.

26. Pique L, Graham S, Pearl M, Kharrazi M, Schrijver I. Cystic fibrosis newborn screening programs: implications of the *CFTR* variant spectrum in non-white patients. Genet Med. 2017;19:36–44.

27. Bishop MD, Freedman SD, Zielenski J, Ahmed N, Dupuis A, Martin S, Ellis L, Shea J, Hopper I, Corey M, Kortan P, Haber G, Ross C, Tzountzouris J, Steele L, Ray PN, Tsui LC, Durie PR. The cystic fibrosis transmembrane conductance regulator gene and ion channel function in patients with idiopathic pancreatitis. Hum Genet. 2005;118:372–81.

28. Drumm ML, Konstan MW, Schluchter MD, Handler A, Pace R, Zou F, Zariwala M, Fargo D, Xu A, Dunn JM, Darrah RJ, Dorfman R, Sandford AJ, Corey M, Zielenski J, Durie P, Goddard K, Yankaskas JR, Wright FA, Knowles MR, Gene Modifier Study G. Genetic modifiers of lung disease in cystic fibrosis. N Engl J Med. 2005;353:1443–53.

29. Cyst. Fibros. Found., Johns Hopkins Univ., Hosp. Sick Child. 2015. Clinical and functional translation of *CFTR* (*CFTR*2). http://*CFTR*2.org; 2019.

30. Jurkuvenaite A, Chen L, Bartoszewski R, Goldstein R, Bebok Z, Matalon S, Collawn JF. Functional stability of rescued delta F508 cystic fibrosis transmembrane conductance regulator in airway epithelial cells. Am J Respir Cell Mol Biol. 2010;42:363–72.

31. Jurkuvenaite A, Varga K, Nowotarski K, Kirk KL, Sorscher EJ, Li Y, Clancy JP, Bebok Z, Collawn JF. Mutations in the amino terminus of the cystic fibrosis transmembrane conductance regulator enhance endocytosis. J Biol Chem. 2006;281:3329–34.

32. Bagdany M, Veit G, Fukuda R, Avramescu RG, Okiyoneda T, Baaklini I, Singh J, Sovak G, Xu H, Apaja PM, Sattin S, Beitel LK, Roldan A, Colombo G, Balch W, Young JC, Lukacs GL. Chaperones rescue the energetic landscape of mutant *CFTR* at single molecule and in cell. Nat Commun. 2017;8:398.

33. Lukacs GL, Verkman AS. *CFTR*: folding, misfolding and correcting the DeltaF508 conformational defect. Trends Mol Med. 2012;18:81–91.

34. Mogayzel PJ Jr, Dunitz J, Marrow LC, Hazle LA. Improving chronic care delivery and outcomes: the impact of the cystic fibrosis Care Center Network. BMJ Qual Saf. 2014;23(Suppl 1):i3–8.

35. Flume PA, O'Sullivan BP, Robinson KA, Goss CH, Mogayzel PJ Jr, Willey-Courand DB, Bujan J, Finder J, Lester M, Quittell L, Rosenblatt R, Vender RL, Hazle L, Sabadosa K, Marshall B, Cystic Fibrosis Foundation PTC. Cystic fibrosis pulmonary guidelines: chronic medications for maintenance of lung health. Am J Respir Crit Care Med. 2007;176:957–69.

36. Elkins MR, Robinson M, Rose BR, Harbour C, Moriarty CP, Marks GB, Belousova EG, Xuan W, Bye PT, National Hypertonic Saline in Cystic Fibrosis Study G. A controlled trial of long-term inhaled hypertonic saline in patients with cystic fibrosis. N Engl J Med. 2006;354:229–40.

37. Elkins M, Dentice R. Timing of hypertonic saline inhalation for cystic fibrosis. Cochrane Database Syst Rev. 2016;12:CD008816.

38. Dentice RL, Elkins MR, Middleton PG, Bishop JR, Wark PA, Dorahy DJ, Harmer CJ, Hu H, Bye PT. A randomised trial of hypertonic saline during hospitalisation for exacerbation of cystic fibrosis. Thorax. 2016;71:141–7.

39. Dentice R, Elkins M. Timing of dornase alfa inhalation for cystic fibrosis. Cochrane Database Syst Rev. 2018;11:CD007923.

40. Dentice R, Elkins M. Timing of dornase alfa inhalation for cystic fibrosis. Cochrane Database Syst Rev. 2016;7:CD007923.

41. Bye PT, Elkins MR. Other mucoactive agents for cystic fibrosis. Paediatr Respir Rev. 2007;8:30–9.

42. Mogayzel PJ Jr, Naureckas ET, Robinson KA, Mueller G, Hadjiliadis D, Hoag JB, Lubsch L, Hazle L, Sabadosa K, Marshall B, Pulmonary Clinical Practice Guidelines C. Cystic fibrosis pulmonary guidelines. Chronic medications for maintenance of lung health. Am J Respir Crit Care Med. 2013;187:680–9.

43. Cogen J, Emerson J, Sanders DB, Ren C, Schechter MS, Gibson RL, Morgan W, Rosenfeld M. Risk factors for lung function decline in a large cohort of young cystic fibrosis patients. Pediatr Pulmonol. 2015;50:763–70.

44. Lund-Palau H, Turnbull AR, Bush A, Bardin E, Cameron L, Soren O, Wierre-Gore N, Alton EW, Bundy JG, Connett G, Faust SN, Filloux A, Freemont P, Jones A, Khoo V, Morales S, Murphy R, Pabary R, Simbo A, Schelenz S, Takats Z, Webb J, Williams HD, Davies JC. Pseudomonas aeruginosa infection in cystic fibrosis: pathophysiological mechanisms and therapeutic approaches. Expert Rev Respir Med. 2016;10:685–97.

45. Jain K, Smyth AR. Current dilemmas in antimicrobial therapy in cystic fibrosis. Expert Rev Respir Med. 2012;6:407–22.

46. Langton Hewer SC, Smyth AR. Antibiotic strategies for eradicating Pseudomonas aeruginosa in people with cystic fibrosis. Cochrane Database Syst Rev. 2014;11:CD004197.

47. Langton Hewer SC, Smyth AR. Antibiotic strategies for eradicating Pseudomonas aeruginosa in people with cystic fibrosis. Cochrane Database Syst Rev. 2017;4:CD004197.

48. Mogayzel PJ Jr, Naureckas ET, Robinson KA, Brady C, Guill M, Lahiri T, Lubsch L, Matsui J, Oermann CM, Ratjen F, Rosenfeld M, Simon RH, Hazle L, Sabadosa K, Marshall BC, Cystic Fibrosis Foundation Pulmonary Clinical Practice Guidelines C. Cystic Fibrosis Foundation pulmonary guideline. Pharmacologic approaches to prevention and eradication of initial Pseudomonas aeruginosa infection. Ann Am Thorac Soc. 2014;11:1640–50.

49. Smyth AR. Pseudomonas eradication in cystic fibrosis: who will join the ELITE? Thorax. 2010;65:281–2.
50. Vanscoy LL, Blackman SM, Collaco JM, Bowers A, Lai T, Naughton K, Algire M, McWilliams R, Beck S, Hoover-Fong J, Hamosh A, Cutler D, Cutting GR. Heritability of lung disease severity in cystic fibrosis. Am J Respir Crit Care Med. 2007;175:1036–43.
51. Cyst. Fibros. Found. Drug development pipeline. CF foundation, www.cff.org/trials/pipeline.
52. Harvey BG, Leopold PL, Hackett NR, Grasso TM, Williams PM, Tucker AL, Kaner RJ, Ferris B, Gonda I, Sweeney TD, Ramalingam R, Kovesdi I, Shak S, Crystal RG. Airway epithelial *CFTR* mRNA expression in cystic fibrosis patients after repetitive administration of a recombinant adenovirus. J Clin Invest. 1999;104:1245–55.
53. Simon RH, Engelhardt JF, Yang Y, Zepeda M, Weber-Pendleton S, Grossman M, Wilson JM. Adenovirus-mediated transfer of the *CFTR* gene to lung of nonhuman primates: toxicity study. Hum Gene Ther. 1993;4:771–80.
54. Wilmott RW, Amin RS, Perez CR, Wert SE, Keller G, Boivin GP, Hirsch R, De Inocencio J, Lu P, Reising SF, Yei S, Whitsett JA, Trapnell BC. Safety of adenovirus-mediated transfer of the human cystic fibrosis transmembrane conductance regulator cDNA to the lungs of nonhuman primates. Hum Gene Ther. 1996;7:301–18.
55. Knowles MR, Hohneker KW, Zhou Z, Olsen JC, Noah TL, Hu PC, Leigh MW, Engelhardt JF, Edwards LJ, Jones KR, et al. A controlled study of adenoviral-vector-mediated gene transfer in the nasal epithelium of patients with cystic fibrosis. N Engl J Med. 1995;333:823–31.
56. Armstrong DK, Cunningham S, Davies JC, Alton EW. Gene therapy in cystic fibrosis. Arch Dis Child. 2014;99:465–8.
57. Maiuri L, Raia V, Kroemer G. Strategies for the etiological therapy of cystic fibrosis. Cell Death Differ. 2017;24:1825–44.
58. Ricciardi AS, Quijano E, Putman R, Saltzman WM, Glazer PM. Peptide nucleic acids as a tool for site-specific gene editing. Molecules (Basel, Switzerland). 2018;23(3) https://doi.org/10.3390/molecules23030632.
59. Faruqi AF, Datta HJ, Carroll D, Seidman MM, Glazer PM. Triple-helix formation induces recombination in mammalian cells via a nucleotide excision repair-dependent pathway. Mol Cell Biol. 2000;20:990–1000.
60. McNeer NA, Chin JY, Schleifman EB, Fields RJ, Glazer PM, Saltzman WM. Nanoparticles deliver triplex-forming PNAs for site-specific genomic recombination in CD34+ human hematopoietic progenitors. Mol Ther. 2011;19:172–80.
61. Fields RJ, Quijano E, McNeer NA, Caputo C, Bahal R, Anandalingam K, Egan ME, Glazer PM, Saltzman WM. Modified poly(lactic-co-glycolic acid) nanoparticles for enhanced cellular uptake and gene editing in the lung. Adv Healthc Mater. 2015;4:361–6.
62. Papapetrou EP, Zoumbos NC, Athanassiadou A. Genetic modification of hematopoietic stem cells with nonviral systems: past progress and future prospects. Gene Ther. 2005;12(Suppl 1):S118–30.
63. McNeer NA, Anandalingam K, Fields RJ, Caputo C, Kopic S, Gupta A, Quijano E, Polikoff L, Kong Y, Bahal R, Geibel JP, Glazer PM, Saltzman WM, Egan ME. Nanoparticles that deliver triplex-forming peptide nucleic acid molecules correct F508del *CFTR* in airway epithelium. Nat Commun. 2015;6:6952.
64. Robinson E, MacDonald KD, Slaughter K, McKinney M, Patel S, Sun C, Sahay G. Lipid nanoparticle-delivered chemically modified mRNA restores chloride secretion in cystic fibrosis. Mol Ther. 2018;26:2034–46.
65. Donnelley M, Parsons DW. Gene therapy for cystic fibrosis lung disease: overcoming the barriers to translation to the clinic. Front Pharmacol. 2018;9:1381.
66. Porteus MH, Carroll D. Gene targeting using zinc finger nucleases. Nat Biotechnol. 2005;23:967–73.
67. Jinek M, Chylinski K, Fonfara I, Hauer M, Doudna JA, Charpentier E. A programmable dual-RNA-guided DNA endonuclease in adaptive bacterial immunity. Science (New York, NY). 2012;337:816–21.
68. Harrison PT, Sanz DJ, Hollywood JA. Impact of gene editing on the study of cystic fibrosis. Hum Genet. 2016;135:983–92.
69. Lee CM, Flynn R, Hollywood JA, Scallan MF, Harrison PT. Correction of the DeltaF508 mutation in the cystic fibrosis transmembrane conductance regulator Gene by zinc-finger nuclease homology-directed repair. Biores Open Access. 2012;1:99–108.
70. Sanz DJ, Hollywood JA, Scallan MF, Harrison PT. Cas9/gRNA targeted excision of cystic fibrosis-causing deep-intronic splicing mutations restores normal splicing of *CFTR* mRNA. PLoS One. 2017;12:e0184009.
71. Van Goor F, Straley KS, Cao D, Gonzalez J, Hadida S, Hazlewood A, Joubran J, Knapp T, Makings LR, Miller M, Neuberger T, Olson E, Panchenko V, Rader J, Singh A, Stack JH, Tung R, Grootenhuis PD, Negulescu P. Rescue of DeltaF508-*CFTR* trafficking and gating in human cystic fibrosis airway primary cultures by small molecules. Am J Physiol Lung Cell Mol Physiol. 2006;290:L1117–30.
72. De Boeck K, Munck A, Walker S, Faro A, Hiatt P, Gilmartin G, Higgins M. Efficacy and safety of ivacaftor in patients with cystic fibrosis and a non-G551D gating mutation. J Cyst Fibros. 2014;13:674–80.
73. Gentzsch M, Mall MA. Ion channel modulators in cystic fibrosis. Chest. 2018;154:383–93.
74. Bompadre SG, Li M, Hwang TC. Mechanism of G551D-*CFTR* (cystic fibrosis transmembrane conductance regulator) potentiation by a high affinity ATP analog. J Biol Chem. 2008;283:5364–9.

75. Van Goor F, Hadida S, Grootenhuis PD, Burton B, Cao D, Neuberger T, Turnbull A, Singh A, Joubran J, Hazlewood A, Zhou J, McCartney J, Arumugam V, Decker C, Yang J, Young C, Olson ER, Wine JJ, Frizzell RA, Ashlock M, Negulescu P. Rescue of CF airway epithelial cell function in vitro by a *CFTR* potentiator, VX-770. Proc Natl Acad Sci U S A. 2009;106:18825–30.

76. Davies JC, Wainwright CE, Canny GJ, Chilvers MA, Howenstine MS, Munck A, Mainz JG, Rodriguez S, Li H, Yen K, Ordonez CL, Ahrens R. Efficacy and safety of ivacaftor in patients aged 6 to 11 years with cystic fibrosis with a G551D mutation. Am J Respir Crit Care Med. 2013;187:1219–25.

77. McKone EF, Borowitz D, Drevinek P, Griese M, Konstan MW, Wainwright C, Ratjen F, Sermet-Gaudelus I, Plant B, Munck A, Jiang Y, Gilmartin G, Davies JC. Long-term safety and efficacy of ivacaftor in patients with cystic fibrosis who have the Gly551Asp-*CFTR* mutation: a phase 3, open-label extension study (PERSIST). Lancet Respir Med. 2014;2:902–10.

78. Ramsey BW, Davies J, McElvaney NG, Tullis E, Bell SC, Drevinek P, Griese M, McKone EF, Wainwright CE, Konstan MW, Moss R, Ratjen F, Sermet-Gaudelus I, Rowe SM, Dong Q, Rodriguez S, Yen K, Ordonez C, Elborn JS. A *CFTR* potentiator in patients with cystic fibrosis and the G551D mutation. N Engl J Med. 2011;365:1663–72.

79. Moss RB, Flume PA, Elborn JS, Cooke J, Rowe SM, McColley SA, Rubenstein RC, Higgins M. Efficacy and safety of ivacaftor in patients with cystic fibrosis who have an Arg117His-*CFTR* mutation: a double-blind, randomised controlled trial. Lancet Respir Med. 2015;3:524–33.

80. Yu H, Burton B, Huang CJ, Worley J, Cao D, Johnson JP Jr, Urrutia A, Joubran J, Seepersaud S, Sussky K, Hoffman BJ, Van Goor F. Ivacaftor potentiation of multiple *CFTR* channels with gating mutations. J Cyst Fibros. 2012;11:237–45.

81. Accurso FJ, Van Goor F, Zha J, Stone AJ, Dong Q, Ordonez CL, Rowe SM, Clancy JP, Konstan MW, Hoch HE, Heltshe SL, Ramsey BW, Campbell PW, Ashlock MA. Sweat chloride as a biomarker of *CFTR* activity: proof of concept and ivacaftor clinical trial data. J Cyst Fibros. 2014;13:139–47.

82. McKone EF, Emerson SS, Edwards KL, Aitken ML. Effect of genotype on phenotype and mortality in cystic fibrosis: a retrospective cohort study. Lancet (London, England). 2003;361:1671–6.

83. Davies JC, Cunningham S, Harris WT, Lapey A, Regelmann WE, Sawicki GS, Southern KW, Robertson S, Green Y, Cooke J, Rosenfeld M. Safety, pharmacokinetics, and pharmacodynamics of ivacaftor in patients aged 2-5 years with cystic fibrosis and a *CFTR* gating mutation (KIWI): an open-label, single-arm study. Lancet Respir Med. 2016;4:107–15.

84. Clancy JP, Rowe SM, Accurso FJ, Aitken ML, Amin RS, Ashlock MA, Ballmann M, Boyle MP, Bronsveld I, Campbell PW, De Boeck K, Donaldson SH, Dorkin HL, Dunitz JM, Durie PR, Jain M, Leonard A, McCoy KS, Moss RB, Pilewski JM, Rosenbluth DB, Rubenstein RC, Schechter MS, Botfield M, Ordonez CL, Spencer-Green GT, Vernillet L, Wisseh S, Yen K, Konstan MW. Results of a phase IIa study of VX-809, an investigational *CFTR* corrector compound, in subjects with cystic fibrosis homozygous for the F508del-*CFTR* mutation. Thorax. 2012;67:12–8.

85. Boyle MP, Bell SC, Konstan MW, McColley SA, Rowe SM, Rietschel E, Huang X, Waltz D, Patel NR, Rodman D. A *CFTR* corrector (lumacaftor) and a *CFTR* potentiator (ivacaftor) for treatment of patients with cystic fibrosis who have a phe508del *CFTR* mutation: a phase 2 randomised controlled trial. Lancet Respir Med. 2014;2:527–38.

86. Flume PA, Liou TG, Borowitz DS, Li H, Yen K, Ordonez CL, Geller DE. Ivacaftor in subjects with cystic fibrosis who are homozygous for the F508del-*CFTR* mutation. Chest. 2012;142:718–24.

87. Wainwright CE, Elborn JS, Ramsey BW. Lumacaftor-ivacaftor in patients with cystic fibrosis homozygous for Phe508del *CFTR*. N Engl J Med. 2015;373:1783–4.

88. Chaudary N. Triplet *CFTR* modulators: future prospects for treatment of cystic fibrosis. Ther Clin Risk Manag. 2018;14:2375–83.

89. Molinski SV, Ahmadi S, Ip W, Ouyang H, Villella A, Miller JP, Lee PS, Kulleperuma K, Du K, Di Paola M, Eckford PD, Laselva O, Huan LJ, Wellhauser L, Li E, Ray PN, Pomes R, Moraes TJ, Gonska T, Ratjen F, Bear CE. Orkambi(R) and amplifier co-therapy improves function from a rare *CFTR* mutation in gene-edited cells and patient tissue. EMBO Mol Med. 2017;9:1224–43.

90. Davies JC, Moskowitz SM, Brown C, Horsley A, Mall MA, McKone EF, Plant BJ, Prais D, Ramsey BW, Taylor-Cousar JL, Tullis E, Uluer A, McKee CM, Robertson S, Shilling RA, Simard C, Van Goor F, Waltz D, Xuan F, Young T, Rowe SM. VX-659-Tezacaftor-Ivacaftor in patients with cystic fibrosis and one or two Phe508del alleles. N Engl J Med. 2018;379:1599–611.

91. Keating D, Marigowda G, Burr L, Daines C, Mall MA, McKone EF, Ramsey BW, Rowe SM, Sass LA, Tullis E, McKee CM, Moskowitz SM, Robertson S, Savage J, Simard C, Van Goor F, Waltz D, Xuan F, Young T, Taylor-Cousar JL. VX-445-Tezacaftor-Ivacaftor in patients with cystic fibrosis and one or two Phe508del alleles. N Engl J Med. 2018;379:1612–20.

92. Rowe SM, Daines C, Ringshausen FC, Kerem E, Wilson J, Tullis E, Nair N, Simard C, Han L, Ingenito EP, McKee C, Lekstrom-Himes J, Davies JC. Tezacaftor-Ivacaftor in residual-function heterozygotes with cystic fibrosis. N Engl J Med. 2017;377:2024–35.

93. Brewington JJ, Filbrandt ET, LaRosa FJ 3rd, Moncivaiz JD, Ostmann AJ, Strecker LM, Clancy

JP. Brushed nasal epithelial cells are a surrogate for bronchial epithelial *CFTR* studies. JCI Insight. 2018;3(13) https://doi.org/10.1172/jci.insight.99385.

94. Cholon DM, Gentzsch M. Recent progress in translational cystic fibrosis research using precision medicine strategies. J Cyst Fibros. 2018;17:S52–s60.

95. Brewington JJ, Filbrandt ET, LaRosa FJ 3rd, Moncivaiz JD, Ostmann AJ, Strecker LM, Clancy JP. Generation of human nasal epithelial cell spheroids for individualized cystic fibrosis transmembrane conductance regulator study. J Vis Exp. 2018;134:e57492.

96. Dekkers JF, Berkers G, Kruisselbrink E, Vonk A, de Jonge HR, Janssens HM, Bronsveld I, van de Graaf EA, Nieuwenhuis EE, Houwen RH, Vleggaar FP, Escher JC, de Rijke YB, Majoor CJ, Heijerman HG, de Winter-de Groot KM, Clevers H, van der Ent CK, Beekman JM. Characterizing responses to *CFTR*-modulating drugs using rectal organoids derived from subjects with cystic fibrosis. Sci Transl Med. 2016;8:344ra384.

97. Hebbring S. Genomic and phenomic research in the 21st century. Trends Genet. 2019;35(1):29–41.

98. McCarthy MI, Abecasis GR, Cardon LR, Goldstein DB, Little J, Ioannidis JP, Hirschhorn JN. Genome-wide association studies for complex traits: consensus, uncertainty and challenges. Nat Rev Genet. 2008;9:356–69.

99. Corvol H, Blackman SM, Boelle PY, Gallins PJ, Pace RG, Stonebraker JR, Accurso FJ, Clement A, Collaco JM, Dang H, Dang AT, Franca A, Gong J, Guillot L, Keenan K, Li W, Lin F, Patrone MV, Raraigh KS, Sun L, Zhou YH, O'Neal WK, Sontag MK, Levy H, Durie PR, Rommens JM, Drumm ML, Wright FA, Strug LJ, Cutting GR, Knowles MR. Genome-wide association meta-analysis identifies five modifier loci of lung disease severity in cystic fibrosis. Nat Commun. 2015;6:8382.

100. Di Paola M, Park AJ, Ahmadi S, Roach EJ, Wu YS, Struder-Kypke M, Lam JS, Bear CE, Khursigara CM. SLC6A14 is a genetic modifier of cystic fibrosis that regulates Pseudomonas aeruginosa attachment to human bronchial epithelial cells. MBio. 2017;8(6):e02073–17.

101. Drumm ML, Konstan MW, Schluchter MD, Handler A, Pace R, Zou F, Zariwala M, Fargo D, Xu A, Dunn JM, Darrah RJ, Dorfman R, Sandford AJ, Corey M, Zielenski J, Durie P, Goddard K, Yankaskas JR, Wright FA, Knowles MR. Genetic modifiers of lung disease in cystic fibrosis. N Engl J Med. 2005;353:1443–53.

102. Li W, Soave D, Miller MR, Keenan K, Lin F, Gong J, Chiang T, Stephenson AL, Durie P, Rommens J, Sun L, Strug LJ. Unraveling the complex genetic model for cystic fibrosis: pleiotropic effects of modifier genes on early cystic fibrosis-related morbidities. Hum Genet. 2014;133:151–61.

103. Knowles MR, Drumm M. The influence of genetics on cystic fibrosis phenotypes. Cold Spring Harb Perspect Med. 2012;2:a009548.

104. Polineni D, Dang H, Gallins PJ, Jones LC, Pace RG, Stonebraker JR, Commander LA, Krenicky JE, Zhou YH, Corvol H, Cutting GR, Drumm ML, Strug LJ, Boyle MP, Durie PR, Chmiel JF, Zou F, Wright FA, O'Neal WK, Knowles MR. Airway mucosal host defense is key to genomic regulation of cystic fibrosis lung disease severity. Am J Respir Crit Care Med. 2018;197:79–93.

105. Dorfman R, Taylor C, Lin F, Sun L, Sandford A, Pare P, Berthiaume Y, Corey M, Durie P, Zielenski J. Modulatory effect of the SLC9A3 gene on susceptibility to infections and pulmonary function in children with cystic fibrosis. Pediatr Pulmonol. 2011;46:385–92.

106. Wright FA, Strug LJ, Doshi VK, Commander CW, Blackman SM, Sun L, Berthiaume Y, Cutler D, Cojocaru A, Collaco JM, Corey M, Dorfman R, Goddard K, Green D, Kent JW Jr, Lange EM, Lee S, Li W, Luo J, Mayhew GM, Naughton KM, Pace RG, Pare P, Rommens JM, Sandford A, Stonebraker JR, Sun W, Taylor C, Vanscoy LL, Zou F, Blangero J, Zielenski J, O'Neal WK, Drumm ML, Durie PR, Knowles MR, Cutting GR. Genome-wide association and linkage identify modifier loci of lung disease severity in cystic fibrosis at 11p13 and 20q13.2. Nat Genet. 2011;43:539–46.

107. Kesimer M, Ehre C, Burns KA, Davis CW, Sheehan JK, Pickles RJ. Molecular organization of the mucins and glycocalyx underlying mucus transport over mucosal surfaces of the airways. Mucosal Immunol. 2013;6:379–92.

108. Orlowski J, Grinstein S. Na+/H+ exchangers. Compr Physiol. 2011;1:2083–100.

109. Kontakioti E, Domvri K, Papakosta D, Daniilidis M. HLA and asthma phenotypes/endotypes: a review. Hum Immunol. 2014;75:930–9.

110. Chauhan B, Santiago L, Hutcheson PS, Schwartz HJ, Spitznagel E, Castro M, Slavin RG, Bellone CJ. Evidence for the involvement of two different MHC Class II regions in susceptibility or protection in allergic bronchopulmonary aspergillosis. J Allergy Clin Immunol. 2000;106:723–9.

111. O'Neal WK, Knowles MR. Cystic fibrosis disease modifiers: complex genetics defines the phenotypic diversity in a monogenic disease. Annu Rev Genomics Hum Genet. 2018;19:201–22.

112. Char JE, Wolfe MH, Cho HJ, Park IH, Jeong JH, Frisbee E, Dunn C, Davies Z, Milla C, Moss RB, Thomas EA, Wine JJ. A little *CFTR* goes a long way: *CFTR*-dependent sweat secretion from G551D and R117H-5T cystic fibrosis subjects taking ivacaftor. PLoS One. 2014;9:e88564.

113. Chu CS, Trapnell BC, Murtagh JJJ, Moss J, Dalemans W, Jallat S, Mercenier A, Pavirani A, Lecocq JP, Cutting GR, et al. Variable deletion of exon 9 coding sequences in cystic fibrosis transmembrane conductance regulator gene mRNA transcripts in normal bronchial epithelium. EMBO J. 1991;10:1355–63.

114. Knowles M, Gatzy J, Boucher R. Increased bioelectric potential difference across respiratory epithelia in cystic fibrosis. N Engl J Med. 1981;305:1489–95.

115. Mall M, Grubb BR, Harkema JR, O'Neal WK, Boucher RC. Increased airway epithelial Na+ absorption produces cystic fibrosis-like lung disease in mice. Nat Med. 2004;10:487–93.

116. Pons G, Marchand MC, d'Athis P, Sauvage E, Foucard C, Chaumet-Riffaud P, Sautegeau A, Navarro J, Lenoir G. French multicenter randomized double-blind placebo-controlled trial on nebulized amiloride in cystic fibrosis patients. The Amiloride-AFLM Collaborative Study Group. Pediatr Pulmonol. 2000;30:25–31.

117. Lennox A, Myerburg MM. SPX-101 is a promising and novel nebulized ENaC inhibitor. Am J Respir Crit Care Med. 2017;196:671–2.

118. Alton E, Armstrong DK, Ashby D, Bayfield KJ, Bilton D, Bloomfield EV, Boyd AC, Brand J, Buchan R, Calcedo R, Carvelli P, Chan M, Cheng SH, Collie DS, Cunningham S, Davidson HE, Davies G, Davies JC, Davies LA, Dewar MH, Doherty A, Donovan J, Dwyer NS, Elgmati HI, Featherstone RF, Gavino J, Gea-Sorli S, Geddes DM, Gibson JSR, Gill DR, Greening AP, Griesenbach U, Hansell DM, Harman K, Higgins TE, Hodges SL, Hyde SC, Hyndman L, Innes JA, Jacob J, Jones N, Keogh BF, Limberis MP, Lloyd-Evans P, Maclean AW, Manvell MC, McCormick D, McGovern M, McLachlan G, Meng C, Montero MA, Milligan H, Moyce LJ, Murray GD, Nicholson AG, Osadolor T, Parra-Leiton J, Porteous DJ, Pringle IA, Punch EK, Pytel KM, Quittner AL, Rivellini G, Saunders CJ, Scheule RK, Sheard S, Simmonds NJ, Smith K, Smith SN, Soussi N, Soussi S, Spearing EJ, Stevenson BJ, Sumner-Jones SG, Turkkila M, Ureta RP, Waller MD, Wasowicz MY, Wilson JM, Wolstenholme-Hogg P, on behalf of the UKCFGTC. Efficacy and Mechanism Evaluation. A randomised, double-blind, placebo-controlled trial of repeated nebulisation of non-viral cystic fibrosis transmembrane conductance regulator (*CFTR*) gene therapy in patients with cystic fibrosis. Southampton (UK): NIHR Journals Library∗Copyright (c) Queen's Printer and Controller of HMSO 2016. This work was produced by Alton et al. under the terms of a commissioning contract issued by the Secretary of State for Health. This issue may be freely reproduced for the purposes of private research and study and extracts (or indeed, the full report) may be included in professional journals provided that suitable acknowledgement is made and the reproduction is not associated with any form of advertising. Applications for commercial reproduction should be addressed to: NIHR Journals Library, National Institute for Health Research, Evaluation, Trials and Studies Coordinating Centre, Alpha House, University of Southampton Science Park, Southampton SO16 7NS, UK.; 2016.

119. Gill DR, Hyde SC. Delivery of genes into the CF airway. Thorax. 2014;69:962–4.

120. Mottais A, Berchel M, Sibiril Y, Laurent V, Gill D, Hyde S, Jaffres PA, Montier T, Le Gall T. Antibacterial effect and DNA delivery using a combination of an arsonium-containing lipophosphoramide with an N-heterocyclic carbene-silver complex – potential benefits for cystic fibrosis lung gene therapy. Int J Pharm. 2018;536:29–41.

121. Marson FAL, Bertuzzo CS, Ribeiro JD. Personalized or precision medicine? The example of cystic fibrosis. Front Pharmacol. 2017;8:390.

122. Dhooghe B, Haaf JB, Noel S, Leal T. Strategies in early clinical development for the treatment of basic defects of cystic fibrosis. Expert Opin Investig Drugs. 2016;25:423–36.

123. Montazersaheb S, Hejazi MS, Nozad Charoudeh H. Potential of peptide nucleic acids in future therapeutic applications. Adv Pharm Bull. 2018;8:551–63.

124. Nishida K, Smith Z, Rana D, Palmer J, Gallicano GI. Cystic fibrosis: a look into the future of prenatal screening and therapy. Birth Defects Res C Embryo Today. 2015;105:73–80.

125. Ricciardi AS, Bahal R, Farrelly JS, Quijano E, Bianchi AH, Luks VL, Putman R, Lopez-Giraldez F, Coskun S, Song E, Liu Y, Hsieh WC, Ly DH, Stitelman DH, Glazer PM, Saltzman WM. In utero nanoparticle delivery for site-specific genome editing. Nat Commun. 2018;9:2481.

Genetics of Idiopathic Pulmonary Fibrosis

6

Susan K. Mathai and David A. Schwartz

Key Point Summary

- Common and rare genetic factors play a significant role in IPF disease risk.
- Biological pathways implicated by findings from IPF genetics studies include those related to surfactants, mucociliary function, cell–cell adhesion, and telomere maintenance.
- Distinct genotypes found in IPF patients may determine clinical phenotypes, although prospective clinical trials are required to translate retrospective observations into findings that can be used in clinical practice.

Introduction

For decades, the cause of Idiopathic Pulmonary Fibrosis (IPF) had been a mystery. Patients often presented after the insidious onset of progressive dyspnea and cough to be diagnosed with extensive irreversibly scarred lungs. However, evolution of genetics and genomics high-throughput technologies over the last two decades have led to rapid growth in our understanding of this enigmatic disease. Indeed, IPF is increasingly being seen as a genetic disease, and novel genetic loci are increasing our understanding of pathophysiology, as well as being identified as therapeutic targets. This chapter summarizes our current understanding of the genetics of IPF and identifies potential avenues for genetic findings to inform precision therapy in this disease.

Clinical Presentation of IPF

Patients with IPF generally present late in the course of their disease—indeed, it is not uncommon for patients to present to specialty centers having spent months or years attempting to find answers as to why their symptoms of shortness of breath and cough have persisted despite courses of therapy for more common pulmonary diseases such as asthma, pneumonia, or bronchitis (Fig. 6.1). The symptoms of pulmonary fibrosis are nonspecific, and therefore, diagnosis can be delayed; patients' symptoms often start with a cough, shortness of breath, and fatigue that persist

S. K. Mathai
Interstitial Lung Disease Program, Center for Advanced Heart & Lung Disease, Baylor University Medical Center at Dallas, Dallas, TX, USA

Department of Internal Medicine, Texas A&M University College of Medicine, Dallas, TX, USA
e-mail: Susan.Mathai@BSWHealth.org

D. A. Schwartz (✉)
Department of Medicine, University of Colorado School of Medicine, Aurora, CO, USA
e-mail: David.Schwartz@ucdenver.edu

© Springer Nature Switzerland AG 2020
J. L. Gomez et al. (eds.), *Precision in Pulmonary, Critical Care, and Sleep Medicine*, Respiratory Medicine, https://doi.org/10.1007/978-3-030-31507-8_6

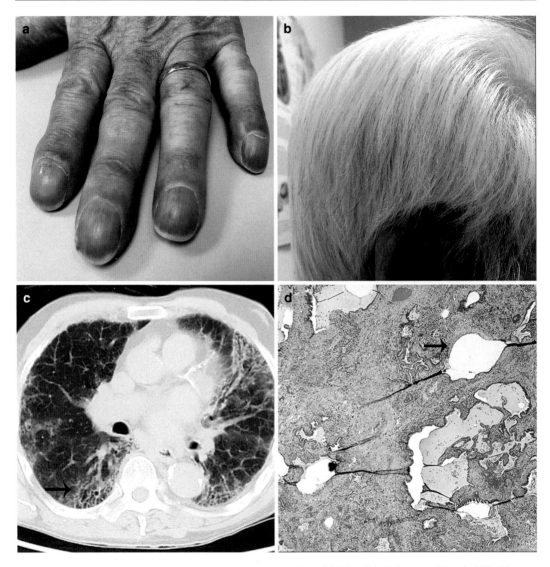

Fig. 6.1 Clinical findings of patients with pulmonary fibrosis. (**a**) Patients with pulmonary fibrosis often present with digital clubbing, as pictured here. This finding is not specific to pulmonary fibrosis and can be seen in other heart and lung diseases. (**b**) Early graying of the hair is often reported in patients with familial forms of pulmonary fibrosis. This patient with familial pulmonary fibrosis had white hair by the time he was early in the fourth decade of life but did not present with pulmonary fibrosis until his seventh decade. (**c**) Axial image from a CT scan of the chest of a patient with Idiopathic Pulmonary Fibrosis (IPF), illustrating some characteristic findings, including peripheral and basilar predominant reticular abnormality, traction bronchiectasis, and honeycombing (arrow). (*Courtesy of Dr. Christopher J.G. Sigakis, Radiology Partners, Dallas, Texas, USA.*) (**d**) High power image of histopathology from a patient with familial pulmonary fibrosis illustrating significant collagen deposition (pink, acellular areas) and characteristic honeycomb change (arrow)

despite treatment for infection and work-up for non-pulmonary causes of exercise limitation. Often, until a careful physical exam is performed revealing inspiratory crackles, or a chest X-ray is performed revealing interstitial abnormalities, the cause of patients' symptoms remains a mystery.

Chest X-ray findings are themselves nonspecific. In patients presenting with a significant burden of disease, radiographs will reveal evidence of volume loss and interstitial abnormalities. These findings often prompt the use of computed tomography (CT) to further characterize the patients' lungs. High resolution computed tomography (HRCT) of the chest is the ideal modality with which to image the chest of patients with Interstitial Lung Diseases (ILDs) like IPF. Classic HRCT findings include peripheral and basilar predominant reticular abnormality with traction bronchiectasis and honeycombing [1] (Fig. 6.1c). Pulmonary function testing pursued to characterize a patient's disease will show decreased total lung capacity (TLC) and residual volume (RV), often with decreased diffusing capacity of the lungs for carbon monoxide (DLCO), indicating a loss in lung volume and a gas exchange impairment.

Clinical Evaluation, Diagnosis, and Treatment of IPF

Diffuse parenchymal lung diseases, also known as interstitial lung diseases (ILDs), are a diverse set of more than 200 parenchymal lung diseases, many of which are rare [2]. The ILDs can present with varied radiologic and clinical findings and have varying etiologies, from autoimmune diseases to environmental exposures, and some of them lead to irreversible scarring of the lung parenchyma known as pulmonary fibrosis. A subset of ILDs have no identifiable cause and are frequently termed idiopathic interstitial pneumonias (IIPs). IPF is the most widely studied and most common IIP and ILD [2]. As a result, many of the breakthroughs in terms of genetic risk and novel therapeutic approaches in ILD have focused on IPF cohorts. Furthermore, the diagnosis of IPF has specific therapeutic implications as currently available anti-fibrotic therapies have been studied and approved for IPF patients, but not for patients with other fibrosing IIPs [3–5].

Therefore, distinguishing IPF from other ILDs is a primary step in the evaluation of a patient presenting with the appropriate radiologic and clinical findings. Radiologic findings on HRCT consistent with the Usual Interstitial Pneumonia (UIP) pattern (i.e., honeycombing, traction bronchiectasis, and peripheral and basilar predominant reticular abnormality with a paucity of ground glass abnormality) are required for an HRCT-based diagnosis of IPF [6] (Fig. 6.1c). When radiologic findings are not specific enough to make this diagnosis, in the appropriate clinical context, lung

biopsy is often pursued. Histopathologic findings of the UIP pattern (i.e., fibroblastic foci, microscopic honeycombing, and a relative paucity of cellular infiltrate) would be consistent with a diagnosis of IPF (Fig. 6.1d). However, ultimately, IPF is a diagnosis of exclusion: Because other conditions can also present with UIP pattern on HRCT or pathology, rheumatologic diseases and environmental/occupational exposures must be ruled out before a diagnosis of IPF can be made [3, 6, 7]. Because there is no simple blood test for the disease, ILD diagnoses, including IPF, are best made in the setting of an experienced center with multidisciplinary conferences where experts in pulmonary medicine, radiology, and pathology discuss individual cases and come to consensus [3, 6–9].

Despite recent advances in approved medical therapies, the prognosis for IPF remains poor. Prior epidemiological studies suggest that the median survival after diagnosis is 3–5 years [10, 11]. Antifibrotic medical therapies (i.e., nintedanib and pirfenidone) that slow the rate of progression of fibrotic change in the lungs now exist, but none are able to reverse existing changes [4, 5]. Additionally, although pooled data from clinical studies suggests that existing therapies have an overall mortality effect, if it does indeed exist, it is small [12, 13]. The differentiation of IPF from other ILDs is critical because in the case of other ILDs, especially those related to systemic autoimmune disorders, immunosuppression is indicated; however, in the case of IPF, analyses of large clinical trial data suggest that immunosuppression is harmful and should be avoided [14]. Lung transplantation remains the only curative therapy for end-stage ILD, including IPF; however, lung transplantation is not available to many patients diagnosed with IPF, and it can itself be a major cause or morbidity and mortality, with a median survival of 5.8 years [15].

Rare Genetic Variants Associated with IPF

Surfactant Proteins

Decades ago, it was observed that cases of pulmonary fibrosis appeared to cluster in families, a clue that there was inherited risk in this disease. As others would argue, one of the most important risk factors for the development of IPF is a family history of pulmonary fibrosis [16]. Studies performed in Europe indicated that familial pulmonary fibrosis accounted for 2–4% of IPF cases [17, 18]. In later years, investigators published data from cohorts suggesting a higher percentage of familial cases [19, 20]. Although familial pulmonary fibrosis cases tended to present younger than their sporadic counterparts, and some cohorts showed evidence of a heterogeneity of radiologic and pathologic findings [21–23], in almost all cases the clinical presentation of familial IPF was indistinguishable from nonfamilial or sporadic presentation of IPF [18, 24].

Geneticists took advantage of familial clusters of pulmonary fibrosis cases to study IPF by utilizing a candidate gene approach. An early hypothesis was that abnormalities in genes encoding surfactant proteins, specifically Surfactant Protein C (*SFTPC*), would be associated with IPF because surfactant proteins, which are expressed in the alveoli by Type 2 alveolar cells and prevent alveolar collapse, are critical to normal pulmonary physiology. In 2001, Nogee and colleagues utilized samples from an infant with a diagnosis of ILD at 1 year of age, as well as samples from multiple family members with respiratory deficiencies, and sequenced *SFTPC* [22]. The investigators identified a coding mutation in *SFTPC* that segregated in an autosomal dominant fashion with disease, as well as decreased surfactant levels in the affected patient's lungs [22]. Numerous subsequent studies identified additional coding and noncoding mutations in *SFTPC* and rare coding mutations in *SFTPA* associated with pulmonary fibrosis in adults [25–28] and with pediatric interstitial lung diseases [29–32] (Fig. 6.2c, d). Other surfactant-related proteins implicated in pulmonary fibrosis risk and pathogenesis include ATP-binding cassette transporter A3 (*ABCA3*), whose mutations have been found in small familial studies to be associated with pediatric disease, though none have linked the gene to adult IPF [33–35].

The mechanism through which surfactant protein mutations may be related to pulmonary fibrosis is aberrant intracellular processing of abnormal pro-proteins [36, 37]. Some *SFTPC* mutations lead to the production of precursor proteins that cannot be processed by the endoplasmic reticulum of the Type 2 alveolar cell, leading to endoplasmic reticulum (ER) stress, cellular injury, and apoptosis [38–40].

Telomerase Pathway Genes

Chromosomes are capped on either end by regions of repetitive noncoding nucleotide repeat segments known as telomeres, which protect coding regions of the chromosomes from deterioration during mitosis. Telomeres are added to chromosomes by the telomerase complex, a group of proteins and RNA sequence, that includes the telomerase reverse transcriptase (*TERT*) and an RNA component (*TERC*). Shortened telomeres are associated with a variety of clinical manifestations, including hematologic abnormalities, liver dysfunction, and pulmonary fibrosis; subjects with numerous affected organ systems are referred to as having "telomeropathies" [41].

Telomerase-pathway genes were recognized as important in pulmonary fibrosis through the study of dyskeratosis congenita (DKC), a syndrome characterized by abnormal skin pigmentation, nail dystrophy, and oral leukoplakia, but which can also affect other organ systems such as bone marrow, and cause pulmonary fibrosis [42]. While X-linked versions of the disease are linked to *DKC1* mutations [43], other forms of disease are linked to mutations in *TERT* and *TERC* [42, 44–46]. Given this mutation–phenotype association, candidate gene studies examining *TERT* and *TERC* were pursued.

An analysis of 73 familial interstitial pneumonia (FIP) families (defined as those in which there were two more cases of IIP) identified coding mutations in *TERT* and *TERC* that were associated with members affected by pulmonary fibrosis, and further analysis revealed both decreased telomerase activity and shortened telomeres in those carrying the mutations [47]. Tsakiri and colleagues reported similar findings in a distinct FIP cohort, for which linkage analysis identified a region of interest on chromosome 5 containing

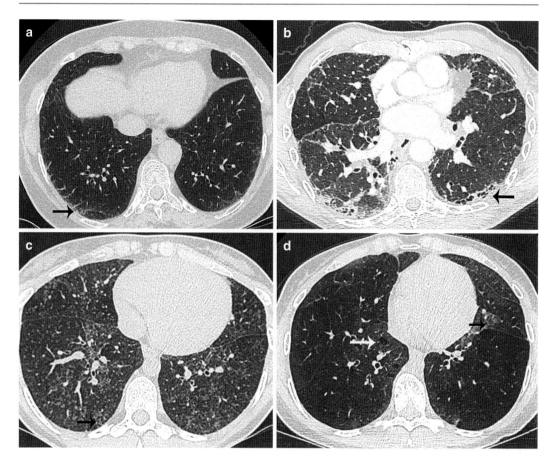

Fig. 6.2 Imaging findings in familial pulmonary fibrosis. (**a**) Axial image from a CT scan of the chest from a patient with subtle reticular abnormality (arrow). This patient was from a family carrying a *TERT* mutation. (**b**) Image of CT scan of the chest from a patient with more advanced fibrotic change, including honeycombing (arrow). This patient also carried a *TERT* mutation. (**c**) This image illustrates a ground glass abnormality and tree-in-bud abnormality (arrow) seen in a patient with a surfactant protein A (*SFPTA1*) mutation. (**d**) This CT image illustrates radiologic changes of ground glass abnormality (black arrow) and pulmonary cysts (white arrow) in a patient who carried an *NKX2-1* gene mutation. (*Images courtesy of Dr. Raphael Borie, Hôpital Bichat – Claude-Bernard (Hôpitaux Universitaires Paris Nord Val de Seine, Paris, France)*)

TERT [48]. Subsequent sequencing of this gene in these families revealed missense and frameshift mutations in two families. Follow-up analysis of 44 additional FIP families identified more *TERT* and *TERC* mutations, and mutation carriers again showed decreased telomerase activity and shortened telomeres [48]. These initial findings suggested that *TERT* or *TERC* mutations may be responsible for up to 10% of FIP cases (Fig. 6.2).

The disease-associated coding mutations in telomerase genes led investigators to question whether telomere length itself was a risk factor for IPF. Subjects with FIP and IPF were recruited, and it was found that regardless of *TERT* or *TERC* mutation status, about one-quarter of those with FIP or IPF had evidence of telomere shortening [47, 49]. Indeed, in a study by Adler and colleagues that examined 100 cases of sporadic IPF, none of the subjects had *TERT* mutations, one had a *TERC* mutation, but the majority of them had telomere lengths shorter than the median in age-matched healthy controls [50]. Additionally, the authors examined type 2 alveolar cells from diseased lung tissue and, using in situ hybridization, determined that telomeres were shorter in those with disease [50].

More recent studies have utilized newer technologies, such as exome sequencing, to find rare variants in other telomere-related genes. Regulator of telomere elongation helicase 1 (*RTEL1*) and poly(A)-specific ribonuclease (*PARN*) are two genes in which exome-sequencing has led to rare-variant discovery [51–53]. As with *TERT* and *TERC* mutations, those with rare variants in *RTEL1* and *PARN* also showed evidence of shortened telomeres [51–53]. Exome sequencing also identified rare *TINF2*, *NAF1*, and novel *DKC1* mutations in FIP cohorts [54–56]. Interestingly, pulmonary fibrosis patients that have hepatic or bone marrow abnormalities are more likely than those without extrapulmonary involvement to have telomerase pathway mutations [57, 58] (Figs. 6.1 and 6.2).

The precise reason that short telomeres lead to the clinical finding of pulmonary fibrosis is not known; however, mouse model-based studies suggest that impaired telomerase function and short telomeres hamper the normal epithelial response to injury [50]. At this time, it is not known whether elongating telomeres would restore appropriate responses to lung injury.

Common Genetic Variants and IPF

Many of the rare variant studies described above utilized candidate-gene sequencing approaches. As genome-wide genotyping technologies evolved, genome-wide association studies (GWAS) of IPF were conducted to examine the role of common variants, often defined as those with a minor allele frequency (MAF) >0.05, in disease risk.

The first IPF GWAS in 2008 identified a common intronic *TERT* variant as a risk factor for IPF [59]. In 2011, a larger study was done utilizing a linkage analysis approach followed by fine mapping that identified a gain-of-function variant (rs35705950) in the promoter region of the Mucin 5B, Oligomeric Mucus/Gel-Forming (*MUC5B*) gene as a strong risk factor for both familial pulmonary fibrosis and sporadic IPF [60]. This was an unexpected finding in that there had been no reason prior to this study to suspect mucin abnormalities would be related to pulmonary fibrosis. *MUC5B* encodes for Mucin-5B, a major component of mucus in many mucosal surfaces including saliva, cervix and lung, and it is critical to the immune function of the lung [61] (Fig. 6.3). The rs35705950 variant is associated with increased *MUC5B* gene expression in the lungs of normal and IPF subjects [60, 62]; when IPF subjects were compared to controls, there was significantly higher *MUC5B* gene expression in IPF subjects regardless of genotype [60].

The *MUC5B* risk variant is common in non-Hispanic whites—approximately 19% of them will carry one or more copies of the risk allele (i.e., T) [60]. Those that were heterozygous (GT) and homozygous (TT) had increased odds ratios (ORs) for pulmonary fibrosis—6.8 (95% confidence interval [CI], 3.9–12.0) and 20.8 (95% CI, 3.8–113.7) for FIP, respectively, and 9.0 (95% CI, 6.2–13.1) and 21.8 (95% CI, 5.1–93.5) for IPF, respectively [60]. The rs35705950 minor allele frequency (MAF) was 0.338 in familial pulmonary fibrosis subjects and 0.375 in sporadic IPF groups, indicating that the risk allele was important in familial and sporadic cases [60]. The high frequency with which rs35705950

Fig. 6.3 Localization of Mucin-5B in human lung tissue. (**a**) 3,3′-Diaminobenzidine (DAB) staining for Mucin 5B (MUC5B) in human lung tissue from a patient with IPF shows strong staining (brown) for the protein in cells lining the airways as well as within the airways themselves (arrow). (**b**) Immunofluorescence (IF) for MUC5B (blue), club cell secretory protein (CCSP) (red), and surfactant protein C (SPC) (green) shows the locations of these proteins in normal human lung tissue. Areas where CCSP and MUC5B are co-expressed, predominantly in the airway epithelia, appear violet. (**c**) IF for MUC5B (blue), CCSP (red), and SPC (green) in fibrotic lung tissue from an IPF patient illustrates extensive MUC5B in the airway spaces as well as co-localization of CCSP and MUC5B in airway epithelia (violet). (*Images courtesy of Mr. Avram Walts, Dr. Yasushi Nakano, and Dr. Evgenia Dobrinskikh, University of Colorado School of Medicine, Aurora, Colorado, USA*)

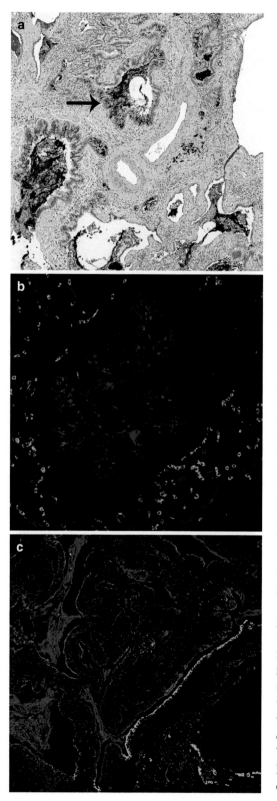

was found in a general non-Hispanic white population suggests that the *MUC5B* variant is neither necessary nor sufficient for the development of IPF—other genetic or nongenetic (e.g., environmental) factors are likely to be at play in determining an individual's disease risk [63].

The association of the *MUC5B* variant with IPF has been replicated numerous times in independent cohorts [60, 64–70], illustrating the strength and reproducibility of these findings. In addition, rs35705950 has been examined in cohorts with other forms of pulmonary fibrosis with differing results. Case–control studies of systemic sclerosis-ILD [64, 66], asbestosis, sarcoidosis [64], chronic obstructive pulmonary disease, and asthma have not shown significant associations between rs35705950 and disease [71]. However, recently, a study of two separate cohorts with chronic hypersensitivity pneumonitis (HP) revealed that rs35705950 was associated with this condition with MAFs similar to what has been described in IPF cohorts [72]. Also, a recent study of rheumatoid arthritis (RA)-related ILD revealed a strong association between rs35705950 and RA-ILD [73, 74]. Therefore, while the *MUC5B* promoter polymorphism is not associated with all forms of ILD or with other advanced lung diseases, it is associated with chronic HP and RA-ILD, two progressive fibrosing ILDs that share common histopathologic and radiologic patterns (i.e., UIP) with IPF [73]. Therefore, it may be the case that the *MUC5B* variant is associated with the UIP fibrosing response to lung injury itself—not just with what physicians have clinically diagnosed as IPF.

The mechanism through which the *MUC5B* promoter polymorphism causes pulmonary fibrosis is hypothesized to be related to impaired mucociliary clearance and subsequent aberrant response to recurrent injury (Fig. 6.3). Data to support this hypothesis was recently published with in vivo and in vitro experiments that illustrated decreased ciliary function in airway cells of *Muc5b*-overexpressing transgenic mice [75]. While the mice expressing excess *Muc5b* in their lungs did not develop spontaneous fibrosis, they exhibited greater fibrosis in response to a commonly utilized model of fibrotic lung injury: intratracheal bleomycin [75]. Use of a mucolytic agent in these mice was shown to ameliorate the fibrotic response to injury, suggesting that the mucus itself could be a target of antifibrotic therapy [75].

A GWAS study published in 2013, examining 1616 fibrotic ILDs versus 4683 controls, confirmed previously identified disease-associated loci (i.e., chromosome 5p15 containing *TERT*; 11p15 containing *MUC5B;* 3q25 near *TERC*), but also identified seven new risk loci, including *FAM13A* (4q22), *DSP* (6p24), *OBFC1* (10q24), *ATP11A* (13q4), *DPP9* (19p13), and regions on chromosomes 7q22 and 15q14–15 [76]. An imputation-based follow-up study also identified the HLA region as strongly associated with disease [77]. These loci and genes are varied in terms of their implicated pathways and biological functions. In general, they can be categorized roughly into host defense (*MUC5B, ATP11A, HLA*-region), cell–cell adhesion (*DSP, DPP9*), and DNA repair (*TERT, TERC, OBFC1*) [63, 76, 78, 79]. These loci, along with the *MUC5B* variant, may account for up to one-third of disease risk [76, 79].

A separate GWAS with similar study design confirmed the *MUC5B* association, but also identified loci in Toll-interacting protein (*TOLLIP*) and peptidase-like 2C (*SPPL2C*) as disease-associated variants [65]. Intriguingly, this manuscript not only described risk variants, but also presented evidence that specific variants (i.e., rs5743890) in *TOLLIP* were associated with differential mortality from disease [65, 80]. More recently, a GWAS performed in a European cohort confirmed *DSP* and *MUC5B* variants' associations with IPF and identified a novel common variant in *AKAP13* that was also associated with differential gene expression in lung tissue [70]. *AKAP13* is a particularly intriguing target for future investigation because it is known to be involved in profibrotic signaling processes, and it localizes to alveolar epithelial cells and lymphoid follicles in IPF patients [70].

Consistent with the association results of the *MUC5B* variant with IPF reported in 2011 [60], the ORs for loci identified by the 2013 GWAS by

Fingerlin and colleagues did not differ between FIP and sporadic IPF cases [76], suggesting that genetic risk factors for fibrotic IIPs, whether recognized as "familial" or not, are similar [63, 81]. The findings described thus far, summarized in Table 6.1, have focused on individual variants and their implications for disease risk, but have not considered the implications of having numerous common and/or rare risk variants. Future studies should examine the interactions between different disease-associated variants and determine the functional relationships between individual variants and disease phenotypes.

Genetic Variants and Clinical Management of IPF

The findings presented above regarding genetic risk and IPF have described potential therapeutic targets and hypotheses regarding disease pathogenesis, but the diversity of biological pathways implicated begs further questions: (1) Are there genetically determined IPF disease endotypes? (2) What are the clinical implications in terms of treatment and prognosis of having specific genetic risk variants? The clinical course of IPF has long been noted to be heterogeneous and unpredictable, yet relentlessly progressive, making these questions central to clinicians. Table 6.2 summarizes the associations of genetic variants with clinical outcomes in IPF described next.

Clinical Phenotypes

To address these critical questions in terms of the common *MUC5B* genetic variant most strongly associated with IPF, a retrospective analysis of clinical trials data was performed by Peljto and colleagues, who found that the *MUC5B* minor allele conferred increased survival [82]. The risk variant in the *TOLLIP* gene associated with IPF was also associated with mortality [65]. Clinical manifestations for pulmonary fibrosis patients with telomerase-pathway gene mutations are heterogeneous—indeed, many do not necessarily carry the clinical diagnosis of IPF, and have been noted to have other forms of fibrosing ILD, including pleuroparenchymal fibroelastosis, chronic HP, and connective tissue disease-related ILD [83]. Based on observational studies of large groups of mutation carriers, those with *TERC* mutations tended to be diagnosed at an earlier age relative to those with *TERT*, *RTEL1* or *PARN* mutations, and they were more likely to have hematologic abnormalities [83]. Additionally, the rate of decline in lung function (as measured by

Table 6.1 Genetic variants associated with IPF

Genes	Gene product functions	Common variants, rare variants, or both?	Type of studies	Key references
Surfactant-related genes				
SFTPC *SFTPA1* *NKX2-1* *ABCA3*	Lung surfactant and surfactant processing	Rare variants	Targeted sequencing, linkage analysis, targeted sequencing	Nogee et al. [22], Thomas et al. [95], Lawson et al. [26], Van Moorsel et al. [35], Ono et al. [96], Wang et al. [27], Hamvas et al. [97], Campo et al. [98], Epaud et al. [99]
Telomere-related genes				
TERT *TERC* *PARN* *RTEL1* *DKC1* *OBFC1*	DNA-repair and senescence	Both	Targeted sequencing, exome sequencing, and genome-wide association studies (GWAS)	de Leon et al. [100], Armanios et al. [44], Armanios et al. [47], Tsakiri et al. [48], Fingerlin et al. [76], Wei et al. [67], Stuart et al. [84], Cogan et al. [52], Kropski et al. [56]
Host defense-related genes				
MUC5B	Mucin	Common variant	Linkage analysis; GWAS	Seibold et al. [60], Zhang et al. [101], Stock et al. [64], Borie et al. [66], Noth et al. [65], Fingerlin et al. [76], Wei et al. [67], Horimasu et al. [68]
TOLLIP	Toll-interacting protein	Common variants	GWAS	Noth et al. [65]
ATP11A	ATPase	Common variant	GWAS	Fingerlin et al. [76]
Cell–cell adhesion				
DSP	Major component of desmosome	Common variant	GWAS	Fingerlin et al. [76], Mathai et al. [102], Allen et al. [70]
Protein cleavage				
DPP9	Serine protease	Common variant	GWAS	Fingerlin et al. [76]
SPPL2C	Intramembrane protease	Common variant	GWAS	Noth et al. [65]
Pro-fibrotic mediator				
AKAP13	RhoA guanine nucleotide exchange factor	Common variant	GWAS	Allen et al. [70]
Unknown function				
FAM13A	Unknown	Common variant	GWAS	Fingerlin et al. [76]
chromosomal region 7q22	Unknown	Common variant	GWAS	Fingerlin et al. [76]
Chromosomal region 15q14–15	Unknown	Common variant	GWAS	Fingerlin et al. [76]

Table 6.2 Genetic variants and markers associated with clinical outcomes in IPF

Genetic variant/ marker	Affected outcome	Key references
MUC5B promoter polymorphism genotype, rs35705950 (minor allele)	Improved survival	Peljto et al. [82]
TOLLIP genotype, rs5743890 (minor allele)	Increased mortality risk	Noth et al. [65]
TOLLIP genotype, rs3750920 (TT genotype)	Clinical response to oral N-acetylcysteine	Oldham et al. [80]
Telomerase-related rare variant	Poor prognosis	Newton et al. [83], Borie et al. [57]
Telomerase-related mutation	Post-transplant complications	Silhan et al. [89]
Telomere length	Transplant-free survival	Stuart et al. [84]
Telomere length	Post-transplant survival	Newton et al. [90]

absolute FVC) noted for telomerase-mutation carriers was higher than the rate of decline observed for IPF patients in general, suggesting that the prognosis for these patients may be poorer than for all-comers diagnosed with disease [83]. Additionally, telomere length, independent of age, sex, and baseline disease severity, was a predictor of transplant-free survival in IPF but not in non-IPF ILD, despite a low prevalence of actual *TERT* mutations in the subjects studied [84]. This finding underscores the evidence that telomerase dysfunction may be central to disease even in subjects with no identifiable coding mutation in telomerase-related genes.

Therapeutic Implications

Prospective clinical trials utilizing genotype-based stratification have not yet been performed in IPF; however, retrospective studies suggest that existing drugs have differential efficacy based on genotype. Retrospective analysis of the PANTHER-IPF trial indicated that patients in the N-acetylcysteine (NAC) treatment group with

TOLLIP rs3750920 TT genotype had increased survival versus those with other genotypes, while those with the CC genotype had worse outcomes [80]. While NAC has not been shown in all-comers with IPF to be an effective treatment [85], these observational findings suggest that therapies may have differential effects based on *TOLLIP* rs3750920 genotype. Recent retrospective analyses of patients with *TERT* and *TERC* mutations treated with pirfenidone suggested that the medication may not have affected the rate of decline in FVC among those with mutations, although the study is limited by its small sample size (given how rare these coding mutations are) and its retrospective design [86]. Currently, there are also limited data to suggest that the approved IPF-specific antifibrotic therapies nintedanib and pirfenidone have differential efficacy based on genotype or coding mutations in telomerase pathway genes. Clinical trials need to be designed and analyzed with these results in mind to determine whether more precise approaches increase clinical effectiveness of existing IPF drugs [79].

Due to the limited availability of medical therapies for IPF, many patients either undergo, or are at least evaluated for, lung transplantation. Post-lung transplantation care involves significant and indefinite immunosuppression that can have toxic effects on other organs, including the bone marrow. Given the extrapulmonary manifestations observed in telomerase-pathway mutation-carrying pulmonary fibrosis patients, cohorts of such patients have been examined for posttransplantation outcomes. Retrospective studies reviewing posttransplant survival in patients with telomerase mutations illustrate a higher incidence of posttransplant complications, driven primarily by hematologic abnormalities and bone marrow dysfunction [87], as well as renal dysfunction and lower respiratory tract infections [88], with telomerase-pathway mutation carriers compared to historic controls [87, 89]. These complications frequently require adjustments to immunosuppressive regimens for posttransplant patients; however, telomerase mutations are not at this time considered a contraindication to lung transplantation [88]. A more recent study of telomere length in posttransplant patients also argues that telomere shortening may be a marker of poor survival and decreased time to lung allograft dysfunction, a poor clinical outcome [90]. Interestingly, though the patients with < 10th percentile telomere length had higher rates of primary graft dysfunction, they did not show higher rates of acute rejection, cytopenias, infection, or renal dysfunction [90].

Our poor ability to prognosticate for our patients diagnosed with a progressive but unpredictable disease, and to know which antifibrotic medication might be better for any given patient, limits our ability to personalize care. Furthermore, at this time, genotyping, especially for common variants, is not part of routine clinical care. The above findings suggest that as genotype information becomes increasingly incorporated into clinical trials and clinical outcomes research, bedside care could be transformed in IPF, allowing clinicians to use genotypes as biomarkers to better understand patient phenotype and to tailor therapeutic choices to the individual [91].

Early Detection of Pulmonary Fibrosis

The fact that there are no existing therapies that reverse established pulmonary fibrosis makes the area of early disease detection an urgent clinically relevant one, particularly because patients are often diagnosed late in the course of their disease, after having been symptomatic for a long period of time. Review of imaging from large cohorts, such as the Framingham Heart Study, have provided evidence that early interstitial abnormalities (ILAs) are common [92]. Specifically, Hunninghake and colleagues found evidence of ILAs in 7% of subjects over 50 years of age without any known ILD, while definitive fibrosis was noted in nearly 2% of all those screened [92], rates higher than had been observed in other studies [79, 92]. Critically, ILAs have been shown in numerous cohorts to progress radiologically in the majority of cases and to be associated with increased all-cause mortality and respiratory-disease-related mortality [93, 94]. In addition, the IPF-associated

MUC5B promoter polymorphism has been associated with ILAs, raising the possibility that common genetic variants could be utilized to counsel patients or to risk-stratify individuals for potential radiologic or other clinical screening [79, 91, 92].

Conclusion

The rapid growth in the field of IPF genetics and the development of novel antifibrotic therapies over the past few decades has led to a sea change in the field. Where once the etiology and prognosis of IPF remained mysterious, and patients were told that they had no real options for effective medical therapies, we are now beginning to appreciate the profound clinical heterogeneity of IPF and can offer patients evidence-based medical therapies. Genetic factors play at least some role in the clinically observed heterogeneity of IPF, and further study will allow us to move known associations and observations into data that can inform shared decision-making with patients. Furthermore, the variety of biological pathways implicated by the genetics of IPF, including pathways related to surfactants, mucus, mucociliary function, and telomere maintenance, raise the possibility that distinct genotypes require specific treatments. Though there are hints of these treatment implications in the literature, prospective clinical trials are required to inform our clinical practice.

Acknowledgments The authors would like to thank Dr. Raphael Borie, Dr. Christopher J.G. Sigakis, Mr. Avram Walts, Dr. Yasushi Nakano, and Dr. Evgenia Dobrinskikh for their assistance in preparing figures for this manuscript.

References

1. Lynch DA, Sverzellati N, Travis WD, Brown KK, Colby TV, Galvin JR, et al. Diagnostic criteria for idiopathic pulmonary fibrosis: a Fleischner Society White Paper. Lancet Respir Med. 2017;6(2):138–53.
2. Cottin V, Hirani NA, Hotchkin DL, Nambiar AM, Ogura T, Otaola M, et al. Presentation, diagnosis and clinical course of the spectrum of progressive-

fibrosing interstitial lung diseases. Eur Respir Rev. 2018;27(150):180076.

3. Raghu G, Remy-Jardin M, Myers JL, Richeldi L, Ryerson CJ, Lederer DJ, et al. Diagnosis of idiopathic pulmonary fibrosis an official ATS/ERS/JRS/ALAT clinical practice guideline. Am J Respir Crit Care Med. 2018;198(5):e44–68.

4. Richeldi L, du Bois RM, Raghu G, Azuma A, Brown KK, Costabel U, et al. Efficacy and safety of nintedanib in idiopathic pulmonary fibrosis. N Engl J Med. 2014;370(22):2071–82.

5. King TE, Bradford WZ, Castro-Bernardini S, Fagan EA, Glaspole I, Glassberg MK, et al. A phase 3 trial of pirfenidone in patients with idiopathic pulmonary fibrosis. N Engl J Med. 2014;370(22):2083–92.

6. Lynch DA, Sverzellati N, Travis WD, Brown KK, Colby TV, Galvin JR, et al. Diagnostic criteria for idiopathic pulmonary fibrosis: a Fleischner Society White Paper. Lancet Respir Med. 2018;6(2):138–53.

7. Castillo D, Walsh S, Hansell DM, Vasakova M, Cottin V, Altinisik G, et al. Validation of multidisciplinary diagnosis in IPF. Lancet Respir Med. 2018;6(2):88–9.

8. Walsh SLF, Maher TM, Kolb M, Poletti V, Nusser R, Richeldi L, et al. Diagnostic accuracy of a clinical diagnosis of idiopathic pulmonary fibrosis: an international case-cohort study. Eur Respir J. 2017;50(2):1700936.

9. Wells AU. Any fool can make a rule and any fool will mind it. BMC Med. 2016;14(1):23.

10. Ley B, Collard HR, King TE. Clinical course and prediction of survival in idiopathic pulmonary fibrosis. Am J Respir Crit Care Med. 2011;183(4):431–40.

11. Ley B, Collard HR. Epidemiology of idiopathic pulmonary fibrosis. Clin Epidemiol. 2013;5:483–92.

12. Richeldi L, Cottin V, du Bois RM, Selman M, Kimura T, Bailes Z, et al. Nintedanib in patients with idiopathic pulmonary fibrosis: combined evidence from the TOMORROW and INPULSIS®trials. Respir Med. 2016;113:74–9.

13. Nathan SD, Albera C, Bradford WZ, Costabel U, Glaspole I, Glassberg MK, et al. Effect of pirfenidone on mortality: pooled analyses and meta-analyses of clinical trials in idiopathic pulmonary fibrosis. Lancet Respir Med. 2017;5(1):33–41.

14. Raghu G, Anstrom KJ, King TE, Lasky JA, Martinez FJ. Prednisone, azathioprine, and N-acetylcysteine for pulmonary fibrosis. N Engl J Med. 2012;366(21):1968–77.

15. Thabut G, Mal H. Outcomes after lung transplantation. J Thorac Dis. 2017;9(8):2684–91.

16. García-Sancho C, Buendía-Roldán I, Fernández-Plata MR, Navarro C, Pérez-Padilla R, Vargas MH, et al. Familial pulmonary fibrosis is the strongest risk factor for idiopathic pulmonary fibrosis. Respir Med. 2011;105(12):1902–7.

17. Hodgson U, Laitinen T, Tukiainen P. Nationwide prevalence of sporadic and familial idiopathic pulmonary fibrosis: evidence of founder effect among multiplex families in Finland. Thorax. 2002;57(4):338–42.

18. Marshall RP, Puddicombe A, Cookson WO, Laurent GJ. Adult familial cryptogenic fibrosing alveolitis in the United Kingdom. Thorax. 2000;55(2):143–6.

19. Lawson WE, Loyd JE. The genetic approach in pulmonary fibrosis: can it provide clues to this complex disease? Proc Am Thorac Soc. 2006;3(4):345–9.

20. Loyd JE. Pulmonary fibrosis in families. Am J Respir Cell Mol Biol. 2003;29(3 Suppl):S47–50.

21. Steele MP, Speer MC, Loyd JE, Brown KK, Herron A, Slifer SH, et al. Clinical and pathologic features of familial interstitial pneumonia. Am J Respir Crit Care Med. 2005;172(9):1146–52.

22. Nogee LM, Dunbar AE, Wert SE, Askin F, Hamvas A, Whitsett JA. A mutation in the surfactant protein C gene associated with familial interstitial lung disease. N Engl J Med. 2001;344(8):573–9.

23. Kropski JA, Pritchett JM, Zoz DF, Crossno PF, Markin C, Garnett ET, et al. Extensive phenotyping of individuals at risk for familial interstitial pneumonia reveals clues to the pathogenesis of interstitial lung disease. Am J Respir Crit Care Med. 2015;191(4):417–26.

24. Lee H-L, Ryu JH, Wittmer MH, Hartman TE, Lymp JF, Tazelaar HD, et al. Familial idiopathic pulmonary fibrosis: clinical features and outcome. Chest. 2005;127(6):2034–41.

25. Fernandez BA, Fox G, Bhatia R, Sala E, Noble B, Denic N, et al. A Newfoundland cohort of familial and sporadic idiopathic pulmonary fibrosis patients: clinical and genetic features. Respir Res. 2012;13(1):64.

26. Lawson WE, Grant SW, Ambrosini V, Womble KE, Dawson EP, Lane KB, et al. Genetic mutations in surfactant protein C are a rare cause of sporadic cases of IPF. Thorax. 2004;59(11):977–80.

27. Wang Y, Kuan PJ, Xing C, Cronkhite JT, Torres F, Rosenblatt RL, et al. Genetic defects in surfactant protein A2 are associated with pulmonary fibrosis and lung cancer. Am J Hum Genet. 2009;84(1):52–9.

28. Maitra M, Wang Y, Gerard RD, Mendelson CR, Garcia CK. Surfactant protein A2 mutations associated with pulmonary fibrosis lead to protein instability and endoplasmic reticulum stress. J Biol Chem. 2010;285(29):22103–13.

29. Hamvas A, Nogee LM, White FV, Schuler P, Hackett BP, Huddleston CB, et al. Progressive lung disease and surfactant dysfunction with a deletion in surfactant protein C gene. Am J Respir Cell Mol Biol. 2004;30(6):771–6.

30. Nogee LM, Dunbar AE, Wert S, Askin F, Hamvas A, Whitsett JA. Mutations in the surfactant protein C gene associated with interstitial lung disease. Chest. 2002;121(3 Suppl):20S–1S.

31. Tredano M, Griese M, Brasch F, Schumacher S, de Blic J, Marque S, et al. Mutation of SFTPC in infantile pulmonary alveolar proteinosis with or without fibrosing lung disease. Am J Med Genet A. 2004;126A(1):18–26.

32. Cameron HS, Somaschini M, Carrera P, Hamvas A, Whitsett JA, Wert SE, et al. A common mutation in the surfactant protein C gene associated with lung disease. J Pediatr. 2005;146(3):370–5.

33. Shulenin S, Nogee LM, Annilo T, Wert SE, Whitsett JA, Dean M. ABCA3 gene mutations in newborns with fatal surfactant deficiency. N Engl J Med. 2004;350(13):1296–303.

34. Young LR, Nogee LM, Barnett B, Panos RJ, Colby TV, Deutsch GH. Usual interstitial pneumonia in an adolescent with ABCA3 mutations. Chest. 2008;134(1):192–5.

35. Van Moorsel CHM, Van Oosterhout MFM, Barlo NP, De Jong PA, Van Der Vis JJ, Ruven HJT, et al. Surfactant protein C mutations are the basis of a significant portion of adult familial pulmonary fibrosis in a dutch cohort. Am J Respir Crit Care Med. 2010;182(11):1419–25.

36. Beers MF, Mulugeta S. Surfactant protein C biosynthesis and its emerging role in conformational lung disease. Annu Rev Physiol. 2005;67:663–96.

37. Whitsett JA, Weaver TE. Hydrophobic surfactant proteins in lung function and disease. N Engl J Med. 2002;347(26):2141–8.

38. Bridges JP, Wert SE, Nogee LM, Weaver TE. Expression of a human surfactant protein C mutation associated with interstitial lung disease disrupts lung development in transgenic mice. J Biol Chem. 2003;278(52):52739–46.

39. Mulugeta S, Nguyen V, Russo SJ, Muniswamy M, Beers MF. A surfactant protein C precursor protein BRICHOS domain mutation causes endoplasmic reticulum stress, proteasome dysfunction, and caspase 3 activation. Am J Respir Cell Mol Biol. 2005;32(6):521–30.

40. Mulugeta S, Maguire JA, Newitt JL, Russo SJ, Kotorashvili A, Beers MF. Misfolded BRICHOS SP-C mutant proteins induce apoptosis via caspase-4- and cytochrome c-related mechanisms. Am J Physiol Lung Cell Mol Physiol. 2007;293(3):L720–9.

41. Armanios M, Blackburn EH. The telomere syndromes. Nat Rev Genet. 2012;13(10):693–704.

42. Vulliamy T, Dokal I. Dyskeratosis congenita. Semin Hematol. 2006;43(3):157–66.

43. Knight SW, Vulliamy TJ, Heiss NS, Matthijs G, Devriendt K, Connor JM, et al. 1.4 Mb candidate gene region for X linked dyskeratosis congenita defined by combined haplotype and X chromosome inactivation analysis. J Med Genet. 1998;35(12):993–6.

44. Armanios M, Chen J-L, Chang Y-PC, Brodsky RA, Hawkins A, Griffin CA, et al. Haploinsufficiency of telomerase reverse transcriptase leads to anticipation in autosomal dominant dyskeratosis congenita. Proc Natl Acad Sci U S A. 2005;102(44):15960–4.

45. Vulliamy TJ, Marrone A, Knight SW, Walne A, Mason PJ, Dokal I. Mutations in dyskeratosis congenita : their impact on telomere length and the diversity of clinical presentation. Blood. 2006;107(7):2680–5.

46. Vulliamy T, Marrone A, Szydlo R, Walne A, Mason PJ, Dokal I. Disease anticipation is associated with progressive telomere shortening in families with dyskeratosis congenita due to mutations in TERC. Nat Genet. 2004;36(5):447–9.

47. Armanios MY, Chen JJ-L, Cogan JD, Alder JK, Ingersoll RG, Markin C, et al. Telomerase mutations in families with idiopathic pulmonary fibrosis. N Engl J Med. 2007;356(13):1317–26.

48. Tsakiri KD, Cronkhite JT, Kuan PJ, Xing C, Raghu G, Weissler JC, et al. Adult-onset pulmonary fibrosis caused by mutations in telomerase. Proc Natl Acad Sci U S A. 2007;104(18):7552–7.

49. Cronkhite J, Xing C, Raghu G. Telomere shortening in familial and sporadic pulmonary fibrosis. Am J Respir Crit Care Med. 2008;178(7):729–37.

50. Alder JK, Barkauskas CE, Limjunyawong N, Stanley SE, Kembou F, Tuder RM, et al. Telomere dysfunction causes alveolar stem cell failure. Proc Natl Acad Sci. 2015;112(16):201504780.

51. Stuart BD, Choi J, Zaidi S, Xing C, Holohan B, Chen R, et al. Exome sequencing links mutations in PARN and RTEL1 with familial pulmonary fibrosis and telomere shortening. Nat Genet. 2015;47(5):512–7.

52. Cogan JD, Kropski JA, Zhao M, Mitchell DB, Rives L, Markin C, et al. Rare variants in RTEL1 are associated with familial interstitial pneumonia. Am J Respir Crit Care Med. 2015;191(6):646–55.

53. Kannengiesser C, Borie R, Menard C, Reocreux M, Nitschke P, Gazal S, et al. Heterozygous RTEL1 mutations are associated with familial pulmonary fibrosis. Eur Respir J. 2015;46(249816): 474–85.

54. Alder JK, Stanley SE, Wagner CL, Hamilton M, Hanumanthu VS, Armanios M. Exome sequencing identifi es mutant TINF2 in a family with pulmonary fibrosis. Chest. 2015;147(5):1361–8.

55. Stanley SE, Gable DL, Wagner CL, Carlile TM, Hanumanthu VS, Podlevsky JD, et al. Loss-of-function mutations in the RNA biogenesis factor NAF1 predispose to pulmonary fibrosis-emphysema. Sci Transl Med. 2016;8(351):351ra107.

56. Kropski JA, Mitchell DB, Markin C, Polosukhin VV, Choi L, Johnson JE, et al. A novel dyskerin (DKC1) mutation is associated with familial interstitial pneumonia. Chest. 2014;146(1):e1–7.

57. Borie R, Tabèze L, Thabut G, Nunes H, Cottin V, Marchand-Adam S, et al. Prevalence and characteristics of TERT and TERC mutations in suspected genetic pulmonary fibrosis. Eur Respir J. 2016;48(6):1721–31.

58. Parry EM, Alder JK, Qi X, Chen JJ-L, Armanios M. Syndrome complex of bone marrow failure and pulmonary fibrosis predicts germline defects in telomerase. Blood. 2011;117(21):5607–11.

59. Mushiroda T, Wattanapokayakit S, Takahashi A, Nukiwa T, Kudoh S, Ogura T, et al. A genome-wide association study identifies an association of a common variant in TERT with susceptibility

to idiopathic pulmonary fibrosis. J Med Genet. 2008;45(10):654–6.

60. Seibold MA, Wise AAL, Speer MCM, Steel MP, Brown KKK, Loyd JE, et al. A common MUC5B promoter polymorphism and pulmonary fibrosis. N Engl J Med. 2011;364(16):1503–12.

61. Roy MG, Livraghi-Butrico A, Fletcher AA, McElwee MM, Evans SE, Boerner RM, et al. Muc5b is required for airway defence. Nature. 2014;505(7483):412–6.

62. Helling BA, Gerber AN, Kadiyala V, Sasse SK, Pedersen BS, Sparks L, et al. Regulation of MUC5B expression in idiopathic pulmonary fibrosis. Am J Respir Cell Mol Biol. 2017;57(1):91–9.

63. Mathai SK, Schwartz DA, Warg LA. Genetic susceptibility and pulmonary fibrosis. Curr Opin Pulm Med. 2014;20(5):429.

64. Stock CJ, Sato H, Fonseca C, Banya WA, Molyneaux PL, Adamali H, et al. Mucin 5B promoter polymorphism is associated with idiopathic pulmonary fibrosis but not with development of lung fibrosis in systemic sclerosis or sarcoidosis. Thorax. 2013;68(5):436–41.

65. Noth I, Zhang Y, Ma S-F, Flores C, Barber M, Huang Y, et al. Genetic variants associated with idiopathic pulmonary fibrosis susceptibility and mortality: a genome-wide association study. Lancet Respir Med. 2013;1(4):309–17.

66. Borie R, Crestani B, Dieude P, Nunes H, Allanore Y, Kannengiesser C, et al. The MUC5B variant is associated with idiopathic pulmonary fibrosis but not with systemic sclerosis interstitial lung disease in the European Caucasian population. PLoS One. 2013;8(8):e70621.

67. Wei R, Li C, Zhang M, Jones-Hall YL, Myers JL, Noth I, et al. Association between MUC5B and TERT polymorphisms and different interstitial lung disease phenotypes. Transl Res. 2014;163(5):494–502.

68. Horimasu Y, Ohshimo S, Bonella F, Tanaka S, Ishikawa N, Hattori N, et al. MUC5B promoter polymorphism in Japanese patients with idiopathic pulmonary fibrosis. Respirology. 2015;20(3):439–44.

69. Peljto AL, Selman M, Kim DS, Murphy E, Tucker L, Pardo A, et al. The MUC5B promoter polymorphism is associated with idiopathic pulmonary fibrosis in a Mexican cohort but is rare among Asian ancestries. Chest. 2015;147(2):460–4.

70. Allen RJ, Porte J, Braybrooke R, Flores C, Fingerlin TE, Oldham JM, et al. Genetic variants associated with susceptibility to idiopathic pulmonary fibrosis in people of European ancestry: a genome-wide association study. Lancet Respir Med. 2017;5(11):869–80.

71. Yang IV, Schwartz DA. Epigenetics of idiopathic pulmonary fibrosis. Transl Res. 2015;165(1):48–60.

72. Ley B, Newton CA, Arnould I, Elicker BM, Henry TS, Vittinghoff E, et al. The MUC5B promoter polymorphism and telomere length in patients with chronic hypersensitivity pneumonitis: an obser-

vational cohort-control study. Lancet Respir Med. 2017;5(8):639–47.

73. Juge P-A, Lee JS, Ebstein E, Furukawa H, Dobrinskikh E, Gazal S, et al. MUC5B promoter variant and rheumatoid arthritis with interstitial lung disease. N Engl J Med. 2018;379:2209.

74. Juge P-A, Borie R, Kannengiesser C, Gazal S, Revy P, Wemeau-Stervinou L, et al. Shared genetic predisposition in rheumatoid arthritis-interstitial lung disease and familial pulmonary fibrosis. Eur Respir J. 2017;49(5):1602314.

75. Hancock LA, Hennessy CE, Solomon GM, Dobrinskikh E, Estrella A, Hara N, et al. Muc5b overexpression causes mucociliary dysfunction and enhances lung fibrosis in mice. Nat Commun. 2018;9(1):5363.

76. Fingerlin TE, Murphy E, Zhang W, Peljto AL, Brown KK, Steele MP, et al. Genome-wide association study identifies multiple susceptibility loci for pulmonary fibrosis. Nat Genet. 2013;45(6):613–20.

77. Fingerlin TE, Zhang W, Yang IV, Ainsworth HC, Russell PH, Blumhagen RZ, et al. Genome-wide imputation study identifies novel HLA locus for pulmonary fibrosis and potential role for autoimmunity in fibrotic idiopathic interstitial pneumonia. BMC Genet. 2016;17(1):74.

78. Yang IV, Fingerlin TE, Evans CM, Schwarz MI, Schwartz DA. MUC5B and idiopathic pulmonary fibrosis. Ann Am Thorac Soc. 2015;12(Suppl 2):S193–9.

79. Mathai SK, Yang IV, Schwarz MI, Schwartz DA. Incorporating genetics into the identification and treatment of idiopathic pulmonary fibrosis. BMC Med. 2015;13(1):191.

80. Oldham JM, Ma SF, Martinez FJ, Anstrom KJ, Raghu G, Schwartz DA, et al. TOLLIP, MUC5B, and the response to N-acetylcysteine among individuals with idiopathic pulmonary fibrosis. Am J Respir Crit Care Med. 2015;192(12):1475–82.

81. Mathai SK, Schwartz DA. Taking the "I" out of IPF. Eur Respir J. 2015;45(6):1539.

82. Peljto AL, Zhang Y, Fingerlin TE, Ma SF, Garcia JG, Richards TJ, et al. Association between the MUC5B promoter polymorphism and survival in patients with idiopathic pulmonary fibrosis. JAMA. 2013;309(21):2232–9.

83. Newton CA, Batra K, Torrealba J, Kozlitina J, Glazer CS, Aravena C, et al. Telomere-related lung fibrosis is diagnostically heterogeneous but uniformly progressive. Eur Respir J. 2016;48(6):1710–20.

84. Stuart BD, Lee JS, Kozlitina J, Noth I, Devine MS, Glazer CS, et al. Effect of telomere length on survival in patients with idiopathic pulmonary fibrosis: an observational cohort study with independent validation. Lancet Respir Med. 2014;2(7):557–65.

85. Idiopathic Pulmonary Fibrosis Clinical Research Network, Martinez FJ, de Andrade JA, Anstrom KJ, King TE, Raghu G. Randomized trial of acetylcyste-

ine in idiopathic pulmonary fibrosis. N Engl J Med. 2014;370(22):2093–101.

86. Justet A, Thabut G, Manali E, Molina Molina M, Kannengiesser C, Cadranel J, et al. Safety and efficacy of pirfenidone in patients carrying telomerase complex mutation. Eur Respir J. 2018;51(3): 1701875.

87. Borie R, Kannengiesser C, Hirschi S, Le Pavec J, Mal H, Bergot E, et al. Severe hematologic complications after lung transplantation in patients with telomerase complex mutations. J Heart Lung Transplant. 2015;34(4):538–46.

88. Tokman S, Singer JP, Devine MS, Westall GP, Aubert JD, Tamm M, et al. Clinical outcomes of lung transplant recipients with telomerase mutations. J Hear Lung Transplant. 2015;34(10):1318–24.

89. Silhan LL, Shah PD, Chambers DC, Snyder LD, Riise GC, Wagner CL, et al. Lung transplantation in telomerase mutation carriers with pulmonary fibrosis. Eur Respir J. 2014;44(1):178–87.

90. Newton CA, Kozlitina J, Lines JR, Kaza V, Torres F, Garcia CK. Telomere length in patients with pulmonary fibrosis associated with chronic lung allograft dysfunction and post–lung transplantation survival. J Hear Lung Transplant. 2017;36(8): 845–53.

91. Mathai SK, Newton CA, Schwartz DA, Garcia CK. Pulmonary fibrosis in the era of stratified medicine. Thorax. 2016;71(12):1154.

92. Hunninghake GM, Hatabu H, Okajima Y, Gao W, Dupuis J, Latourelle JC, et al. MUC5B promoter polymorphism and interstitial lung abnormalities. N Engl J Med. 2013;368(23):2192–200.

93. Araki T, Putman RK, Hatabu H, Gao W, Dupuis J, Latourelle JC, et al. Development and progression of interstitial lung abnormalities in the Framingham Heart Study. Am J Respir Crit Care Med. 2016;194:1514.

94. Putman RK, Hatabu H, Araki T, Gudmundsson G, Gao W, Nishino M, et al. Association between interstitial lung abnormalities and all-cause mortality. JAMA. 2016;315(7):672.

95. Thomas AQ, Lane K, Phillips J 3rd, Prince M, Markin C, Speer M, et al. Heterozygosity for a surfactant protein C gene mutation associated with usual interstitial pneumonitis and cellular nonspecific interstitial pneumonitis in one kindred. Am J Respir Crit Care Med. 2002;165(9):1322–8.

96. Ono S, Tanaka T, Ishida M, Kinoshita A, Fukuoka J, Takaki M, et al. Surfactant protein C G100S mutation causes familial pulmonary fibrosis in Japanese kindred. Eur Respir J. 2011;38(4):861–9.

97. Hamvas A, Deterding RR, Wert SE, White FV, Dishop MK, Alfano DN, et al. Heterogeneous pulmonary phenotypes associated with mutations in the thyroid transcription factor gene NKX2-1. Chest. 2013;144(3):794–804.

98. Campo I, Zorzetto M, Mariani F, Kadija Z, Morbini P, Dore R, et al. A large kindred of pulmonary fibrosis associated with a novel ABCA3 gene variant. Respir Res. 2014;15:43.

99. Epaud R, Delestrain C, Louha M, Simon S, Fanen P, Tazi A. Combined pulmonary fibrosis and emphysema syndrome associated with ABCA3 mutations. Eur Respir J. 2014;43(2):638–41.

100. Diaz de Leon A, Cronkhite JT, Katzenstein AL, Godwin JD, Raghu G, Glazer CS. Telomere lengths, pulmonary fibrosis and telomerase (TERT) mutations. PLoS One. 2010;5(5):e10680.

101. Zhang Y, Noth I, Garcia JG, Kaminski N. A variant in the promoter of MUC5B and idiopathic pulmonary fibrosis. N Engl J Med. 2011;364(16):1576–7.

102. Mathai SK, Pedersen BS, Smith K, Russell P, Schwarz MI, Brown KK, et al. Desmoplakin variants are associated with idiopathic pulmonary fibrosis. Am J Respir Crit Care Med. 2016;193(10):1151–60.

Genetics of Lung Cancer

Katrina Steiling and Joshua D. Campbell

Key Point Summary
- Lung cancer is primarily caused by environmental exposures, such as tobacco smoke, that cause non-inherited somatic mutations. However, other genetic factors may influence individual response to these environmental exposures and risk for lung cancer, and heritable genetic factors may play a direct role in a minority of lung cancer cases.
- Testing of specific mutations that drive lung tumorigenesis is recommended in cases where there is a chemotherapeutic drug available to target cells that harbor that mutation. Examples include mutations of *EGFR*, *ALK*, and *ROS1* genes.
- Lung tumors evolve over time through the accumulation of new mutations, and even early stage lung tumors show a high level of intratumor heterogeneity that may drive response to therapy and risk for recurrence. More studies are needed to determine how to integrate measures of tumor evolution into precision approaches to therapy for patients with lung cancer.

K. Steiling (✉)
Division of Computational Biomedicine, Department of Medicine, Boston University Medical Center, Bioinformatics Program, Boston University, The Pulmonary Center, Boston University Medical Center, Boston, MA, USA
e-mail: steiling@bu.edu

J. D. Campbell
Division of Computational Biomedicine, Department of Medicine, Boston University Medical Center, Bioinformatics Program, Boston University, Boston, MA, USA
e-mail: camp@bu.edu

Introduction

Lung cancer is the leading cause of cancer-related deaths worldwide [1]. Lung cancer is classified, treated, and studied based on the morphologic appearance of cancerous cells. The two major types of lung cancer are non-small cell lung cancer (NSCLC) and small cell lung cancer (SCLC). NSCLC is the most common type, accounting for approximately 85% of all cases [2]. NSCLC is further subdivided into the subtypes adenocarcinoma and squamous cell carcinoma, with adenocarcinoma being the most common [3]. While both squamous cell carcinoma and adenocarcinoma are strongly associated with cigarette smoking, only a subset of cigarette smokers (10–20%) develops lung cancer [4]. Furthermore, approximately 10–15% of nonsmokers develop adenocarcinoma [4]. These observations together suggest that both environmental and genetic factors influence susceptibility to lung cancer. Specific molecular alterations that occur in lung tumors form the basis of precision therapy for select subsets of patients with lung cancer whose tumors harbor drug-targetable mutations.

Role of Mutations in Lung Cancer

Different types of genetic factors play important roles in susceptibility to lung cancer, tumorigenesis, tumor progression, and response to therapy. For other lung diseases, such as cystic fibrosis, inherited genetic variation is a major factor that influences the risk of disease. In contrast, lung cancer is a disease primarily caused by environmental exposures or errors in DNA replication that induce non-inherited somatic mutations [5]. Somatic mutations are mutations that are acquired by cells and that can be passed on to progeny cells. In the United States, 90% of lung cancer cases are attributable to tobacco smoke [5], an exposure which induces somatic mutations. However, heritable genetic variants are thought to influence individual variability in the susceptibility to environmental perturbagens, and a heritable genetic risk alone may be the predominant factor in a small number of lung cancer cases [5].

Lung cancer development, or tumorigenesis, is the process whereby a somatic mutation alters a molecular pathway and causes a cell to grow and proliferate in an unregulated manner [6]. Driver mutations alter key cellular pathways that give a cancer cell a survival advantage compared to normal cells. Driver mutations differ from passenger mutations, that is, mutations in cancer cells that do not confer a growth or survival advantage. When a single cell with a driver mutation proliferates, it forms a clone of cells that share that driver mutation. Over time, the progeny of that original cell may accumulate additional somatic alterations, acquire new cancer hallmarks, and expand into a novel cancer clone [7]. In the right environment, these clones of cells can proliferate sufficiently to form a lung tumor [6]. The key cellular pathways that comprise the hallmarks of cancer are resistance to cell death, sustained proliferative signaling, evading of growth suppressors, enabled replicative immortality, invasion and metastasis, induced angiogenesis, deregulated cellular energetics, avoidance of immune destruction, genome instability, and tumor-promoting inflammation [3, 8]. Detection of mutations that contribute to lung cancer development and progression has been enabled by high-throughput next-generation sequencing (NGS) [9]. Hundreds to thousands of mutations occur in most cancers [7], but only a small number of these mutations are driver mutations.

Types of Genomic Alterations in Lung Cancer

Several types of genetic alterations can be detected in lung tumors (Fig. 7.1). Mutations are frequently divided between those that are smaller (≤1 kilobase) and larger (>1 kilobase) in scale [10]. There are several types of smaller-scale mutations observed in lung cancer. Single base-pair changes compared to a reference genome are called single nucleotide variants (SNVs). Another type of mutation termed insertions or deletions (indels) are sites at which one or more nucleotides are added to, or subtracted from, the DNA sequence compared to a reference genome [11]. A third type of genetic alteration called a copy number variation (CNV) occurs when a large segment of the genome is either deleted or duplicated [12]. When the number of copies increases, this is called a "gain." When the number of copies decreases, it is called a "loss."

Larger-scale chromosomal and structural abnormalities (>1 kilobase) can also occur in lung tumors (Fig. 7.2). When one portion of a chromosome fuses with a portion of another chromosome, this is called a translocation or rearrangement mutation [12]. Similarly, a duplication may occur, where a large portion of a chromosome is duplicated one or more times [12]. If the entire chromosome is present in an abnormal number, this is called aneuploidy, while poly-

Fig. 7.1 Types of small-scale mutations found in lung cancer

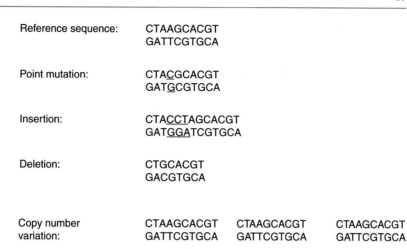

Reference sequence:	CTAAGCACGT GATTCGTGCA
Point mutation:	CTA<u>C</u>GCACGT GAT<u>G</u>CGTGCA
Insertion:	CTA<u>CCT</u>AGCACGT GAT<u>GGA</u>TCGTGCA
Deletion:	CTGCACGT GACGTGCA
Copy number variation:	CTAAGCACGT GATTCGTGCA CTAAGCACGT GATTCGTGCA CTAAGCACGT GATTCGTGCA

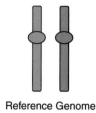

Reference Genome

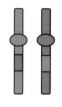

Translocation

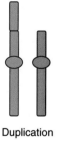

Duplication

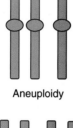

Aneuploidy

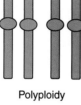

Polyploidy

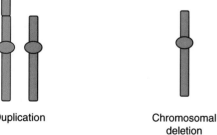

Chromosomal deletion

Fig. 7.2 Types of large-scale genomic alterations found in lung cancer

ploidy is an abnormal copy number of all the chromosomes. Deletions of entire chromosomes are also possible, leading to the loss of all genes on that chromosome. In cancer cells, these abnormalities can arise during mitosis if there is abnormal chromosomal segregation.

Causes of Somatic Mutations That Lead to Lung Cancer

Much of lung cancer is environmental in etiology, and the primary risk factor for developing lung cancer is cigarette smoking [5]. Cigarette smoke contains more than 7000 chemicals, many of which are carcinogens [13]. The mechanism by which cigarette smoke causes lung cancer is the introduction of somatic mutations in key cellular pathways that drive tumorigenesis, a link that has been well established [14]. Smoking increases the risk of lung cancer by 15–30 fold [13]. The persistent risk of lung cancer in individuals that have quit smoking may be a result of accumulated somatic mutations during the time when they smoked.

Other environmental exposures also increase the rate of mutations in the respiratory tract and lung tissue, and, thereby, also increase the risk of lung cancer. For example, it has been well established that exposure to environmental tobacco smoke (ETS) increases lung cancer risk [5, 15]. ETS contains numerous carcinogenic and genotoxic compounds that are also found in mainstream cigarette smoke [16, 17]. These include tar and other particulate matter, nicotine, volatile hydrocarbons, aromatic compounds, and nitrosamines [16, 17]. Constituents of tobacco can be found in the blood and urine of nonsmokers, including the carcinogen 4-(methylnitrosamino)-1-(3-pyridyl)-1-butanol (NNAL) [18]. Heavy exposure to ETS in childhood and adolescence doubles the risk of lung cancer [19]. Nonsmokers with heavy secondhand smoke exposure from their spouse have a 1.27-fold increased risk for lung cancer [20]. In addition to ETS, other exposures that increase lung cancer risk include radon, outdoor air pollution, exposure to occupational carcinogens such as asbestos, and exposure to metals such as arsenic, chromium, and nickel [5]. Multiple exposures can have synergistic effects in terms of risk for lung cancer. For example, individuals with both tobacco smoke exposure and exposure to either asbestos or silica have a substantially higher risk of lung cancer than individuals with either exposure alone [5, 21].

Beyond inhaled exposures, other medical conditions may increase the rate of lung cancer by promoting mutagenesis via chronic inflammation. Among these conditions is HIV infection, which increases the risk of lung cancer by approximately 2–3.5-fold [22, 23]. Prior exposure to radiation therapy, for example, during treatment for breast cancer, increases lung cancer risk by over tenfold [24]. Pulmonary fibrosis increases lung cancer risk by over sevenfold even after adjusting for smoking status [25]. The presence of COPD and emphysema also are independent risk factors for lung cancer [5]. Environmental exposures and comorbid medical conditions, combined with individual susceptibility and genetic risk, together create the conditions necessary to establish a lung tumor via introduction of a driver mutation [6].

Genetics of Lung Cancer

Although the primary risks for lung cancer are related to environmental exposures that lead to somatic mutations, individual susceptibility to these mutagens is thought to be influenced by inherited genetic variants. While cigarette smoking is the cause of >90% of lung cancers, only 10–20% of cigarette smokers ultimately develop lung cancer [26], suggesting that genetic background contributes to individual susceptibility to the carcinogens in tobacco smoke. In addition to the many cases of lung cancer linked to cigarette smoking, approximately 300,000 lung cancer

cases per year are not attributable to tobacco exposure [21]. This corresponds to an incidence of lung cancer in nonsmokers of 4.8–20.8 per 100,000 [21], a risk that may be related to individual differences in the susceptibility to other environmental exposures or to heritable genetic factors. Relatives of patients with lung cancer are at a 1.7–2-fold increased risk of lung cancer compared to those without relatives with early-onset lung cancer [21, 27, 28]. Risk of lung cancer in nonsmokers with a family history of lung cancer is related to the number of affected relatives and early age of diagnosis [29]. This risk may be further elevated in African Americans [27]. Familial risk is challenging to interpret because it is unclear whether having first-degree relatives with lung cancer increases an individual's risk due to shared genetics or shared environmental exposures [29]. However, the above observations suggest a possible genetic basis for lung cancer risk and/or susceptibility to environmental carcinogens.

Candidate Gene Studies

Candidate single-nucleotide polymorphism (SNP) studies evaluate a small set of SNPs for association with a trait of interest, such as lung cancer. SNPs are usually selected based on prior knowledge of gene function or from hypothesis-generating studies using SNP arrays that measure thousands of SNPs but that are potentially limited by high false discovery rates. Candidate SNP approaches have identified several gene candidates that may modulate the risk of lung cancer (Table 7.1). For example, SNPs in colony-stimulating factor (CSF1R), tumor protein p63 (TP63), and a corepressor that interacts with retinoblastoma protein J1 (RBPJ1) were significantly associated with lung cancer in nonsmoking women [30].

Polymorphisms in genes involved in detoxification or mismatch repair might also be important in lung cancer risk. In one study, suboptimal DNA repair capacity in nonsmokers was associated with a 1.92-fold increased risk of lung cancer [31]. Lung cancer risk is further increased in individuals

Table 7.1 Genes and loci associated with lung cancer risk

Type of study	Genes/loci associated with lung cancer risk
Candidate gene	*CSF1R* *TP63* *RBPJ1* *MLH1* *MSH2* *CYP1A1* *CYP1B1* *GSTM1* *GSTP1*
GWAS	15q24–25.1 5p15 6q 6q23–25 6p22.1 6p21.33 18p11.22 12q13.13
Pedigree analysis	*HER2* *EGFR*

A number of individual genes and genetic loci have been found to be associated with lung cancer risk. Study designs used to identify these lung cancer risk loci include candidate gene studies, genome-wide association studies, and pedigree analyses of familial lung cancer syndromes. While these candidates provide important insights into possible factors that might influence lung cancer risk, none have been adequately validated and, therefore, are not recommended for routine clinical testing

with both secondhand smoke exposure and suboptimal DNA repair capacity [31], suggesting that the ability to metabolize and neutralize the chemicals and carcinogens in cigarette smoke is an important factor that contributes to lung cancer risk. Specific genes involved in DNA mismatch repair, such as mutL homolog 1 (*MLH1*) and mutS homolog 2 (*MSH2*), have been linked to lung adenocarcinoma in nonsmokers [32], with polymorphisms in *MSH2* associated with lung cancer risk [33]. Other genes involved in drug metabolism, such as the members of the cytochrome P450 oxidase family *CYP1A1* [34–36] and *CYP1B1* [35], are also associated with elevated lung cancer risk in never smokers. Genes involved in detoxification of polycyclic aromatic hydrocarbons found in cigarette smoke, such as glutathione S transferases [37], have also been linked to lung cancer risk. Homozygous carriers of the glutathione S-transferase mu 1 (*GSTM1*) null allele had a 2.3-fold increased risk of lung cancer in the context of long-term exposure to ETS [37] though this association has not been replicated in other studies [36]. Lung cancer risk was further elevated in nonsmokers with both the *GSTM1* null allele in addition to a polymorphism in another glutathione S-transferase gene (GSTP1val allele) [37]. These observations suggest that individual polymorphisms together with environmental exposures, such as ETS, work together to increase susceptibility to lung cancer and that multiple polymorphisms have a synergistic effect.

While candidate SNP studies have provided valuable insights into the possible mechanisms by which genetic factors influence the response to environmental exposures to increase lung cancer risk, none of these polymorphisms have been sufficiently studied and validated in order to recommend routine testing in patients. Furthermore, the relative contributions of these polymorphisms to lung cancer risk compared to environmental exposures such as tobacco smoke are small. Routine testing for these polymorphisms is not currently recommended for patients with lung cancer, or for relatives of patients with lung cancer.

Genome-Wide Association Studies of Lung Cancer Risk

Genome-wide association studies (GWAS) evaluate the association of thousands or millions of SNPs with a trait such as lung cancer. These studies are challenged by the absence of a large number of environmental variables and comorbidities (e.g., COPD) that may additionally influence lung cancer risk but are often not included in GWAS as well as the large sample sizes needed to reliably detect associations at a genome-wide scale. Despite these limitations, GWAS have been successful in identifying several chromosomal regions that might be important determinants of lung cancer susceptibility though results have been inconsistent across populations (Table 7.1) [21].

A series of studies identified a region on the long arm of chromosome 15 (15q24–25.1) to be associated with heritable lung cancer risk [21, 38, 39], an association that was particularly strong for individuals diagnosed with lung cancer at an early age [38]. However, other studies did not replicate this finding [40]. Loci on 5p15 have been associated with lung cancer in both white and Asian populations [38, 41] and never smokers [39, 40]. Two SNPs on chromosome 5 have been associated with lung cancer although this association was diminished after accounting for the effect of COPD [42]. A locus on the long arm of chromosome 6 may be associated with lung cancer risk in light smokers and never smokers [43]. However, other studies have not replicated this association [38, 40]. A germline susceptibility locus on 6q23-25 was also identified from analysis of high risk family pedigrees [21] although the causative gene was unclear. Other groups have described loci on the short arm of chromosome 6 (6p21.33 and 6p21.1) as being associated with lung cancer risk [39, 44]. Other potential regions of interest that have not been validated include a locus on the short arm of chromosome 18 (18p11.22), which is associated with lung cancer in Korean never smokers [45] and a SNP at 12q13.13 associated with lung cancer risk in Asian populations [44].

Familial Lung Cancer Syndromes

Another approach to identifying genetic susceptibility loci for lung cancer is to examine families in which multiple members develop lung cancer. While heritable lung cancer represents an extremely small proportion of total lung cancer cases, this unique population provides a window into identifying and understanding driver mutations that influence heritable lung cancer risk. Many of the germline mutations described using pedigree analyses occur in genes that frequently also have somatic mutations in lung cancer (Table 7.1). For example, the germline mutation in the human epidermal growth factor receptor 2 (*HER2*) gene associated with lung cancer risk has been identified in a family of Japanese descent [46]. Germline mutations in the epidermal growth factor receptor (*EGFR*) have also been described,

including the T790M mutation, which is associated with lung cancer risk and also confers resistance to EGFR tyrosine kinase inhibitors [47, 48], and the V843I mutation, which is associated with multicentric adenomatous hyperplasia and lung adenocarcinoma, as well as familial lung cancer [49, 50]. The *EGFR*-activating mutation R776H has been linked to NSCLC with squamous differentiation in a mother and daughter with NSCLC [51].

Genetics of Lung Cancer Survival

Beyond its role in lung cancer susceptibility, genetics may also play a role in lung cancer survival. The SNP rs4324798 has been identified as an independent prognostic factor for overall survival in SCLC [42]. SNPs located at the locus 4q12 have been associated with progression free survival in NSCLC [52]. Interestingly, these SNPs were associated with *EGFR* expression but not with *EGFR* mutation status, suggesting a mechanism via which they influence survival [52]. Two additional SNPs (rs4237904 and rs7976914) were associated with overall survival in NSCLC, although the function of these SNPs is not known [53]. Further study is needed to identify and validate the association of SNPs with lung cancer prognosis and survival.

Driver Mutations in NSCLC

While surgical resection is the mainstay of treatment for early-stage NSCLC, the majority of lung cancers are diagnosed at a later stage where chemotherapy is used either alone or in addition to surgical resection. Significant progress has been made in personalized cancer therapy owing to the identification of driver mutations and drugs that selectively target cells that harbor these mutations (Table 7.2). For patients with lung tumors who are candidates for chemotherapy, therapies targeted at specific molecular alterations have improved treatment options for patients with advanced disease [54]. Many of these mutations occur in genes in the Ras/Raf/

Table 7.2 Lung cancer driver mutations

Lung cancer type	Genes with known driver mutations
NSCLC	EGFR
	ALK
	ROS1
	BRAF
	NTRK
	HER2/ERBB2
	MET
	RET
	KRAS
SCLC	TP53
	PTEN
	MYC
	RB1

RTK pathway. However, the majority of lung tumors harbor mutations that are not yet targetable and, thus, are treated with conventional chemotherapy [54].

Epidermal Growth Factor Receptor (*EGFR*) Mutations

EGFR encodes a tyrosine kinase target in the ERBB family and exists as a monomer on the cell surface [52]. Mutations in this gene activate phosphoinositide 3-kinase (PI3K)/AKT signaling through the *ERBB3* receptor tyrosine kinase [55]. Activating *EGFR* mutations lead to sustained proliferative signaling and cellular growth, which are a hallmark of cancer. *EGFR* mutations are found in ~15% of lung adenocarcinomas in the United States [3, 56] and are more common in Asian populations [57], never smokers [56], and women [56]. *EGFR* mutations, which are generally found in adenocarcinomas rather than squamous cell carcinomas [3], include exon 19 deletions and exon 21 (L858R) mutations [58].

EGFR mutations are clinically important because tumors harboring these mutations can be targeted with EGFR tyrosine kinase inhibitors (TKIs) such as erlotinib, gefitinib, or afatinib [59]. Guidelines recommend prioritizing testing for *EGFR* mutations over other molecular tests because of the availability of precision therapies targeted to this mutation [60]. Patients receiving EGFR TKIs can develop resistance to them. A common mechanism for resistance to EGFR

TKIs is the development of a T790M mutation [61–63], which consists of a substitution of a methionine for threonine at position 790 of the *EGFR* gene. This mutation occurs in as many as half of lung tumors that develop resistance to first-line EGFR TKIs [62, 64]. Another mechanism of resistance to EGFR TKI therapy is amplification of the *MET* oncogene, which occurs in 5–20% of tumors that progress on an EGFR TKI [55, 63–65]. A third mechanism of resistance to EGFR TKI therapy is transformation of the NSCLC tumor into a high-grade large cell neuroendocrine tumor [66] or SCLC [67].

Anaplastic Lymphoma Kinase (*ALK*) Fusion Mutation

The ALK translocation mutation is an inversion that occurs on chromosome 2 [68] and results in the joining of the echinoderm microtubule-associated protein-like 4 (*EML4*) gene to the anaplastic lymphoma kinase (*ALK*) gene [69]. This creates the fusion oncogene *EMR4–ALK*, which causes upregulation of *ALK* expression and unregulated cell growth [68]. This mutation is far more common in adenocarcinomas and rarely seen in squamous cell carcinomas [68]. Like *EGFR* mutations, the *ALK* fusion mutation is more commonly detected in lung tumors from never smokers [69]. *ALK* fusions, which are present in 3–5% of lung adenocarcinomas in the United States [68, 70–72], can be treated with targeted medications such as crizotinib [73], ceritinib [74], and alectinib [75]. Guidelines recommend prioritizing testing for *ALK* fusions, in addition to testing for *EGFR* mutations, because of the availability of precision therapies targeted to the mutation [60].

Progression of a lung tumor being treated with the ALK inhibitor crizotinib may indicate development of a secondary mutation conferring resistance. One such mutation is G1202R, which is located at the front of the *ALK* gene's kinase domain [75]. Another such mutation is F1174V, which is an activating substitution mutation at the phenylalanine residue at position 1174 [75]. The F1174V mutation is thought to decrease the size of the side chain involved in the hydrophobic core next to the activation loop of the ALK protein, which favors an active conformation of the protein [75].

ROS Proto-Oncogene 1, Receptor Tyrosine Kinase (*ROS1*) Mutations

ROS1, located on the long arm of chromosome 6 (6q22) [72], is a transmembrane tyrosine kinase receptor [69]. Little is known about the function of the extracellular domain of this protein, but it is thought to be tied to multiple downstream signaling pathways involved in cell proliferation and cell cycle [69]. Like *ALK* fusion events, *ROS1* mutations are more commonly observed in lung tumors from patients who are younger and never smokers [69]. *ROS1* mutations, observed in 0.7–2% of NSCLC tumors [69, 71, 76], can be gene fusion events or point mutations. *ROS1* fusions observed in NSCLC, which lead to constitutive activation of *ROS1*, include *CD74–ROS1*, *SLC34A2–ROS*, *CD74–ROS1*, and *FIG–ROS1* [71]. Similar to *ALK* fusion events, *ROS1* fusion events promote cellular proliferation [72]. Because the *ROS1* kinase domain has a high degree of homology with the *ALK* kinase domain [69], tumors with *ROS1* mutations can be targeted by treatment with medications such as crizotinib [72, 76] or other ALK inhibitors [69].

B-Raf Proto-Oncogene, Serine/Threonine Kinase (*BRAF*) Mutations

BRAF, one of three RAF isoforms [77], is a serine/threonine kinase that is part of the MAPK pathway [78]. Activating mutations of *BRAF* promote cellular proliferation [78]. *BRAF* mutations occur in 1–3% of lung adenocarcinomas [77–80] and are much more common in lung tumors from patients with a history of heavy smoking [80, 81]. As such, these mutations are usually mutually exclusive of *EGFR* or *ALK* mutations [78, 81]. Patients with lung tumors harboring *BRAF* mutations frequently develop second primary lung tumors with KRAS Proto-Oncogene, GTPase

(*KRAS*) mutations [81]. *BRAF* mutations, which seem to occur with equal frequency in men and women [80], are usually point mutations. Genotypes described, along with their estimated frequencies, include V600E (30–57%) [77, 79–81], G469A (22–39%) [77, 79, 81], K601E (15.4%) [77], D469V (13%) [81], D594G (6–11%) [79, 81], and V600M (2%) [81]. Mutations in *BRAF* can be targeted with RAF inhibitors such as vemurafenib [82] or dabrafenib plus trametinib [78, 83] although lung tumors with non-V600 mutations may be less sensitive to them [81].

Neurotrophic Receptor Tyrosine Kinase (NTRK) Gene Fusions

There are three NTRK genes which encode the three tropomyosin receptor kinases (*NTRK1*, *NTRK2*, *NTRK3*) [84]. While expression of these genes is usually limited to the nervous system, fusion events can occur that cause the proteins to be expressed as a chimeric protein in a variety of cancers [84]. Mutations in these genes occur in approximately 1% of all solid tumors [84], including lung cancers [85]. Gene fusions described include *MPRIP–NTRK1* and *CD74–NTRK1*, which cause constitutive activation of *NTRK1* (a.k.a., *TRKA*) [85]. Tumors with these fusions can be treated with the oral TRK-inhibitor larotrectinib [84].

MET Proto-Oncogene, Receptor Tyrosine Kinase (*MET*) Amplification and Mutation

MET is receptor tyrosine kinase [64, 65] proto-oncogene [55] located on chromosome 7q21-31 [65]. The ligand for *MET* is hepatocyte growth factor (*HGF*) [65]. Perturbation of the HGF-MET pathway leads to cellular proliferation, angiogenesis, and metastasis [65] via multiple downstream pathways including PI3K/AKT and ERK [65]. *MET* was first identified as a potential novel target in a large study of matched tumor and normal tissues profiled using whole exome sequencing [54]. Overall, about 5% of lung adenocarcinomas harbor *MET* mutations [86]. Dysregulation of *MET* can occur via amplification of the receptor or by mutations that affect its function [65]. *MET* amplification leads to first-generation EGFR TKI resistance [55, 63–65]. *MET/EGFR* co-mutations occur in approximately 5–20% of *EGFR*-mutated tumors with resistance to EGFR TKIs [67]. Higher *MET* copy number has been associated with worse prognosis [87]. *MET* has a juxtamembrane domain whose deletion leads to *MET* activation [86]. Mutations in this domain may involve skipping of exon 14 and subsequent activation of *MET* [54, 88, 89], a mutation that occurs in approximately 3–4% of lung adenocarcinomas [86, 88, 90], and is associated with older age [88]. *MET* mutations can be targeted with *MET* inhibitors such as crizotinib and cabozantinib [88, 90].

Erb-B2 Receptor Tyrosine Kinase 2 (*ERBB2*) Mutations

ERBB2, also known as human epidermal growth factor receptor 2 (*HER2*), is a receptor tyrosine kinase in the ERBB family [91, 92]. Its activation results in downstream activation of several pathways involved in cellular proliferation, cellular differentiation, migration, and survival [91, 92]. *HER2/ERBB2* mutations in lung cancer, which were initially identified in a large study of matched lung tumor and normal tissue profiled using whole exome sequencing [54], are estimated to occur in 1.7–4% of NSCLC [91–93]. When a *HER2/ERBB2* mutation is present in a lung tumor, there are rarely other targetable driver mutations [93]. Mutations in this gene are more common in lung tumors occurring in never smokers [91, 93] and women [93] and are almost exclusively described in adenocarcinomas [54, 92, 93]. Therapies targeting *HER2/ERBB2* are commonly used in breast cancers, another tumor which commonly harbors *HER2/ERBB2* mutations. These drugs might also be used to target *HER2/ERBB2* mutations in lung tumors [93], but further investigations are needed to determine their efficacy.

Ret Proto-Oncogene (*RET*) Fusions

The *RET* (also known as Rearranged during Transfection) gene is a cell surface receptor tyrosine kinase [94] located on the long arm of chromosome 10 [95]. *RET* can be fused with *KIF5B* (located on the short arm of chromosome 10) via a genomic inversion event or with *CCDC6* via a translocation [96]. These fusions lead to abnormal activation of *RET* [97], which results in increased downstream signaling of the RAS–ERK and PI3K/AKT pathways that regulate cell proliferation and survival [96]. *RET* fusion occurs in 1–2% of lung adenocarcinomas [94, 96, 97] and is associated with tumors that are less well differentiated [94]. *RET* fusions are more likely to be observed in tumors from patients that are younger [94] and never smokers [94, 98]. Patients with tumors that harbor this mutation may respond to targeted therapies such as cabozantinib [98] or vandetanib [99].

KRAS Proto-Oncogene, GTPase (*KRAS*) Mutations

KRAS is part of the RAS family of oncogenes [100]. RAS proteins are small GTPases involved in downstream signaling through multiple pathways involved in cellular proliferation, differentiation, and survival, including PI3K/AKT, RAF–MEK–ERK, RAL–GEF [100]. *KRAS* is a downstream signaling molecule of the EGFR pathway [58]. *KRAS* mutations are commonly found in lung tumors of individuals who have smoked cigarettes and are rarely seen in never smokers [56]. A higher frequency of *KRAS* mutations is associated with greater smoking history and higher body mass index [56]. *KRAS* mutations are also associated with a poorer prognosis [100]. *KRAS* mutations are present in 15–20% of lung adenocarcinomas but rarely in squamous cell carcinomas [58, 100]. In theory, KRAS inhibitors could be used to target lung tumors with these mutations, and although clinical trials to test them are ongoing, there are currently no such approved therapies.

Other NSCLC-Related Mutations

While several individual NSCLC driver mutations have been identified that can lead to dramatic responses to specific therapies targeted at cells harboring these mutations (i.e., *EGFR*, *ALK*, *ROS1*), only a minority of tumors harbor such mutations. Recent efforts have attempted to more broadly profile tumors to identify new drivers of cancer initiation and progression that might also serve as targets for new therapies. This approach has been facilitated by advances in NGS, and the creation of consortiums able to acquire large study sample sizes necessary to reach the statistical power required to differentiate driver mutations from passenger mutations.

In a large comparison of adenocarcinoma and squamous cell carcinoma lung tumors, there were distinct patterns of gene mutations and somatic copy number alterations [101]. This study identified several new focal amplifications in protein coding genes as well as multiple mutations in the RTK–Ras–Raf pathway [101]. One example is the novel driver gene *SOS1*, a guanine nucleotide exchange factor (GEF) that catalyzes the exchange of GDP for GTP, resulting in activation of Ras [102]. Recurrent *SOS1* mutations were observed in lung adenocarcinomas without other mutations in the RTK–Ras–Raf pathway. Further, these mutations could transform cells in vitro and were sensitive to MEK, but not EGFR, inhibition.

Squamous cell carcinomas have a high overall mutation rate with a near-universal mutation of *TP53* and mutations in pathways related to cell cycle control, response to oxidative stress, apoptotic signaling, and cellular differentiation, including CKDN2A/RB1, NFE2L2/KEAP1/CUL3, PI3K/AKT, and SOX2/TP53/NOTCH1 pathways [103]. *EGFR* and *KRAS* mutations were rare in squamous cell carcinomas and common in adenocarcinomas [103]. Some of the highly recurrent mutations were predicted to cause new epitopes to be presented on cancer cells [101], suggesting a potential role for cancer vaccine development.

Another approach to finding novel patterns of somatic mutations that might have implications for tumorigenesis, tumor progression, or therapy includes using NGS to identify mutational signatures [104]. Over 30 distinct mutational signatures have been identified [104], including one that was enriched for the C > A transversions caused by carcinogens in cigarette smoke. Besides environmental mutagens, endogenous biological processes can also contribute to the mutational load observed in lung cancers. Members of the APOBEC family have been implicated in several cancers, including lung cancer [7, 105, 106]. APOBEC cytidine deaminases convert cytosine to uracil during RNA editing and are hypothesized to induce mutation clusters in tumors [105] as well as a large proportion of subclonal mutations [107]. In addition to APOBEC, lung tumors also demonstrated mutational signatures related to an elevated rate of spontaneous deamination of 5-methyl-cytosine residues, which is associated with aging, or the so-called molecular clock [107].

Driver Mutations in SCLC

SCLC, which comprises approximately 15% of all lung cancers, is characterized by rapid growth, early metastasis, and a very low 2-year survival rate [108, 109]. The development of SCLC is very strongly linked to cigarette smoking [109]. Compared with NSCLC, SCLC has a much faster doubling time and higher propensity to metastasize early. Reflecting this clinical divergence between the two major lung cancer cell types, the genomic landscapes of SCLC and NSCLC also differ substantially. SCLC is highly complex at the molecular level and characterized by a large number of mutations in each tumor [109]. For example, one study of a SCLC cell line using NGS identified 22,910 somatic substitutions, 65 indels, 334 CNVs, and 58 structural variants [108]. Common tumor suppressor genes that are inactivated in SCLC include *TP53* [108–110] (>75–90% of SCLC) and *PTEN* [108] (Table 7.2). There can also be amplification of *MYC* (~20% of SCLC), and while the retinoblastoma tumor suppressor gene (*RB1*) is nearly universally mutated in SCLC [108–110] it is mutated in a minority of NSCLC [110]. 3p deletion is also commonly observed in SCLC [109]. Less commonly, there are activating mutations in *PIK3CA*, *EGFR*, and *KRAS* [108]. *KRAS* is rarely mutated in SCLC although it is frequently altered in NSCLC [110], while *MET* mutations have been detected in SCLC cell lines and tumors [65].

Evolution of Lung Cancer

While much progress has been made in identifying driver mutations that are responsible for lung cancer development and can be targets for personalized lung cancer therapy, one of the ongoing challenges in treating patients with lung cancer is the evolution of individual lung tumors. Every lung tumor changes over time, a process driven by cell-level evolution, in which natural selection drives the selection of subclonal populations that harbor alleles conferring a survival advantage [111]. Similar to Darwinian evolution, lung tumor evolution occurs due to genetic variation combined with replicative and environmental pressures leading to selection of the fittest clones for survival and growth [112]. This branched evolution, where surviving subclones in various parts of the tumor are derived from a parent cancer cell, leads to variable intratumor heterogeneity [106].

Both genetic drift, or the changes in allele frequencies from one generation of cells to the next, and the rate at which new mutations appear play important roles in how lung tumors change over time and how they respond to therapy [111].

Phylogenetic methods are often used to understand tumor evolution. In these analyses, the tumor is depicted as a tree (Fig. 7.3) [111]. The trunk of the tree represents mutations that are shared/ubiquitous across all cancer cells within the entire tumor specimen that was sampled. Clones are cells that share a particular alteration. Through the process of clonal divergence, new genetic lesions are acquired over time, and subclones with these new mutations descend from their common ancestor cell. A branch on the tree thus indicates a set of mutations present specifically in that subclone. The branch length is proportional to the number of mutations, while the degree of intratumoral heterogeneity is proportional to the number of branches and distance between them.

Tumor evolution is responsible for tumorigenesis and for the development of resistance to chemotherapy agents [111, 112]. Tumors vary in the rates in which new clones appear and extinguish, and in the rate of clonal development [111]. Because each subclone harbors the mutations of ancestral clones, as well as a new set of mutations,

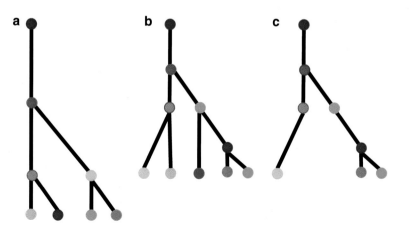

Fig. 7.3 Depiction of lung tumor evolution using phylogenetic trees. Each dot represents a clone with a specific set of mutations. The start of each trunk represents the parent clone, or original cancer cell, for each tumor. Each branchpoint represents the development of a new mutation that leads to a new subclone. The length of the branches indicates time. Compared to tumor (**a**), tumor (**b**) has a faster mutation rate (shorter branches) and a higher level of intratumor heterogeneity (more subclones present in the final tumor). Tumor (**c**) has a similar mutation rate to tumor (**b**) but has less intratumor heterogeneity

the new mutations serve as a reservoir from which a growth or survival advantage might be conferred. The larger the diversity of subclones within a tumor, the greater the capacity of that tumor to respond to selective pressures such as the introduction of a new chemotherapeutic agent. It is this intratumoral heterogeneity that drives natural selection within the tumor itself [111]. Therefore, while lung tumors sampled at a single point in time might appear to have very similar clonal structures, one tumor may have accumulated its mutations over a long period of time, whereas a second tumor may have accumulated its mutations over a short period of time [111]. These factors have implications for lung cancer therapy and the development of resistance to chemotherapy.

Lung tumor evolution is intertwined with the tumor's environment. The cells and factors that surround the cancer help determine which mutations are advantageous and confer a survival or growth advantage [112]. Because the tumor environment plays an equally important role in tumor evolution, the diversity of a primary tumor might differ from the diversity of its metastases, and the diversity of an untreated tumor might differ from that of a recurrent tumor in the same patient.

The initial studies examining lung tumor heterogeneity suggest that understanding and profiling tumor evolution is likely to play an important role in the future for precision lung cancer therapy. For example, in an early study using multi-region exome sequencing and whole-exome sequencing of NSCLC prior to adjuvant chemotherapy, spatial heterogeneity was identified in all tumors with a median of 30% heterogeneous mutations [107]. Each lung tumor showed both ubiquitous and heterogeneous driver mutations, but the heterogeneous driver mutations were often dominant in only a portion of the tumor [107]. In another study, NGS demonstrated intraregional subclonal populations in lung adenocarcinomas [106], suggesting that analysis of a single biopsy specimen does not fully represent the mutational spectrum present in lung tumors. More recent studies using single cell sequencing have shown that intratumoral heterogeneity is present even in early stage lung cancers, which are usually treated with surgical resection and

without systemic chemotherapy [113]. In fact, higher levels of lung tumor heterogeneity were associated with a higher risk of disease recurrence and death [113]. Chromosomal instability, rather than point mutations, mediated much of this heterogeneity [113]. Driver mutations were almost always clonal, and more than 75% of tumors had subclonal driver mutations [113].

The best way to integrate these important observations of tumor evolution into clinical practice has not yet been determined, and, thus, multi-region sampling is not yet routinely recommended outside the context of clinical trials or research studies. However, it is easy to envision a future where lung cancer pathology reports contain not only information about a tumor's cell type, stage, and the presence or absence of specific targetable driver mutations, but also information on a lung tumor's heterogeneity and evolution. For example, information on the amount of genomic instability and propensity to develop new clones might impact prognostication as information on the amount of subclonal diversity present within the lung tumor might affect the propensity to develop resistance to chemotherapeutic agents. Monitoring this in advance could help physicians better anticipate how an individual lung tumor will respond and evolve to therapies so that future therapies can target the evolving tumor.

Because current mutation testing is usually performed on tumor tissue, it is necessary to balance the risk of obtaining greater amount of tissue or sequential biopsies with its potential benefit. Circulating tumor DNA (ctDNA) testing is a rapidly evolving technology and area of research [114, 115] that might have future utility as a less invasive method of monitoring lung tumor evolution and detecting residual or recurrent disease that will facilitate the tailoring of therapies to evolving tumors.

Conclusion

Lung cancer is primarily caused by tobacco smoke and other environmental exposures that cause non-inherited somatic mutations, but it is also influenced by inherited genetic factors that modify individual response to environmental exposures. Personalized therapies for lung cancer exist for some specific mutations that drive lung tumorigenesis for which chemotherapeutic drugs have been developed, most notably, those involving mutations of *EGFR*, *ALK*, and *ROS1*. Future efforts to improve precision medicine in lung cancer should focus on understanding SCLC, identifying a broader range of mutations in NSCLC, and monitoring the evolution of lung tumors.

References

1. Jemal A, Bray F, Center MM, Ferlay J, Ward E, Forman D. Global cancer statistics. CA Cancer J Clin. 2011;61(2):69–90.
2. Molina JR, Yang P, Cassivi SD, Schild SE, Adjei AA. Non-small cell lung cancer: epidemiology, risk factors, treatment, and survivorship. Mayo Clin Proc. 2008;83(5):584–94.
3. Imielinski M, Berger AH, Hammerman PS, Hernandez B, Pugh TJ, Hodis E, et al. Mapping the hallmarks of lung adenocarcinoma with massively parallel sequencing. Cell. 2012;150(6):1107–20.
4. Shields PG. Molecular epidemiology of lung cancer. Ann Oncol Off J Eur Soc Med Oncol ESMO. 1999;10(Suppl 5):S7–11.
5. Alberg AJ, Samet JM. Epidemiology of lung cancer. Chest. 2003;123(1 Suppl):21S–49S.
6. Robles AI, Zenklusen JC. Seeing the forest through the phylogenetic tree. N Engl J Med. 2017;376(22):2190–1.
7. Burns MB, Temiz NA, Harris RS. Evidence for APOBEC3B mutagenesis in multiple human cancers. Nat Genet. 2013;45(9):977–83.
8. Hanahan D, Weinberg RA. Hallmarks of cancer: the next generation. Cell. 2011;144(5):646–74.
9. Meyerson M, Gabriel S, Getz G. Advances in understanding cancer genomes through second-generation sequencing. Nat Rev Genet. 2010;11(10):685–96.
10. The Wellcome Trust Case Control Consortium, Conrad DF, Pinto D, Redon R, Feuk L, Gokcumen O, et al. Origins and functional impact of copy number variation in the human genome. Nature. 2010;464(7289):704–12.
11. Mills RE, Luttig CT, Larkins CE, Beauchamp A, Tsui C, Pittard WS, et al. An initial map of insertion and deletion (INDEL) variation in the human genome. Genome Res. 2006;16(9):1182–90.
12. Feuk L, Carson AR, Scherer SW. Structural variation in the human genome. Nat Rev Genet. 2006;7(2):85–97.
13. What are the risk factors for lung cancer? [Internet]. Center for disease control and prevention; 2018. Available from: https://www.cdc.gov/cancer/lung/basic_info/risk_factors.htm.
14. United States. Surgeon General's Advisory Committee on Smoking and Health, and United States. Public Health Service. Office of the Surgeon General. Smoking and Health [Internet]. United States. Public Health Service. Office of the Surgeon General.; 1964 [cited 2019 Feb 5]. Available from: https://profiles.nlm.nih.gov/ps/access/NNBBMQ.pdf.
15. Samet JM, Avila-Tang E, Boffetta P, Hannan LM, Olivo-Marston S, Thun MJ, et al. Lung cancer in never smokers: clinical epidemiology and environmental risk factors. Clin Cancer Res. 2009;15(18):5626–45.
16. Löfroth G. Environmental tobacco smoke: overview of chemical composition and genotoxic components. Mutat Res. 1989;222(2):73–80.
17. Claxton LD, Morin RS, Hughes TJ, Lewtas J. A genotoxic assessment of environmental tobacco smoke using bacterial bioassays. Mutat Res. 1989;222(2):81–99.
18. Hecht SS, Carmella SG, Murphy SE, Akerkar S, Brunnemann KD, Hoffmann D. A tobacco-specific lung carcinogen in the urine of men exposed to cigarette smoke. N Engl J Med. 1993;329(21):1543–6.
19. Lung cancer and exposure to tobacco smoke in the household. N Engl J Med. 1991;324(6):412–5.
20. Taylor R, Najafi F, Dobson A. Meta-analysis of studies of passive smoking and lung cancer: effects of study type and continent. Int J Epidemiol. 2007;36(5):1048–59.
21. Alberg AJ, Brock MV, Ford JG, Samet JM, Spivack SD. Epidemiology of lung cancer: diagnosis and management of lung cancer, 3rd ed: American College of Chest Physicians evidence-based clinical practice guidelines. Chest. 2013;143(5 Suppl):e1S–e29S.
22. Kirk GD, Merlo C, O'Driscoll P, Mehta SH, Galai N, Vlahov D, et al. HIV infection is associated with an increased risk for lung cancer, independent of smoking. Clin Infect Dis. 2007;45(1):103–10.
23. Chaturvedi AK, Pfeiffer RM, Chang L, Goedert JJ, Biggar RJ, Engels EA. Elevated risk of lung cancer among people with AIDS. AIDS Lond Engl. 2007;21(2):207–13.
24. Huang Y-J, Huang T-W, Lin F-H, Chung C-H, Tsao C-H, Chien W-C. Radiation therapy for invasive breast cancer increases the risk of second primary lung cancer: a nationwide population-based cohort analysis. J Thorac Oncol Off Publ Int Assoc Study Lung Cancer. 2017;12(5):782–90.
25. Hubbard R, Venn A, Lewis S, Britton J. Lung cancer and cryptogenic fibrosing alveolitis. A population-based cohort study. Am J Respir Crit Care Med. 2000;161(1):5–8.
26. Steiling K, Ryan J, Brody JS, Spira A. The field of tissue injury in the lung and airway. Cancer Prev Res. 2008;1(6):396–403.
27. Naff JL, Coté ML, Wenzlaff AS, Schwartz AG. Racial differences in cancer risk among rela-

tives of patients with early onset lung cancer. Chest. 2007;131(5):1289–94.

28. Schwartz AC, Ruckdechel JC. Familial lung cancer: genetic susceptibility and relationship to chronic obstructive pulmonary disease. Am J Respir Crit Care Med. 2006;173:16–22.

29. Matakidou A, Eisen T, Houlston RS. Systematic review of the relationship between family history and lung cancer risk. Br J Cancer. 2005;93(7):825–33.

30. Kang H-G, Lee SY, Jeon H-S, Choi YY, Kim S, Lee WK, et al. A functional polymorphism in CSF1R gene is a novel susceptibility marker for lung cancer among never-smoking females. J Thorac Oncol Off Publ Int Assoc Study Lung Cancer. 2014;9(11):1647–55.

31. Gorlova OY, Weng S-F, Zhang Y, Amos CI, Spitz MR, Wei Q. DNA repair capacity and lung cancer risk in never smokers. Cancer Epidemiol Biomark Prev Publ Am Assoc Cancer Res Cosponsored Am Soc Prev Oncol. 2008;17(6):1322–8.

32. Lo Y-L, Hsiao C-F, Jou Y-S, Chang G-C, Tsai Y-H, Su W-C, et al. Polymorphisms of MLH1 and MSH2 genes and the risk of lung cancer among never smokers. Lung Cancer Amst Neth. 2011;72(3):280–6.

33. Jung CY, Choi JE, Park JM, Chae MH, Kang H-G, Kim KM, et al. Polymorphisms in the hMSH2 gene and the risk of primary lung cancer. Cancer Epidemiol Biomark Prev Publ Am Assoc Cancer Res Cosponsored Am Soc Prev Oncol. 2006;15(4):762–8.

34. Taioli E, Gaspari L, Benhamou S, Boffetta P, Brockmoller J, Butkiewicz D, et al. Polymorphisms in CYP1A1, GSTM1, GSTT1 and lung cancer below the age of 45 years. Int J Epidemiol. 2003;32(1):60–3.

35. Wenzlaff AS, Cote ML, Bock CH, Land SJ, Santer SK, Schwartz DR, et al. CYP1A1 and CYP1B1 polymorphisms and risk of lung cancer among never smokers: a population-based study. Carcinogenesis. 2005;26(12):2207–12.

36. Raimondi S, Boffetta P, Anttila S, Bröckmoller J, Butkiewicz D, Cascorbi I, et al. Metabolic gene polymorphisms and lung cancer risk in non-smokers. An update of the GSEC study. Mutat Res. 2005;592(1–2):45–57.

37. Wenzlaff AS, Cote ML, Bock CH, Land SJ, Schwartz AG. GSTM1, GSTT1 and GSTP1 polymorphisms, environmental tobacco smoke exposure and risk of lung cancer among never smokers: a population-based study. Carcinogenesis. 2005;26(2):395–401.

38. Truong T, Hung RJ, Amos CI, Wu X, Bickeböller H, Rosenberger A, et al. Replication of Lung Cancer Susceptibility Loci at Chromosomes 15q25, 5p15, and 6p21: a pooled analysis from the International Lung Cancer Consortium. JNCI J Natl Cancer Inst. 2010;102(13):959–71.

39. Wang Y, Broderick P, Webb E, Wu X, Vijayakrishnan J, Matakidou A, et al. Common 5p15.33 and 6p21.33 variants influence lung cancer risk. Nat Genet. 2008;40(12):1407–9.

40. Wang Y, Broderick P, Matakidou A, Eisen T, Houlston RS. Role of 5p15.33 (TERT-CLPTM1L), 6p21.33 and 15q25.1 (CHRNA5-CHRNA3) variation and lung cancer risk in never-smokers. Carcinogenesis. 2010;31(2):234–8.

41. Hsiung CA, Lan Q, Hong Y-C, Chen C-J, Hosgood HD, Chang I-S, et al. The 5p15.33 locus is associated with risk of lung adenocarcinoma in never-smoking females in Asia. PLoS Genet. 2010;6(8):e1001051.

42. Yang P, Li Y, Jiang R, Cunningham JM, Li Y, Zhang F, et al. A rigorous and comprehensive validation: common genetic variations and lung cancer. Cancer Epidemiol Biomark Prev Publ Am Assoc Cancer Res Cosponsored Am Soc Prev Oncol. 2010;19(1):240–4.

43. Amos CI, Pinney SM, Li Y, Kupert E, Lee J, de Andrade MA, et al. A susceptibility locus on chromosome 6q greatly increases lung cancer risk among light and never smokers. Cancer Res. 2010;70(6):2359–67.

44. Wang Z, Seow WJ, Shiraishi K, Hsiung CA, Matsuo K, Liu J, et al. Meta-analysis of genome-wide association studies identifies multiple lung cancer susceptibility loci in never-smoking Asian women. Hum Mol Genet. 2016;25(3):620–9.

45. Ahn M-J, Won H-H, Lee J, Lee S-T, Sun J-M, Park YH, et al. The 18p11.22 locus is associated with never smoker non-small cell lung cancer susceptibility in Korean populations. Hum Genet. 2012;131(3):365–72.

46. Yamamoto H, Higasa K, Sakaguchi M, Shien K, Soh J, Ichimura K, et al. Novel germline mutation in the transmembrane domain of HER2 in familial lung adenocarcinomas. J Natl Cancer Inst. 2014;106(1):djt338.

47. Bell DW, Gore I, Okimoto RA, Godin-Heymann N, Sordella R, Mulloy R, et al. Inherited susceptibility to lung cancer may be associated with the T790M drug resistance mutation in EGFR. Nat Genet. 2005;37(12):1315–6.

48. Prudkin L, Tang X, Wistuba II. Germ-line and somatic presentations of the EGFR T790M mutation in lung cancer. J Thorac Oncol Off Publ Int Assoc Study Lung Cancer. 2009;4(1):139–41.

49. Ikeda K, Nomori H, Mori T, Sasaki J, Kobayashi T. Novel germline mutation: EGFR V843I in patient with multiple lung adenocarcinomas and family members with lung cancer. Ann Thorac Surg. 2008;85(4):1430–2.

50. Ohtsuka K, Ohnishi H, Kurai D, Matsushima S, Morishita Y, Shinonaga M, et al. Familial lung adenocarcinoma caused by the EGFR V843I germ-line mutation. J Clin Oncol Off J Am Soc Clin Oncol. 2011;29(8):e191–2.

51. van Noesel J, van der Ven WH, van Os TAM, Kunst PWA, Weegenaar J, Reinten RJA, et al. Activating germline R776H mutation in the epidermal growth factor receptor associated with lung cancer with squamous differentiation. J Clin Oncol Off J Am Soc Clin Oncol. 2013;31(10):e161–4.

52. Chang I-S, Jiang SS, Yang JC-H, Su W-C, Chien L-H, Hsiao C-F, et al. Genetic modifiers of progression-free survival in never-smoking lung adenocarcinoma patients treated with first-line tyrosine kinase inhibitors. Am J Respir Crit Care Med. 2017;195(5):663–73.

53. Wu X, Wang L, Ye Y, Aakre JA, Pu X, Chang G-C, et al. Genome-wide association study of genetic predictors of overall survival for non-small cell lung cancer in never smokers. Cancer Res. 2013;73(13):4028–38.

54. Collisson EA, Campbell JD, Brooks AN, Berger AH, Lee W, Chmielecki J, et al. Comprehensive molecular profiling of lung adenocarcinoma. Nature. 2014;511(7511):543–50.

55. Engelman JA, Zejnullahu K, Mitsudomi T, Song Y, Hyland C, Park JO, et al. MET amplification leads to gefitinib resistance in lung cancer by activating ERBB3 signaling. Science. 2007;316(5827):1039–43.

56. Kawaguchi T, Koh Y, Ando M, Ito N, Takeo S, Adachi H, et al. Prospective analysis of oncogenic driver mutations and environmental factors: Japan molecular epidemiology for lung cancer study. J Clin Oncol. 2016;34(19):2247–57.

57. Shi Y, JS-K A, Thongprasert S, Srinivasan S, Tsai C-M, Khoa MT, et al. A prospective, molecular epidemiology study of EGFR mutations in Asian patients with advanced non-small-cell lung cancer of adenocarcinoma histology (PIONEER). J Thorac Oncol Off Publ Int Assoc Study Lung Cancer. 2014;9(2):154–62.

58. Ai X, Guo X, Wang J, Stancu AL, Joslin PMN, Zhang D, et al. Targeted therapies for advanced non-small cell lung cancer. Oncotarget. 2018;9(101):37589–607.

59. Mayekar MK, Bivona TG. Current landscape of targeted therapy in lung cancer. Clin Pharmacol Ther. 2017;102(5):757–64.

60. Lindeman NI, Cagle PT, Beasley MB, Chitale DA, Dacic S, Giaccone G, et al. Molecular testing guideline for selection of lung cancer patients for EGFR and ALK tyrosine kinase inhibitors: guideline from the College of American Pathologists, International Association for the Study of Lung Cancer, and Association for Molecular Pathology. J Thorac Oncol Off Publ Int Assoc Study Lung Cancer. 2013;8(7):823–59.

61. Kosaka T, Yatabe Y, Endoh H, Yoshida K, Hida T, Tsuboi M, et al. Analysis of epidermal growth factor receptor gene mutation in patients with non-small cell lung cancer and acquired resistance to gefitinib. Clin Cancer Res. 2006;12(19):5764–9.

62. Balak MN, Gong Y, Riely GJ, Somwar R, Li AR, Zakowski MF, et al. Novel D761Y and common secondary T790M mutations in epidermal growth factor receptor-mutant lung adenocarcinomas with acquired resistance to kinase inhibitors. Clin Cancer Res. 2006;12(21):6494–501.

63. Yu HA, Arcila ME, Rekhtman N, Sima CS, Zakowski MF, Pao W, et al. Analysis of tumor specimens at the time of acquired resistance to EGFR-TKI therapy in 155 patients with EGFR-mutant lung cancers. Clin Cancer Res. 2013;19(8):2240–7.

64. Bean J, Brennan C, Shih J-Y, Riely G, Viale A, Wang L, et al. MET amplification occurs with or without T790M mutations in EGFR mutant lung tumors with acquired resistance to gefitinib or erlotinib. Proc Natl Acad Sci U S A. 2007;104(52):20932–7.

65. Cipriani NA, Abidoye OO, Vokes E, Salgia R. MET as a target for treatment of chest tumors. Lung Cancer. 2009;63(2):169–79.

66. Baglivo S, Ludovini V, Sidoni A, Metro G, Ricciuti B, Siggillino A, et al. Large cell neuroendocrine carcinoma transformation and EGFR -T790M mutation as coexisting mechanisms of acquired resistance to EGFR-TKIs in lung cancer. Mayo Clin Proc. 2017;92(8):1304–11.

67. Sequist LV, Waltman BA, Dias-Santagata D, Digumarthy S, Turke AB, Fidias P, et al. Genotypic and histological evolution of lung cancers acquiring resistance to EGFR inhibitors. Sci Transl Med. 2011;3(75):75ra26.

68. Boland JM, Erdogan S, Vasmatzis G, Yang P, Tillmans LS, Johnson MRE, et al. Anaplastic lymphoma kinase immunoreactivity correlates with ALK gene rearrangement and transcriptional up-regulation in non–small cell lung carcinomas. Hum Pathol. 2009;40(8):1152–8.

69. Chin LP, Soo RA, Soong R, Ou S-HI. Targeting ROS1 with anaplastic lymphoma kinase inhibitors: a promising therapeutic strategy for a newly defined molecular subset of non-small-cell lung cancer. J Thorac Oncol Off Publ Int Assoc Study Lung Cancer. 2012;7(11):1625–30.

70. Pikor LA, Ramnarine VR, Lam S, Lam WL. Genetic alterations defining NSCLC subtypes and their therapeutic implications. Lung Cancer. 2013;82(2):179–89.

71. Rimkunas VM, Crosby KE, Li D, Hu Y, Kelly ME, Gu T-L, et al. Analysis of receptor tyrosine kinase ROS1-positive tumors in non-small cell lung cancer: identification of a FIG-ROS1 fusion. Clin Cancer Res. 2012;18(16):4449–57.

72. Bergethon K, Shaw AT, Ignatius Ou S-H, Katayama R, Lovly CM, McDonald NT, et al. ROS1 rearrangements define a unique molecular class of lung cancers. J Clin Oncol. 2012;30(8):863–70.

73. Solomon BJ, Mok T, Kim D-W, Wu Y-L, Nakagawa K, Mekhail T, et al. First-line crizotinib versus chemotherapy in ALK -positive lung cancer. N Engl J Med. 2014;371(23):2167–77.

74. Soria J-C, Tan DSW, Chiari R, Wu Y-L, Paz-Ares L, Wolf J, et al. First-line ceritinib versus platinum-based chemotherapy in advanced ALK-rearranged non-small-cell lung cancer (ASCEND-4): a randomised, open-label, phase 3 study. Lancet Lond Engl. 2017;389(10072):917–29.

75. Ignatius Ou S-H, Azada M, Hsiang DJ, Herman JM, Kain TS, Siwak-Tapp C, et al. Next-generation sequencing reveals a Novel NSCLC ALK F1174V mutation and confirms ALK G1202R mutation confers high-level resistance to alectinib (CH5424802/RO5424802) in ALK-rearranged NSCLC patients who progressed on crizotinib. J Thorac Oncol Off Publ Int Assoc Study Lung Cancer. 2014;9(4):549–53.

76. Zeng L, Li Y, Xiao L, Xiong Y, Liu L, Jiang W, et al. Crizotinib presented with promising efficacy but for concomitant mutation in next-generation sequencing-identified ROS1-rearranged non-small-cell lung cancer. OncoTargets Ther. 2018;11:6937–45.

77. Kinno T, Tsuta K, Shiraishi K, Mizukami T, Suzuki M, Yoshida A, et al. Clinicopathological features of nonsmall cell lung carcinomas with BRAF mutations. Ann Oncol. 2014;25(1):138–42.

78. Planchard D, Besse B, Groen HJM, Souquet P-J, Quoix E, Baik CS, et al. Dabrafenib plus trametinib in patients with previously treated BRAF(V600E)-mutant metastatic non-small cell lung cancer: an open-label, multicentre phase 2 trial. Lancet Oncol. 2016;17(7):984–93.

79. Paik PK, Arcila ME, Fara M, Sima CS, Miller VA, Kris MG, et al. Clinical characteristics of patients with lung adenocarcinomas harboring *BRAF* mutations. J Clin Oncol. 2011;29(15):2046–51.

80. Villaruz LC, Socinski MA, Abberbock S, Berry LD, Johnson BE, Kwiatkowski DJ, et al. Clinicopathologic features and outcomes of patients with lung adenocarcinomas harboring *BRAF* mutations in the lung cancer mutation consortium: *BRAF* mutations in lung adenocarcinomas. Cancer. 2015;121(3):448–56.

81. Litvak AM, Paik PK, Woo KM, Sima CS, Hellmann MD, Arcila ME, et al. Clinical characteristics and course of 63 patients with BRAF mutant lung cancers. J Thorac Oncol. 2014;9(11):1669–74.

82. Hyman DM, Puzanov I, Subbiah V, Faris JE, Chau I, Blay J-Y, et al. Vemurafenib in multiple nonmelanoma cancers with *BRAF* V600 mutations. N Engl J Med. 2015;373(8):726–36.

83. Planchard D, Smit EF, Groen HJM, Mazieres J, Besse B, Helland Å, et al. Dabrafenib plus trametinib in patients with previously untreated BRAFV600E-mutant metastatic non-small-cell lung cancer: an open-label, phase 2 trial. Lancet Oncol. 2017;18(10):1307–16.

84. Drilon A, Laetsch TW, Kummar S, DuBois SG, Lassen UN, Demetri GD, et al. Efficacy of larotrectinib in *TRK* fusion–positive cancers in adults and children. N Engl J Med. 2018;378(8):731–9.

85. Vaishnavi A, Capelletti M, Le AT, Kako S, Butaney M, Ercan D, et al. Oncogenic and drug-sensitive NTRK1 rearrangements in lung cancer. Nat Med. 2013;19(11):1469–72.

86. Onozato R, Kosaka T, Kuwano H, Sekido Y, Yatabe Y, Mitsudomi T. Activation of MET by gene amplification or by splice mutations deleting the juxta-membrane domain in primary resected lung cancers. J Thorac Oncol Off Publ Int Assoc Study Lung Cancer. 2009;4(1):5–11.

87. Okuda K, Sasaki H, Yukiue H, Yano M, Fujii Y. Met gene copy number predicts the prognosis for completely resected non-small cell lung cancer. Cancer Sci. 2008;99(11):2280–5.

88. Awad MM, Oxnard GR, Jackman DM, Savukoski DO, Hall D, Shivdasani P, et al. *MET* exon 14 mutations in non–small-cell lung cancer are associated with advanced age and stage-dependent *MET* genomic amplification and c-met overexpression. J Clin Oncol. 2016;34(7):721–30.

89. Frampton GM, Ali SM, Rosenzweig M, Chmielecki J, Lu X, Bauer TM, et al. Activation of MET via diverse exon 14 splicing alterations occurs in multiple tumor types and confers clinical sensitivity to MET inhibitors. Cancer Discov. 2015;5(8):850–9.

90. Paik PK, Drilon A, Fan P-D, Yu H, Rekhtman N, Ginsberg MS, et al. Response to MET inhibitors in patients with stage IV lung adenocarcinomas harboring MET mutations causing exon 14 skipping. Cancer Discov. 2015;5(8):842–9.

91. Arcila ME, Chaft JE, Nafa K, Roy-Chowdhuri S, Lau C, Zaidinski M, et al. Prevalence, clinico-pathologic associations, and molecular spectrum of ERBB2 (HER2) tyrosine kinase mutations in lung adenocarcinomas. Clin Cancer Res. 2012;18(18):4910–8.

92. Pillai RN, Behera M, Berry LD, Rossi MR, Kris MG, Johnson BE, et al. *HER2* mutations in lung adenocarcinomas: a report from the lung cancer mutation consortium: *HER2* mutations in lung adenocarcinomas. Cancer. 2017;123(21):4099–105.

93. Mazières J, Peters S, Lepage B, Cortot AB, Barlesi F, Beau-Faller M, et al. Lung cancer that harbors an *HER2* mutation: epidemiologic characteristics and therapeutic perspectives. J Clin Oncol. 2013;31(16):1997–2003.

94. Wang R, Hu H, Pan Y, Li Y, Ye T, Li C, et al. *RET* fusions define a unique molecular and clinicopathologic subtype of non–small-cell lung cancer. J Clin Oncol. 2012;30(35):4352–9.

95. Ju YS, Lee W-C, Shin J-Y, Lee S, Bleazard T, Won J-K, et al. A transforming KIF5B and RET gene fusion in lung adenocarcinoma revealed from whole-genome and transcriptome sequencing. Genome Res. 2012;22(3):436–45.

96. Li F, Feng Y, Fang R, Fang Z, Xia J, Han X, et al. Identification of RET gene fusion by exon array analyses in "pan-negative" lung cancer from never smokers. Cell Res. 2012;22(5):928–31.

97. Kohno T, Ichikawa H, Totoki Y, Yasuda K, Hiramoto M, Nammo T, et al. KIF5B-RET fusions in lung adenocarcinoma. Nat Med. 2012;18(3):375–7.

98. Mukhopadhyay S, Pennell NA, Ali SM, Ross JS, Ma PC, Velcheti V. RET-rearranged lung adenocarcinomas with lymphangitic spread, psammoma bodies, and clinical responses to cabozantinib. J Thorac Oncol. 2014;9(11):1714–9.

99. Takeuchi K, Soda M, Togashi Y, Suzuki R, Sakata S, Hatano S, et al. RET, ROS1 and ALK fusions in lung cancer. Nat Med. 2012;18(3):378–81.

100. Moran DM, Trusk PB, Pry K, Paz K, Sidransky D, Bacus SS. KRAS mutation status is associated with enhanced dependency on folate metabolism pathways in non-small cell lung cancer cells. Mol Cancer Ther. 2014;13(6):1611–24.

101. Campbell JD, Alexandrov A, Kim J, Wala J, Berger AH, Pedamallu CS, et al. Distinct patterns of somatic genome alterations in lung adenocarcinomas and squamous cell carcinomas. Nat Genet. 2016;48(6):607–16.

102. Cai D, Choi PS, Gelbard M, Meyerson M. Identification and characterization of oncogenic SOS1 mutations in lung adenocarcinoma. Mol Cancer Res MCR. 2019;17(4):1002–12.

103. The Cancer Genome Atlas Research Network. Comprehensive genomic characterization of squamous cell lung cancers. Nature. 2012 Sep;489(7417):519–25.

104. Australian Pancreatic Cancer Genome Initiative, ICGC Breast Cancer Consortium, ICGC MMML-Seq Consortium, ICGC PedBrain, Alexandrov LB, Nik-Zainal S, et al. Signatures of mutational processes in human cancer. Nature. 2013;500(7463):415–21.

105. Roberts SA, Lawrence MS, Klimczak LJ, Grimm SA, Fargo D, Stojanov P, et al. An APOBEC cytidine deaminase mutagenesis pattern is widespread in human cancers. Nat Genet. 2013;45(9):970–6.

106. Zhang J, Fujimoto J, Zhang J, Wedge DC, Song X, Zhang J, et al. Intratumor heterogeneity in localized lung adenocarcinomas delineated by multiregion sequencing. Science. 2014;346(6206):256–9.

107. de Bruin EC, McGranahan N, Mitter R, Salm M, Wedge DC, Yates L, et al. Spatial and temporal diversity in genomic instability processes defines lung cancer evolution. Science. 2014;346(6206):251–6.

108. Pleasance ED, Stephens PJ, O'Meara S, McBride DJ, Meynert A, Jones D, et al. A small-cell lung cancer genome with complex signatures of tobacco exposure. Nature. 2010;463(7278):184–90.

109. Byers LA, Rudin CM. Small cell lung cancer: where do we go from here?: SCLC: where do we go from here? Cancer. 2015;121(5):664–72.

110. Wistuba I. Molecular genetics of small cell lung carcinoma. Semin Oncol. 2001;28:3–13.

111. Maley CC, Aktipis A, Graham TA, Sottoriva A, Boddy AM, Janiszewska M, et al. Classifying the evolutionary and ecological features of neoplasms. Nat Rev Cancer. 2017;17(10):605–19.

112. Greaves M, Maley CC. Clonal evolution in cancer. Nature. 2012;481(7381):306–13.

113. Jamal-Hanjani M, Wilson GA, McGranahan N, Birkbak NJ, Watkins TBK, Veeriah S, et al. Tracking the evolution of non-small-cell lung cancer. N Engl J Med. 2017;376(22):2109–21.

114. Merker JD, Oxnard GR, Compton C, Diehn M, Hurley P, Lazar AJ, et al. Circulating tumor DNA analysis in patients with cancer: American Society of Clinical Oncology and College of American Pathologists Joint Review. J Clin Oncol. 2018;36(16):1631–41.

115. Abbosh C, Birkbak NJ, Wilson GA, Jamal-Hanjani M, Constantin T, Salari R, et al. Phylogenetic ctDNA analysis depicts early-stage lung cancer evolution. Nature. 2017;545(7655):446–51.

Part III

Biomarkers

Chest Imaging for Precision Medicine

Samuel Y. Ash, Raúl San José Estépar,
and George R. Washko

Introduction

Thoracic imaging has become an integral part of clinical care for patients with acute and chronic respiratory conditions. This care includes everything from population-based public health efforts such as lung cancer screening, to evermore sophisticated and individualized approaches that enable providers to leverage specific clinical images to guide a single patient's care [1, 2]. This broad deployment includes an ever-growing number of imaging tools, developed and validated by a robust research community, that can be used for disease detection and risk stratification as well as for prognostication and the monitoring of response to therapeutic intervention. The ability of medical imaging to provide a detailed view of an individual patient's anatomy, and in some case of some modalities, their physiology, makes it a key component in the advancement of precision medicine, and the medical images themselves may yield additional insight

into a patient's genes, environment, and lifestyle [3]. More generally, imaging may help to enable the so-called "deep-phenotyping" and stratification by providing information that is not readily available from the traditional "signs and symptoms" approach to medical diagnosis [4].

In the following chapter we will briefly review the introduction of medical imaging to clinical care, discuss how research efforts have shaped the clinical utilization of such technology and then provide some discussion on where imaging will take us in the next 10–20 years. Although it may be argued where "standard medical care" ends and "precision medicine" begins, we suggest that medical imaging in general, and thoracic imaging in particular, is already helping to provide precision medicine in day-to-day medical care, and that recent and coming advances in imaging technologies, especially quantitative approaches to image post-processing, are likely to continue to continue to expand the role of medical imaging in precision medicine in the decades to come.

S. Y. Ash (✉) · G. R. Washko
Pulmonary and Critical Care Medicine, Brigham and
Women's Hospital, Boston, MA, USA
e-mail: syash@bwh.harvard.edu; gwashko@bwh.harvard.edu

R. S. J. Estépar
Radiology, Brigham and Women's Hospital,
Boston, MA, USA
e-mail: rsanjose@bwh.harvard.edu

Chest X-Ray

The discovery of the X-ray by Wilhelm Conrad Rontgen was first reported in 1895, and physicians quickly co-opted the technology to make new observations in thoracic disease [5]. Reports soon appeared describing the change in the shape

© Springer Nature Switzerland AG 2020
J. L. Gomez et al. (eds.), *Precision in Pulmonary, Critical Care, and Sleep Medicine*,
Respiratory Medicine, https://doi.org/10.1007/978-3-030-31507-8_8

of the heart with contraction, motion of the diaphragms with respiration and possibly one of the first examples of imaging-enabled precision medicine, the utility of X-rays to plan the surgical extraction of bullets from soldiers with gunshot wounds [5]. As technology evolved to make X-ray equipment more available, X-ray imaging of the chest became a commonplace part of the clinical evaluation of disease. Although we may not always recognize an individual chest X-ray's role in advancing personalized medical care, its role in providing clues as to a patient's genes, environment, and lifestyle cannot be overstated [3].

Part of the strength of chest X-ray in particular is the ability to quickly identify features of multiple thoracic structures that are associated with underlying pathology. This includes not only the lungs but also the heart and the major vessels, as well as the bony structures and soft tissues. For example, a young patient with recurrent respiratory infections, sputum production, and shortness of breath may carry diagnoses that range from asthma to cystic fibrosis. However, a simple chest X-ray revealing dextrocardia suggests she is more likely to have a genetic disorder related to ciliary function than another disease with a similar phenotype (Fig. 8.1) [6]. This finding therefore clearly allows further evaluation and therapy to be tailored to that individual.

More recently, the growth of artificial intelligence and advances in computer vision have led to exciting developments in the analysis of chest X-rays that may ultimately improve the precision with which care is provided on a large scale. For example, Lakhani et al. recently developed a technique that enables the automated detection of tuberculosis on chest X-ray [7]. This approach utilizes deep convolutional neural networks (DCNN), a form of machine learning that has proven to be well suited to image analysis. More specifically, using a combination of two DCNN models, AlexNet and GooLeNet, the authors developed a network that was able to identify tuberculosis with 96% accuracy [7]. This work and similar approaches to identify other pathologies on chest X-rays is an area of active investigation that many research groups are currently working to advance into more routine clinical care. This would enable clinicians and patients to have fast access to results and information about a patient's diagnosis and exposures that might not otherwise be quickly available in a resource limited setting.

Computed Tomography

One of the next great leaps in medical imaging came in the 1970s with the introduction of computed tomographic imaging [8]. Physicians were no longer limited to the 2-D superimposition of features, and they could now obtain in-vivo 3-D images of solid organs in their native physiologic state. Not only did this enable clinicians to "see" structures more clearly and easily, but also because CT uses a relatively standardized display to represent the attenuation properties of tissues (measured in Hounsfield Units), the research community quickly appreciated that quantitative approaches to image processing could provide new objective measures to compliment visual interpretation [8]. Over the following sections we will discuss the current use of thoracic CT in enabling precision medicine, which primarily includes the use of qualitative or visual analysis of CT images, and also highlight several new and innovative quantitative approaches that have the potential to transform our approach to individual patients and conditions.

It is difficult to overstate the importance of thoracic CT imaging for providing information that enables the tailoring of medical care. Its utility has led to a ubiquity that makes it easy to forget its

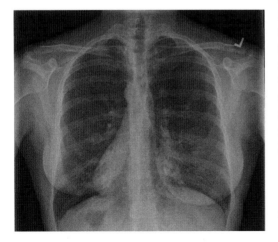

Fig. 8.1 Dextrocardia

importance in patient stratification, and in fact one could argue that it has become a part of "standard" patient evaluation, and because of that, it should not be considered as part of deep phenotyping at all. Putting that argument aside, it is worth remembering the incredible volume of information that it provides is critically important in targeting therapy and often not readily available from other common means of clinical evaluation.

As a case example, consider a patient presenting to the emergency department with shortness of breath and chest pain. Frequently even a detailed history and exam may not reveal the underlying cause, and findings from other standard studies such as electrocardiograms and laboratory studies may be nonspecific or otherwise unrevealing. A single chest CT in such a case can reveal everything from a pulmonary embolism, to a pneumothorax, to a pericardial effusion, each of which leads to a different and specific targeted set of therapies; imaging therefore immediate distinguishes "a given patient from other patients with [a] similar clinical presentation" [9, 10].

Even in the absence of acute findings, the CT imaging study may show chronic findings like emphysema, pulmonary fibrosis, or coronary calcification that help phenotype the patient and inform additional testing [11, 12]. In addition, specific features related to findings like emphysema may be useful for gaining insight into an individual patient's genetic risk factors for a disease and possibly even help direct therapy. For example, basilar predominant, panlobular emphysema on chest CT imaging is strongly suggestive of alpha-1-antitrypsin (AAT) deficiency, an autosomal dominant inherited disorder the treatment for which includes intravenous augmentation of the proteinase inhibitor AAT [13, 14]. Thus, thoracic CT imaging may not only help provide clues as to a patient's genotype, but also inform therapy [3, 10].

More recently, it has been recognized that beyond establishing a diagnosis, utilizing additional ancillary findings on chest CT may also help guide therapeutic decisions even within a particular condition. For example, not only is chest CT far more accurate than combined history and physical scores such as the Wells Score and the Revised Geneva Score for the diagnosis of pulmonary embolism, but also additional findings on chest CT in patients with pulmonary emboli may help with risk stratification and guide therapeutic decisions [15, 16]. For example, Piazza et al. found that catheter-directed fibrinoloysis in patients with massive and sub-massive pulmonary emboli decreased RV dilation, reduced pulmonary hypertension, and decreased anatomic thrombus burden without increasing the risk of intracranial hemorrhage. The criteria they utilized to identify patients for their study included pulmonary embolism as well as an increased ratio of the right ventricular to left ventricular size on CT [17]. Fig. 8.2 shows sample cardiac models based on volumetric non-contrast CT images of the right (blue) and left (red) ventricles in three subjects with varying degrees of respiratory disease. For example, the subject on the far left is a smoker without COPD who has a right ventricular to left ventricular ratio (RV/LV) of 0.5, a right ventricular systolic pressure (RVSP) of of 20 and no evidence of ventricular dysfunction. The middle image is from a subject with GOLD 3 COPD who has an RV/LV of 0.8, RV dilation and an elevated RVSP of 47. Finally, the subject on the far right has GOLD 3 COPD with LV dilation and an ejection fraction of 35%. However, recent research has shown that novel statistical techniques can be used to perform automated, volumetric measures of ventricular size, even on non-electrocardiogram gated, non-contrast chest CT scans, potentially enabling these measures to become part of routine care in the future and providing additional insights into the disparate cardiac implications of a variety of chest diseases (Fig. 8.2) [18]. Thus, chest CT may be of use not only in making the diagnosis of pulmonary embolism but also in guiding therapy.

Perhaps one of the biggest potential areas of growth for precision medicine in CT imaging is growing recognition of the importance and power of "incidental" findings on chest CT. One of the greatest fears associated with the broader adoption of large-scale CT screening programs for diseases like lung cancer has been the explosion of incidental findings on these studies and how to manage them [1]. While this remains a concern, it also represents a significant opportunity for both the research and clinical communities in terms of deep phenotyping and patient stratification. From a research standpoint, the large, multicenter, lon-

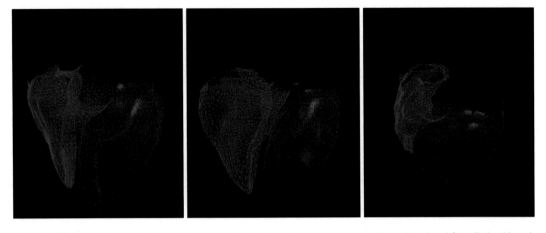

Fig. 8.2 Elevated right ventricular to left ventricular size in acute pulmonary embolism. (Reprinted from Rahaghi et al. [18] with permission from Elsevier)

gitudinal CT databases created as part of the National Lung Cancer Screening Trial (NLST) and Nederland-Leuvens Longkanker Screenings Onderzoek (NELSON) are tremendous resources for the identification of novel imaging biomarkers that may ultimately inform patient stratification and care. Combined with studies from other large research cohorts, incidental findings from NLST and NELSON have also begun to inform clinical research and care [1, 19].

For example, multiple studies have now demonstrated that up to 10% of current and former smokers have subtle, high density changes in the lung parenchyma seen on chest CT [20, 21]. These changes, often termed interstitial lung abnormalities, have been associated with lower lung function, worse exercise capacity, an increased risk of death and with a single nucleotide polymorphism associated with idiopathic pulmonary fibrosis [22–30]. Combined, these findings suggest that interstitial lung abnormalities may, in some instances, represent early or subtle evidence of pulmonary fibrosis. This is particularly exciting because pulmonary fibrosis is associated with extremely high mortality, and the only currently available pharmacologic treatments slow the disease's progression but do not reverse damage that has already been done [31, 32]. Thus, earlier diagnosis of the disease could be beneficial. Ongoing work is seeking to better define these interstitial lung abnormalities, and, potentially in conjunction with other protein or genetic biomarkers, to identify those individuals with inter-

stitial lung abnormalities at the highest risk for pulmonary fibrosis with the hope of eventually determining if anti-fibrotic medications are useful in those individuals. These incidental findings on a lung cancer screening chest CT may therefore ultimately be of significant utility in phenotyping a patient and advancing precision medicine.

In addition to high density changes such as interstitial lung abnormalities, low density changes, particularly emphysema, on chest CT have also shown promise for personalizing medical care for patients. For example, the National Emphysema Treatment Trial (NETT) evaluated the effect of lung volume reduction surgery on outcomes in patients with COPD. [33] It found that the procedure most benefitted patients with severe upper lobe predominant emphysema who had a decreased exercise capacity. Subsequent work has focused on the use of alternative methods for lung volume reduction, such as using bronchoscopically placed valves and coils, some of which have recently been approved by the Food and Drug Administration (FDA) for clinical use [34, 35]. Appropriate stratification using CT imaging is central to the evaluation of patients for both surgical and bronchoscopic lung volume reduction, including not only upper lobe predominant disease, but also, in the case of the bronchoscopic devices, complete fissures to ensure minimal collateral air flow and ensure adequate deflation of the upper lobes [36, 37]. Thus CT imaging is key to applying these interventions in a suitably precise way.

In addition to the largely visual analysis performed on the CT images as part of NETT, additional work has been done to take advantage of potential quantitative measurements of emphysema and other lung imaging findings on CT. There are several objective approaches to detect and quantify emphysema, and some of the most straightforward are based on selecting a HU threshold that demarcates emphysema from non-emphysematous tissue [38, 39]. These methods have been extensively benchmarked against histologic investigation, and the ensuing application of such techniques demonstrated that emphysema scored by CT is related to lung function but that there is a broad range of emphysema present for a given degree of airflow obstruction [40–44].

These approaches may also allow for the precise application and monitoring of pharmacologic interventions. For example, in 2016 investigators reported the results of a multicenter study of augmentation therapy in patients with alpha-1 antitrypsin deficiency called RAPID [13]. Those study participants receiving augmentation therapy had significantly less progression of emphysema than their placebo-controlled counterparts. There was no significant effect of augmentation therapy on other clinical parameters such as decline in lung function. Emphysema progression on CT scan is now being evaluated by the COPD Biomarker Qualification Consortium for qualification as an accepted biomarker by the United States Food and Drug Administration (FDA) for use in clinical investigation [13, 45, 46].

The objective detection and quantification of low attenuation areas on CT has also been expanded and applied to chronic conditions characterized by cystic destruction of the lung parenchyma. One of the best examples of this are the increasing number of efforts focused on LAM. LAM is a chronic progressive disease characterized by upper lobe predominant cysts in the lung tissue [47]. It is believed that these cysts contribute to lung dysfunction and are therefore a target of pharmacologic therapy [48, 49]. Like COPD, the great heterogeneity of presentation and progression of LAM makes the completion of trials with definitive clinical outcomes challenging. Unlike COPD, LAM is a relatively rare disease and even with a highly motivated network of patients, physicians, and advocates, large placebo-controlled trials with definitive clinical outcomes are not feasible [50]. For this reason, the biomedical community is keenly interested in using imaging to identify subsets of disease and use features such as cyst size and count as intermediate endpoints for interventional studies. For example, Argula et al. have developed a measure of both cyst size and number and shown that it is correlated with the response to treatment of LAM [51]. Additional work may ultimately reveal if certain imaging features predict treatment response in multiple cystic lung disease, allowing treatment to be tailored to the individual patient.

Magnetic Resonance Imaging

Although not as widely employed in pulmonary disease as CT imaging, magnetic resonance imaging (MRI) has proven exceedingly useful for the phenotyping of other chest diseases such as cardiac disease [52]. The breadth of cardiac MRI imaging and its role in precision medicine is beyond the scope of this review. However, it is worth noting the role of cardiac MRI in one particular area with regard to disease stratification: sarcoidosis. Clinically, the prevalence of cardiac involvement in patients with systemic sarcoidosis has been estimated to be between 20% and 27% in the United States and as high as 58% in Japan [53, 54]. However, autopsy studies suggest this may be a significant underestimate of the disease burden [53–55]. While some patients with cardiac involvement in sarcoidosis present with dramatic signs and symptoms including syncope or even sudden cardiac death, many others may have vague symptoms of dyspnea or fatigue or may be entirely asymptomatic [56]. Given the significant risk of sudden cardiac death associated with cardiac sarcoidosis and the need to consider placement of an automatic internal cardioverter-defibrillator (AICD), identifying those patients with sarcoidosis who have cardiac involvement is of great importance [57]. Although due to cost and access, it has not yet become the primary screening tool for cardiac sarcoidosis, cardiac MRI has been shown to be highly accurate, with a sensitivity of likely greater than 90% for cardiac involvement, and if its cost were to improve then it may ultimately become a more routine part of sarcoid evaluation [58].

While, the use of MRI remains in respiratory care remains limited because the expansive air–liquid interface that makes the lung so exceptional at gas exchange also creates an artifact which degrades standard proton image quality, it does have several potential advantages compared to CT imaging for certain forms of lung imaging, including the lack of ionizing radiation, higher resolution and functional information [8, 59, 60, 61]. Investigational MRI studies using hyperpolarized oxygen and noble gases have leveraged these advantages to enable the in vivo assessments of distal airspace micro-architecture, regional ventilation, and microvascular perfusion [61]. A prime example of this and the potential role of MRI in precision pulmonary medicine is in the planning of bronchial thermoplasty. In a small investigational study, Thomen et al. performed both hyperpolarized (Helium 3) enhanced MRI and chest CT imaging of 6 healthy volunteers and 10 patients with severe asthma [62]. Seven of the patients with severe asthma then received bronchial thermoplasty and were imaged a second time. By combining the functional information obtained from MRI with structural information from CT, the investigators were able to measure and compare segment to segment differences in ventilation between the groups and found significant differences between controls and those with severe asthma [62]. This use of multiple imaging modalities highlights not only the strength of MRI, but also the potential benefits to combining the information gained by using multiple types of imaging.

Positron Emission Tomography

Another imaging modality that has been used in combination with CT imaging is positron emission tomography (PET). While there are a wide range of radiopharmaceuticals used in PET imaging, we will focus on [18F]fluorodeoxyglucose (FDG) PET imaging as it is the most commonly used in clinical imaging. FDG-PET uses radiola-

beled glucose (FDG) to provide three-dimensional information on glucose metabolism [63]. This thereby enables the evaluation of local or tissue-specific metabolic features. Used in combination with co-registered CT imaging, areas of with evidence of increased glucose metabolism can then be precisely located within the chest or the rest of the body [63]. Clinically, FDG-PET is best known for its role in the evaluation of known or suspected malignancy, and in some ways this use can be seen as a type of precision medicine approach by helping to stage patients: FDG-PET enables them to be stratified based on pathophysiology not readily apparent through based on signs and symptoms, ultimately directly impacting their planned care and clinical course [64].

From a research standpoint, these same PET techniques can be applied to the lung to ascertain the regional distribution of metabolic activity in parenchymal lung diseases such as emphysema or pulmonary fibrosis [65, 66]. This information may in turn provide insight into the pathobiology of disease or be prognostic for response to therapeutic intervention. As with MRI, PET is also amenable to the use of multiple imaging agents and the potential additional information that can be obtained from PET is best exemplified through its extensive application in the assessment of lung perfusion in health and disease [67].

Ultrasound

Similar to MRI and PET, ultrasound is another imaging modality that is well suited to providing functional information about chest diseases. It should be noted that cardiac ultrasound, referred to as echocardiography, is clearly a very well-established imaging modality. Although the breadth of echocardiography is beyond the scope of this review, it is difficult to overstate its importance in the phenotyping of patients with cardiac disease [68, 69]. From a pulmonary standpoint, ultrasound has found widespread clinical use in the evaluation of the pleura and pleural space, especially with identifying and localizing pleural effusions and pneumothoraces [70, 71]. However, prior and ongoing research have increasingly shown that ultrasonography may be useful in the evaluation of the lung parenchyma itself. For example, specific ultrasound protocols may be able to help differentiate between areas of lung consolidation and atelectasis [72]. These techniques are of particular interest because of the lack of ionizing radiation associated with ultrasound. In addition, its relatively low cost and portability means that it can be used by the clinician at the bedside both in the developed as well as in the developing world, potentially improving the ability to sub-stratify patients in more resource limited settings [73].

Conclusion and Future Directions

Over the past 125 years, advances in chest imaging, including chest radiography, CT, MRI, PET, and ultrasound, have dramatically changed our practice of medicine and yielded countless insights into the etiology and manifestations of chest diseases. In many ways chest imaging is already fulfilling the mission of precision medicine to be able to target treatments to the needs of individual patients based on information not available from the traditional "signs and symptoms" approach, applying knowledge gained from large-scale research studies on diseases that include pulmonary vascular disease, emphysema, and interstitial lung disease, to identify patients who may respond to particular therapies. The growth of artificial intelligence and computer vision raises the possibility of rapidly obtaining even more information from medical imaging of the chest and further refining the phenotyping that imaging allows in order to identify true "deep phenotypes" with specific genetic and clinical associations. Because of this, imaging may ultimately become even more important in the care of patients with chest diseases than it already is today.

References

1. National Lung Screening Trial Research T, Aberle DR, Adams AM, Berg CD, Black WC, Clapp JD, et al. Reduced lung-cancer mortality with low-dose computed tomographic screening. N Engl J Med. 2011;365(5):395–409.
2. Agusti A, Bafadhel M, Beasley R, Bel EH, Faner R, Gibson PG, et al. Precision medicine in airway diseases: moving to clinical practice. Eur Respir J. 2017;50(4):1701655.
3. The Precision Medicine Initiative. Available from: https://obamawhitehouse.archives.gov/precision-medicine.
4. Konig IR, Fuchs O, Hansen G, von Mutius E, Kopp MV. What is precision medicine? Eur Respir J. 2017;50(4):1700391.
5. Morgan RH, Lewis I. The roentgen ray: its past and future. Dis Chest. 1945;11:502–10.
6. Knowles MR, Zariwala M, Leigh M. Primary ciliary dyskinesia. Clin Chest Med. 2016;37(3):449–61.
7. Lakhani P, Sundaram B. Deep learning at chest radiography: automated classification of pulmonary tuberculosis by using convolutional neural networks. Radiology. 2017;284(2):574–82. 162326.
8. Brooks RA, Di Chiro G. Theory of image reconstruction in computed tomography. Radiology. 1975;117(3 Pt 1):561–72.
9. White CS, Kuo D. Chest pain in the emergency department: role of multidetector CT. Radiology. 2007;245(3):672–81.
10. Jameson JL, Longo DL. Precision medicine–personalized, problematic, and promising. N Engl J Med. 2015;372(23):2229–34.
11. Koo HK, Jin KN, Kim DK, Chung HS, Lee CH. Association of incidental emphysema with annual lung function decline and future development of airflow limitation. Int J Chron Obstruct Pulmon Dis. 2016;11:161–6.
12. Washko GR, Lynch DA, Matsuoka S, Ross JC, Umeoka S, Diaz A, et al. Identification of early interstitial lung disease in smokers from the COPDGene Study. Acad Radiol. 2010;17(1):48–53.
13. Chapman KR, Burdon JG, Piitulainen E, Sandhaus RA, Seersholm N, Stocks JM, et al. Intravenous augmentation treatment and lung density in severe alpha1 antitrypsin deficiency (RAPID): a randomised, double-blind, placebo-controlled trial. Lancet. 2015;386(9991):360–8.
14. Tarkoff MP, Kueppers F, Miller WF. Pulmonary emphysema and alpha 1-antitrypsin deficiency. Am J Med. 1968;45(2):220–8.
15. Teigen CL, Maus TP, Sheedy PF, Johnson CM, Stanson AW, Welch TJ. Pulmonary embolism: diagnosis with electron-beam CT. Radiology. 1993;188(3):839–45.
16. Shen JH, Chen HL, Chen JR, Xing JL, Gu P, Zhu BF. Comparison of the Wells score with the revised Geneva score for assessing suspected pulmonary embolism: a systematic review and meta-analysis. J Thromb Thrombolysis. 2016;41(3):482–92.
17. Piazza G, Hohlfelder B, Jaff MR, Ouriel K, Engelhardt TC, Sterling KM, et al. A prospective, single-arm, multicenter trial of ultrasound-facilitated, catheter-directed, low-dose fibrinolysis for acute massive and submassive pulmonary embolism: The SEATTLE II Study. JACC Cardiovasc Interv. 2015;8(10):1382–92.

18. Rahaghi FN, Sanchez-Ferrero GV, Minhas JK, Come CE, De La Bruere IA, Wells JM, et al. Ventricular geometry from non-contrast non-ECG gated CT scans: an imaging maker of cardiopulmonary disease in smokers. Acad Radiol. 2017;24(5):594–602.

19. Ru Zhao Y, Xie X, de Koning HJ, Mali WP, Vliegenthart R, Oudkerk M. NELSON lung cancer screening study. Cancer Imaging. 2011;11 Spec No A:S79–84.

20. Ash SY, Harmouche R, Ross JC, Diaz AA, Hunninghake GM, Putman RK, et al. The objective identification and quantification of interstitial lung abnormalities in smokers. Acad Radiol. 2017;24(8):941–6.

21. Jin GY, Lynch D, Chawla A, Garg K, Tammemagi MC, Sahin H, et al. Interstitial lung abnormalities in a CT lung cancer screening population: prevalence and progression rate. Radiology. 2013;268(2):563–71.

22. Putman RK, Hunninghake GM, Dieffenbach PB, Barragan-Bradford D, Serhan K, Adams U, et al. Interstitial lung abnormalities are associated with acute respiratory distress syndrome. Am J Respir Crit Care Med. 2017;195(1):138–41.

23. Ash SY, Harmouche R, Putman RK, Ross JC, Diaz AA, Hunninghake GM, et al. Clinical and genetic associations of objectively identified interstitial changes in smokers. Chest. 2017;152(4):780–91.

24. Putman RK, Hatabu H, Araki T, Gudmundsson G, Gao W, Nishino M, et al. Association between interstitial lung abnormalities and all-cause mortality. JAMA. 2016;315(7):672–81.

25. Doyle TJ, Dellaripa PF, Batra K, Frits ML, Iannaccone CK, Hatabu H, et al. Functional impact of a spectrum of interstitial lung abnormalities in rheumatoid arthritis. Chest. 2014;146(1):41–50.

26. Hunninghake GM, Hatabu H, Okajima Y, Gao W, Dupuis J, Latourelle JC, et al. MUC5B promoter polymorphism and interstitial lung abnormalities. N Engl J Med. 2013;368(23):2192–200.

27. Doyle TJ, Washko GR, Fernandez IE, Nishino M, Okajima Y, Yamashiro T, et al. Interstitial lung abnormalities and reduced exercise capacity. Am J Respir Crit Care Med. 2012;185(7):756–62.

28. Doyle TJ, Hunninghake GM, Rosas IO. Subclinical interstitial lung disease: why you should care. Am J Respir Crit Care Med. 2012;185(11):1147–53.

29. Washko GR, Hunninghake GM, Fernandez IE, Nishino M, Okajima Y, Yamashiro T, et al. Lung volumes and emphysema in smokers with interstitial lung abnormalities. N Engl J Med. 2011;364(10):897–906.

30. Lederer DJ, Enright PL, Kawut SM, Hoffman EA, Hunninghake G, van Beek EJ, et al. Cigarette smoking is associated with subclinical parenchymal lung disease: the Multi-Ethnic Study of Atherosclerosis (MESA)-lung study. Am J Respir Crit Care Med. 2009;180(5):407–14.

31. Azuma A, Nukiwa T, Tsuboi E, Suga M, Abe S, Nakata K, et al. Double-blind, placebo-controlled trial of pirfenidone in patients with idiopathic pulmonary fibrosis. Am J Respir Crit Care Med. 2005;171(9):1040–7.

32. Richeldi L, Cottin V, du Bois RM, Selman M, Kimura T, Bailes Z, et al. Nintedanib in patients with idiopathic pulmonary fibrosis: combined evidence from the TOMORROW and INPULSIS((R)) trials. Respir Med. 2016;113:74–9.

33. Fishman A, Martinez F, Naunheim K, Piantadosi S, Wise R, Ries A, et al. A randomized trial comparing lung-volume-reduction surgery with medical therapy for severe emphysema. N Engl J Med. 2003;348(21):2059–73.

34. Herth FJ, Noppen M, Valipour A, Leroy S, Vergnon JM, Ficker JH, et al. Efficacy predictors of lung volume reduction with Zephyr valves in a European cohort. Eur Respir J. 2012;39(6):1334–42.

35. Kemp SV, Slebos DJ, Kirk A, Kornaszewska M, Carron K, Ek L, et al. A multicenter randomized controlled trial of zephyr endobronchial valve treatment in heterogeneous emphysema (TRANSFORM). Am J Respir Crit Care Med. 2017;196(12):1535–43.

36. Schuhmann M, Raffy P, Yin Y, Gompelmann D, Oguz I, Eberhardt R, et al. Computed tomography predictors of response to endobronchial valve lung reduction treatment. Comparison with Chartis. Am J Respir Crit Care Med. 2015;191(7):767–74.

37. Sciurba FC, Ernst A, Herth FJ, Strange C, Criner GJ, Marquette CH, et al. A randomized study of endobronchial valves for advanced emphysema. N Engl J Med. 2010;363(13):1233–44.

38. Muller NL, Staples CA, Miller RR, Abboud RT. "Density mask". An objective method to quantitate emphysema using computed tomography. Chest. 1988;94(4):782–7.

39. Castaldi PJ, San Jose Estepar R, Mendoza CS, Hersh CP, Laird N, Crapo JD, et al. Distinct quantitative computed tomography emphysema patterns are associated with physiology and function in smokers. Am J Respir Crit Care Med. 2013;188(9):1083–90.

40. Castaldi PJ, San José Estépar R, Mendoza CS, Hersh CP, Laird N, Crapo JD, et al. Distinct quantitative computed tomography emphysema patterns are associated with physiology and function in smokers. Am J Respir Crit Care Med. 2013;188(9):1083–90.

41. Diaz AA, Bartholmai B, San Jose Estepar R, Ross J, Matsuoka S, Yamashiro T, et al. Relationship of emphysema and airway disease assessed by CT to exercise capacity in COPD. Respir Med. 2010;104(8):1145–51.

42. Haruna A, Muro S, Nakano Y, Ohara T, Hoshino Y, Ogawa E, et al. CT scan findings of emphysema predict mortality in COPD. Chest. 2010;138(3):635–40.

43. Schroeder JD, McKenzie AS, Zach JA, Wilson CG, Curran-Everett D, Stinson DS, et al. Relationships between airflow obstruction and quantitative CT measurements of emphysema, air trapping, and airways in subjects with and without chronic obstructive pulmonary disease. AJR Am J Roentgenol. 2013;201(3):W460–70.

44. Wang Z, Gu S, Leader JK, Kundu S, Tedrow JR, Sciurba FC, et al. Optimal threshold in CT quantification of emphysema. Eur Radiol. 2013;23(4):975–84.

45. Parr DG, Dirksen A, Piitulainen E, Deng C, Wencker M, Stockley RA. Exploring the optimum approach to the use of CT densitometry in a randomised placebo-controlled study of augmentation therapy in alpha 1-antitrypsin deficiency. Respir Res. 2009;10:75.

46. Stockley RA, Parr DG, Piitulainen E, Stolk J, Stoel BC, Dirksen A. Therapeutic efficacy of alpha-1 anti-trypsin augmentation therapy on the loss of lung tissue: an integrated analysis of 2 randomised clinical trials using computed tomography densitometry. Respir Res. 2010;11:136.

47. Sclafani A, VanderLaan P. Lymphangioleiomyomatosis. N Engl J Med. 2018;378(23):2224.

48. McCormack FX, Inoue Y, Moss J, Singer LG, Strange C, Nakata K, et al. Efficacy and safety of sirolimus in lymphangioleiomyomatosis. N Engl J Med. 2011;364(17):1595–606.

49. Takada T, Mikami A, Kitamura N, Seyama K, Inoue Y, Nagai K, et al. Efficacy and safety of long-term Sirolimus therapy for Asian patients with Lymphangioleiomyomatosis. Ann Am Thorac Soc. 2016;13(11):1912–22.

50. Ingelfinger JR, Drazen JM. Patient organizations and research on rare diseases. N Engl J Med. 2011;364(17):1670–1.

51. Argula RG, Kokosi M, Lo P, Kim HJ, Ravenel JG, Meyer C, et al. A novel quantitative computed tomographic analysis suggests how Sirolimus stabilizes progressive air trapping in Lymphangioleiomyomatosis. Ann Am Thorac Soc. 2016;13(3):342–9.

52. Magnetic resonance imaging of the cardiovascular system. Present state of the art and future potential. Council on Scientific Affairs. Report of the magnetic resonance imaging panel. JAMA. 1988;259(2):253–9.

53. Silverman KJ, Hutchins GM, Bulkley BH. Cardiac sarcoid: a clinicopathologic study of 84 unselected patients with systemic sarcoidosis. Circulation. 1978;58(6):1204–11.

54. Matsui Y, Iwai K, Tachibana T, Fruie T, Shigematsu N, Izumi T, et al. Clinicopathological study of fatal myocardial sarcoidosis. Ann N Y Acad Sci. 1976;278:455.

55. Yigla M, Badarna-Abu-Ria N, Tov N, Ravell-Weiller D, Rubin AH. Sarcoidosis in northern Israel; clinical characteristics of 120 patients. Sarcoidosis Vasc Diffuse Lung Dis. 2002;19(3):220–6.

56. Kandolin R, Lehtonen J, Airaksinen J, Vihinen T, Miettinen H, Ylitalo K, et al. Cardiac sarcoidosis: epidemiology, characteristics, and outcome over 25 years in a nationwide study. Circulation. 2015;131(7):624–32.

57. Paz HL, McCormick DJ, Kutalek SP, Patchefsky A. The automated implantable cardiac defibrillator. Prophylaxis in cardiac sarcoidosis. Chest. 1994;106(5):1603–7.

58. Smedema JP, Snoep G, van Kroonenburgh MP, van Geuns RJ, Dassen WR, Gorgels AP, et al. Evaluation of the accuracy of gadolinium-enhanced cardiovascular magnetic resonance in the diagnosis of cardiac sarcoidosis. J Am Coll Cardiol. 2005;45(10):1683–90.

59. Berrington de Gonzalez A, Mahesh M, Kim KP, Bhargavan M, Lewis R, Mettler F, et al. Projected cancer risks from computed tomographic scans performed in the United States in 2007. Arch Intern Med. 2009;169(22):2071–7.

60. Brenner DJ, Hall EJ. Computed tomography–an increasing source of radiation exposure. N Engl J Med. 2007;357(22):2277–84.

61. Wielputz M, Kauczor HU. MRI of the lung: state of the art. Diagn Interv Radiol. 2012;18(4):344–53.

62. Thomen RP, Sheshadri A, Quirk JD, Kozlowski J, Ellison HD, Szczesniak RD, et al. Regional ventilation changes in severe asthma after bronchial thermoplasty with (3)he MR imaging and CT. Radiology. 2015;274(1):250–9.

63. Basu S, Kwee TC, Surti S, Akin EA, Yoo D, Alavi A. Fundamentals of PET and PET/CT imaging. Ann N Y Acad Sci. 2011;1228:1–18.

64. de Groot PM, Carter BW, Betancourt Cuellar SL, Erasmus JJ. Staging of lung cancer. Clin Chest Med. 2015;36(2):179–96, vii–viii.

65. Groves AM, Win T, Screaton NJ, Berovic M, Endozo R, Booth H, et al. Idiopathic pulmonary fibrosis and diffuse parenchymal lung disease: implications from initial experience with 18F-FDG PET/CT. J Nucl Med. 2009;50(4):538–45.

66. Subramanian DR, Jenkins L, Edgar R, Quraishi N, Stockley RA, Parr DG. Assessment of pulmonary neutrophilic inflammation in emphysema by quantitative positron emission tomography. Am J Respir Crit Care Med. 2012;186(11):1125–32.

67. Sanders KJ, Ash SY, Washko GR, Mottaghy FM, Schols A. Imaging approaches to understand disease complexity: chronic obstructive pulmonary disease as a clinical model. J Appl Physiol (1985). 2018;124(2):512–20:jap 00143 2017.

68. Popp RL. Echocardiographic assessment of cardiac disease. Circulation. 1976;54(4):538–52.

69. Woods B, Hawkins N, Mealing S, Sutton A, Abraham WT, Beshai JF, et al. Individual patient data network meta-analysis of mortality effects of implantable cardiac devices. Heart. 2015;101(22):1800–6.

70. Lichtenstein DA, Menu Y. A bedside ultrasound sign ruling out pneumothorax in the critically ill. Lung sliding. Chest. 1995;108(5):1345–8.

71. Ravin CE. Thoracocentesis of loculated pleural effusions using grey scale ultrasonic guidance. Chest. 1977;71(5):666–8.

72. Lichtenstein D, Meziere G, Seitz J. The dynamic air bronchogram. A lung ultrasound sign of alveolar consolidation ruling out atelectasis. Chest. 2009;135(6):1421–5.

73. Harvey H, Ahn R, Price D, Burke T. Innovating for the developing world : meeting the affordability challenge. AJR Am J Roentgenol. 2014;203(4):835–7.

Julia Winkler and Erica L. Herzog

Introduction

Next-generation analytics have exponentially increased the application of translational medicine approaches to human disease. Advances in genomics, transcriptomics, proteomics, and metabolomics have facilitated the development of personalized approaches to the treatment of many conditions including malignancies such as lung cancer [1], rare diseases such as cystic fibrosis [2], and conditions such as asthma [3]. While the development of associated with allergies precision medicine–based strategies for the majority of pulmonary, critical care, and sleep medicine (PCCSM) domains remains nascent, the last decade has seen great evolution in the understanding of these disorders [4–7]. Crucial to this progress is the study of biospecimens obtained from patients with the diseases being studied.

The practice of biobanking involves the systematic collection, processing, storage, and dissemination of various biospecimens and their associated clinical data [8]. These specimens, which form the basis for personalized molecular medicine, are stored for current and future studies in which they may serve as a cohort for discovery or validation. The development of methods allowing in-depth, "omics"-based approaches place biobanks at that center of translational research [9]. Thus, any discussion of precision medicine requires adequate understanding of best practices in biobanking [10]. The following chapter presents an overview of biobanking as it relates to PCCSM. Definitions and historical aspects will be introduced along with an overview of repository components, ethics, management, regulatory aspects, and best practices. Considerations relevant to unique PCCSM-related specimen types and data are provided. We end with a brief discussion of emerging challenges and opportunities in this important and growing field.

Biobanking: History and Definitions

Since the late 1800s, specimens obtained from patients have been stored at institutions around the world. Whereas many of these collections began with tissues obtained for clinical purposes, modern biobanks have evolved to support specific research goals such as epidemiologic studies, mechanism-based studies of disease, support of clinical trials, and development of precision-based medical interventions to improve human health and disease management [8]. Concomitant

J. Winkler · E. L. Herzog (✉)
Section of Pulmonary, Critical Care and Sleep Medicine, Department of Internal Medicine, Yale School of Medicine, New Haven, CT, USA
e-mail: julia.winkler@yale.edu; erica.herzog@yale.edu

© Springer Nature Switzerland AG 2020
J. L. Gomez et al. (eds.), *Precision in Pulmonary, Critical Care, and Sleep Medicine*, Respiratory Medicine, https://doi.org/10.1007/978-3-030-31507-8_9

with this evolution has been the development of a biobank taxonomy, with classifications aligning with the area of interest. In addition to the classical model of investigator-driven, single-center biobanking, newer approaches include those that are population based like the Kaiser Permanente Biobank [11], multi-center disease focused like the Lung Tissue Research Consortium [12], privately operated like the NDRI [13], nationalized, biobanks like the expansive UK Biobank [14], and most recently "virtual," which curate data and specimen information from other sites to create an electronic repository [15]. All of these models have their place in the PCCSM realm. For example, a small, investigator-driven biobank would likely be established to answer a specific question related to pathogenesis of a specific disease process. In contrast, a population-based or nationalized biobank might be more amenable to the pursuit of questions that are only answerable in cohorts of thousands of patients, and a virtual biobank would be appropriate for obtaining samples from multiple sites.

Biobank Components

Regardless of their size and scope, biobanks require systematic methods for the collection, processing, and dissemination of specimens. All these components must be standardized to ensure operational integrity and validity of data. The repository design rests on the premise of a long-term commitment to continuous collection, storage, and maintenance and requires a stable organizational and financial model to ensure adequate function over time [16]. The central components of a biobank include the subjects and the associated legal and ethical issues related to participation and informed consent; the plan for and implementation of measures for data protection and confidentiality; the involvement of the stakeholders; the procurement, transport, processing, and dissemination of samples; and the handling of clinical data [9] as shown in Fig. 9.1. The unique challenges inherent in each component will be discussed below.

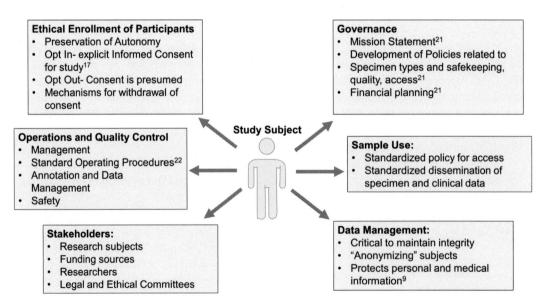

Fig. 9.1 Biobank components: Describes the various components of the biobank system. This includes governances, participants Opt In, Opt Out enrollment, standardization of processing, storage and distribution of samples and corresponding data, stakeholders and confidentiality. Participants' awareness and consent in the enrollment of a study are critical to the foundation of a biobank because the study subject is the central component and, therefore, the protection of subject data and medical information is a necessity. Stakeholders and governances' role and contribution to biobank must be determined because of their importance to the overall function of the biobank system

Participants: Opt In, Opt Out, and Informed Consent

The biobanking process begins with the research subject. Two forms of biobanks exist. One is an "opt-in" biobank, which requires explicit informed consent from the patient. In this model, when potential subjects are approached for entry, the critical process of informed consent occurs [17]. Potential participants are first assessed for their competence to make the decision to enroll. Once this is achieved, subjects are then informed of study objectives, importance of their involvement, potential risks and benefits of involvement, and the voluntary nature of enrollment. In addition, it should be made clear as to whether subjects are able to withdraw from the study. For enrollment into biobanks, a provision is included that allows the use or sharing of samples and its linked clinical data in future research efforts. The physician or researcher should be clear and explicit regarding the nature of the research study, any potential adverse events, and the autonomy to decline or withdraw from the study without repercussions/penalty [18]. The physician or researcher needs to be protective of special populations such as minors, elderly, and cognitively impaired or mentally ill individuals [18]. Enrolled subjects are provided with a copy of their signed consent form, and their consent document is retained at the biobank.

A newer model is the "opt-out" biobank. This method refers to participants recruited from large health care or public sample collections in which medical records are linked to residual specimens collected during study visits. In contrast to the "opt-in" method, in which patients provide explicit informed consent for inclusion, the "opt-out" process informs patients of the study with the ability to actively remove themselves from participation. This method may allow more rapid and robust enrollment with less bias [6] and enthusiasm may be growing for this type of endeavor [15]. However, when compared to the traditional model this approach carries several negatives. Most importantly, it may inadvertently enroll subjects who do not in fact wish to proceed with the study. In addition, it creates logistical and administrative challenges given the large number of potential subjects to be studied. Last, the passive nature of enrollment may undermine subject retention, making serial sampling and longitudinal follow up more difficult [17]. It remains to be seen whether the opt-in or opt-out model is better for personalized research in the PCCSM domains.

Confidentiality, Privacy, and Data Protection

Once the subject is enrolled in the study, the protection of privacy and confidentiality become paramount. Confidentiality and patient privacy require that no unauthorized individual will gain access to personal medical information in the biobank system [9]. Study personnel are responsible for "anonymizing" or assigning unique identifiers to a study subject that deidentifies their protected health information. The master list of study subject numbers, or "key," should be kept secure and only accessible to approved and necessary medical and/or research professionals in the biobank [19]. Maintaining patient privacy is a legal and ethical consideration that must be taken seriously to uphold trust of patients, investors and institutions [9].

Biobank Stakeholders and Governance

Stakeholders The immediate stakeholders of a biobank include the research subjects, funding sources, and the researchers and ethics committee at the housing institution. All of these parties have an interest in biobank function and integrity though their levels of involvement may vary. In terms of the subjects, the traditional model of an institutional facility in which patient involvement is limited to specimen donation has evolved such that patients are now increasingly active. In fact, some research subjects are increasingly assuming a more active role in biobanking, from recruiting and publicity to design and operations and even, in some cases, to initiation and management [20].

This increased awareness and involvement perhaps reflect that the participants assume the largest risk (loss of confidentiality and small potential for physical harm during specimen donation) with the smallest immediate reward. It might also reflect the change in how patients involved in research are viewed, no longer simply as passive "subjects" but more active "participants" [20].

Governance Governance and operational aspects of repositories are handled separately. Governance is shared between individuals of the scientific advisory committee at the host institution and, at time, the ethics committee and funding agencies [9, 21]. According to the 2012 ISBER Best Practices document [19], the governance plan should include provisions addressing the repository mission, specimen types, safekeeping provisions related to sample maintenance, security and integrity, policies regarding access and disposition of samples, plans regarding management of samples and their linked clinical data both during routine operation and in the event of funding lapses, donor withdrawal, repository closure, and natural disasters [19]. These governance aspects require a sound financial model, which will vary depending on the type and scope of services [16]. Despite these differences, adherence to a core set of principles will help ensure financial stability and optimize value. Most recommendations propose a 5-year funding plan based on cost estimates. These costs might involve facilities, personnel and salaries, processing and storage, equipment, inventory management, service contracts, and consumables among others. Allowances should be made for unforeseen changes, and costs should be reviewed periodically to ensure accuracy of projections and uninterrupted function [19].

Operations and Management

The biobank director operates the biobank to execute the governance principles. These responsibilities involve operational aspects related to regulatory compliance, SOP adherence and quality assurance, quality assurance, sample access, personnel management, and data management.

This individual also serves as the link between the stakeholders and the repository function. Staffing for biobanks may involve personnel involved in managerial or technical tasks, administration, and various support capacities [19].

Operational Aspects

Operational components of the biobank relate to the practical aspects and day-to-day functions of sample procurement, transport, intake, labeling, processing, storage, removal, and shipping. Quality assurance and safety are additional considerations at this stage. These aspects are presented below and outlined in Fig. 9.2.

Procurement and Transport of Samples Once the subject agrees to participate, the next step is the procurement of samples. Here, strong communication and coordination between the clinical and laboratory personnel are crucial to allow the appropriate and timely transfer of biological specimens. For the prospective drawing of blood, a qualified phlebotomist must follow a standardized protocol for acquisition and handling of the specimen and prevent any changes to clinical environment during the study [21]. For BAL, pleural, and tissue samples obtained from the clinical setting, every effort should be made to deliver the specimens within a short time frame in order to minimize degradation of RNA, protein, and metabolites [21]. The transfer of samples from clinic to laboratory setting should occur by an appropriate, sample-specific transport, for example, dry ice, cool pack, or ambient packaging [22]. The sample should be temporarily stored in an environment that will best maintain the integrity of that sample to limit external exposure and avoid acute environmental changes.

Sample Intake An accurate record should be maintained of the acceptance, transfer, and return of samples that enter and leave the biorepository. The laboratory personnel who accept the clinical samples should record the type of study, subject identification number, sample type, date, and time received. Because processing variables

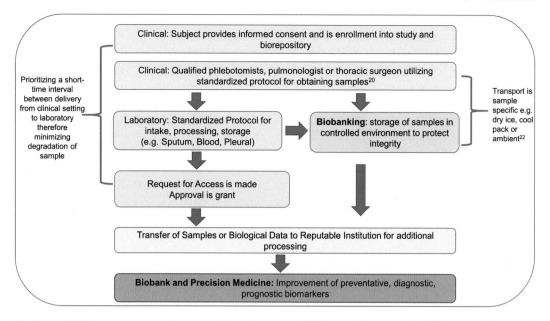

Fig. 9.2 PCCSM procurement and transport of samples: The pulmonary critical care and sleep medicine (PCCSM) translation research process begins with the procurement of samples that takes place within the clinical environment. Subjects of representative disease population are enrolled into study and specific, protocol-driven extraction of samples is performed by a certified phlebotomist, pulmonologist, or thoracic surgeon [21]. The samples are transfer to the lab, prioritizing a timely and appropriate (dry ice, ice bath, ambient [22]) manner by qualified personnel. The samples are processed by a standard protocol or directly transferred into a biobank storage center that consists of controlled, sample-specific environment. The biospecimen can either be analyzed through various laboratory techniques or disseminated to other reputable institutions for further processing. A potential goal for the biobank system is to utilize samples in order to determine biological targets such as preventative, diagnostic, and/or prognostic biomarkers to improve effectiveness of therapies and the overall health of patient populations

might affect sample performance, detailed records regarding the collection, processing, and storage are required. This includes the generation of logs with all of the relevant "times" (time of procurement, time delivered to the lab, time processing began, time processed samples were ultimately stored, etc.) [22]. The biospecimen records are best updated in real time and managed using a secure database with routine backup [19]. Any inconsistency of sample intake, processing, and storage may become a confounding factor affecting the accuracy of research outcomes [23]. Therefore, establishing and maintaining standard and organized processing, storage, and analysis of biological samples are essential for the expansion of biomedical and clinical research from biorepositories.

Sample Labeling While it sounds simple, specimen labeling is critical to the biobanking effort. If at all possible, the method used should minimize the chance of errors including those due to human error (mislabeled at the time of processing), label failure (label separates during storage), or identification failure (inability to read label when the specimen is retrieved) [22]. While older biobanks used handwritten approaches, newer options include computer-generated labels or barcodes that link back to an informatics-based identification system [22] readable by both human eye and computer equipment (i.e., alphanumeric and bar code) [19]. The sample database at the very least should contain specimen characteristics (date, volume, number of aliquots, etc.) though more sophisticated systems may be linked to the clinical database as well [21, 23]. However, the complex the system the more potential for error so each biobank should consider their needs and plan accordingly.

Processing Once in the laboratory environment, quality control is of the utmost importance (reviewed extensively by Grizzle and Sexton [22]). The laboratory personnel are trained to precisely adhere to a standard operating procedure to minimize sample variability and ensure rigor. The laboratory must consider other important elements when working with biospecimens. This includes maintaining a sterile working space, avoiding contamination, disinfecting cell culture areas, expiration of tubes/materials, and the usage of sterile reagents. Additionally, the laboratory personnel are also trained in the proper handling of biological specimen and waste complying with environmental health and safety standards. In the laboratory environment there must be up to date, temperature-regulated, and fully functional storage machines for long-term biobanking storage; this includes ultra-cold liquid nitrogen tanks for vapor phase storage, freezers, refrigerators, etc. This equipment should be routinely monitored to detect changes to the internal storage environment. The constant care and maintenance of laboratory equipment including centrifuges, cell culture, and chemical hoods are also required for adequate sample processing.

Long-Term Storage Depending on the specimen type, storage options are chilling/hypothermic (2–8 °C), low subzero (−4 °C to 0 °C), freezing (−20 °C to −150 °C) in mechanical/electrical freezers, or vapor-phase liquid nitrogen (to a minimum of −196 °C). Repeated free–thaw and warm temperature exposure can stress samples and render them unsuitable for further analysis. For example, failure to achieve sample-type-specific freezing and storage might allow plasma proteases to degrade essential proteins and, in turn, affect proteomics or metabolomics data. To maintain viability of samples thawed from long-term storage (−80 °C), the researcher must follow proper cell thawing protocol and avoid multiple freeze thawing cycles. Last, when samples are removed, the biobank records must be updated immediately.

Removal and Transfer The decision to distribute samples can be at times complex. The different stakeholders in a particular biobank might have competing interests that affect access policy. For example, the institution that has invested significant time and resources in the development of a biobank may require some form of compensation for use. The researchers who enrolled the subjects have a more personal connection to the samples and would likely seek academic credit. Biobanks that are funded by public or private efforts have an interest in samples being utilized as do the patients who enrolled in the study and donated their specimens and clinical data [24]. In order to merge these interests, most biobanks have a written access policy based in some way on the "best practices" document published by the International Society for Biological and Environmental Repositories [25, 26]. These policies weigh the scientific merit, potential value/impact, and ethical nature of applications though the criteria are by no means standardized across disciplines [24].

Shipping Once a request for samples has been approved, preparation begins for transfer of samples. In noncommercial settings, the next step is the generation of a material transfer agreement (MTA) to formalize the transfer of materials and their linked annotation between investigators and institutions. MTAs are legal documents designed to clarify the rights and responsibilities of both parties related to the samples being transferred. They generally address proper use, indemnification, and restriction of third-party dissemination [22].

The actual transfer of samples between sites generally involves the use of couriers. These shipments must adhere to regulations regarding the use of hazardous shipping items (chemicals and dry ice as well safe handling of potentially infectious substances of human origin). Because the use of a courier does not absolve the sender of liability, the individual preparing the shipment must be trained in International Air Transport Association (IATA) requirements [22].

Quality Assurance Given their important role in biomedical research, biobanks are subject to high levels of scrutiny and quality assurance to the

Table 9.1 PCCSM biobank: quality assurance according to ISBER best practices

General operations level	Standard operating procedures (SOP) [22]	Explicit, direct protocols that can be utilized by new and experienced personnel
	Financial plan [19]	Financial plan that predicts potential cost of biobank [19] Monitor biobanks budget and adjust accordingly [19] Budget for maintenance and repairs for equipment
	Organizational planning [19]	Policies in place that apply to entire life span of the biobank [19]
	Communication [19]	Procedures, goals, and policies accessible to stakeholders [19]
	Termination plan	Establishing a trajectory for study and what to do with biobank samples, data, and medical information once finished
Quality control level	Good laboratory practice (GLP) [27]	Standard method of process, storing, and transferring samples
	Regular audits [22]	Inspects SOPs [22], inventory, and recorded data, equipment management
	Facilities [19]	Temperature, sufficient space for processing and storage, proper lighting, generators [19]
	Storage and processing equipment [19]	Storage suits the specimen [19] Regular maintenance and monitoring of equipment Personnel trained to use equipment properly Regular decontamination [19] Temperature record [19]
	Management of data [19]	Secure databases containing records of samples and data
Employee level	Employee education and competency	Trained and educated personnel that adhere to SOPs [22], uphold GLP [27], and subject privacy
	Training [19]	Examples: (if applicable) Handling of hazardous/chemical materials and waste Biological safety level training Handling of human or animal specimen training HIPAA Good laboratory and/or clinical practice training
	Packaging and shipping [19]	Courier services *Air*: Abide by IATA regulations [19] *Ground*: Abide by national/institutional conditions for preparing sample shipment
	Personal safety	Enforce federal/institutional safety policies and protocols that avoid injury to subjects and personnel [19] Personal protective equipment (PPE) Lab emergency equipment and protocols available

adequate quality control. These efforts, which are summarized in Table 9.1, begin with the development of standard operating procedures (SOPs), or highly detailed protocols that operationalize all aspects of the repository and its activities. The SOP should be written clearly and directions that are detailed enough to direct even a first-time user. Changes to the SOPs should only occur with the approval of the relevant stakeholders, and deviations should be documented clearly in the processing logs. As with all laboratory protocols, SOPs should be maintained at the bench in an accessible procedure manual [22]. Personnel should adhere to the universally accepted stan-

dards of good laboratory practice (GLP) [27]. Repository activities benefit from periodic audits of operational aspects including adherence to SOPs, record keeping, equipment maintenance, inventory, and freezer logs [22]. They also benefit from regular evaluations of quality control related to specimens of interest. While for bodily fluids this might be restricted to documentation of processing times, storage times, and temperatures, more sophisticated laboratories might assess reproducibility of assays across randomly selected duplicate aliquots [8, 22]. Quality control for tissues can be more complex, and it has been reported that up to 15% of tissue procured for research are unsuitable for use [28]. This failure may result from sampling of a relatively "normal" area of diseased tissues or an unacceptably long time between procurement and processing [22]. Several methods have been proposed to address these challenges; however, no consensus exists. Last, and perhaps, the most important for biobank function is the education and engagement of employees. Personnel must be trained in good laboratory practice, adherence to SOPs, and human subjects' protection [19, 22, 27].

Safety By virtue of collecting human specimens, a repository is by definition a collection of hazardous material. All human samples are handled with universal precautions [29] with the use of personal protective equipment (PPE) and assumed to be potentially infectious, even if the donor is known to have tested negative for major bloodborne pathogens. This is critical to the safety of personnel working in the laboratory and receiving the samples. These individuals should undergo Hepatitis B vaccination and receive training and yearly recertification in work with bloodborne pathogens [21]. They should also be competent in the handling of chemical hazards as many of the compounds used in storage and processing are known to be biological and reproductive hazards. Shipment of these materials requires specialized training as does the handling of spills, contamination, and disposal of toxic waste. Last, the freezers, hoods, and laboratory spaces used for work with human specimens should be labeled as such [19].

Types of Biobank Specimens in PCCSM Research

Biobanks developed using the above approaches may house a wide variety of biological specimens that can be used in research studies. In addition to peripheral blood, which is an easily accessed specimen that is obtainable from nearly all subjects, PCCSM studies may also involve the study of sputum, bronchoalveolar lavage fluid, induced sputum, pleural fluid, and lung tissue. The importance of these samples is discussed briefly below and depicted in Fig. 9.3.

Peripheral Blood Due to its minimally invasive, time-efficient, inexpensive, and easily repeatable nature, peripheral blood is a key sample in precision-based PCCSM studies. Specimens of interest may include the study of fluid components such as unseparated whole blood, plasma, and cellular components such as leukocytes, erythrocytes, and platelets.

In this method, a certified phlebotomist collects blood into either anticoagulant fortified tubes (for plasma and cells) and noncoagulating tubes (for serum). The needle should be at least 23 gauge to avoid hemolysis and the blood drawing should occur slowly and smoothly [21]. The plasma and serum can also be collected in non-gel or gel (polymeric) tubes [31]. The polymeric tubes possess Ficoll abilities, blood layer separation by a density gradient during centrifugation, that is useful for the isolation of different components of blood such as leukocytes, monocytes, erythrocytes, and plasma. The tubes associated with a plasma draw are specified by its anticoagulant nature and include heparin, citrate, or potassium ethylenediaminetetraacetic acid (EDTA) [31]. Prior to initiation of sample collection, it is important to determine the ultimate application as this will dictate the proper anticoagulant as some anticoagulants are not compatible with certain analytic methods. Anticoagulants may also alter the activation state of cells so it is important to understand the optimal collection matrix for a given application [32]. Leukocytes are generally isolated using density gradient based methods to isolated peripheral blood mononuclear cells (PBMCs) while neutrophils, erythrocytes, and platelets require more specialized techniques. The cell-free fraction (plasma or serum) can be used for measurements of soluble mediators that include proteins [33], metabolites [34], nucleic acids [35] and are also amenable for the generation of conditioned media. Similarly, once the cells are obtained, they are then appropriate for immediate use in fluorescence-activated cell sorting (FACS) [36], genomics and transcriptomics [37], proteomics, metabolomics, and cell culture [38]. They may also be cryopreserved and banked for future studies [39]. As with the choice of anticoagulation,

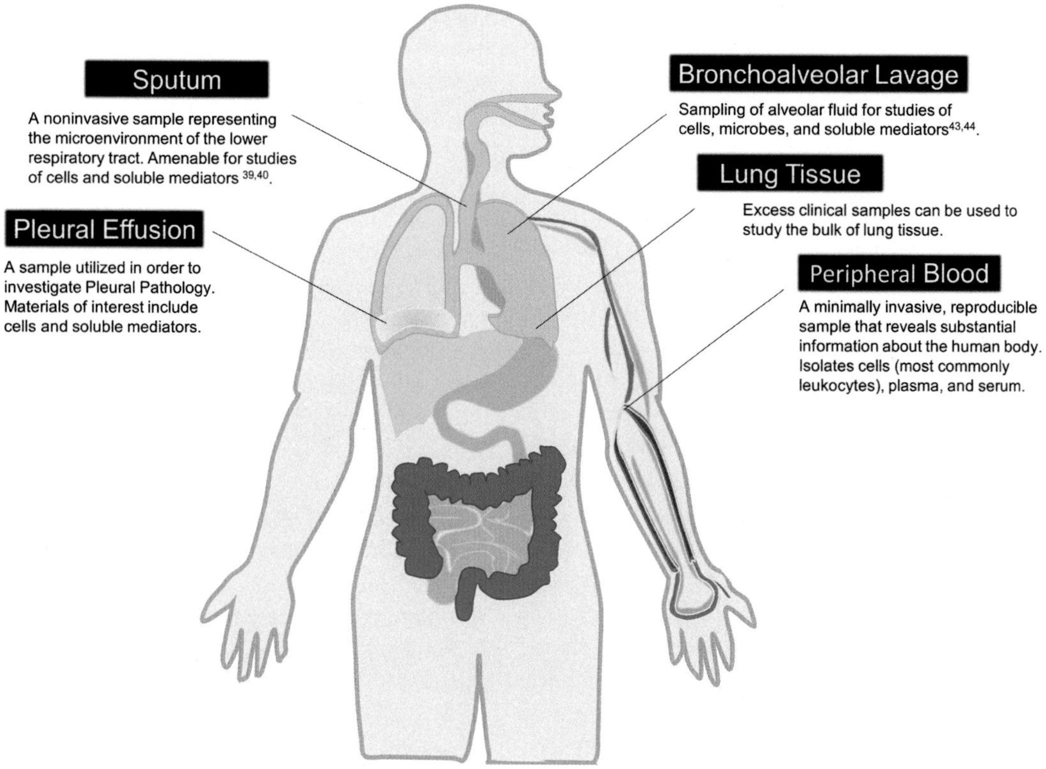

Sputum

A noninvasive sample representing the microenvironment of the lower respiratory tract. Amenable for studies of cells and soluble mediators [39,40].

Pleural Effusion

A sample utilized in order to investigate Pleural Pathology. Materials of interest include cells and soluble mediators.

Bronchoalveolar Lavage

Sampling of alveolar fluid for studies of cells, microbes, and soluble mediators [43,44].

Lung Tissue

Excess clinical samples can be used to study the bulk of lung tissue.

Peripheral Blood

A minimally invasive, reproducible sample that reveals substantial information about the human body. Isolates cells (most commonly leukocytes), plasma, and serum.

Fig. 9.3 Commonly studied biobank specimen in PCCSM Research: This image illustrates the types of biobank specimen utilized in pulmonary critical care and sleep medicine (PCCSM) research. The following specimens are pleural effusion, sputum, bronchoalveolar lavage, lung tissue, and peripheral blood. Pleural effusion can be useful in order to investigate pleural pathology. Sputum is a noninvasive, easily reproducible sample that represents the microenvironment of the lower respiratory tract. Bronchoalveolar lavage is a more invasive but useful tool in sampling the alveolar fluid for cells, microbes, and soluble mediators [30]. Lung tissue can be utilized for many different types of laboratory examinations and assays. Peripheral blood is an important biobank specimen because it is minimally invasive, easily reproducible, and inexpensive while conveying a substantial amount of information about the lungs and body. (Adapted with permission from Super Teacher Worksheets)

it is important to consider the downstream application when choosing the storage method.

Sputum In addition to their clinical utility in diagnosing infections, sputum samples possess great value in the study of lung disorders [40]. Sputum induction is a noninvasive, repeatable method of obtaining information on the microenvironment of the lower respiratory tract. The standard protocol for sputum induction begins with the patient taking bronchodilators followed by inhaling nebulized hypertonic saline to induce expectoration of sputum into a collection container. The sample can then be processed [40] and cells subject to classical evaluations such as manual cell counts and more sophisticated studies such as mass cytometry [41] and transcriptional profiling [42].

Bronchoalveolar Lavage Bronchoalveolar lavage refers to a procedure in which a sedated patient undergoes bronchoscopic sampling of alveolar fluid via the instillation and controlled removal of isotonic saline [43]. In the clinical setting, aliquots extracted from the procedure are utilized for microbial (initial aliquot) and cellular examination (subsequent aliquot denote the alveolar space). When BAL samples are used in research, they are either procured under a research protocol or obtained from excess clinical samples that would have otherwise been discarded [30]. When this method is performed for research purposes, it is important to determine the differential cell count of the fluid pellet, which can then be used for FACS-based or transcriptional studies [44]. The fluid, in contrast, is typically centrifuged and stored in aliquots for further use in studies of protein composition [45], metabolic properties [46], nucleic acid content [35], microbial content [47], and lipid composition [40].

Pleural Effusions Studies of pleural pathology frequently involve the analysis of pleural effusions obtained at the time of thoracentesis. Because transudates are believed to arise from an imbalance of hydrostatic forces that arise from extrapulmonary conditions, exudates – which arise due to pathologies affecting the lung or pleural space mechanism [48] – are more likely to be studied by PCCSM investigators. The pleural space is easily accessible during routine clinical procedures, and fluid is typically removed in excess of the volume required for clinical analysis. Multiple endpoints of interest can be studied in these specimens [49] including cell-based studies for flow cytometry [50], microarray or sequencing [51], mechanical responses [52], and biochemical evaluation of fluid composition using proteomics [53] or ELISA [54]-based methods.

Lung Tissue Surgical lung samples obtained through excess clinical samples obtained at lung biopsy, transplant, or autopsy may also be housed in a PCCSM biobank. These specimens, which are used clinically for the histologic study of the lung in health and disease, are also amenable for research purposes. For studies of bulk genomics such as transcriptional or proteomic work, snap frozen samples may be adequate [55] but for more complex single-cell evaluations, preparation of single-cell suspensions followed by cryopreservation is usually required [56]. Tissues can also be processed for the isolation of parenchymal and immune populations [36]. Explanted or resected lungs can also be used for the generation of ex vivo mimetics of the pulmonary microenvironment such as decellularized matrices [57] and precision cut lung slices [58].

Other Samples As science progresses it is likely that additional specimens such as oral or stool specimens, for study of the microbiome [47], or the recently reported presence of lung disease–associated biomarkers in the urine [59], will become more widespread.

In summary, the uniquely assessable nature of the lung creates multiple opportunities for the sampling of specimens. Proper handling and storage of these specimens may yield new insights into both common and rare disorders affecting the respiratory system.

Clinical Data Considerations in PCCSM Research

Another crucial factor in biobank management is the handling of clinical data. Because the samples will be used for studies of human disease, it is imperative that the linked clinical information be well curated and easily accessible [21]. In terms of the medical history, demographics such as age, sex, race, weight, and BMI are nearly mandatory components as are diagnosis, comorbid conditions, medications, and smoking status. Because many pulmonary conditions are associated with exposures, occupational history may be relevant. Physiology assessments such as absolute and percent-predicted spirometry values, lung volumes, and diffusion capacity are helpful parameters to include, especially when the goal is to study associations with disease severity. The results of imaging exams such as chest X-rays, CT scans, and echocardiograms might be relevant in forms of chronic lung diseases [60]. In some settings, the results of 6-minute walk testing and oxygen desaturations may be relevant. For longitudinal studies, serial measurements of both the biomarker and its linked biologic parameter over time are required so the clinical phenotyping requires a way to enter serial values [4, 5, 61]. If the endpoint of interest is a categorical outcome such as hospitalization, transplantation, or death, the data management requires a method to both capture this information and to enter it into the database [62]. For studies of the critically ill, multiple clinical variables are available and the investigators must decide which attributes are most relevant [7]. It is here that a link to the electronic medical record might be useful [63]. For studies of sleep-related disorders, data regarding PSG results and CPAP adherence may be included along with comorbid conditions and outcomes [6].

Challenges

As can be seen, the optimal operation of PCCSM biobanks requires adherence to a set of well-defined criteria to optimize the ethical collection of specimens and data. However, even in the best situations unforeseen challenges may arise. Most of these issues relate to the use, relevance, and ownership of specimens. A description of potential pitfalls is outlined below and summarized in Table 9.2.

Table 9.2 Challenges that emerge with establishing and running a PCCSM Biobank

Challenge	Description	Potential solutions
Underuse of samples [64]	Study growth exceeds resources support	Clear goals and regular monitoring of sample intake and output [22]
Variability	Reproducibility of samples among institutions	Follow standardized operational [22] and laboratory procedures
Bias	Enrollment not representative Accept everyone [65], accept no one	Subject enrollment is representative of disease population
Shortage and relevance of samples	Clinically based shortages due to changes in approaches to diagnosis and disease [66]	Constantly adapting to advancements in medicine and techniques
Ownership of samples	Ambiguity of ownership between institution and investigator	Legal and ethical contract established before study [8]

Underuse of Samples A common problem encountered by some biobanks is the underuse of samples [64]. As sample collection progresses, unless there is a constant outflow of specimens, the repository size and complexity may grow to overwhelm the resources available for their maintenance. This concern can be alleviated to some extent with rational design based on clear goals and periodic inventory matching intake with output [22]. The growth of national and international efforts and virtual biobanking may offset these concerns.

Variability Inherent in the development of precision-based methods is the need for derivation and replication cohorts. This principle requires that a finding be reproduced in at least one independent cohort. Very robust findings might be able to withstand the lab-to-lab variability in processing and output but some situations [33], particularly those related to heterogeneous disease situations such as cancer or fibrosis, might be more challenging to reproduce. Thus, when a repository-supplied sample cohort fails to confirm the original finding, it will be up to the investigators to determine whether technical or biological limitations account for the finding.

Bias A third challenge to the use and importance of biobanks is bias. Bias might arise in the enrollment phase to result in the participants being unrepresentative of the intended study population. For example, the UK Biobank which seeks to enroll across a spectrum of demographics and conditions has recently published a "healthy volunteer bias," in which enrolled subjects showed statistically significant differences in age, sex, socioeconomic status, rates of smoking, and alcohol use than people in the general population [65]. Similar forms of bias likely exist in disease-specific biobanks, which due to recruiting from academic medical centers are more likely to enroll complex and advanced patients than are followed by community practitioners. Bias may also arise in the laboratory-based aspects of a biobank where variation in day-to-day practice, storage, freeze–thaw, and other factors might influence the performance of a given sample in a particular analytic [21].

Shortage and Relevance of Samples Another challenge faced by repositories is shortage of samples due to changes in clinical practice. One example of this is the situation in the field of lung fibrosis in which excess portions of clinically indicated lung biopsies were once robust of tissue from patients with early-stage disease. However, as imaging technology has progressed, lung biopsies are now quite rare and only performed in patients with a somewhat atypical presentation [66]. In addition, the clinical criteria for the disease have continued to evolve with a less restrictive diagnostic algorithm, and the introduction of new therapies has changed the management and clinical outcomes for patients with this condition [66]. It is the responsibility of the receiving researcher, and not the biobank, to deal with the scientific implications of the latter concern.

Ownership of Samples One little mentioned aspect of biobanks is that the samples belong to the institution and not the individuals. This concept can lead to conflict when an investigator that founded or operated a successful banking operation leaves the institution. In such events, legal agreements are required to arrive at a suitable compromise [8]. Similar problems can arise when funding or approval for a biobank lapses and the fate of thousands of specimens is put in jeopardy. Here, it would be hoped that an agreement with a third party can be reached to assume operation and ownership of the biomaterials and their linked clinical data. Such was the case with the Lung Tissue Research Consortium, which successfully transitioned from being managed by academic investigators to a third party CRO [12]. It cannot be stressed enough that any change in sample ownership must occur in a legal and ethical manner that is consistent with the consent form signed by the patient.

The rapidly changing nature of the scientific landscape renders it impossible to anticipate the future challenges in biobanking. Adherence to best practices and close communication between stakeholders and legal entities are the best approaches to support and protect repository efforts.

Conclusion

Biospecimens are the cornerstone of any attempt at precision medicine. The changing landscape of PCCSM research has required new approaches to enrollment and retention of subjects, stakeholder involvement, financing, specimen handling and storage, data transfer, and quality control, and the ability to face new and unforeseen challenges. Assiduous attention to these aspects will ensure the success and sustainability of current and future banking efforts to promote respiratory health for future generations.

References

1. Mok TS. Personalized medicine in lung cancer: what we need to know. Nat Rev Clin Oncol. 2011;8:661–8.
2. Marson FAL, Bertuzzo CS, Ribeiro JD. Personalized or precision medicine? The example of cystic fibrosis. Front Pharmacol. 2017;8:390.
3. Canonica GW, Ferrando M, Baiardini I, et al. Asthma: personalized and precision medicine. Curr Opin Allergy Clin Immunol. 2018;18:51–8.
4. Brownell R, Kaminski N, Woodruff PG, et al. Precision medicine: the new frontier in idiopathic pulmonary fibrosis. Am J Respir Crit Care Med. 2016;193:1213–8.
5. Sidhaye VK, Nishida K, Martinez FJ. Precision medicine in COPD: where are we and where do we need to go? Eur Respir Rev. 2018;27:180022.
6. Khalyfa A, Gileles-Hillel A, Gozal D. The challenges of precision medicine in obstructive sleep apnea. Sleep Med Clin. 2016;11:213–26.
7. Maslove DM, Lamontagne F, Marshall JC, Heyland DK. A path to precision in the ICU. Crit Care. 2017;21:79.
8. De Souza YG, Greenspan JS. Biobanking past, present and future: responsibilities and benefits. AIDS. 2013;27:303–12.
9. Patil S, Majumdar B, Awan KH, et al. Cancer oriented biobanks: a comprehensive review. Oncol Rev. 2018;12:357.
10. Vaught J, Lockhart NC. The evolution of biobanking best practices. Clin Chim Acta. 2012;413:1569–75.
11. Kaiser Permanente Research Bank Kaiser Permanente Northern California Multimedia Communications. https://researchbank.kaiserpermanente.org/. Accessed 7 Jan 2019.
12. Lung Tissue Research Consortium. https://ltrcpublic.com/. Accessed 7 Jan 2019.
13. National Disease Research Interchange. https://ndri-resource.org/about-us. Accessed 7 Jan 2019.
14. Biobank UK. 2018. https://www.ukbiobank.ac.uk/. Accessed 7 Jan 2019.

15. van Draanen J, Davidson P, Bour-Jordan H, et al. Assessing researcher needs for a virtual biobank. Biopreserv Biobank. 2017;15:203–10.

16. Gee S, Oliver R, Corfield J, Georghiou L, Yuille M. Biobank finances: a socio-economic analysis and review. Biopreserv Biobank. 2015;13:435–51.

17. Kaufman D, Bollinger J, Dvoskin R, Scott J. Preferences for opt-in and opt-out enrollment and consent models in biobank research: a national survey of veterans administration patients. Genet Med. 2012;14:787–94.

18. Kinkorova J. Biobanks in the era of personalized medicine: objectives, challenges, and innovation: overview. EPMA J. 2015;7:4.

19. Campbell LD, Astrin JJ, DeSouza Y, Giri J, Patel AA, Rawley-Payne M, Rush A, Sieffert N. The 2018 revision of the ISBER best practices: summary of changes and the editorial team's development process. In: Campbell LD, editor. 4th ed. 2018;16(1):1–103.

20. Mitchell D, Geissler J, Parry-Jones A, et al. Biobanking from the patient perspective. Res Involv Engagem. 2015;1:4.

21. Grizzle WE, Bell WC, Sexton KC. Issues in collecting, processing and storing human tissues and associated information to support biomedical research. Cancer Biomark. 2010;9:531–49.

22. Grizzle WE, Sexton KC. Commentary on improving biospecimen utilization by classic biobanks: identifying past and minimizing future mistakes. Biopreserv Biobank. 2019;17:243–7.

23. Benner J. Establish a transparent chain-of-custody to mitigate risk and ensure quality of specialized samples. Biopreserv Biobank. 2009;7:151–3.

24. Langhof H, Kahrass H, Sievers S, Strech D. Access policies in biobank research: what criteria do they include and how publicly available are they? A cross-sectional study. Eur J Hum Genet. 2017;25:293–300.

25. 2012 best practices for repositories collection, storage, retrieval, and distribution of biological materials for research international society for biological and environmental repositories. Biopreserv Biobank. 2012;10:79–161.

26. Campbell LD, Astrin JJ, DeSouza Y, et al. The 2018 revision of the ISBER best practices: summary of changes and the editorial team's development process. Biopreserv Biobank. 2018;16:3–6.

27. World Health Organization. Handbook: good laboratory practices. 2nd ed. Geneva: World Health Organization; 2009.

28. Grizzle WE, Aamodt R, Clausen K, LiVolsi V, Pretlow TG, Qualman S. Providing human tissues for research: how to establish a program. Arch Pathol Lab Med. 1998;122:1065–76.

29. Heathcare Wide Hazards: (Lack of) Universal Precautions. https://www.osha.gov/SLTC/etools/hospital/hazards/univprec/univ.html. Accessed 7 Jan 2019.

30. Moller DR, Koth LL, Maier LA, et al. Rationale and design of the genomic research in alpha-1 antitrypsin deficiency and sarcoidosis (GRADS) study. Sarcoidosis protocol. Ann Am Thorac Soc. 2015;12:1561–71.

31. Kirwan JA, Brennan L, Broadhurst D, et al. Preanalytical processing and biobanking procedures of biological samples for metabolomics research: a white paper, community perspective (for "precision medicine and pharmacometabolomics task group"- The metabolomics society initiative). Clin Chem. 2018;64:1158–82.

32. Duvigneau JC, Sipos W, Hartl RT, et al. Heparin and EDTA as anticoagulant differentially affect cytokine mRNA level of cultured porcine blood cells. J Immunol Methods. 2007;324:38–47.

33. Tzouvelekis A, Herazo-Maya JD, Slade M, et al. Validation of the prognostic value of MMP-7 in idiopathic pulmonary fibrosis. Respirology. 2017;22:486–93.

34. Rindlisbacher B, Schmid C, Geiser T, Bovet C, Funke-Chambour M. Serum metabolic profiling identified a distinct metabolic signature in patients with idiopathic pulmonary fibrosis – a potential biomarker role for LysoPC. Respir Res. 2018;19:7.

35. Ryu C, Sun H, Gulati M, et al. Extracellular mitochondrial DNA is generated by fibroblasts and predicts death in idiopathic pulmonary fibrosis. Am J Respir Crit Care Med. 2017;196:1571–81.

36. Reilkoff RA, Peng H, Murray LA, et al. Semaphorin 7a+ regulatory T cells are associated with progressive idiopathic pulmonary fibrosis and are implicated in transforming growth factor-beta1-induced pulmonary fibrosis. Am J Respir Crit Care Med. 2013;187:180–8.

37. Herazo-Maya JD, Sun J, Molyneaux PL, et al. Validation of a 52-gene risk profile for outcome prediction in patients with idiopathic pulmonary fibrosis: an international, multicentre, cohort study. Lancet Respir Med. 2017;5:857–68.

38. Zhou Y, Peng H, Sun H, et al. Chitinase 3-like 1 suppresses injury and promotes fibroproliferative responses in mammalian lung fibrosis. Sci Transl Med. 2014;6:240ra76.

39. Herazo-Maya JD, Noth I, Duncan SR, et al. Peripheral blood mononuclear cell gene expression profiles predict poor outcome in idiopathic pulmonary fibrosis. Sci Transl Med. 2013;5:205ra136.

40. Freeman CM, Crudgington S, Stolberg VR, et al. Design of a multi-center immunophenotyping analysis of peripheral blood, sputum and bronchoalveolar lavage fluid in the Subpopulations and Intermediate Outcome Measures in COPD Study (SPIROMICS). J Transl Med. 2015;13:19.

41. Yao Y, Welp T, Liu Q, et al. Multiparameter single cell profiling of airway inflammatory cells. Cytometry B Clin Cytom. 2017;92:12–20.

42. Yan X, Chu JH, Gomez J, et al. Noninvasive analysis of the sputum transcriptome discriminates clinical phenotypes of asthma. Am J Respir Crit Care Med. 2015;191:1116–25.

43. Bronchoscopy. https://www.hopkinsmedicine.org/healthlibrary/test_procedures/pulmonary/bronchoscopy_92,P07743. Accessed 25 Sept 2018.

44. Prasse A, Binder H, Schupp JC, et al. BAL cell gene expression is indicative of outcome and airway basal cell involvement in IPF. Am J Respir Crit Care Med. 2019;199:622–30.
45. Schiller HB, Mayr CH, Leuschner G, et al. Deep proteome profiling reveals common prevalence of MZB1-positive plasma B cells in human lung and skin fibrosis. Am J Respir Crit Care Med. 2017;196:1298–310.
46. Wolak JE, Esther CR Jr, O'Connell TM. Metabolomic analysis of bronchoalveolar lavage fluid from cystic fibrosis patients. Biomarkers. 2009;14:55–60.
47. Han MK, Zhou Y, Murray S, et al. Lung microbiome and disease progression in idiopathic pulmonary fibrosis: an analysis of the COMET study. Lancet Respir Med. 2014;2:548–56.
48. Feller-Kopman D, Light R. Pleural disease. N Engl J Med. 2018;378:740–51.
49. Nishioka Y. Malignant pleural effusion: further translational research is crucial. Transl Lung Cancer Res. 2012;1:167–9.
50. Ceyhan BB, Demiralp E, Celikel T. Analysis of pleural effusions using flow cytometry. Respiration. 1996;63:17–24.
51. Hou Z, Wen Y, Wang Y, Xing Z, Liu Z. Microarray expression profile and analysis of circular RNA regulatory network in malignant pleural effusion. Cell Cycle. 2018;17:2819–32.
52. Tse HT, Gossett DR, Moon YS, et al. Quantitative diagnosis of malignant pleural effusions by single-cell mechanophenotyping. Sci Transl Med. 2013;5:212ra163.
53. Li H, Tang Z, Zhu H, Ge H, Cui S, Jiang W. Proteomic study of benign and malignant pleural effusion. J Cancer Res Clin Oncol. 2016;142:1191–200.
54. Wang Y, Chen Z, Chen J, et al. The diagnostic value of apolipoprotein E in malignant pleural effusion associated with non-small cell lung cancer. Clin Chim Acta. 2013;421:230–5.
55. Bauer Y, Tedrow J, de Bernard S, et al. A novel genomic signature with translational significance for human idiopathic pulmonary fibrosis. Am J Respir Crit Care Med. 2015;52:217–31.
56. Xu Y, Mizuno T, Sridharan A, et al. Single-cell RNA sequencing identifies diverse roles of epithelial cells in idiopathic pulmonary fibrosis. JCI Insight. 2016;1:e90558.
57. Sun H, Zhu Y, Pan H, et al. Netrin-1 regulates fibrocyte accumulation in the decellularized fibrotic sclerodermatous lung microenvironment and in bleomycin-induced pulmonary fibrosis. Arthritis Rheumatol. 2016;68:1251–61.
58. Alsafadi HN, Staab-Weijnitz CA, Lehmann M, et al. An ex vivo model to induce early fibrosis-like changes in human precision-cut lung slices. Am J Physiol Lung Cell Mol Physiol. 2017;312:L896–902.
59. Stockley RA. Biomarkers in chronic obstructive pulmonary disease: confusing or useful? Int J Chron Obstruct Pulmon Dis. 2014;9:163–77.
60. Depeursinge A, Vargas A, Platon A, Geissbuhler A, Poletti PA, Muller H. Building a reference multimedia database for interstitial lung diseases. Comput Med Imaging Graph. 2012;36:227–38.
61. Savale L, Guignabert C, Weatherald J, Humbert M. Precision medicine and personalising therapy in pulmonary hypertension: seeing the light from the dawn of a new era. Eur Respir Rev. 2018;27:180004.
62. Vestbo J. Natural experiments and large databases in respiratory and cardiovascular disease. Eur Respir Rev. 2016;25:130–4.
63. Martin GS. The essential nature of healthcare databases in critical care medicine. Crit Care. 2008;12:176.
64. Paradiso AV, Daidone MG, Canzonieri V, Zito A. Biobanks and scientists: supply and demand. J Transl Med. 2018;16:136.
65. Fry A, Littlejohns TJ, Sudlow C, et al. Comparison of sociodemographic and health-related characteristics of UK biobank participants with those of the general population. Am J Epidemiol. 2017;186:1026–34.
66. Raghu G, Remy-Jardin M, Myers JL, et al. Diagnosis of idiopathic pulmonary fibrosis. An official ATS/ERS/JRS/ALAT clinical practice guideline. Am J Respir Crit Care Med. 2018;198:e44–68.

Biomarkers in Obstructive Airway Diseases

10

Rachel S. Kelly, Kathleen A. Stringer, and Chris H. Wendt

Key Point Summary

- Obstructive lung diseases, including asthma, COPD, and ACO, are well suited to precision medicine initiatives given their heterogeneous nature, the existence of clinically relevant phenotypes, and the lack of therapeutic options specifically targeted at their endotypes.
- Despite some lack of standardization and replication across several efforts, omics-based biomarker studies have shown impressive results for the identification of endotypes and for the guidance of targeted therapeutics in obstructive lung diseases.

R. S. Kelly
Systems Genetics and Genomics Unit, Channing Division of Network Medicine, Brigham and Women's Hospital, Harvard Medical School, Boston, MA, USA
e-mail: hprke@channing.harvard.edu

K. A. Stringer
Department of Clinical Pharmacy, College of Pharmacy and Division of Pulmonary and Critical Care Medicine, Department of Medicine, School of Medicine, University of Michigan, Ann Arbor, MI, USA
e-mail: stringek@umich.edu

C. H. Wendt (✉)
Pulmonary, Critical Care and Sleep Medicine, University of Minnesota, Minneapolis VAMC, Minneapolis, MN, USA
e-mail: wendt005@umn.edu

Introduction

Chronic obstructive pulmonary disease (COPD) and asthma are the two most common obstructive lung diseases [1–3]. Both individually and combined, these diseases have a significant impact on human morbidity and mortality worldwide. Although COPD and asthma differ in etiology and pathophysiology and are considered distinct diseases, they share clinical manifestations, such as airway inflammation and obstruction. Consequently, the therapies used to manage these diseases overlap as they are directed toward reducing airway inflammation and reversing bronchoconstriction. The overlap of asthma and COPD, referred to as asthma–COPD overlap (ACO), further contributes to the heterogeneity and the difficulty of management and treatment of obstructive lung diseases [4].

Early treatment approaches for asthma and COPD led to an initial improvement in symptoms, exacerbation rates, and hospitalizations. Unfortunately, most available pharmacotherapy is still limited to treating airway inflammation and bronchoconstriction, and despite early promise, the initial decline in asthma hospitalizations has flattened, while COPD hospitalizations are on the rise [5, 6]. This, in part, reflects the fact that most clinical trials have not been designed to capture heterogeneity in response to therapy in large heterogeneous populations, and, therefore, their outcomes are driven by a subset of patients. Consequently, the number needed to treat often exceeds 10 patients for one patient to benefit. This underlines the need for new approaches to improve health benefits and limit costs for individual patients. Precision medicine, the tailoring of therapies to individual patients and patient groups based on genetic, biomarker, and/or phenotypic characteristics that distinguish them from other patients with similar clinical presentations, has great potential to improve health [7]. A number of different asthma and COPD endotypes (i.e., subtypes of disease defined by distinct functional or pathobiological mechanisms) have been identified, and, as such, these diseases are often considered a collection of disorders rather than single diseases. However, to date, there are few options for diagnostic testing to identify specific endotypes or targeted therapeutics to treat them.

A promising approach to precision medicine for obstructive lung diseases is the use of biomarker-defined endotypes to guide focused treatment as evidenced by existing applications of biomarkers, such as eosinophils, to predict therapeutic response and guide treatment in both asthma and COPD [8–10]. With the advent of high-throughput genomics, proteomics, and metabolomics technologies, we are now on the threshold of rapidly advancing endotype-specific biomarkers for the implementation of precision medicine for obstructive pulmonary diseases.

Asthma

Asthma affects nearly 340 million people worldwide across all age groups and is responsible for an estimated 1000 deaths every day [11]. Asthma arises from complex, and as of yet not fully understood, nonlinear dynamic interactions between genetics and the environment, with the vast majority of cases (~95%) estimated to begin in childhood. The term "asthma" derives from the ancient Greek to mean "short-drawn breath, hard breathing, or death rattle," and it was in 1698 that Sir John Floyer first hypothesized that bronchial constriction was the cause for these symptoms. By the late nineteenth century, more formalized definitions of asthma incorporating an association with allergy and environmental triggers were being developed, although treatments such as epinephrine, anticholinergics, methylxanthines, and inhaled β_2-agonists were not introduced until the first half of the twentieth century. From this point onwards, there was an explosion in the development of treatments for asthma, including corticosteroids in the 1950s.

With these therapeutic opportunities came the realization of the heterogeneous nature of asthma. While for many years it was conceptualized as a single disease, it is now considered to be a broad "umbrella" for a group of distinct but related disease phenotypes, largely based on differing responses to the same therapeutics [12]. Initially, patients determined to be asthmatic were all treated in a similar manner, chiefly with bronchodilators and corticosteroids, despite variability in therapeutic success. Thoughts then turned to phenotyping as a means to guide treatment. In particular, two phenotypic characteristics of great importance were considered to be "age at onset" and atopy [13]. Although asthma continues to often be defined by either allergic status, or childhood- versus adulthood-onset, such broad groupings are of limited use, particularly with regards to the concept of precision medicine.

Despite some phenotype-driven therapeutic success, it has become increasingly evident that there are multiple characteristics of great importance for defining asthma and that even within the same phenotype not all cases are alike [13]. These characteristics include differing levels of severity, progression and therapeutic response. Furthermore, phenotypes are not mutually exclusive; several phenotypes can exist within a patient while differing phenotypes may in fact show the same response to a therapeutic intervention. Confounding comorbidities and coexisting conditions, such as sleep apnea, obesity, pregnancy, vaccinations, and smoking, all contribute to this complexity, and there is currently no unified system of classification [12]. Consequently, despite a number of attempts to identify and define the most prevalent phenotypes, including notable initiatives such as the global Asthma Phenotype Task Force, there is currently no definitive list of asthma phenotypes [14]. Therefore, a phenotypic approach is currently insufficient to predict, monitor or guide the treatment of asthma [15]. Further, phenotypic characteristics of asthma do not necessarily relate to, or provide any insight into, the underlying pathogenesis or biological mechanisms [16]. Consequently, the field is now beginning to move toward linking clinical phenotypes to molecular processes [13, 17, 18], in other words, to move from phenotype to endotype.

Asthma Endotypes

One of the best examples of an asthma endotype is what was initially broadly categorized as "allergic" asthma. Approximately 60% of asthma is considered to be allergic, and it is particularly common among early-onset asthma and milder cases [12, 19]. The allergic definition, which is diagnosed through testing skin prick reactivity to allergens and/or by measuring the serum levels of specific immunoglobulin E (IgE), is based on airway inflammation caused by antigen-presenting cells that promote the production of type 2 T helper (Th2) cells from naïve T lymphocytes. Th2 cells then mediate an allergic cascade through pro-inflammatory Th2 cytokines, that is, interleukin (IL)-4, IL-5, IL-9, and IL-13, which trigger the activation and recruitment of IgE antibody producing B cells and the subsequent release of pro-inflammatory mediators, including tryptase, histamine, prostaglandins, and leukotrienes [12, 15]. As our understanding of the role of Th2 cells increased, the term "allergic" asthma largely gave way to "Th2-high expression profile" [13]. However, it was subsequently shown that cytokines including IL-4, IL-5 and IL-13 could also be produced by non-Th2 cells, such as basophils, mast cells, and eosinophils. Consequently, this

condition is now characterized by many as "Type 2 asthma" to reflect its more diverse immunologic origin [13]. Although the terms allergic and Th2 asthma are still commonly used, the term Type 2 (or Th2-high) asthma more accurately reflects a biologically informative endotype while the remaining patients are characterized by what they are not, that is, non-Type 2 asthma [20]. Nevertheless, Type 2 asthma itself can, and should, be further subdivided into more meaningful groups as it encompasses both childhood and adult onset asthma, high and low levels of IgE/atopy, mild-to-severe cases and importantly, differing responses to therapeutics, ranging from excellent to poor, which likely implicate differing pathologies [21]. The complexity of the underlying mechanisms of asthma, involving interactions, regulatory feedback, and multiple competing and complementary pathways is highlighted in Fig. 10.1. This figure also illustrates a number of components involved in the manifestation of asthma that have been utilized as biomarkers or therapeutic targets. As the evolving concept of allergic asthma demonstrates, the definition of asthma endotypes is not trivial and remains a developing concept.

Accurate and reproducible endotyping would be of great utility for the study and management of asthma. One of the key reasons to define an endotype is to enable the development of more "precise" treatments that target specific pathways known to be dysregulated in that particular endotype. Biomarkers have a crucial role to play in every stage of this process; they can be utilized to predict, define or diagnose an endotype, to monitor disease progression or severity, and, as has been most commonly done to date, to assess response to treatment. In fact, many of the currently used asthma biomarkers have been proposed to fill several of these roles.

Interestingly, two of the first biomarkers of asthma, that is, blood levels of IgE and eosinophils, which correlate with the presence and severity of asthma [20], continue to be among the most widely used biomarkers and have driven the development of biologics like omalizumab, which prevents the interaction of IgE with the high-affinity receptor FcεRI on mast cells, eosin-

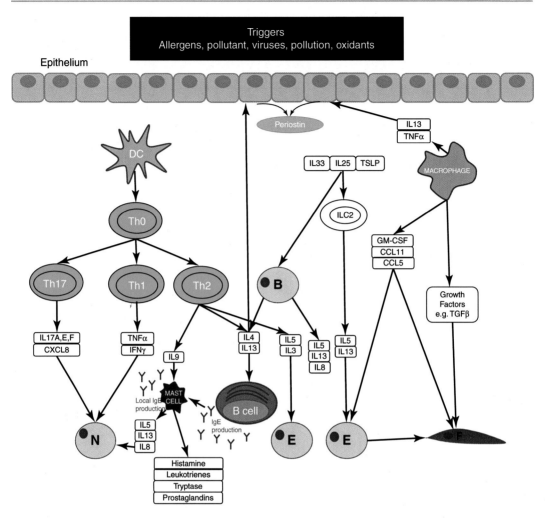

Fig. 10.1 Pathways involved in the pathogenesis of asthma and the constituent variables within them that have been utilized to guide therapeutics or define endotypes. B Basophil, CCL CC chemokine ligand, DC Dendritic cell, E Eosinophil, F Fibroblast, IgE Immunoglobulin E, IL Interleukin, ILC2 Type 2 innate lymphoid, N Neutrophil, Th T Helper, TGF Transforming growth factor, TNF tumor necrosis factor, TSLP thymic stromal lymphopoietin

ophils, basophils, and dendritic cells [22]. However, the way in which these biomarkers are used has evolved as the understanding of asthma endotypes has increased. In particular, blood eosinophilia has been crucial in the identification of Type 2 immune response–driven inflammation in asthma patients as well as in the response to the anti-IL-4/IL-13 and anti-IL-5–targeted treatments (e.g., mepolizumab) [15]. However, eosinophil levels alone cannot identify a single distinct endotype: in addition to the eosinophilic inflammation endotype, there is a mixed granulocytic endotype that is characterized by elevated levels of both eosinophils and neutrophils, as well as a neutrophilic inflammation endotype, and a pauci-granulocytic inflammation endotype that is characterized by normal neutrophil and eosinophil levels [15]. Furthermore, it has been noted that there is little correlation between systemic blood eosinophilia with local sputum or bronchial eosinophilia. Therefore, the eosinophil levels in these differing biosamples cannot be used interchangeably as they may reflect further subdivisions of the Type 2 endotypes [12, 15].

As alluded to above, neutrophils have also been commonly used as biomarkers in asthma. Neutrophils are triggered by IL-8 and contribute to eosinophilic activity; however, they have been reported to have some independent biomarker ability, related to FEV$_1$ and response to methacholine challenge [15]. Other commonly used, "classic" biomarkers of disease, severity and therapeutic response include fractional exhaled nitric oxide (FeNO), leukotrienes and lipoxins, which can act as markers of inflammation. However, as with eosinophils and neutrophils, there is some contradictory evidence regarding their clinical utility [23, 24].

Despite the uncertainty surrounding Type 2 endotypes and their appropriate biomarkers, progress is still far beyond that for non-Type 2 asthma [17]. This largely stems from the fact that the pathological pathways that contribute to non-Type 2 asthma are more complex and less well-understood [13]. As such, there are less existing precision medicine initiatives, and to date no endotype-driven interventions have been proven effective for non-Type 2 asthma [13]. Non-Type 2 asthma, with prevalence estimates that range from 10–33%, tends to develop later in life, to be more common in women, and to be associated with obesity and infection [25]. Importantly, it also appears to correlate with more severe asthma and a lower responsiveness to standard therapy [15]. Therefore, new precision approaches to better characterize, understand, and treat non-Type2 asthma are urgently needed.

Moving beyond classic biomarkers, most of which fall along the inflammatory cascade, novel biomarkers have an important and growing role in the era of precision medicine. In particular, the use of omics technologies for the high-throughput profiling of genetic variation, gene transcripts, proteins, and metabolites to identify biomarkers are beginning to come to the fore. The most prominent of these are genome-wide gene expression studies. A number of genes including *chloride channel, calcium-activated, family member 1 (CLCA1), periostin (POSTN)*, and *serpin family B member 2 (SERPINB2)* have all been found to be upregulated in people with asthma and downregulated by corticosteroid treatment, while increased expression of *CLCA1, periostin*, and *SERPINB2* have been associated with good clinical response to corticosteroids, and *FK506-binding protein 51 (FKBP51)* with a poor response [13, 26, 27]. Similarly, *dipeptidyl peptidase 4 (DPP4)* expression has been indicated as a biomarker of response to anti-IL-13 therapies [28]. Thus, gene expression signatures offer diagnostic, endotyping, and therapeutic guidance and response biomarker potential [26]. MicroRNAs (miRNAs), small noncoding single-strand RNA chains that are involved in post-transcriptional regulation processes, are also of particular interest due to their effects in the immune system. They have demonstrated utility in the diagnosis and characterization of asthma, while also revealing new biological insights. In particular, serum levels of miRNA-1248 were shown to differ between people with and without asthma, and this miRNA was subsequently found to interact with, and increase expression of, IL-5, which was not previously known to be post-transcriptionally regulated [29]. Epigenetic mechanisms, including DNA methylation, histone modifications, and noncoding RNAs, may also regulate gene expression, and epigenetic regulation has indeed been shown for a number of genes involved in the effector pathways regulating T cell activation, such as interferon (IFN)-γ, IL-4, IL-13, and IL-1. However, there is still a significant gap in the understanding of how epigenetic marks influence asthma [30].

The genetic landscape of asthma has been widely studied [31]. Genes such as *HLA, IL13, IL33*, thymic stromal lymphopoietin (*TSLP*), and IL-1 receptor like 1 (*IL1RL1*), which encode the receptor for IL-33, are associated with asthma onset, while a 17q21 locus, which contains both *ORMDL3* and *GSDML* genes, remains one of the most replicated regions for childhood onset asthma. Initiatives such as the Beta Adrenergic Response by Genotype (BARGE) study have identified variants in *ADRB2* that are associated with response to short-acting β$_2$-agonist therapy, but results have been variable in other studies. Although genetic findings have provided crucial insights into asthma biology, aided with the identification of potential therapeutic targets and likely play a critical role in the determination of asthma endotypes, they have offered little in the way of clinically translatable biomarker development. This may be due to the fact that as a polygenic disorder, a single genetic variant is insufficient for prediction, diagnosis, or monitoring. Rather, one would need to characterize and understand a large proportion of an individual's genome to truly quantify and assess these factors, and, even then, this would not be sufficient without a detailed knowledge of the exogenous and environmental factors that interact with this genome. This suggests that asthma precision medicine is still likely decades away from being achieved for the management of asthma, if indeed it is possible at all.

The *omes* that are downstream of the genome, including the proteome, metabolome, and microbiome, are often heralded for their closer relationship to phenotype, and, therefore, the mechanistic understanding they can impart in addition to their ability to act as biomarkers. They also have the benefit of being relatively easy and inexpensive to measure noninvasively. Results of metabolomics studies are particularly promising [32], with volatile organic compounds measured in exhaled breath arising as potential biomarkers for the prediction or presence of asthma in children [33, 34]. The focus on exhaled compounds has been awarded its own "breathomics" subspecialty. Proteomics findings have been similarly encouraging. For example, bronchial levels of Galectin-3 have been shown to correspond to improvement in respiratory function following treatment with the anti-IgE monoclonal antibody, omalizumab [35]. However, although international efforts are ongoing to address the issue, the lack of standardization and validation in metabolomics and proteomics studies has hampered the ability of biomarkers to reach the stage of clinical translation [32, 36]. The microbiome is in the earliest stages of development in terms of biomarkers and although it has been shown that bacterial diversity and burden are greater in people with asthma than those without it, and that the microbiome is critical in asthma susceptibility and development, there is little evidence to suggest

that microbial taxa can play a role in asthma precision medicine [37]. In many ways omics candidate biomarkers reflect or confirm what is already known of asthma biology: candidate biomarkers are regulators or products of pathogenic pathways in asthma such as immunity and inflammation, hypoxia and oxidative stress, and complement cascades. Nonetheless, they also offer novel insights into specific mechanisms and will likely play a critical role in the era of asthma precision medicine moving forward.

COPD

Chronic obstructive pulmonary disease (COPD) is an umbrella term to describe a heterogeneous disease that includes multiple phenotypes and endotypes. These entities are unified by the common physiology of airflow obstruction that is not completely reversible. Since the term COPD was first coined in the mid-1960s [38], little has changed in this oversimplified method of diagnosis or in the characterization of the disease. While initial classification of COPD consisted of those with emphysema (termed *pink puffers*) or chronic bronchitis (termed *blue bloaters*), we have come to realize that COPD is far more complex in its etiology and pathophysiology. Traditionally, FEV_1, FVC, and their ratio are used to define and quantify COPD severity, although this measurement is inadequate in describing COPD heterogeneity, predicting clinical course, or directing therapy. Hence, there has been a drive to identify COPD phenotypes with unique characteristics that correlate with clinically meaningful outcomes, such as symptoms, exacerbations and/or mortality. Ideally, these phenotypes would be linked to an underlying biological process and represent a true endotype with directed therapy. With the exception of COPD related to alpha1-antitrypsin deficiency (AAT) deficiency, no COPD-specific endotypes with clinically relevant treatments exist. Several broad clinically relevant phenotypes have been identified, along with phenotype-directed therapies, which have been mostly limited to long-acting bronchodilators and nonspecific anti-inflammatory medications.

Commonly recognized clinical phenotypes consist of the frequent exacerbator, rapid decliner, asthmatic with "fixed" obstruction, and asthma/COPD overlap. With the advent of quantitative computed tomography imaging, which provides high resolution of anatomy, we can now identify imaging-based phenotypes consisting of emphysema and/or small airway thickness. However, without understanding the underlying pathobiology of these various phenotypes, phenotype-specific treatments are limited.

Progress in the identification of COPD phenotype biomarkers has been made by recent observational studies and clinical trials. In 2010, the COPD Foundation with backing from the U.S. FDA, established the *COPD Biomarker Qualification Consortium* (*CBQC*), which included pharmaceutical representatives and academic investigators, to identify and evaluate COPD biomarkers. Through their recommendations, plasma fibrinogen qualified as the first FDA-approved biomarker for COPD to be used for patient selection for enrollment into clinical trials to enrich for those who are at risk for disease worsening [39]. While identifying elevated plasma levels of fibrinogen as a biomarker is a step forward, fibrinogen lacks disease specificity and does not establish an endotype. Biomarkers best facilitate the implementation of precision medicine if they are endotype specific and have the potential to identify novel targeted therapies [40]. Over the last two decades, clinical trials focused on treating airway inflammation and obstruction demonstrated only incremental improvements in exacerbation rates with each additional new therapy [6]. Therefore, there is an urgent need to identify biomarkers for unique COPD endotypes to develop and direct new therapies to improve symptoms, prevent decline in lung function, prevent exacerbations and improve quality of life.

Genomic Biomarkers of COPD

Although cigarette smoking is the most common risk factor for COPD, there remains significant variation in susceptibility amongst those who smoke. This observation, along with the fact COPD often occurs in individuals without identifiable risk factors, and several studies showing an increased prevalence of airflow obstruction in first-degree relatives of individuals with COPD, suggests that genetic factors contribute to COPD susceptibility [41–44].

Alpha1-antitrypsin (AAT) deficiency is a well-described genetic disorder that predisposes individuals to develop emphysema and COPD. AAT deficiency results from the inheritance of two severe deficiency alleles encoding for the AAT protein and accounts for approximately 1% of individuals with COPD. The deficiency is fairly common among populations of European ancestry with an estimated prevalence of 1 per 3000–5000 persons born in the United States [45]. The diagnosis of AAT deficiency is made by measuring serum or plasma AAT levels in addition to AAT protein phenotyping and genotyping of the serpin family A member 1 (*SERPINA1*) gene, which encodes AAT. The AAT deficiency endotype is a classic example where augmentation therapy is directed at the genetic defect, that is low circulating levels of AAT. Augmentation therapy consists of injections of partially purified plasma enriched for AAT. Several observational studies suggest that AAT augmentation therapy slows the rate of decline in moderate-to-severe COPD. However, there is no definitive randomized trial confirming this observation, and the long-term impact of replacement therapy remains unknown [46–50]. In addition, there remains heterogeneity in disease presentation and in the response to therapy suggesting that additional genetic modifiers influence disease in the setting of AAT deficiency.

COPD is a heterogeneous disease and as such likely has complex genetic determinants. With the advent of high-throughput genotyping techniques, investigators have performed genome-wide association studies (GWAS) on large populations to measure the association of single-nucleotide polymorphisms (SNPs) with COPD phenotypes. These studies require large populations with well-defined phenotypes. Although COPD GWAS studies have been relatively underpowered, a number of genes have been associated with COPD, and some of these associations have been further validated with functional studies. To determine if COPD phenotypic biomarkers were linked to genetic variants, three large cohorts (ECLIPSE, ICGN, and COPDGene) were combined to perform a study that measured the association of SNPs on several lung-specific proteins (pneumoproteins) with systemic inflammatory biomarkers previously associated with COPD severity and exacerbations [51]. Two pneumoprotein biomarkers, club cell secretory protein (CCSP) and surfactant protein D (SPD), had distant genetic loci that were associated with circulating levels of these proteins; however, the link between their SNPs and COPD severity and exacerbations remains unknown [51]. Transforming growth factor beta-2 (*TGFB2*) and matrix metalloproteinase 12 (*MMP12*) have been strongly associated with COPD and lung function [52, 53]. Variants associated with lung function in adult smokers include a protective variant of *MMP12*, a region near the cholinergic receptor nicotinic alpha 3 subunit (*CHRNA3*) and cholinergic receptor nicotinic alpha 5 subunit (*CHRNA5*) genes on chromosome 15, and hedgehog interacting protein (*HHIP*), a gene on chromosome 4q31 that is essential for lung development and is involved in signal transduction [53–59]. Despite the statistical and biological evidence for these associations, none has yet been translated into a therapeutic target or clinical use.

COPD Exacerbations

An acute exacerbation of COPD (AECOPD) is defined as "a sustained worsening of the patient's condition, from the stable state and beyond normal day-to-day variations, that is acute in onset and necessitates a change in regular medication in a patient with underlying COPD" [60, 61]. This definition is challenging as it lacks specificity and requires interpretation by the provider and/or patient. The frequent exacerbator phenotype has various definitions relating to number and severity of annual AECOPD episodes, often defined as two or more AECOPD per year.

Despite not having a precise definition, the frequent exacerbator phenotype has been a focus of multiple clinical trials, as frequent AECOPD episodes are associated with significant morbidity and increased mortality. The pathobiology underlying frequent exacerbations remains unknown, thereby limiting directed therapy. Hence, there has been significant effort to identify biomarkers that distinguish an AECOPD and/or are linked to the frequent exacerbator phenotype.

COPD is a disease characterized by inflammatory changes in the small airways due to both airway neutrophilia and lung parenchymal T cell activation [62–64]. Therefore, although the best predictor for AECOPD is prior history of exacerbations [65], many studies have sought to identify inflammatory biomarkers as predictors of AECOPD, including white blood cell count, C-reactive protein (CRP) and fibrinogen (Table 10.1) [66–71]. Early studies revealed that sputum neutrophilia was associated with a rapid decline in FEV_1, and it could act as a biomarker for COPD [72, 73]. Although pulmonary neutrophilia correlates with airway disease, especially chronic bronchitis, the lung parenchyma in COPD is characterized by a predominance of macrophages, $CD4^+$ and $CD8^+$ T cells, which all contribute to the inflammatory state [62]. Several biomarker studies have thus identified cytokines in plasma that are linked to activated macrophages and T cells, such as IL-6, IL-8, IL-15, and TNF-α (Fig. 10.2).

Those with frequent AECOPD often demonstrate a more rapid decline in lung function, presumably due to irreversible airway injury. Indicative of injury during AECOPD are elevated levels of matrix metalloproteinase-9 (MMP9) and its cognate inhibitor tissue inhibitor of metalloproteinase 1 (TIMP-1) [74]. Surfactant D, which also plays a role in innate immunity and is lung specific, is altered during AECOPD. Lomas et al. reported elevated serum levels of surfactant D in COPD, with the highest levels in those at increased risk of AECOPD. Surfactant D levels subsequently declined with steroid treatment, suggesting it could be a biomarker for AECOPD [75]. However, a lack of validation studies and contradictory findings of reduced levels of sur-

Table 10.1 COPD biomarker candidates

Biomarker	Biospecimen	Family	Ref
AECOPD			
White blood cell	Blood	Inflammation	[66]
CRP	Blood	Inflammation	[66–70]
Fibrinogen	Blood	Inflammation	[66, 68]
TNF-α	Blood	Inflammation	[68, 159]
IL-6	Blood, sputum, exhaled breath	Inflammation	[68, 69]
IL-8	Blood	Inflammation	[68, 69]
sRAGE	Blood	Inflammation	[160]
IL-17A	Sputum	Inflammation	[159, 161, 162]
IL-1β	Sputum	Inflammation	[159]
IL-10	Blood	Inflammation	[161]
IL-15	Lung tissue	Inflammation	[163]
Eosinophils	Blood	Inflammation	[8, 9]
Serum amyloid A	Blood	Metabolism	[70]
Adiponectin	Blood	Metabolism	[69]
MMP 9/TIMP-1	Sputum	Lung injury	[74]
Surfactant D	Blood	Pneumoprotein	[75]
COPD decline			
sRAGE	Blood	Inflammation	[6]
CRP	Blood	Inflammation	[81]
IL-6	Blood	Inflammation	[77]
INF-γ	Blood	Inflammation	[77]
MMP 9	Blood	Lung injury	[81]
CCSP	Blood	Pneumoprotein	[79]
COPD mortality			
CRP	Blood	Inflammation	[68, 71]
Fibrinogen	Blood	Inflammation	[68, 71]
IL-6	Blood, sputum, exhaled breath	Inflammation	[68, 71]
IL-8	Blood	Inflammation	[68, 71]
WBC, neutrophil	Blood	Inflammation	[71]
CCSP	Blood	Pneumoprotein	[68, 71]
Surfactant D	Blood	Pneumoprotein	[71]
PARC/CCL18	Blood	Inflammation, Pneumoprotein	[100]
Emphysema			
sRAGE	Blood	Inflammation	[6, 83–85]
CCSP	Blood	Pneumoprotein	[71]
Osteopontin	Sputum	Apoptosis	[164]
COPD severity			
sRAGE	Blood	Inflammation	[64, 82, 90–92]
EN-RAGE	Blood	Inflammation	[64]
NGAL	Blood	Inflammation	[64]
Fibrinogen	Blood	Inflammation	[64]
MPO	Blood	Inflammation	[64]
TGF-β	Blood	Inflammation	[64]
HB-EGF	Blood	Inflammation	[64]
IL-6	Blood	Inflammation	[96]
TNF-α	Blood	Inflammation	[96]

(continued)

Table 10.1 (continued)

Biomarker	Biospecimen	Family	Ref
VEGF	Blood	Inflammation	[96]
MCP1	Blood	Inflammation	[96]
CCSP	Blood	Pneumoprotein	[94, 95]
MMP-9	Blood	Lung injury	[96]
Desmosine	Blood	Lung injury	[93, 97]

PARC/CCL18 pulmonary and activation regulated chemokines

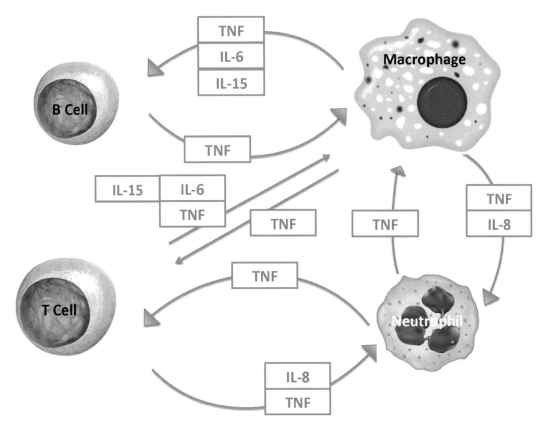

Fig. 10.2 Pathways reflecting biomarkers associated with acute exacerbations of COPD. IL Interleukin, TNF Tumor necrosis factor

factant D in bronchoalveolar lavage fluid in smokers with and without COPD currently preclude the use of surfactant D as a clinical biomarker [76].

Lung Function Decline in COPD

COPD is not only heterogeneous in its presentation but also its clinical course. Some individuals with COPD have relatively stable to mild loss in lung function over time, while others experience a rapid decline in lung function. It would be advantageous to identify people with a "rapid decliner" phenotype and treat them with targeted therapies to preserve lung function. Since most biomarker studies have been cross-sectional rather than longitudinal, few biomarkers have been related to lung function decline (Table 10.1). Bhavani and colleagues performed a 5-year prospective longitudinal study of 224 smokers and found that among active smokers, increased

IFN-γ and IL-6 T-cell responses were positively associated with the annual rate of emphysema progression [77]. In a 9-year longitudinal study, reduced serum levels of club cell secretory protein (CCSP) were associated with an accelerated decline in FEV$_1$ [78, 79]. CCSP is a member of the secretoglobulin family that is secreted by non-ciliated bronchial club cells and plays a role in anti-inflammatory and anti-oxidative stress responses. Distant genetic loci for CCSP affect its circulating levels but have a weak association with COPD [51], while morphometric analysis reveal decreased immunostaining of CCSP in endobronchial biopsies in COPD [80]. In addition to these biomarkers, inflammatory markers, such as CRP and soluble receptor for advanced glycation end products (sRAGE), have been associated with a rapid decline in lung function, along with MMP9 marking lung injury [71, 81].

Emphysema

COPD is defined by airflow obstruction due to varying degrees of small airway disease and emphysema. High-resolution chest computed tomography allows the quantification of emphysema with a high degree of correlation to histopathology, but it is costly and requires exposure to radiation and, thus, is not amenable to frequent repeat testing to follow disease progression. Emphysema-specific biomarkers would be helpful to characterize histopathological heterogeneity and provide new therapeutic targets. There is increasing evidence that the soluble, circulating form of sRAGE is a useful biomarker for the presence and/or progression of emphysema in COPD [82]. RAGE is a transmembrane receptor that regulates inflammatory signaling through its interaction with ligands of the damage-associated molecular pattern molecules. RAGE signaling plays a role in lung development and structure while soluble forms of the receptor block signaling. Genetic variants near the RAGE gene, *AGER*, have been associated with emphysema in the presence of airflow obstruction, and low levels of sRAGE correlate with emphysema severity, suggesting the RAGE axis may be a potential therapeutic target [83–89].

COPD Severity

Because quantity of emphysema is associated with airflow obstruction severity, the association of sRAGE levels with emphysema severity implies that sRAGE is also associated with COPD severity as measured by FEV$_1$ [64, 82, 90–92]. Similarly, because those with frequent AECOPD tend to have more severe COPD and are at risk for more rapid decline in FEV$_1$, biomarkers of AECOPD and rapid decline in FEV$_1$, such as fibrinogen, IL-6, TNF-α and MMP9, are also associated with COPD severity. Potential biomarkers of COPD severity reflect biological processes that include (1) inflammation, such as monocyte chemotactic protein 1 (MCP1) promoting neutrophil recruitment, and (2) tissue remodeling and destruction, such as MMP9 and desmosine (Fig. 10.3) [64, 93–97]. Desmosine, which is composed of four lysine amino acid residues and functions as a crosslinking molecule in elastin that is released upon elastin degradation, is a promising biomarker, as both urine and serum levels of desmosine are associated with diseases involving elastin degradation, including COPD and emphysema [98].

COPD Mortality

C-C Motif Chemokine Ligand 18 (CCL18; also known as pulmonary and activation-regulated chemokine (PARC)) is an attractive COPD biomarker that is constitutively expressed at high levels by lung monocytes, macrophages, and dendritic cells and is measurable in serum [99]. Combining two large longitudinal cohorts, Evaluation of COPD Longitudinally to Identify Predictive Surrogate Endpoints (ECLIPSE) and Lung Health Study (LHS), Sin and colleagues found that CCL18 levels were elevated in COPD and tracked clinical outcomes, including risk of cardiovascular hospitalization and mortality [100]. This is particularly important since AECOPD episodes are associated with increased risk of cardiovascular events [101]. Other pneumoproteins, such as CCSP and surfactant D, along with inflammatory markers are also associated with mortality outcomes (Table 10.1) [68,

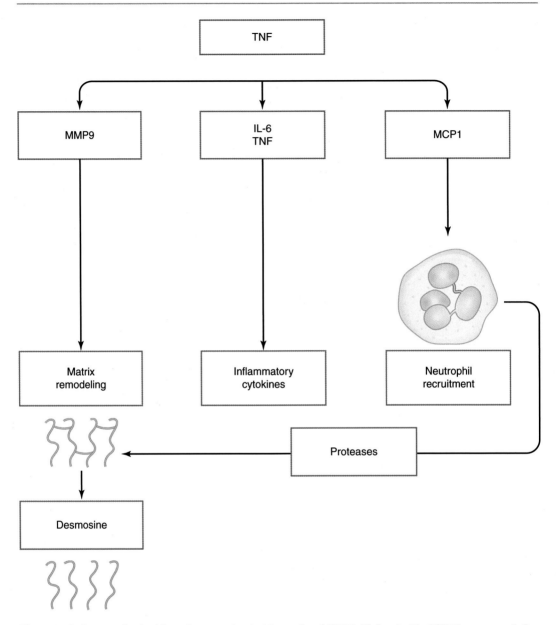

Fig. 10.3 Pathways reflecting biomarkers associated with severity of COPD. IL-Interleukin, TNF Tumor necrosis factor, MMP Matrix metalloproteinase, MCP Monocyte chemoattractant protein

71]. To date, none have been validated sufficiently to establish their utility for clinical use.

Future Omics-Based COPD Biomarker Studies

Recent advances in spectrometry and chromatography have enabled investigators to measure hundreds to thousands of metabolites and/or proteins in biological samples simultaneously. Approaches include global profiling of metabolites and/or proteins, and a targeted measurement of multiple species simultaneously. Both untargeted and targeted metabolomic studies of ECLIPSE participants' serum identified lipoproteins and amino acids that are differentially observed in people with COPD compared to healthy smokers [102,

103]. Lipids, particularly sphingolipids, have been implicated in the pathobiology of COPD. Sphingolipids play a role in lung inflammation, while ceramide (a sphingolipid metabolite) upregulation leads to emphysema in a murine model and its increased levels associate with emphysema in humans [104–106]. Sphingolipids, however, are complex, and multiple species are detectable in plasma. Bowler and colleagues performed sphingolipid profiling on 69 sphingolipid species in COPDGene participant plasma and identified five sphingomyelins associated with emphysema and several ceramide species associated with AECOPD [107].

Proteolysis is a hallmark of COPD, particularly emphysema, and elevated levels of peptides, along with elastin degradation products, have been reported in COPD [108]. One novel peptide, N-acetyl Pro-Gly-Pro (PGP), is a product of extracellular matrix breakdown and is elevated in sputum and plasma of people with COPD [109, 110]. Interestingly, PGP functions as a CXCR ligand and, thus, participates as a neutrophil chemoattractant. Elevated levels of PGP correlate with AECOPD, and its levels drop with effective treatment [111]. Thus, PGP functions both as a biomarker of AECOPD and as a potential therapeutic target. The metabolite tryptophan is an essential amino acid whose depletion is found in those with AECOPD [112]. Tryptophan metabolism occurs through the enzyme indoleamine 2,3-dioxygenase (IDO) that produces metabolites of the kynurenine pathway. The accumulation of kynurenine and its metabolites lead to both immune tolerance and anti-inflammatory effects. Activation of IDO as depicted by increased kynurenine/tryptophan levels is observed in AECOPD [112] and has also been linked to lung cancer [113].

The microbiome is in its earliest stages of development regarding its role in COPD pathogenesis and serving as a technique to identify endotype biomarkers. No unique COPD microbiome has been identified, but it is clear that the microbiome in COPD is altered compared to healthy controls, is influenced by steroids and antibiotics, and becomes less diverse with severe disease [114–118]. Microbiome and other ongoing omics studies are encouraging and suggest that future investigations will define pathobiological pathways and give insight into targeted treatment approaches for newly defined COPD endotypes.

Asthma–COPD Overlap (ACO)

Asthma–COPD overlap has a reported prevalence that ranges from 15% to 55% and represents a particularly clinically challenging problem because it is ill-defined, as it comprises elements of asthma and COPD that progress disproportionately over time in any given patient [119]. While COPD is more common than asthma in adults, COPD patients, particularly older COPD patients, can manifest asthmatic symptoms. ACO has been reported to be associated with lower health-related quality of life, more frequent exacerbations and higher mortality rates compared with COPD [120, 121]. These differences were not explained by patient demographics, lung function or the presence of emphysema on CT. The complexity of ACO is illustrated by a range of recent descriptions and criteria from the Global Initiatives for Asthma (GINA; ginasthma.org) and COPD (GOLD; goldcopd.org) [122], the American Thoracic Society (ATS) [123] and COPDGene [124] (Table 10.2). While a consensus definition does not exist, it is generally accepted in practice that ACO consists of a similar number of features of asthma and COPD [4, 125].

The Precision Medicine Initiative, launched by President Obama in 2015 with the intent to more fully understand mechanistic underpinnings of disease heterogeneity and advance drug discovery, has renewed interest in ACO [126]. However, like asthma and COPD, ACO is a heterogeneous illness. Absence of definitive diagnostic criteria has hindered ACO biomarker discovery and the identification of targeted pharmacotherapy. In particular, biomarkers to direct treatment are absent in ACO and there are no biomarkers that capture the underlying biological mechanisms [126]. As is the case for asthma and COPD, there are different ACO endotypes that include predominant neutrophilic or eosinophilic

Table 10.2 Asthma–COPD overlap (ACO) definitions

GINA/GOLD[a]	ATS Roundtable Diagnostic Criteria[b]	COPD gene
1. ACO is characterized by persistent airflow limitation with several features usually associated with asthma and several features usually associated with COPD 2. ACO includes several different phenotypes that are likely driven by different underlying mechanisms	*Major* 1. Persistent airflow limitation (post-bronchodilator FEV_1/FVC <0.70 or LLN) 2. At least a 10-pack year history of tobacco smoking OR equivalent indoor or outdoor air pollution exposure 3. Documented history of asthma before the age of 40 or BDR >400 ml in FEV_1 *Minor* 1. Documented history of atopy or allergic rhinitis 2. BDR of FEV_1 ≥200 mL and 12% from baseline values on 2 or more visits 3. Peripheral blood eosinophil count of ≥300 cells·uL^{-1}	1. A history of asthma or hay fever, evidence of obstructive lung disease noted on spirometry (FEV_1/FVC, 0.7) with improvement in FEV_1 greater than 200 ml and greater than 12% following bronchodilator administration, and less than 15% emphysema on HRCT 2. Evidence of obstructive lung disease noted on spirometry with improvement in FEV_1 greater than 400 ml and greater than 15% following bronchodilator administration, regardless of history of asthma or hay fever; and less than 15% emphysema on the basis of HRCT

FEV_1 forced expiratory volume in 1 s, *FVC* forced vital capacity, *BDR* bronchodilator response using 400 ug of albuterol/salbutamol (or equivalent), *LLN* lower limit of normal, *HRCT* high-resolution computed tomography
[a]GINA/GOLD advises that "syndrome" not be used to describe ACO since it implies a single disease
[b]The presence of all three major criteria and at least on minor criterion is recommended for diagnosis

inflammation, a mix of both, or neither [127]. Based on these findings, assessment of sputum cellularity or use of biomarkers of Th2 inflammation (e.g., sputum and/or blood eosinophils, FeNO, IgE) have been proposed as strategies to distinguish these groups [123, 128, 129].

Candidate ACO Biomarkers

ACO patients often meet exclusion criteria for clinical trials of asthma and COPD, so the effectiveness of therapeutic interventions in this group of patients is unclear [130]. Even fewer biomarker discovery studies have been performed that include distinct asthma, COPD, and ACO groups [131]. Evidence that a shared genetic predisposition exists for COPD and asthma has been established, but genetics studies, such as GWAS, have not been performed specifically for ACO [41, 44]. The strongest evidence for the existence of an ACO phenotype are airway epithelial cell gene expression data showing that a Th2 signature score obtained from people with asthma was correlated with asthma-related features and differential response to corticoisteroids among people with COPD [132]. Specifically, the epithelial

gene expression changes that best reflected ACO were evident in both the large and small airway epithelium and were associated with markers of Th2 inflammation, increased airway wall, blood eosinophils and bronchodilator responsiveness, and improvement in hyperinflammation with inhaled corticosteroid treatment [132]. To date, however, there are no definitive biomarkers of ACO. Interestingly, a number of biological pathways such as tryptophan and sphingolipid metabolism have been identified as dysregulated in both asthma and COPD [112, 133–135], suggesting that technologies such as proteomics and metabolomics will provide a compelling avenue beyond genetics to explore ACO endotypes.

FeNO, which has been used to gauge the extent of airway inflammation, particularly eosinophilic inflammation [136], has been studied as a potential biomarker to differentiate ACO from COPD [137]. Although FeNO levels have been observed to be higher in ACO than COPD, rigorous studies testing range of specificity and sensitivity have not been conducted, and FeNO alone has not been shown to adequately distinguish ACO.

Sputum is the biofluid that has provided the most differentiating information about ACO, asthma and COPD. In an exploratory study of five pre-selected markers, sputum concentration of neutrophil-gelatinase-associated lipocalin (NGAL) was the only candidate biomarker that differentiated ACO from either asthma or COPD [138]. This study was limited as it focused only on sputum IL-13 (selected for its potential role in asthma), myeloperoxidase and NGAL (selected for their potential role in COPD) and chitinase-like protein and IL-6 (selected for their potential role in ACO). Similar results for NGAL were obtained in a smaller, separate cohort of patients by this same group [139]. Larger prospective validation studies are needed to determine whether NGAL is a predictive biomarker for ACO.

Lung Function Decline in ACO and Implications for Pharmacotherapy

In a subgroup of asthma patients, disease progression includes worsening irreversible airway obstruction, while in some COPD patients, disease progression includes reversible airway obstruction. Notably, both COPD and asthma are characterized by accelerated age-related decline in lung function, but the extent of this decline does not differentiate the diseases. Asthma patients who develop ACO are more likely to be patients with a prolonged history of asthma or those with severe asthma, and COPD patients that develop ACO are more prone to bronchial hyperresponsiveness that contributes to increased airway inflammation [4]. Because the prevalence of ACO increases with age, it may represent a more progressive and severe form of obstructive lung disease than either COPD or asthma alone.

The stepwise approaches to therapeutics used for COPD and asthma do not apply to ACO. Because there have not been any randomized clinical trials of pharmacotherapy specific to ACO, there are no ACO-specific therapeutic guidelines. Given the heterogeneous nature of ACO, including variability in airway inflammation type (e.g., neutrophils, eosinophils), treatment is aimed at symptoms and clinical observations that include, for example, the extent

of irreversible airway obstruction, frequency of exacerbations, and blood levels of eosinophils. Treatment may include use of an anti-IL-5 antibody (e.g., mepolizumab) that targets eosinophilic airway inflammation as well as traditional therapies of asthma and COPD (i.e., glucocorticoids, β_2-agonists, long-acting muscarinic antagonists) [4, 140].

In summary, ACO is prevalent in patients with obstructive lung disease, but its etiology remains incompletely understood. To determine whether genetic factors predispose asthma or COPD patients to ACO or how the duration and severity of asthma predisposes asthma patients to ACO requires further study. As basic features of ACO become clearer, the identification of predictive and prognostic biomarkers may be possible. This, in turn, would enable the discovery of drug targets to bring precision medicine to ACO.

Future Directions

Biomarker studies of asthma and COPD have made evident that no single gene or molecular biomarker will be sufficient to differentiate endotypes of these complex and multi-factorial diseases. In fact, biomarker panels incorporating multiple markers in combination have shown increased efficacy over single biomarkers. For example, in asthma, a composite biomarker including blood eosinophils, periostin, and FeNO outperformed its single constituent parts in the identification of anti-IgE omalizumab responders [141]. In the large COPD ECLIPSE cohort, white blood cell count, along with levels of IL-6, CRP, IL-8, fibrinogen, CCL18, and surfactant protein D, significantly improved the ability to predict mortality [71]. Similarly, it is likely that the optimal strategy to identify endotypes is to consider multiple variables, both omics-based and more traditional (e.g., interleukins).

In addition to the technological developments required to measure these biomarkers, novel statistical methodologies are required to analyze and interpret them. To this end, data-driven machine learning and clustering approaches that are objective by design are becoming increasingly popular. For example, the Severe Asthma Research Program (SARP) identified six biologically and clinically meaningful asthma patient clusters using over 100 variables, including both phenotypic and molecular data [141]. Similarly, the Unbiased BIOmarkers in PREDiction of respiratory disease outcomes (U-BIOPRED) project used clinical and physiological variables to identify four asthma patient clusters that shared some overlapping clinical and biomarker features with the SARP clusters [142, 143]. Integrated omics data are ideal for defining endotypes as the natural interactions and structure of the data can help to identify subtype-specific processes and pathways. In numerous cancer types, integrated omics data have been shown to improve the definition of clinically relevant tumor subtypes [144], and similarly promising results are emerging for respiratory diseases [145]. In a proof of principle experiment, nine omics datasets were integrated by similarity network fusion (SNF), an iterative, unsupervised approach, that yielded 100% correct classification of certain COPD phenotypes [145]. Although the few asthma studies utilizing purely omics data to derive clusters have had small sample sizes, intriguing results support the existence of multiple heterogeneous subtypes with differing omics profiles and pathophysiological pathways, including differences in atopic status, eosinophil count, and cytokine count [142, 146–151]. The choice of variables to be included in such analyses is critical and should ideally include classic and omics markers in diverse populations as well as demographic and environmental factors, such as age, diet, and BMI [152].

While unsupervised clustering approaches have been the method of choice to identify potential asthma and COPD endotypes, a number of other approaches are being applied as investigators try to make sense of highly complex and multidimensional data. These include latent class analysis, multivariate regression splines, topological data analysis, which has shown to be particularly well suited to the definition of endotypes [153], and Bayesian networks [154, 155]. Whether these approaches can identify biologically and clinically meaningful endotypes that, crucially, can be validated is as yet unknown. As with the biomarkers

themselves, it is likely that a variety of complementary analytical approaches will be required to achieve the identification and understanding of endotypes, a step that would represent a vital leap forward for precision medicine.

Challenges for Precision Medicine in Obstructive Pulmonary Diseases

Increasing evidence suggests that treatment and disease management strategies based on underlying pathobiological mechanisms, rather than a "one-size-fits-all" approach, are more effective to improve outcomes and optimize use of healthcare resources for obstructive lung diseases. However, developing and enacting precision medicine poses a large number of challenges.

A key issue in the development of biomarkers, and thus in precision medicine, is not only their validation, but also establishing their practicality, availability, and cost-effectiveness. It has been stated that "the practicality of a biomarker test is inversely proportional to its invasiveness" [12]. Therefore, a key factor is the bio-sample in which the biomarker is measured. With a few notable exceptions, including blood eosinophils, many biomarkers for lung-related diseases require specialized equipment, training or assays. For example, bronchoscopy/biopsy and bronchoalveolar lavage are well suited for the detection of lung-related biomarkers; however, despite their demonstrated safety, the invasive nature of these procedures renders them of little use for regular and ongoing monitoring. Biomarkers in exhaled breath are entirely noninvasive and have a proximal relationship to the lung. Technologies such as the electric nose (eNose) potentially offer new opportunities for dynamic monitoring of asthma and ACO via exhaled breath; however, there are still a number of breath-specific challenges to overcome, including the absence of a valid dilution factor for exhaled breath, that have hampered large-scale translation [156]. Induced sputum is similarly noninvasive, but is associated with high costs and a large technical demand [12].

Another challenge to address is the lack of knowledge regarding the temporal stability of either endotypes or most measured candidate biomarkers identified thus far. Omics studies are likely to play an increasingly important role to address this issue, as the cost of such studies has decreased. To date, relatively few omics studies have been truly integrative or multi-omic in nature, but this is another necessary next step that will increase our understanding of obstructive lung diseases. Furthermore, multiple large-scale studies that capture both multiple endotypes and diverse patients are required to generate data necessary to develop and validate integrative biomarker panels. Finally, there is a particular need for studies focused on non-Type-2 asthma, COPD as a whole, and ACO to help bridge understanding in the management and treatment of endotypes of these conditions that have distinct underlying pathobiological processes yet lead to overlapping clinical features.

Conclusion

Obstructive airway diseases remain a significant hazard to human health. Despite this threat, a full understanding of the mechanistic and biological underpinnings that explain the heterogeneity of asthma, COPD and ACO has not yet been achieved. As such, biomarkers that reliably identify specific endotypes of these diseases for which targeted pharmacotherapy could be provided remains elusive. Nevertheless, progress is being made. The definition of asthma has evolved over the last decade and is being pushed beyond phenotypes to endotypes. This is evidenced by distinct differences attributable to Th2 inflammation among some people with asthma and the advancements made by using composite biomarkers (e.g., blood eosinophils, periostin, FeNO) to identify emerging asthma endotypes. This has fueled the development of biologic therapeutics for Th2 asthma, including the anti-IL-5 monoclonal antibody mepolizumab. In targeted studies, asthma patients with a severe eosinophil endotype derived greater benefit from mepolizumab than other asthma patients [157]. In the eosinophilic endotypes of asthma, IgE has been shown to be a viable and effective drug target for

anti-IgE antibodies like omalizumab. In fact, since the eosinophilic endotype spans all obstructive airway diseases, including ACO, it may foster redirection of how obstructive airway disease is characterized and diagnosed and fuel the development of drugs aimed at other specific biological targets. In COPD, the AAT endotype has the potential to direct the development of targeted gene-modifying therapies while phosphodiesterase-4 inhibitors (e.g. roflumilast) may be effective as targeted treatment for the frequent exacerbator phenotype. In aggregate, while much work remains to be done, there are promising signs that precision medicine can be achieved in obstructive airway disease. Continued progress will require robust research efforts in systems biology, pharmacology and statistics to drive biomarker and drug target discoveries. A large initiative aimed at driving precision medicine is the U.S. National Heart, Lung, and, Blood Institute's Trans-Omics for Precision Medicine (TOPMed) Program. The early phase of this program includes the generation of whole-genome sequencing data for patients with well-defined clinical phenotypes and outcomes from earlier NHLBI-funded studies [158]. As the program advances, it is expected that its results, along with those of other biomarker discovery efforts, will lead to the validation of endotypes for asthma, COPD, and ACO.

References

1. Hurd S. The impact of COPD on lung health worldwide: epidemiology and incidence. Chest. 2000;117(2 Suppl):1S–4S.
2. Afonso AS, Verhamme KM, Sturkenboom MC, Brusselle GG. COPD in the general population: prevalence, incidence and survival. Respir Med. 2011;105(12):1872–84.
3. Subbarao P, Mandhane PJ, Sears MR. Asthma: epidemiology, etiology and risk factors. CMAJ. 2009;181(9):E181–90.
4. Postma DS, Rabe KF. The asthma-COPD overlap syndrome. N Engl J Med. 2015;373(13):1241–9.
5. Akinbami LJ, Moorman JE, Bailey C, Zahran HS, King M, Johnson CA, et al. Trends in asthma prevalence, health care use, and mortality in the United States, 2001–2010. NCHS Data Brief. 2012;(94):1–8.
6. Vestbo J, Hurd SS, Agusti AG, Jones PW, Vogelmeier C, Anzueto A, et al. Global strategy for the diagnosis,

management, and prevention of chronic obstructive pulmonary disease: GOLD executive summary. Am J Respir Crit Care Med. 2013;187(4):347–65.

7. Ashley EA. The precision medicine initiative: a new national effort. JAMA. 2015;313(21):2119–20.

8. Vedel-Krogh S, Nielsen SF, Lange P, Vestbo J, Nordestgaard BG. Blood eosinophils and exacerbations in chronic obstructive pulmonary disease. The Copenhagen General Population Study. Am J Respir Crit Care Med. 2016;193(9):965–74.

9. Bafadhel M, Greening NJ, Harvey-Dunstan TC, Williams JE, Morgan MD, Brightling CE, et al. Blood eosinophils and outcomes in severe hospitalized exacerbations of COPD. Chest. 2016;150(2):320–8.

10. Pavord ID, Korn S, Howarth P, Bleecker ER, Buhl R, Keene ON, et al. Mepolizumab for severe eosinophilic asthma (DREAM): a multicentre, double-blind, placebo-controlled trial. Lancet. 2012;380(9842):651–9.

11. 2018 TGAR. http://globalasthmareport.org. Auckland, New Zealand: World Health Organization; 2018. Available from: http://globalasthmareport.org/Global%20Asthma%20Report%202018.pdf.

12. Kim H, Ellis AK, Fischer D, Noseworthy M, Olivenstein R, Chapman KR, et al. Asthma biomarkers in the age of biologics. Allergy Asthma Clin Immunol. 2017;13:48.

13. Gauthier M, Ray A, Wenzel SE. Evolving concepts of asthma. Am J Respir Crit Care Med. 2015;192(6):660–8.

14. Skloot GS. Asthma phenotypes and endotypes: a personalized approach to treatment. Curr Opin Pulm Med. 2016;22(1):3–9.

15. Guilleminault L, Ouksel H, Belleguic C, Le Guen Y, Germaud P, Desfleurs E, et al. Personalised medicine in asthma: from curative to preventive medicine. Eur Respir Rev. 2017;26(143):160010.

16. Lotvall J, Akdis CA, Bacharier LB, Bjermer L, Casale TB, Custovic A, et al. Asthma endotypes: a new approach to classification of disease entities within the asthma syndrome. J Allergy Clin Immunol. 2011;127(2):355–60.

17. Muraro A, Lemanske RF Jr, Hellings PW, Akdis CA, Bieber T, Casale TB, et al. Precision medicine in patients with allergic diseases: airway diseases and atopic dermatitis-PRACTALL document of the European Academy of Allergy and Clinical Immunology and the American Academy of Allergy, Asthma & Immunology. J Allergy Clin Immunol. 2016;137(5):1347–58.

18. Brown HM. Asthma, allergy and steroids. Br J Clin Pract. 1961;15:1001–17.

19. Robinson D, Humbert M, Buhl R, Cruz AA, Inoue H, Korom S, et al. Revisiting Type 2-high and Type 2-low airway inflammation in asthma: current knowledge and therapeutic implications. Clin Exp Allergy. 2017;47(2):161–75.

20. Fahy JV. Asthma was talking, but we weren't listening. Missed or ignored signals that have slowed treatment progress. Ann Am Thorac Soc. 2016;13(Suppl 1):S78–82.

21. Wenzel SE. Emergence of biomolecular pathways to define novel asthma phenotypes. Type-2 immunity and beyond. Am J Respir Cell Mol Biol. 2016;55(1):1–4.

22. Berry A, Busse WW. Biomarkers in asthmatic patients: has their time come to direct treatment? J Allergy Clin Immunol. 2016;137(5):1317–24.

23. Fitzpatrick AM. Biomarkers of asthma and allergic airway diseases. Ann Allergy Asthma Immunol. 2015;115(5):335–40.

24. Chung KF, Wenzel SE, Brozek JL, Bush A, Castro M, Sterk PJ, et al. International ERS/ATS guidelines on definition, evaluation and treatment of severe asthma. Eur Respir J. 2014;43(2):343–73.

25. Fahy JV. Type 2 inflammation in asthma--present in most, absent in many. Nat Rev Immunol. 2015;15(1):57–65.

26. Woodruff PG, Boushey HA, Dolganov GM, Barker CS, Yang YH, Donnelly S, et al. Genome-wide profiling identifies epithelial cell genes associated with asthma and with treatment response to corticosteroids. Proc Natl Acad Sci U S A. 2007;104(40):15858–63.

27. Chung KF. Asthma phenotyping: a necessity for improved therapeutic precision and new targeted therapies. J Intern Med. 2016;279(2):192–204.

28. Colice G, Price D, Gerhardsson de Verdier M, Rabon-Stith K, Ambrose C, Cappell K, et al. The effect of DPP-4 inhibitors on asthma control: an administrative database study to evaluate a potential pathophysiological relationship. Pragmat Obs Res. 2017;8:231–40.

29. Panganiban RP, Pinkerton MH, Maru SY, Jefferson SJ, Roff AN, Ishmael FT. Differential microRNA expression in asthma and the role of miR-1248 in regulation of IL-5. Am J Clin Exp Immunol. 2012;1(2):154–65.

30. Chogtu B, Bhattacharjee D, Magazine R. Epigenetics: the new frontier in the landscape of asthma. Scientifica. 2016;2016:4638949.

31. Vicente CT, Revez JA, Ferreira MAR. Lessons from ten years of genome-wide association studies of asthma. Clin Transl Immunology. 2017;6(12):e165.

32. Kelly RS, Dahlin A, McGeachie MJ, Qiu W, Sordillo J, Wan ES, et al. Asthma metabolomics and the potential for integrative omics in research and the clinic. Chest. 2017;151(2):262–77.

33. Smolinska A, Klaassen EM, Dallinga JW, van de Kant KD, Jobsis Q, Moonen EJ, et al. Profiling of volatile organic compounds in exhaled breath as a strategy to find early predictive signatures of asthma in children. PLoS One. 2014;9(4):e95668.

34. Motta A, Paris D, D'Amato M, Melck D, Calabrese C, Vitale C, et al. NMR metabolomic analysis of exhaled breath condensate of asthmatic patients at two different temperatures. J Proteome Res. 2014;13(12):6107–20.

35. Riccio AM, Mauri P, De Ferrari L, Rossi R, Di Silvestre D, Benazzi L, et al. Galectin-3: an early predictive biomarker of modulation of airway remodeling in patients with severe asthma treated with omalizumab for 36 months. Clin Transl Allergy. 2017;7:6.

36. Teran LM, Montes-Vizuet R, Li X, Franz T. Respiratory proteomics: from descriptive studies to personalized medicine. J Proteome Res. 2015;14(1):38–50.

37. Sokolowska M, Frei R, Lunjani N, Akdis CA, O'Mahony L. Microbiome and asthma. Asthma Res Pract. 2018;4:1.

38. Petty TL. The history of COPD. Int J Chron Obstruct Pulmon Dis. 2006;1(1):3–14.

39. Miller BE, Tal-Singer R, Rennard SI, Furtwaengler A, Leidy N, Lowings M, et al. Plasma fibrinogen qualification as a drug development tool in chronic obstructive pulmonary disease. Perspective of the chronic obstructive pulmonary disease biomarker qualification consortium. Am J Respir Crit Care Med. 2016;193(6):607–13.

40. Brightling CE, Bleecker ER, Panettieri RA Jr, Bafadhel M, She D, Ward CK, et al. Benralizumab for chronic obstructive pulmonary disease and sputum eosinophilia: a randomised, double-blind, placebo-controlled, phase 2a study. Lancet Respir Med. 2014;2(11):891–901.

41. DeMeo DL, Carey VJ, Chapman HA, Reilly JJ, Ginns LC, Speizer FE, et al. Familial aggregation of FEF(25–75) and FEF(25–75)/FVC in families with severe, early onset COPD. Thorax. 2004;59(5):396–400.

42. Kueppers F, Miller RD, Gordon H, Hepper NG, Offord K. Familial prevalence of chronic obstructive pulmonary disease in a matched pair study. Am J Med. 1977;63(3):336–42.

43. Larson RK, Barman ML, Kueppers F, Fudenberg HH. Genetic and environmental determinants of chronic obstructive pulmonary disease. Ann Intern Med. 1970;72(5):627–32.

44. Silverman EK, Chapman HA, Drazen JM, Weiss ST, Rosner B, Campbell EJ, et al. Genetic epidemiology of severe, early-onset chronic obstructive pulmonary disease. Risk to relatives for airflow obstruction and chronic bronchitis. Am J Respir Crit Care Med. 1998;157(6 Pt 1):1770–8.

45. Silverman EK, Sandhaus RA. Clinical practice. Alpha1-antitrypsin deficiency. N Engl J Med. 2009;360(26):2749–57.

46. Survival and FEV1 decline in individuals with severe deficiency of alpha1-antitrypsin. The Alpha-1-Antitrypsin Deficiency Registry Study Group. Am J Respir Crit Care Med. 1998;158(1):49–59.

47. Seersholm N, Wencker M, Banik N, Viskum K, Dirksen A, Kok-Jensen A, et al. Does alpha1-antitrypsin augmentation therapy slow the annual decline in FEV1 in patients with severe hereditary alpha1-antitrypsin deficiency? Wissenschaftliche Arbeitsgemeinschaft zur Therapie von Lungenerkrankungen (WATL) alpha1-AT study group. Eur Respir J. 1997;10(10):2260–3.

48. Wencker M, Fuhrmann B, Banik N, Konietzko N, Wissenschaftliche Arbeitsgemeinschaft zur Therapie von Lungenerkrankungen. Longitudinal follow-up of patients with alpha(1)-protease inhibitor deficiency before and during therapy with IV alpha(1)-protease inhibitor. Chest. 2001;119(3):737–44.

49. Dirksen A, Dijkman JH, Madsen F, Stoel B, Hutchison DC, Ulrik CS, et al. A randomized clinical trial of alpha(1)-antitrypsin augmentation therapy. Am J Respir Crit Care Med. 1999;160(5 Pt 1):1468–72.

50. Dirksen A, Piitulainen E, Parr DG, Deng C, Wencker M, Shaker SB, et al. Exploring the role of CT densitometry: a randomised study of augmentation therapy in alpha1-antitrypsin deficiency. Eur Respir J. 2009;33(6):1345–53.

51. Kim DK, Cho MH, Hersh CP, Lomas DA, Miller BE, Kong X, et al. Genome-wide association analysis of blood biomarkers in chronic obstructive pulmonary disease. Am J Respir Crit Care Med. 2012;186(12):1238–47.

52. Hunninghake GM, Cho MH, Tesfaigzi Y, Soto-Quiros ME, Avila L, Lasky-Su J, et al. MMP12, lung function, and COPD in high-risk populations. N Engl J Med. 2009;361(27):2599–608.

53. Cho MH, McDonald ML, Zhou X, Mattheisen M, Castaldi PJ, Hersh CP, et al. Risk loci for chronic obstructive pulmonary disease: a genome-wide association study and meta-analysis. Lancet Respir Med. 2014;2(3):214–25.

54. Pillai SG, Ge D, Zhu G, Kong X, Shianna KV, Need AC, et al. A genome-wide association study in chronic obstructive pulmonary disease (COPD): identification of two major susceptibility loci. PLoS Genet. 2009;5(3):e1000421.

55. Hardin M, Zielinski J, Wan ES, Hersh CP, Castaldi PJ, Schwinder E, et al. CHRNA3/5, IREB2, and ADCY2 are associated with severe chronic obstructive pulmonary disease in Poland. Am J Respir Cell Mol Biol. 2012;47(2):203–8.

56. Wilk JB, Shrine NR, Loehr LR, Zhao JH, Manichaikul A, Lopez LM, et al. Genome-wide association studies identify CHRNA5/3 and HTR4 in the development of airflow obstruction. Am J Respir Crit Care Med. 2012;186(7):622–32.

57. Wilk JB, Chen TH, Gottlieb DJ, Walter RE, Nagle MW, Brandler BJ, et al. A genome-wide association study of pulmonary function measures in the Framingham Heart Study. PLoS Genet. 2009;5(3):e1000429.

58. Van Durme YM, Eijgelsheim M, Joos GF, Hofman A, Uitterlinden AG, Brusselle GG, et al. Hedgehog-interacting protein is a COPD susceptibility gene: the Rotterdam Study. Eur Respir J. 2010;36(1):89–95.

59. Zhou X, Baron RM, Hardin M, Cho MH, Zielinski J, Hawrylkiewicz I, et al. Identification of a chronic obstructive pulmonary disease genetic determinant that regulates HHIP. Hum Mol Genet. 2012;21(6):1325–35.

60. Rodriguez-Roisin R. Toward a consensus definition for COPD exacerbations. Chest. 2000;117(5 Suppl 2):398S–401S.

61. Burge S, Wedzicha JA. COPD exacerbations: definitions and classifications. Eur Respir J Suppl. 2003;41:46s–53s.

62. Hogg JC, Chu F, Utokaparch S, Woods R, Elliott WM, Buzatu L, et al. The nature of small-airway obstruction in chronic obstructive pulmonary disease. N Engl J Med. 2004;350(26):2645–53.

63. Cosio MG, Saetta M, Agusti A. Immunologic aspects of chronic obstructive pulmonary disease. N Engl J Med. 2009;360(23):2445–54.

64. Cockayne DA, Cheng DT, Waschki B, Sridhar S, Ravindran P, Hilton H, et al. Systemic biomarkers of neutrophilic inflammation, tissue injury and repair in COPD patients with differing levels of disease severity. PLoS One. 2012;7(6):e38629.

65. Hurst JR, Anzueto A, Vestbo J. Susceptibility to exacerbation in COPD. Lancet Respir Med. 2017;5(9):e29.

66. Thomsen M, Ingebrigtsen TS, Marott JL, Dahl M, Lange P, Vestbo J, et al. Inflammatory biomarkers and exacerbations in chronic obstructive pulmonary disease. JAMA. 2013;309(22):2353–61.

67. Hurst JR, Donaldson GC, Perera WR, Wilkinson TM, Bilello JA, Hagan GW, et al. Use of plasma biomarkers at exacerbation of chronic obstructive pulmonary disease. Am J Respir Crit Care Med. 2006;174(8):867–74.

68. Agusti A, Edwards LD, Rennard SI, MacNee W, Tal-Singer R, Miller BE, et al. Persistent systemic inflammation is associated with poor clinical outcomes in COPD: a novel phenotype. PLoS One. 2012;7(5):e37483.

69. Chan KH, Yeung SC, Yao TJ, Ip MS, Cheung AH, Chan-Yeung MM, et al. Elevated plasma adiponectin levels in patients with chronic obstructive pulmonary disease. Int J Tuberc Lung Dis. 2010;14(9):1193–200.

70. Bozinovski S, Hutchinson A, Thompson M, Macgregor L, Black J, Giannakis E, et al. Serum amyloid a is a biomarker of acute exacerbations of chronic obstructive pulmonary disease. Am J Respir Crit Care Med. 2008;177(3):269–78.

71. Celli BR, Locantore N, Yates J, Tal-Singer R, Miller BE, Bakke P, et al. Inflammatory biomarkers improve clinical prediction of mortality in chronic obstructive pulmonary disease. Am J Respir Crit Care Med. 2012;185(10):1065–72.

72. Stanescu D, Sanna A, Veriter C, Kostianev S, Calcagni PG, Fabbri LM, et al. Airways obstruction, chronic expectoration, and rapid decline of FEV1 in smokers are associated with increased levels of sputum neutrophils. Thorax. 1996;51(3):267–71.

73. Singh D, Edwards L, Tal-Singer R, Rennard S. Sputum neutrophils as a biomarker in COPD: findings from the ECLIPSE study. Respir Res. 2010;11:77.

74. Mercer PF, Shute JK, Bhowmik A, Donaldson GC, Wedzicha JA, Warner JA. MMP-9, TIMP-1 and inflammatory cells in sputum from COPD patients during exacerbation. Respir Res. 2005;6:151.

75. Lomas DA, Silverman EK, Edwards LD, Locantore NW, Miller BE, Horstman DH, et al. Serum surfactant protein D is steroid sensitive and associated with exacerbations of COPD. Eur Respir J. 2009;34(1):95–102.

76. More JM, Voelker DR, Silveira LJ, Edwards MG, Chan ED, Bowler RP. Smoking reduces surfactant protein D and phospholipids in patients with and without chronic obstructive pulmonary disease. BMC Pulm Med. 2010;10:53.

77. Bhavani S, Tsai CL, Perusich S, Hesselbacher S, Coxson H, Pandit L, et al. Clinical and immunological factors in emphysema progression. Five-year prospective longitudinal exacerbation study of chronic obstructive pulmonary disease (LES-COPD). Am J Respir Crit Care Med. 2015;192(10):1171–8.

78. Broeckaert F, Bernard A. Clara cell secretory protein (CC16): characteristics and perspectives as lung peripheral biomarker. Clin Exp Allergy. 2000;30(4):469–75.

79. Park HY, Churg A, Wright JL, Li Y, Tam S, Man SF, et al. Club cell protein 16 and disease progression in chronic obstructive pulmonary disease. Am J Respir Crit Care Med. 2013;188(12):1413–9.

80. Gamez AS, Gras D, Petit A, Knabe L, Molinari N, Vachier I, et al. Supplementing defect in club cell secretory protein attenuates airway inflammation in COPD. Chest. 2015;147(6):1467–76.

81. Higashimoto Y, Iwata T, Okada M, Satoh H, Fukuda K, Tohda Y. Serum biomarkers as predictors of lung function decline in chronic obstructive pulmonary disease. Respir Med. 2009;103(8):1231–8.

82. Yonchuk JG, Silverman EK, Bowler RP, Agusti A, Lomas DA, Miller BE, et al. Circulating soluble receptor for advanced glycation end products (sRAGE) as a biomarker of emphysema and the RAGE axis in the lung. Am J Respir Crit Care Med. 2015;192(7):785–92.

83. Cheng DT, Kim DK, Cockayne DA, Belousov A, Bitter H, Cho MH, et al. Systemic soluble receptor for advanced glycation endproducts is a biomarker of emphysema and associated with AGER genetic variants in patients with chronic obstructive pulmonary disease. Am J Respir Crit Care Med. 2013;188(8):948–57.

84. Carolan BJ, Hughes G, Morrow J, Hersh CP, O'Neal WK, Rennard S, et al. The association of plasma biomarkers with computed tomography-assessed emphysema phenotypes. Respir Res. 2014;15:127.

85. Miniati M, Monti S, Basta G, Cocci F, Fornai E, Bottai M. Soluble receptor for advanced glycation end products in COPD: relationship with emphysema and chronic cor pulmonale: a case-control study. Respir Res. 2011;12:37.

86. Hancock DB, Eijgelsheim M, Wilk JB, Gharib SA, Loehr LR, Marciante KD, et al. Meta-analyses of genome-wide association studies identify multiple loci associated with pulmonary function. Nat Genet. 2010;42(1):45–52.

87. Repapi E, Sayers I, Wain LV, Burton PR, Johnson T, Obeidat M, et al. Genome-wide association study identifies five loci associated with lung function. Nat Genet. 2010;42(1):36–44.

88. Castaldi PJ, Cho MH, San Jose Estepar R, McDonald ML, Laird N, Beaty TH, et al. Genome-wide association identifies regulatory Loci associated with distinct local histogram emphysema patterns. Am J Respir Crit Care Med. 2014;190(4):399–409.

89. Manichaikul A, Hoffman EA, Smolonska J, Gao W, Cho MH, Baumhauer H, et al. Genome-wide study of percent emphysema on computed tomography in the general population. The Multi-Ethnic Study of Atherosclerosis Lung/SNP Health Association Resource Study. Am J Respir Crit Care Med. 2014;189(4):408–18.

90. Gopal P, Reynaert NL, Scheijen JL, Schalkwijk CG, Franssen FM, Wouters EF, et al. Association of plasma sRAGE, but not esRAGE with lung function impairment in COPD. Respir Res. 2014;15:24.

91. Gopal P, Rutten EP, Dentener MA, Wouters EF, Reynaert NL. Decreased plasma sRAGE levels in COPD: influence of oxygen therapy. Eur J Clin Investig. 2012;42(8):807–14.

92. Iwamoto H, Gao J, Pulkkinen V, Toljamo T, Nieminen P, Mazur W. Soluble receptor for advanced glycation end-products and progression of airway disease. BMC Pulm Med. 2014;14:68.

93. Luisetti M, Ma S, Iadarola P, Stone PJ, Viglio S, Casado B, et al. Desmosine as a biomarker of elastin degradation in COPD: current status and future directions. Eur Respir J. 2008;32(5):1146–57.

94. Lomas DA, Silverman EK, Edwards LD, Miller BE, Coxson HO, Tal-Singer R, et al. Evaluation of serum CC-16 as a biomarker for COPD in the ECLIPSE cohort. Thorax. 2008;63(12):1058–63.

95. Braido F, Riccio AM, Guerra L, Gamalero C, Zolezzi A, Tarantini F, et al. Clara cell 16 protein in COPD sputum: a marker of small airways damage? Respir Med. 2007;101(10):2119–24.

96. Pinto-Plata V, Casanova C, Mullerova H, de Torres JP, Corado H, Varo N, et al. Inflammatory and repair serum biomarker pattern: association to clinical outcomes in COPD. Respir Res. 2012;13:71.

97. Ma S, Lieberman S, Turino GM, Lin YY. The detection and quantitation of free desmosine and isodesmosine in human urine and their peptide-bound forms in sputum. Proc Natl Acad Sci U S A. 2003;100(22):12941–3.

98. Turino GM, Ma S, Lin YY, Cantor JO, Luisetti M. Matrix elastin: a promising biomarker for chronic obstructive pulmonary disease. Am J Respir Crit Care Med. 2011;184(6):637–41.

99. Atamas SP, Luzina IG, Choi J, Tsymbalyuk N, Carbonetti NH, Singh IS, et al. Pulmonary and activation-regulated chemokine stimulates collagen production in lung fibroblasts. Am J Respir Cell Mol Biol. 2003;29(6):743–9.

100. Sin DD, Miller BE, Duvoix A, Man SF, Zhang X, Silverman EK, et al. Serum PARC/CCL-18 concentrations and health outcomes in chronic obstructive pulmonary disease. Am J Respir Crit Care Med. 2011;183(9):1187–92.

101. Kunisaki KM, Dransfield MT, Anderson JA, Brook RD, Calverley PMA, Celli BR, et al. Exacerbations of chronic obstructive pulmonary disease and cardiac events. A post hoc cohort analysis from the SUMMIT randomized clinical trial. Am J Respir Crit Care Med. 2018;198(1):51–7.

102. Faner R, Tal-Singer R, Riley JH, Celli B, Vestbo J, MacNee W, et al. Lessons from ECLIPSE: a review of COPD biomarkers. Thorax. 2014;69(7):666–72.

103. Ubhi BK, Cheng KK, Dong J, Janowitz T, Jodrell D, Tal-Singer R, et al. Targeted metabolomics identifies perturbations in amino acid metabolism that sub-classify patients with COPD. Mol BioSyst. 2012;8(12):3125–33.

104. Ghidoni R, Caretti A, Signorelli P. Role of sphingolipids in the pathobiology of lung inflammation. Mediat Inflamm. 2015;2015:487508.

105. Petrache I, Kamocki K, Poirier C, Pewzner-Jung Y, Laviad EL, Schweitzer KS, et al. Ceramide synthases expression and role of ceramide synthase-2 in the lung: insight from human lung cells and mouse models. PLoS One. 2013;8(5):e62968.

106. Petrache I, Natarajan V, Zhen L, Medler TR, Richter AT, Cho C, et al. Ceramide upregulation causes pulmonary cell apoptosis and emphysema-like disease in mice. Nat Med. 2005;11(5):491–8.

107. Bowler RP, Jacobson S, Cruickshank C, Hughes GJ, Siska C, Ory DS, et al. Plasma sphingolipids associated with chronic obstructive pulmonary disease phenotypes. Am J Respir Crit Care Med. 2015;191(3):275–84.

108. Wendt CH, Nelsestuen G, Harvey S, Gulcev M, Stone M, Reilly C. Peptides in bronchoalveolar lavage in chronic obstructive pulmonary disease. PLoS One. 2016;11(5):e0155724.

109. O'Reilly P, Jackson PL, Noerager B, Parker S, Dransfield M, Gaggar A, et al. N-alpha-PGP and PGP, potential biomarkers and therapeutic targets for COPD. Respir Res. 2009;10:38.

110. Weathington NM, van Houwelingen AH, Noerager BD, Jackson PL, Kraneveld AD, Galin FS, et al. A novel peptide CXCR ligand derived from extracellular matrix degradation during airway inflammation. Nat Med. 2006;12(3):317–23.

111. O'Reilly PJ, Jackson PL, Wells JM, Dransfield MT, Scanlon PD, Blalock JE. Sputum PGP is reduced by azithromycin treatment in patients with COPD and correlates with exacerbations. BMJ Open. 2013;3(12):e004140.

112. Gulcev M, Reilly C, Griffin TJ, Broeckling CD, Sandri BJ, Witthuhn BA, et al. Tryptophan catabolism in acute exacerbations of chronic obstructive pulmonary disease. Int J Chron Obstruct Pulmon Dis. 2016;11:2435–46.

113. Engin AB, Ozkan Y, Fuchs D, Yardim-Akaydin S. Increased tryptophan degradation in patients with bronchus carcinoma. Eur J Cancer Care (Engl). 2010;19(6):803–8.

114. Barker BL, Haldar K, Patel H, Pavord ID, Barer MR, Brightling CE, et al. Association between pathogens detected using quantitative polymerase chain reaction with airway inflammation in COPD at stable state and exacerbations. Chest. 2015;147(1):46–55.

115. Martinez FJ, Erb-Downward JR, Huffnagle GB. Significance of the microbiome in chronic obstructive pulmonary disease. Ann Am Thorac Soc. 2013;10(Suppl):S170–9.

116. Garcia-Nunez M, Millares L, Pomares X, Ferrari R, Perez-Brocal V, Gallego M, et al. Severity-related changes of bronchial microbiome in chronic

obstructive pulmonary disease. J Clin Microbiol. 2014;52(12):4217–23.

117. Pragman AA, Kim HB, Reilly CS, Wendt C, Isaacson RE. Chronic obstructive pulmonary disease lung microbiota diversity may be mediated by age or inhaled corticosteroid use. J Clin Microbiol. 2015;53(3):1050.

118. Pragman AA, Lyu T, Baller JA, Gould TJ, Kelly RF, Reilly CS, et al. The lung tissue microbiota of mild and moderate chronic obstructive pulmonary disease. Microbiome. 2018;6(1):7.

119. Postma DS, Weiss ST, van den Berge M, Kerstjens HA, Koppelman GH. Revisiting the Dutch hypothesis. J Allergy Clin Immunol. 2015;136(3):521–9.

120. Kauppi P, Kupiainen H, Lindqvist A, Tammilehto L, Kilpelainen M, Kinnula VL, et al. Overlap syndrome of asthma and COPD predicts low quality of life. J Asthma. 2011;48(3):279–85.

121. Hardin M, Silverman EK, Barr RG, Hansel NN, Schroeder JD, Make BJ, et al. The clinical features of the overlap between COPD and asthma. Respir Res. 2011;12:127.

122. GOLD Ga. Diagnosis and initial treatment of asthma, COPD and asthma-COPD overlap. 2017. Available from: https://ginasthma.org/.

123. Sin DD, Miravitlles M, Mannino DM, Soriano JB, Price D, Celli BR, et al. What is asthma-COPD overlap syndrome? Towards a consensus definition from a round table discussion. Eur Respir J. 2016;48(3):664–73.

124. Cosentino J, Zhao H, Hardin M, Hersh CP, Crapo J, Kim V, et al. Analysis of asthma-chronic obstructive pulmonary disease overlap syndrome defined on the basis of bronchodilator response and degree of emphysema. Ann Am Thorac Soc. 2016;13(9):1483–9.

125. Barrecheguren M, Esquinas C, Miravitlles M. The asthma-COPD overlap syndrome: a new entity? COPD Res Pract. 2015;1:8.

126. Maselli DJ, Hardin M, Christenson SA, Hanania NA, Hersh CP, Adams SG, et al. Clinical approach to the therapy of asthma-COPD overlap. Chest. 2019;155:168–77.

127. Ghebre MA, Bafadhel M, Desai D, Cohen SE, Newbold P, Rapley L, et al. Biological clustering supports both "Dutch" and "British" hypotheses of asthma and chronic obstructive pulmonary disease. J Allergy Clin Immunol. 2015;135(1):63–72.

128. Barnes PJ. Therapeutic approaches to asthma-chronic obstructive pulmonary disease overlap syndromes. J Allergy Clin Immunol. 2015;136(3):531–45.

129. Cosio BG, Perez de Llano L, Lopez Vina A, Torrego A, Lopez-Campos JL, Soriano JB, et al. Th-2 signature in chronic airway diseases: towards the extinction of asthma-COPD overlap syndrome? Eur Respir J. 2017;49(5):1602397.

130. Gibson PG, Simpson JL. The overlap syndrome of asthma and COPD: what are its features and how important is it? Thorax. 2009;64(8):728–35.

131. Kobayashi S, Hanagama M, Yamanda S, Ishida M, Yanai M. Inflammatory biomarkers in asthma-COPD overlap syndrome. Int J Chron Obstruct Pulmon Dis. 2016;11:2117–23.

132. Christenson SA, Steiling K, van den Berge M, Hijazi K, Hiemstra PS, Postma DS, et al. Asthma-COPD overlap. Clinical relevance of genomic signatures of type 2 inflammation in chronic obstructive pulmonary disease. Am J Respir Crit Care Med. 2015;191(7):758–66.

133. Gostner JM, Becker K, Kofler H, Strasser B, Fuchs D. Tryptophan metabolism in allergic disorders. Int Arch Allergy Immunol. 2016;169(4):203–15.

134. Magnus MC, Karlstad O, Midtun O, Haberg SE, Tunheim G, Parr CL, et al. Maternal plasma total neopterin and kynurenine/tryptophan levels during pregnancy in relation to asthma development in the offspring. J Allergy Clin Immunol. 2016;138(5):1319–25.e4.

135. Zinellu A, Fois AG, Zinellu E, Sotgiu E, Sotgia S, Arru D, et al. Increased kynurenine plasma concentrations and kynurenine-tryptophan ratio in mild-to-moderate chronic obstructive pulmonary disease patients. Biomark Med. 2018;12(3):229–37.

136. Dweik RA, Boggs PB, Erzurum SC, Irvin CG, Leigh MW, Lundberg JO, et al. An official ATS clinical practice guideline: interpretation of exhaled nitric oxide levels (FENO) for clinical applications. Am J Respir Crit Care Med. 2011;184(5):602–15.

137. Mostafavi-Pour-Manshadi SM, Naderi N, Barrecheguren M, Dehghan A, Bourbeau J. Investigating fractional exhaled nitric oxide in chronic obstructive pulmonary disease (COPD) and asthma-COPD overlap (ACO): a scoping review. COPD. 2018;15(4):377–91.

138. Gao J, Iwamoto H, Koskela J, Alenius H, Hattori N, Kohno N, et al. Characterization of sputum biomarkers for asthma-COPD overlap syndrome. Int J Chron Obstruct Pulmon Dis. 2016;11:2457–65.

139. Iwamoto H, Gao J, Koskela J, Kinnula V, Kobayashi H, Laitinen T, et al. Differences in plasma and sputum biomarkers between COPD and COPD-asthma overlap. Eur Respir J. 2014;43(2):421–9.

140. Chong J, Leung B, Poole P. Phosphodiesterase 4 inhibitors for chronic obstructive pulmonary disease. Cochrane Database Syst Rev. 2017;(9):Cd002309.

141. Hanania NA, Wenzel S, Rosen K, Hsieh HJ, Mosesova S, Choy DF, et al. Exploring the effects of omalizumab in allergic asthma: an analysis of biomarkers in the EXTRA study. Am J Respir Crit Care Med. 2013;187(8):804–11.

142. Lefaudeux D, De Meulder B, Loza MJ, Peffer N, Rowe A, Baribaud F, et al. U-BIOPRED clinical adult asthma clusters linked to a subset of sputum omics. J Allergy Clin Immunol. 2017;139(6):1797–807.

143. Kuo CS, Pavlidis S, Loza M, Baribaud F, Rowe A, Pandis I, et al. A transcriptome-driven analysis of epithelial brushings and bronchial biopsies to define

asthma phenotypes in U-BIOPRED. Am J Respir Crit Care Med. 2017;195(4):443–55.

144. Zhu B, Song N, Shen R, Arora A, Machiela MJ, Song L, et al. Integrating clinical and multiple omics data for prognostic assessment across human cancers. Sci Rep. 2017;7(1):16954.

145. Li CX, Wheelock CE, Skold CM, Wheelock AM. Integration of multi-omics datasets enables molecular classification of COPD. Eur Respir J. 2018;51(5):1701930.

146. Reinke SN, Gallart-Ayala H, Gomez C, Checa A, Fauland A, Naz S, et al. Metabolomics analysis identifies different metabotypes of asthma severity. Eur Respir J. 2017;49(3):1601740.

147. Moore WC, Meyers DA, Wenzel SE, Teague WG, Li H, Li X, et al. Identification of asthma phenotypes using cluster analysis in the Severe Asthma Research Program. Am J Respir Crit Care Med. 2010;181(4):315–23.

148. Peters MC, Mekonnen ZK, Yuan S, Bhakta NR, Woodruff PG, Fahy JV. Measures of gene expression in sputum cells can identify TH2-high and TH2-low subtypes of asthma. J Allergy Clin Immunol. 2014;133(2):388–94.

149. Sinha A, Desiraju K, Aggarwal K, Kutum R, Roy S, Lodha R, et al. Exhaled breath condensate metabolome clusters for endotype discovery in asthma. J Transl Med. 2017;15(1):262.

150. Howrylak JA, Moll M, Weiss ST, Raby BA, Wu W, Xing EP. Gene expression profiling of asthma phenotypes demonstrates molecular signatures of atopy and asthma control. J Allergy Clin Immunol. 2016;137(5):1390–7.e6.

151. Blighe K, Chawes BL, Kelly RS, Mirzakhani H, McGeachie M, Litonjua AA, et al. Vitamin D prenatal programming of childhood metabolomics profiles at age 3 y. Am J Clin Nutr. 2017;106(4):1092–9.

152. Wenzel SE, Schwartz LB, Langmack EL, Halliday JL, Trudeau JB, Gibbs RL, et al. Evidence that severe asthma can be divided pathologically into two inflammatory subtypes with distinct physiologic and clinical characteristics. Am J Respir Crit Care Med. 1999;160(3):1001–8.

153. Hinks T, Zhou X, Staples K, Dimitrov B, Manta A, Petrossian T, et al. Multidimensional endotypes of asthma: topological data analysis of cross-sectional clinical, pathological, and immunological data. Lancet. 2015;385(Suppl 1):S42.

154. Kelly RS, McGeachie MJ, Lee-Sarwar KA, Kachroo P, Chu SH, Virkud YV, et al. Partial least squares discriminant analysis and Bayesian networks for metabolomic prediction of childhood asthma. Meta. 2018;8(4):68.

155. Agache I, Akdis CA. Endotypes of allergic diseases and asthma: an important step in building blocks for the future of precision medicine. Allergol Int. 2016;65(3):243–52.

156. Bowler RP, Wendt CH, Fessler MB, Foster MW, Kelly RS, Lasky-Su J, et al. New strategies and challenges in lung proteomics and metabolomics. An official American Thoracic Society workshop report. Ann Am Thorac Soc. 2017;14(12):1721–43.

157. McCracken JL, Tripple JW, Calhoun WJ. Biologic therapy in the management of asthma. Curr Opin Allergy Clin Immunol. 2016;16(4):375–82.

158. Institute NHLaB. Trans-omics for Precision Medicine (TOPMed) Program. 2014. Available from: https://www.nhlbi.nih.gov/science/trans-omics-precision-medicine-topmed-program.

159. Zou Y, Chen X, Liu J, Zhou DB, Kuang X, Xiao J, et al. Serum IL-1beta and IL-17 levels in patients with COPD: associations with clinical parameters. Int J Chron Obstruct Pulmon Dis. 2017;12:1247–54.

160. Smith DJ, Yerkovich ST, Towers MA, Carroll ML, Thomas R, Upham JW. Reduced soluble receptor for advanced glycation end-products in COPD. Eur Respir J. 2011;37(3):516–22.

161. Zhang L, Cheng Z, Liu W, Wu K. Expression of interleukin (IL)-10, IL-17A and IL-22 in serum and sputum of stable chronic obstructive pulmonary disease patients. COPD. 2013;10(4):459–65.

162. Roos AB, Sethi S, Nikota J, Wrona CT, Dorrington MG, Sanden C, et al. IL-17A and the promotion of neutrophilia in acute exacerbation of chronic obstructive pulmonary disease. Am J Respir Crit Care Med. 2015;192(4):428–37.

163. Muro S, Taha R, Tsicopoulos A, Olivenstein R, Tonnel AB, Christodoulopoulos P, et al. Expression of IL-15 in inflammatory pulmonary diseases. J Allergy Clin Immunol. 2001;108(6):970–5.

164. Papaporfyriou A, Loukides S, Kostikas K, Simoes DCM, Papatheodorou G, Konstantellou E, et al. Increased levels of osteopontin in sputum supernatant in patients with COPD. Chest. 2014;146(4):951–8.

Biomarkers in Interstitial Lung Diseases

11

Isis E. Fernandez and Oliver Eickelberg

Key Point Summary
- There is an urgent need to identify and validate ILD biomarkers for early diagnosis, and monitoring of disease progression and outcomes.
- Pivotal fibrosis pathophysiology pathways for which biomarker candidates exist are epithelial and immune dysfunction, and ECM remodeling and fibroproliferation.
- Analysis of genomic, proteomic, and other omics data will drive discovery of ILD subphenotypes and enable the development of tailored, pathway-driven therapeutic approaches.

I. E. Fernandez (✉)
Comprehensive Pneumology Center, Ludwig-Maximilians-University and Helmholtz Zentrum München, Member of the German Center for Lung Research, Munich, Germany
e-mail: isis.fernandez@helmholtz-muenchen.de

O. Eickelberg
Division of Pulmonary Sciences and Critical Care Medicine, Department of Medicine, University of Colorado, Aurora, CO, USA
e-mail: oliver.eickelberg@ucdenver.edu

Introduction

Diffuse parenchymal lung diseases (DPLD) are a diverse group of clinical entities, where reversible or irreversible scarring and interstitial fibrosis of the lung occurs. So far, more than 150 causes of DPLD are recognized. For the majority of patients, it is possible to identify a DPLD trigger, such as mold, bird exposure, or an underlying autoimmune disease. However, when no cause is identified, the diagnosis of idiopathic interstitial pneumonia (IIP) is considered. Idiopathic pulmonary fibrosis (IPF) is the most common and lethal type of all IIPs [1–3]. Other types of DPLD that are not IIP, broadly called interstitial lung disease (ILD), include disorders with known causes of fibrosis associated with collagen tissue disorders and autoimmune diseases, granulomatous diseases, and other forms of ILD [4]. DPLD affect the interstitium of the lung, distort pulmonary architecture, and alter the gas exchange ability of the lung. Whether or not associated causes of ILD are identified, once scarring of the lung occurs, it is irreversible. The heterogeneity of ILD is extremely complex, with multiple common features and high overlap in clinical, radiological, and pathological patterns, requiring a multidisciplinary team for diagnosis, and in some cases, open surgical lung biopsy, a procedure with relatively high mortality risk [5]. Thus, there is an urgent need to identify molecu-

© Springer Nature Switzerland AG 2020
J. L. Gomez et al. (eds.), *Precision in Pulmonary, Critical Care, and Sleep Medicine*,
Respiratory Medicine, https://doi.org/10.1007/978-3-030-31507-8_11

lar fingerprints and corresponding biomarkers to improve diagnostic accuracy in ILD.

Idiopathic pulmonary fibrosis (IPF) is a devastating and lethal disease, with a median survival of 2–3 years after diagnosis. It is chronic, progressive, and occurs predominantly in middle aged and older adults. The direct cause of IPF is unknown. People with genetic susceptibility and life-long exposure to known risk factors account for up to a third of all patients [6]. To date, while the key initiating triggers are unidentified, it is known that pulmonary fibrosis develops as an abnormal response to various lung insults that trigger aberrant wound-healing [7], epithelial apoptosis and senescence [8, 9], uncontrolled fibroblast proliferation and activation [10], excessive extracellular matrix deposition [11], and a fibrotic-related immune reaction [12]. Several environmental risk factors and life-long exposures contribute to initiate microinjuries in the lung, including familial susceptibility [13, 14], cigarette smoking [15] and other environmental exposures [16], chronic silent microaspiration [17], and chronic viral infection [18], especially by herpes virus [19, 20].

Despite advances in understanding the molecular mechanisms, genetic factors, and clinical features of IPF, there are several unmet needs. Currently, the two drugs available for IPF treatment, pirfenidone and nintedanib, slow lung function decline and disease progression, but they are unable to cure IPF. As is the case for non-IPF ILD of idiopathic origin, lung transplantation is the only curative IPF treatment, although it has a median survival of approximately 5 years and is accessible only to a highly selected patient population. Furthermore, there are no clinically approved prognostic or predictive biomarker tests to guide patient care.

Because IPF is a disease that primarily affects older individuals with severely compromised respiratory function, the quest for biomarkers has focused on easily accessible peripheral blood biomarkers, rather than invasive measurements in bronchoalveolar lavage (BAL) or lung tissue. Nevertheless, obtaining samples to detect invasive biomarkers may significantly improve our understanding of the pathogenesis of fibrotic lung diseases, and thus, should not be discounted.

Biomarkers are by definition objective, quantifiable characteristics of biological processes. They may, but do not necessarily, correlate with a patient's experience and sense of well-being. There are several types of biomarkers, including diagnostic and prognostic, which help to discriminate between those with and without a particular disease, and predict disease severity or outcomes, respectively [21]. Predictive biomarkers can help determine responsiveness to pharmacological therapy, and thus, be used to stratify patients for clinical trials. Ideally, biomarkers should have an additive value to well-established clinical or functional disease criteria, or serve as a substitute for invasive diagnostic or prognostic procedures (Fig. 11.1) [22].

To date, there are no molecular biomarkers in widespread use for IPF or non-IPF ILD. Although several exciting candidates are under study, none of them have reached clinical practice. For both IPF and non-IPF ILD, there is an urgent need to identify and validate biomarkers to predict disease diagnosis, progression and outcomes [23]. Currently, detection of interstitial lung abnormalities via imaging is the best, albeit limited, approach for early detection of fibrosis [24, 25]. Recent studies of subclinical interstitial lung abnormalities detected by computed tomography (CT) scans in large cohorts have provided independent and reproducible evidence that interstitial lung abnormalities are present in the general population [25–28], are more common in smokers [25], are associated with *MUC5B* promoter polymorphisms and pulmonary function decline [27], progress into a definitive fibrotic disease over time [26], and are associated with increased risk of mortality [28]. Therefore, it is hypothesized that interstitial lung abnormalities could represent the preclinical form of IPF. More broadly, these findings support the feasibility of identifying early biomarkers to aid in the diagnosis of idiopathic forms of fibrosis.

IPF is a highly complex molecular disorder, where multiple lung structural cell types (e.g.,

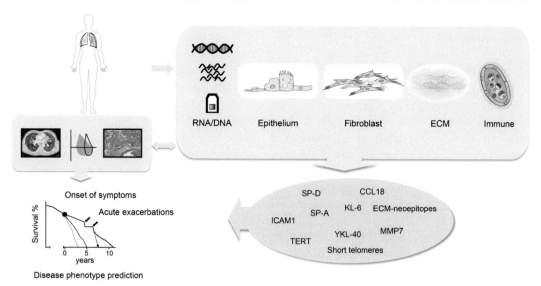

Modified from Greiffo FR, Fernandez IE. ERR 2017

Fig. 11.1 Biomarker analysis of ILD patients. Comprehensive compartmental biomarkers analysis includes clinical data, functional lung parameters, imaging, as well as biological components as, e.g., RNA, epithelium-, fibroblast-, ECM-, and immune-derived targets. (Adapted from Greiffo et al. [22])

Table 11.1 Potential biomarkers in IPF

Compartment	Biomarker	Predisposition	Diagnosis	Prognosis	Therapy monitoring
Alveolar epithelial cell	SP-A + SP-D	−	−	+	−
	KL-6	−	−	++	+
	Telomere shortening	++	−	−	−
	Compiled signature	−	+	+	−
Extracellular matrix and fibroproliferation	MMP7	−	+	++	−
	Neoepitopes	−	−	+	−
	Fibrocytes	−	−	+	−
Immune dysregulation/ inflammation	YKL-40	−	−	+	±
	CCL18	−	−	+	−
	52 gene signature	−	−	++	−

Notes: Markers are rated as follows: ++ denotes relatively strong evidence for the biomarker based on multiple studies or on large single studies; + denotes small single-study evidence for biomarker utility; ± denotes candidate biomarkers with equivocal evidence; − denotes candidate biomarkers without data

Abbreviations: *SP* surfactant protein, *KL-6* Krebs von den Lungen 6, *MMP7* matrix metalloproteinase-7, *CCL18* chemokine (C-C motif) ligand 18, *IL-8* interleukin-8, *ICAM-1* intercellular adhesion molecule-1

epithelial, fibroblast, mesenchymal) interact with innate and adaptive immune cells to impair organ function, increase extracellular matrix (ECM) deposition, and ultimately, destroy the lung architecture. To comprehensively cover different pathways involved in the pathogenesis of IPF, and the diverse nature of molecules involved in disease, we next present candidate biomarkers categorized according to the compartment and processes they are related to epithelial dysfunction, ECM remodeling and fibroproliferation, and immune dysfunction observed in peripheral blood and lung (Table 11.1) [23].

Epithelial Dysfunction Candidate Biomarkers

Surfactant Proteins

Surfactant proteins (SPs), which are synthesized and secreted by alveolar epithelial type II (AEC II) cells, facilitate the transport and function of surfactant lipids that reduce alveolar surface tension and prevent lung collapse, as well as serve as host defense against infectious agents in the terminal airways [29]. Levels of surfactant proteins A (SP-A) and D (SP-D) were elevated in serum and BAL of patients with IPF and other ILDs [30–32]. Increased serum SP-A and SP-D levels predicted mortality in a cohort of IPF patients [33], and SP-D levels were associated with deteriorating lung function values [34, 35] and acute exacerbations [36]. A meta-analysis studying the use of SP-A and SP-D as biomarkers for the diagnosis and prognosis of IPF reported that patients with IPF had higher levels of SP-A compared to patients with other ILDs, and that SP-D was associated with the prognosis and frequency of acute exacerbations. Additionally, genetic variants of the surfactant protein A2 (*SFTPA2*) and surfactant protein C (*SFTPC*) genes were associated with the development of lung fibrosis [37], while variants of the gene encoding SP-A1 (*SFTPA1*) and *SFTPA2* were associated with a disease phenotype of IPF that coexisted with lung cancer [38]. Thus, surfactant proteins may serve as biomarkers of abnormal function, injury, apoptosis, or proliferation of type II AECs, although their ability to reflect disease activity over time and their clinical utility have not yet been established.

Krebs von den Lungen-6 (KL-6)

KL-6 is a mucin-like high-molecular-weight glycoprotein expressed on the surface membrane of alveolar epithelial cells. It is released into the bloodstream when alveolar epithelial cells proliferate, are activated, or are injured. Increased serum levels of KL-6 have been observed in people with IPF [39], as well as other forms of interstitial lung fibrosis and malignancies [40].

Interestingly, KL-6 levels are also increased in IPF patients with coexistent emphysema or Chronic Obstructive Pulmonary Disease (COPD) [41], implying that it broadly reflects epithelial damage. Serum concentrations of KL-6 above 1000 U/mL were also associated with increased mortality [42, 43] and acute exacerbations of IPF [44]. In two recently published retrospective studies of IPF patients, serial increase in serum concentration of KL-6 in 6-month intervals was associated with increased mortality, even after adjustment for lung function parameters and KL-6 concentration at baseline [45]. Increased levels of KL-6 have been also reported in BAL [46] and in sputum of patients with IPF [47].

Telomeres

Telomeres are repetitive noncoding nucleotide sequences at the end of chromosomes that protect them from progressive shortening during the normal cell replication process [48]. Activation of apoptosis occurs when telomeres reach a critical length, and telomere truncation characterizes cell senescence. In IPF, telomere shortening is associated with cell death of airway epithelial cells and could explain the occurrence of disease in older individuals [49]. Telomerase reverse transcriptase (encoded by the *TERT* gene) and telomerase RNA (encoded by *TERC*) are the two major components of telomerases, ribonucleoproteins that restore telomere length. Mutations in *TERT* and *TERC* that lead to abnormal telomere shortening have been observed in 8–15% of patients with familial pulmonary fibrosis [50, 51], and up to 3% of sporadic cases of IPF [52]. Apart from variants in *TERT* and *TERC*, variants in genes responsible for telomere stabilization (e.g., *RTEL1*, *PARN*, and *DKC1*) have also been implicated in the pathogenesis of familial and, to a lesser extent sporadic, fibrosis [53, 54]. IPF transplant patients with telomerase mutations have an increased risk of hematologic complications [55]. Short telomeres have also been found in leucocytes of 25% of sporadic IPF and 37% of familial pulmonary fibrosis cases in the absence of known telomerase mutations [56].

Other Proteins Reflecting Epithelial Damage

Serum samples from subjects with IPF participating in the Prospective Observation of Fibrosis in the Lung Clinical Endpoints (PROFILE) study, a prospective, multicenter, observational cohort study of treatment-naïve, incident cases of fibrotic ILD, were collected at baseline and at multiple time points up to 3 years. Using a two-stage approach and based on protein measures obtained with a multiplex platform, the authors identified ten proteins that were associated with increased mortality in IPF. Of the ten proteins, four had the highest discriminatory ability for important clinical outcomes: SP-D and matrix metallopeptidase 7 (MMP-7) could best discriminate between IPF patients and controls; Cancer Antigen 19-9 (CA 19-9) could best discriminate between progressive and stable disease; and Cancer Antigen 125 (CA-125) could best discriminate between death and survival [57]. Tissue localization of CA 19-9 and CA-125 by immunochemistry showed that they were abundant in the metaplastic IPF epithelium, suggesting they are involved in IPF pathogenesis. In a validation cohort, SP-D, CA 19-9, and CA-125 could discriminate between stable and progressive disease. For example, in patients with progressive IPF, serum concentration of CA-125 increased significantly after 3 months compared to baseline. Taken together, markers of epithelial damage may reflect ongoing injury and are promising biomarkers for disease monitoring in IPF.

ECM Remodeling and Fibropoliferation Candidate Biomarkers

Matrix Metallopeptidase 7 (MMP7)

Matrix metallopeptidases (MMPs) play an important role in the pathogenesis of organ fibrosis by regulating ECM turnover. MMP7 is the most studied and validated biomarker in IPF [58–62], and its elevated levels are associated with disease in multiple compartments (e.g., BAL, serum, lung tissue). In a cohort of 74 patients, Rosas and colleagues described for the first time the elevation of MMP7, along with MMP1, in plasma, serum, and BAL in people with IPF [58]. Other studies reported that MMP7 levels were associated with progression and mortality among IPF patients [59, 60, 63]. For example, the Bosentan Use in Interstitial Lung Disease (BUILD-3) study found that baseline levels of MMP7 could predict early lung function decline, and that its increases over time reflected worsening of lung function [59]. Interestingly, increased MMP7 levels have also been reported in early disease [58, 64]. In participants of the multi-ethnic study of atherosclerosis (MESA), baseline MMP7 levels were associated with reduced lung function, future development of interstitial lung abnormalities, and increased all-cause mortality [64]. Thus, MMP7 measures may be helpful for early ILD detection. Despite all the promising data that supports MMP7 as a potential biomarker in IPF, its use in the clinic has been challenged by the lack of uniform cut-off points used in different studies, and consistent protocols to measure its levels, which include different collection matrices (e.g., serum, EDTA, and heparin plasma). Future studies to determine its clinical utility are now warranted.

Combined Protein Biomarkers

Combined biomarker approaches with multiple variable scoring systems have also shown promise [61]. Richards and colleagues measured levels of 92 proteins in plasma from 241 IPF patients (140 for derivation and 101 for validation cohort) and found that high levels of MMP7, ICAM1, IL-8, VCAM1, and S100A12 were predictive of poor overall survival in the derivation cohort. Although ICAM1 was the only predictor of poor survival in the validation cohort, all five proteins were correlated with poorer transplant-free survival. White and colleagues reported that a biomarker index based on three plasma proteins was able to distinguish IPF from other forms of ILD [62].

Specifically, using a 35-protein multiplex panel, the authors found that plasma levels of SP-D>31 ng/ml, MMP-7>1.75 ng/ml, and osteopontin>6 ng/ml each significantly distinguished patients with IPF from patients with other forms of ILD, both individually and in a combined index.

ECM Neoepitopes

During ECM turnover, MMPs cleave collagen fibers and thereby generate neoepitopes, soluble fragments of ECM that are released into the systemic circulation. In the PROFILE study, the largest IPF biomarker cohort studied globally, authors showed that in 189 prospectively recruited, and longitudinally followed patients with IPF, serum concentrations of neoepitopes were associated with IPF progression and survival rate [65]. In particular, the 3-month change in serum levels of six neoepitopes was associated with progressive disease and increased risk of subsequent mortality.

Fibrocytes

Circulating fibrocytes are bone marrow-derived cells that express hematopoietic (CD45, CD34) and mesenchymal markers (Col-1, fibronectin) that are hypothesized to provide a fibroblast pool to tissues needing repair [66]. They are thought to participate in the pathogenesis of lung fibrosis because they have been observed in the lungs of people with IPF, but not in healthy lungs, and they are recruited via CXCL12 by alveolar epithelial cells [67]. Elevated numbers of circulating fibrocytes have been found in patients with stable IPF, with further increases in IPF patients with acute exacerbations; additionally, having >5% of circulating fibrocytes was associated with worse survival [68, 69].

Immune Dysregulation Candidate Biomarkers

It has become evident that immune dysregulation is a key contributor to fibrogenesis in a num-ber of organs, including the lung. The innate and adaptive immune system can enhance the secretion of pro-fibrotic factors that direct the healing/scarring response toward a fibrotic outcome [12]. The recent literature has provided increasing evidence for a pro-inflammatory signature in peripheral blood and lung tissue of IPF patients, including aberrantly activated cellular populations, supporting a driver immunopathogenic mechanism [70].

Chitinase 3 Like 1 (CHI3L1)

CHI3L1, also known as YKL-40, is a chitinase-like protein produced by alveolar macrophages and AEC II that regulates proliferation in different cell types. Increased YKL-40 levels have been reported in numerous ILD, such as asbestos-related lung disease, hypersensitivity pneumonitis, polymyositis-dermatomyositis ILD, and idiopathic interstitial pneumonia [71–74]. In IPF and in hypersensitivity pneumonitis, increased serum levels were also associated with worse functional status and survival [72, 75].

C-C Motif Chemokine Ligand 18 (CCL18)

Levels of CCL18, a chemoattractant produced by alveolar macrophages, were found to be predictive of outcome in a 6-month follow-up study of 72 patients: Its increased levels were associated with forced vital capacity (FVC) and total lung capacity (TLC) decline [76]. Additionally, CCL18 concentration above 150 ng/ml was associated with increased mortality and disease progression among patients with IPF [76]. More recently, in the Clinical Studies Assessing Pirfenidone in IPF: Research of Efficacy and Safety Outcomes (CAPACITY) 1 and 2, and Assessment of Pirfenidone to Confirm Efficacy and Safety in IPF (ASCEND) trials, plasma concentrations of CCL18 were the most consistent predictor of disease progression [77].

Immune-Related Gene Expression Signatures

Genome-wide gene expression profiling of peripheral blood from IPF patients has been recently performed. Yang and colleagues demonstrated that the peripheral blood transcriptome in IPF patients differed from that of normal individuals, specifically, 1428 and 2790 genes were differentially expressed in mild and severe IPF, respectively, compared to controls [78]. Extending this observation, Herazo-Maya and colleagues showed that gene expression profiles in peripheral blood mononuclear cells (PBMCs) predicted outcomes in IPF patients: A gene signature composed of 52 differentially expressed genes effectively categorized patients as having high versus low mortality risk over a 4-year follow-up period, and the gene expression signature was a better outcome predictor than clinical data alone [79]. Their findings have been validated in multiple cohorts in the U.S. and Europe [80]. Because many of the genes that are part of the signature are critical to immunologic activation, their results suggest that dysregulation of the immune response contributes to IPF progression.

Conclusion

Rapid advances in our understanding of IPF and ILD pathogenesis and the identification of clinically useful biomarkers are expected over the next few years, as the analysis of genomic, proteomic, and other omics data will drive discovery of ILD subphenotypes and enable the development of tailored, pathway-driven therapeutic approaches. We anticipate that genotyping and biomarker testing will soon become routine for patient stratification and personalized treatment of IPF and other ILD, following the conduct of clinical trials and studies demonstrating the effectiveness of the most promising biomarker/therapy candidates. Based on our current knowledge, the three pivotal fibrosis pathophysiology pathways that will correspond to such candidates are epithelial and immune dysfunction, as well as ECM remodeling and fibroproliferation.

References

1. Travis WD, Costabel U, Hansell DM, King TE Jr, Lynch DA, Nicholson AG, Ryerson CJ, Ryu JH, Selman M, Wells AU, Behr J, Bouros D, Brown KK, Colby TV, Collard HR, Cordeiro CR, Cottin V, Crestani B, Drent M, Dudden RF, Egan J, Flaherty K, Hogaboam C, Inoue Y, Johkoh T, Kim DS, Kitaichi M, Loyd J, Martinez FJ, Myers J, Protzko S, Raghu G, Richeldi L, Sverzellati N, Swigris J, Valeyre D, ATS/ERS Committee on Idiopathic Interstitial Pneumonias. An official American Thoracic Society/European Respiratory Society statement: update of the international multidisciplinary classification of the idiopathic interstitial pneumonias. Am J Respir Crit Care Med. 2013;188:733–48.
2. American Thoracic S, European Respiratory S. American Thoracic Society/European Respiratory Society International Multidisciplinary Consensus Classification of the Idiopathic Interstitial Pneumonias. This joint statement of the American Thoracic Society (ATS), and the European Respiratory Society (ERS) was adopted by the ATS board of directors, June 2001 and by the ERS Executive Committee, June 2001. Am J Respir Crit Care Med. 2002;165:277–304.
3. Raghu G, Collard HR, Egan JJ, Martinez FJ, Behr J, Brown KK, Colby TV, Cordier JF, Flaherty KR, Lasky JA, Lynch DA, Ryu JH, Swigris JJ, Wells AU, Ancochea J, Bouros D, Carvalho C, Costabel U, Ebina M, Hansell DM, Johkoh T, Kim DS, King TE Jr, Kondoh Y, Myers J, Muller NL, Nicholson AG, Richeldi L, Selman M, Dudden RF, Griss BS, Protzko SL, Schunemann HJ, Fibrosis AEJACoIP. An official ATS/ERS/JRS/ALAT statement: idiopathic pulmonary fibrosis: evidence-based guidelines for diagnosis and management. Am J Respir Crit Care Med. 2011;183:788–824.
4. Antoniou KM, Margaritopoulos GA, Tomassetti S, Bonella F, Costabel U, Poletti V. Interstitial lung disease. Eur Respir Rev. 2014;23:40–54.
5. Hutchinson JP, McKeever TM, Fogarty AW, Navaratnam V, Hubbard RB. Surgical lung biopsy for the diagnosis of interstitial lung disease in England: 1997–2008. Eur Respir J. 2016;48:1453–61.
6. Raghu G, Rochwerg B, Zhang Y, Garcia CA, Azuma A, Behr J, Brozek JL, Collard HR, Cunningham W, Homma S, Johkoh T, Martinez FJ, Myers J, Protzko SL, Richeldi L, Rind D, Selman M, Theodore A, Wells AU, Hoogsteden H, Schunemann HJ, American Thoracic Society, European Respiratory society, Japanese Respiratory Society, Latin American Thoracic Association. An official ATS/ERS/JRS/ALAT clinical practice guideline: treatment of idiopathic pulmonary Fibrosis. An update of the 2011 clinical practice guideline. Am J Respir Crit Care Med. 2015;192:e3–e19.
7. Scotton CJ, Krupiczojc MA, Konigshoff M, Mercer PF, Lee YC, Kaminski N, Morser J, Post JM, Maher TM, Nicholson AG, Moffatt JD, Laurent GJ, Derian

CK, Eickelberg O, Chambers RC. Increased local expression of coagulation factor X contributes to the fibrotic response in human and murine lung injury. J Clin Invest. 2009;119:2550–63.

8. Lehmann M, Korfei M, Mutze K, Klee S, Skronska-Wasek W, Alsafadi HN, Ota C, Costa R, Schiller HB, Lindner M, Wagner DE, Gunther A, Konigshoff M. Senolytic drugs target alveolar epithelial cell function and attenuate experimental lung fibrosis ex vivo. Eur Respir J. 2017;50:1602367.

9. Minagawa S, Araya J, Numata T, Nojiri S, Hara H, Yumino Y, Kawaishi M, Odaka M, Morikawa T, Nishimura SL, Nakayama K, Kuwano K. Accelerated epithelial cell senescence in IPF and the inhibitory role of SIRT6 in TGF-beta-induced senescence of human bronchial epithelial cells. Am J Physiol Lung Cell Mol Physiol. 2011;300:L391–401.

10. Vancheri C. Idiopathic pulmonary fibrosis: an altered fibroblast proliferation linked to cancer biology. Proc Am Thorac Soc. 2012;9:153–7.

11. Upagupta C, Shimbori C, Alsilmi R, Kolb M. Matrix abnormalities in pulmonary fibrosis. Eur Respir Rev. 2018;27:180033.

12. Desai O, Winkler J, Minasyan M, Herzog EL. The role of immune and inflammatory cells in idiopathic pulmonary fibrosis. Front Med. 2018;5:43.

13. Kropski JA, Pritchett JM, Zoz DF, Crossno PF, Markin C, Garnett ET, Degryse AL, Mitchell DB, Polosukhin VV, Rickman OB, Choi L, Cheng DS, McConaha ME, Jones BR, Gleaves LA, McMahon FB, Worrell JA, Solus JF, Ware LB, Lee JW, Massion PP, Zaynagetdinov R, White ES, Kurtis JD, Johnson JE, Groshong SD, Lancaster LH, Young LR, Steele MP, Phillips Iii JA, Cogan JD, Loyd JE, Lawson WE, Blackwell TS. Extensive phenotyping of individuals at risk for familial interstitial pneumonia reveals clues to the pathogenesis of interstitial lung disease. Am J Respir Crit Care Med. 2015;191:417–26.

14. Nogee LM, Dunbar AE 3rd, Wert SE, Askin F, Hamvas A, Whitsett JA. A mutation in the surfactant protein C gene associated with familial interstitial lung disease. N Engl J Med. 2001;344:573–9.

15. Baumgartner KB, Samet JM, Stidley CA, Colby TV, Waldron JA. Cigarette smoking: a risk factor for idiopathic pulmonary fibrosis. Am J Respir Crit Care Med. 1997;155:242–8.

16. Baumgartner KB, Samet JM, Coultas DB, Stidley CA, Hunt WC, Colby TV, Waldron JA. Occupational and environmental risk factors for idiopathic pulmonary fibrosis: a multicenter case-control study. Collaborating Centers. Am J Epidemiol. 2000;152:307–15.

17. Lee JS. The role of gastroesophageal reflux and microaspiration in idiopathic pulmonary fibrosis. Clin Pulm Med. 2014;21:81–5.

18. Arase Y, Suzuki F, Suzuki Y, Akuta N, Kobayashi M, Kawamura Y, Yatsuji H, Sezaki H, Hosaka T, Hirakawa M, Saito S, Ikeda K, Kumada H. Hepatitis C virus enhances incidence of idiopathic pulmonary fibrosis. World J Gastroenterol. 2008;14:5880–6.

19. Lawson WE, Crossno PF, Polosukhin VV, Roldan J, Cheng DS, Lane KB, Blackwell TR, Xu C, Markin C, Ware LB, Miller GG, Loyd JE, Blackwell TS. Endoplasmic reticulum stress in alveolar epithelial cells is prominent in IPF: association with altered surfactant protein processing and herpesvirus infection. Am J Physiol Lung Cell Mol Physiol. 2008;294:L1119–26.

20. Tang YW, Johnson JE, Browning PJ, Cruz-Gervis RA, Davis A, Graham BS, Brigham KL, Oates JA Jr, Loyd JE, Stecenko AA. Herpesvirus DNA is consistently detected in lungs of patients with idiopathic pulmonary fibrosis. J Clin Microbiol. 2003;41:2633–40.

21. Biomarkers Definitions Working G. Biomarkers and surrogate endpoints: preferred definitions and conceptual framework. Clin Pharmacol Ther. 2001;69:89–95.

22. Greiffo FR, Eickelberg O, Fernandez IE. Systems medicine advances in interstitial lung disease. Eur Respir Rev. 2017;26:170021.

23. Ley B, Brown KK, Collard HR. Molecular biomarkers in idiopathic pulmonary fibrosis. Am J Physiol Lung Cell Mol Physiol. 2014;307:L681–91.

24. Sack CS, Doney BC, Podolanczuk AJ, Hooper LG, Seixas NS, Hoffman EA, Kawut SM, Vedal S, Raghu G, Barr RG, Lederer DJ, Kaufman JD. Occupational exposures and subclinical interstitial lung disease. The MESA (Multi-Ethnic Study of Atherosclerosis) air and lung studies. Am J Respir Crit Care Med. 2017;196:1031–9.

25. Washko GR, Hunninghake GM, Fernandez IE, Nishino M, Okajima Y, Yamashiro T, Ross JC, Estepar RS, Lynch DA, Brehm JM, Andriole KP, Diaz AA, Khorasani R, D'Aco K, Sciurba FC, Silverman EK, Hatabu H, Rosas IO, Investigators CO. Lung volumes and emphysema in smokers with interstitial lung abnormalities. N Engl J Med. 2011;364:897–906.

26. Araki T, Putman RK, Hatabu H, Gao W, Dupuis J, Latourelle JC, Nishino M, Zazueta OE, Kurugol S, Ross JC, San Jose Estepar R, Schwartz DA, Rosas IO, Washko GR, O'Connor GT, Hunninghake GM. Development and progression of interstitial lung abnormalities in the Framingham Heart Study. Am J Respir Crit Care Med. 2016;194:1514–22.

27. Hunninghake GM, Hatabu H, Okajima Y, Gao W, Dupuis J, Latourelle JC, Nishino M, Araki T, Zazueta OE, Kurugol S, Ross JC, San Jose Estepar R, Murphy E, Steele MP, Loyd JE, Schwarz MI, Fingerlin TE, Rosas IO, Washko GR, O'Connor GT, Schwartz DA. MUC5B promoter polymorphism and interstitial lung abnormalities. N Engl J Med. 2013;368:2192–200.

28. Putman RK, Hatabu H, Araki T, Gudmundsson G, Gao W, Nishino M, Okajima Y, Dupuis J, Latourelle JC, Cho MH, El-Chemaly S, Coxson HO, Celli BR, Fernandez IE, Zazueta OE, Ross JC, Harmouche R, Estepar RS, Diaz AA, Sigurdsson S, Gudmundsson EF, Eiriksdottir G, Aspelund T, Budoff MJ, Kinney GL, Hokanson JE, Williams MC, Murchison JT, MacNee W, Hoffmann U, O'Donnell CJ, Launer LJ, Harrris

TB, Gudnason V, Silverman EK, O'Connor GT, Washko GR, Rosas IO, Hunninghake GM, Evaluation of CLtIPSEI, Investigators CO. Association between interstitial lung abnormalities and all-cause mortality. JAMA. 2016;315:672–81.

29. Mulugeta S, Nureki S, Beers MF. Lost after translation: insights from pulmonary surfactant for understanding the role of alveolar epithelial dysfunction and cellular quality control in fibrotic lung disease. Am J Physiol Lung Cell Mol Physiol. 2015;309:L507–25.

30. Honda Y, Kuroki Y, Matsuura E, Nagae H, Takahashi H, Akino T, Abe S. Pulmonary surfactant protein D in sera and bronchoalveolar lavage fluids. Am J Respir Crit Care Med. 1995;152:1860–6.

31. Greene KE, Wright JR, Steinberg KP, Ruzinski JT, Caldwell E, Wong WB, Hull W, Whitsett JA, Akino T, Kuroki Y, Nagae H, Hudson LD, Martin TR. Serial changes in surfactant-associated proteins in lung and serum before and after onset of ARDS. Am J Respir Crit Care Med. 1999;160:1843–50.

32. Gunther A, Schmidt R, Nix F, Yabut-Perez M, Guth C, Rosseau S, Siebert C, Grimminger F, Morr H, Velcovsky HG, Seeger W. Surfactant abnormalities in idiopathic pulmonary fibrosis, hypersensitivity pneumonitis and sarcoidosis. Eur Respir J. 1999;14:565–73.

33. McCormack FX, King TE Jr, Bucher BL, Nielsen L, Mason RJ. Surfactant protein A predicts survival in idiopathic pulmonary fibrosis. Am J Respir Crit Care Med. 1995;152:751–9.

34. Takahashi H, Fujishima T, Koba H, Murakami S, Kurokawa K, Shibuya Y, Shiratori M, Kuroki Y, Abe S. Serum surfactant proteins A and D as prognostic factors in idiopathic pulmonary fibrosis and their relationship to disease extent. Am J Respir Crit Care Med. 2000;162:1109–14.

35. Takahashi H, Shiratori M, Kanai A, Chiba H, Kuroki Y, Abe S. Monitoring markers of disease activity for interstitial lung diseases with serum surfactant proteins A and D. Respirology. 2006;11(Suppl):S51–4.

36. Collard HR, Calfee CS, Wolters PJ, Song JW, Hong SB, Brady S, Ishizaka A, Jones KD, King TE Jr, Matthay MA, Kim DS. Plasma biomarker profiles in acute exacerbation of idiopathic pulmonary fibrosis. Am J Physiol Lung Cell Mol Physiol. 2010;299:L3–7.

37. Nathan N, Giraud V, Picard C, Nunes H, Dastot-Le Moal F, Copin B, Galeron L, De Ligniville A, Kuziner N, Reynaud-Gaubert M, Valeyre D, Couderc LJ, Chinet T, Borie R, Crestani B, Simansour M, Nau V, Tissier S, Duquesnoy P, Mansour-Hendili L, Legendre M, Kannengiesser C, Coulomb-L'Hermine A, Gouya L, Amselem S, Clement A. Germline SFTPA1 mutation in familial idiopathic interstitial pneumonia and lung cancer. Hum Mol Genet. 2016;25:1457–67.

38. Wang Y, Kuan PJ, Xing C, Cronkhite JT, Torres F, Rosenblatt RL, DiMaio JM, Kinch LN, Grishin NV, Garcia CK. Genetic defects in surfactant protein A2 are associated with pulmonary fibrosis and lung cancer. Am J Hum Genet. 2009;84:52–9.

39. Yokoyama A, Kohno N, Hamada H, Sakatani M, Ueda E, Kondo K, Hirasawa Y, Hiwada K. Circulating KL-6 predicts the outcome of rapidly progressive idiopathic pulmonary fibrosis. Am J Respir Crit Care Med. 1998;158:1680–4.

40. Okamoto T, Fujii M, Furusawa H, Tsuchiya K, Miyazaki Y, Inase N. The usefulness of KL-6 and SP-D for the diagnosis and management of chronic hypersensitivity pneumonitis. Respir Med. 2015;109:1576–81.

41. Xu L, Bian W, Gu XH, Shen C. Differing expression of cytokines and tumor markers in combined pulmonary fibrosis and emphysema compared to emphysema and pulmonary fibrosis. COPD. 2017;14:245–50.

42. Hamai K, Iwamoto H, Ishikawa N, Horimasu Y, Masuda T, Miyamoto S, Nakashima T, Ohshimo S, Fujitaka K, Hamada H, Hattori N, Kohno N. Comparative study of circulating MMP-7, CCL18, KL-6, SP-A, and SP-D as disease markers of idiopathic pulmonary fibrosis. Dis Markers. 2016;2016:4759040.

43. Yokoyama A, Kondo K, Nakajima M, Matsushima T, Takahashi T, Nishimura M, Bando M, Sugiyama Y, Totani Y, Ishizaki T, Ichiyasu H, Suga M, Hamada H, Kohno N. Prognostic value of circulating KL-6 in idiopathic pulmonary fibrosis. Respirology. 2006;11:164–8.

44. Ohshimo S, Ishikawa N, Horimasu Y, Hattori N, Hirohashi N, Tanigawa K, Kohno N, Bonella F, Guzman J, Costabel U. Baseline KL-6 predicts increased risk for acute exacerbation of idiopathic pulmonary fibrosis. Respir Med. 2014;108:1031–9.

45. Sokai A, Tanizawa K, Handa T, Kanatani K, Kubo T, Ikezoe K, Nakatsuka Y, Tokuda S, Oga T, Hirai T, Nagai S, Chin K, Mishima M. Importance of serial changes in biomarkers in idiopathic pulmonary fibrosis. ERJ Open Res. 2017;3:00019.

46. Kohno N, Awaya Y, Oyama T, Yamakido M, Akiyama M, Inoue Y, Yokoyama A, Hamada H, Fujioka S, Hiwada K. KL-6, a mucin-like glycoprotein, in bronchoalveolar lavage fluid from patients with interstitial lung disease. Am Rev Respir Dis. 1993;148:637–42.

47. Guiot J, Henket M, Corhay JL, Moermans C, Louis R. Sputum biomarkers in IPF: evidence for raised gene expression and protein level of IGFBP-2, IL-8 and MMP-7. PLoS One. 2017;12:e0171344.

48. Stanley SE, Armanios M. Short telomeres: a repeat offender in IPF. Lancet Respir Med. 2014;2:513–4.

49. Naikawadi RP, Disayabutr S, Mallavia B, Donne ML, Green G, La JL, Rock JR, Looney MR, Wolters PJ. Telomere dysfunction in alveolar epithelial cells causes lung remodeling and fibrosis. JCI Insight. 2016;1:e86704.

50. Armanios MY, Chen JJ, Cogan JD, Alder JK, Ingersoll RG, Markin C, Lawson WE, Xie M, Vulto I, Phillips JA 3rd, Lansdorp PM, Greider CW, Loyd JE. Telomerase mutations in families with idiopathic pulmonary fibrosis. N Engl J Med. 2007;356:1317–26.

51. Tsakiri KD, Cronkhite JT, Kuan PJ, Xing C, Raghu G, Weissler JC, Rosenblatt RL, Shay JW, Garcia CK. Adult-onset pulmonary fibrosis caused by mutations in telomerase. Proc Natl Acad Sci U S A. 2007;104:7552–7.

52. Alder JK, Chen JJ, Lancaster L, Danoff S, Su SC, Cogan JD, Vulto I, Xie M, Qi X, Tuder RM, Phillips JA 3rd, Lansdorp PM, Loyd JE, Armanios MY. Short telomeres are a risk factor for idiopathic pulmonary fibrosis. Proc Natl Acad Sci U S A. 2008;105:13051–6.

53. Petrovski S, Todd JL, Durheim MT, Wang Q, Chien JW, Kelly FL, Frankel C, Mebane CM, Ren Z, Bridgers J, Urban TJ, Malone CD, Finlen Copeland A, Brinkley C, Allen AS, O'Riordan T, McHutchison JG, Palmer SM, Goldstein DB. An exome sequencing study to assess the role of rare genetic variation in pulmonary fibrosis. Am J Respir Crit Care Med. 2017;196:82–93.

54. Kropski JA, Mitchell DB, Markin C, Polosukhin VV, Choi L, Johnson JE, Lawson WE, Phillips JA 3rd, Cogan JD, Blackwell TS, Loyd JE. A novel dyskerin (DKC1) mutation is associated with familial interstitial pneumonia. Chest. 2014;146:e1–7.

55. Borie R, Kannengiesser C, Hirschi S, Le Pavec J, Mal H, Bergot E, Jouneau S, Naccache JM, Revy P, Boutboul D, Peffault de la Tour R, Wemeau-Stervinou L, Philit F, Cordier JF, Thabut G, Crestani B, Cottin V, Groupe d'Etudes et de Recherche sur les Maladies "Orphelines" Pulmonaires (GERM"O"P). Severe hematologic complications after lung transplantation in patients with telomerase complex mutations. J Heart Lung Transplant. 2015;34:538–46.

56. Cronkhite JT, Xing C, Raghu G, Chin KM, Torres F, Rosenblatt RL, Garcia CK. Telomere shortening in familial and sporadic pulmonary fibrosis. Am J Respir Crit Care Med. 2008;178:729–37.

57. Maher TM, Oballa E, Simpson JK, Porte J, Habgood A, Fahy WA, Flynn A, Molyneaux PL, Braybrooke R, Divyateja H, Parfrey H, Rassl D, Russell AM, Saini G, Renzoni EA, Duggan AM, Hubbard R, Wells AU, Lukey PT, Marshall RP, Jenkins RG. An epithelial biomarker signature for idiopathic pulmonary fibrosis: an analysis from the multicentre PROFILE cohort study. Lancet Respir Med. 2017;5:946–55.

58. Rosas IO, Richards TJ, Konishi K, Zhang Y, Gibson K, Lokshin AE, Lindell KO, Cisneros J, Macdonald SD, Pardo A, Sciurba F, Dauber J, Selman M, Gochuico BR, Kaminski N. MMP1 and MMP7 as potential peripheral blood biomarkers in idiopathic pulmonary fibrosis. PLoS Med. 2008;5:e93.

59. Bauer Y, White ES, de Bernard S, Cornelisse P, Leconte I, Morganti A, Roux S, Nayler O. MMP-7 is a predictive biomarker of disease progression in patients with idiopathic pulmonary fibrosis. ERJ Open Res. 2017;3:00074.

60. Tzouvelekis A, Herazo-Maya JD, Slade M, Chu JH, Deiuliis G, Ryu C, Li Q, Sakamoto K, Ibarra G, Pan H, Gulati M, Antin-Ozerkis D, Herzog EL, Kaminski N. Validation of the prognostic value of MMP-7 in idiopathic pulmonary fibrosis. Respirology. 2017;22:486–93.

61. Richards TJ, Kaminski N, Baribaud F, Flavin S, Brodmerkel C, Horowitz D, Li K, Choi J, Vuga LJ, Lindell KO, Klesen M, Zhang Y, Gibson KF. Peripheral blood proteins predict mortality in idiopathic pulmonary fibrosis. Am J Respir Crit Care Med. 2012;185:67–76.

62. White ES, Xia M, Murray S, Dyal R, Flaherty CM, Flaherty KR, Moore BB, Cheng L, Doyle TJ, Villalba J, Dellaripa PF, Rosas IO, Kurtis JD, Martinez FJ. Plasma surfactant protein-D, matrix metalloproteinase-7, and osteopontin index distinguishes idiopathic pulmonary fibrosis from other idiopathic interstitial pneumonias. Am J Respir Crit Care Med. 2016;194:1242–51.

63. Song JW, Do KH, Jang SJ, Colby TV, Han S, Kim DS. Blood biomarkers MMP-7 and SP-A: predictors of outcome in idiopathic pulmonary fibrosis. Chest. 2013;143:1422–9.

64. Armstrong HF, Podolanczuk AJ, Barr RG, Oelsner EC, Kawut SM, Hoffman EA, Tracy R, Kaminski N, McClelland RL, Lederer DJ. Serum matrix metalloproteinase-7, respiratory symptoms, and mortality in community-dwelling adults. MESA (Multi-Ethnic Study of Atherosclerosis). Am J Respir Crit Care Med. 2017;196:1311–7.

65. Jenkins RG, Simpson JK, Saini G, Bentley JH, Russell AM, Braybrooke R, Molyneaux PL, McKeever TM, Wells AU, Flynn A, Hubbard RB, Leeming DJ, Marshall RP, Karsdal MA, Lukey PT, Maher TM. Longitudinal change in collagen degradation biomarkers in idiopathic pulmonary fibrosis: an analysis from the prospective, multicentre PROFILE study. Lancet Respir Med. 2015;3:462–72.

66. Bucala R, Spiegel LA, Chesney J, Hogan M, Cerami A. Circulating fibrocytes define a new leukocyte subpopulation that mediates tissue repair. Mol Med. 1994;1:71–81.

67. Andersson-Sjoland A, de Alba CG, Nihlberg K, Becerril C, Ramirez R, Pardo A, Westergren-Thorsson G, Selman M. Fibrocytes are a potential source of lung fibroblasts in idiopathic pulmonary fibrosis. Int J Biochem Cell Biol. 2008;40:2129–40.

68. Moeller A, Gilpin SE, Ask K, Cox G, Cook D, Gauldie J, Margetts PJ, Farkas L, Dobranowski J, Boylan C, O'Byrne PM, Strieter RM, Kolb M. Circulating fibrocytes are an indicator of poor prognosis in idiopathic pulmonary fibrosis. Am J Respir Crit Care Med. 2009;179:588–94.

69. Alhamad EH, Shakoor Z, Al-Kassimi FA, Almogren A, Gad ElRab MO, Maharaj S, Kolb M. Rapid detection of circulating fibrocytes by flowcytometry in idiopathic pulmonary fibrosis. Ann Thorac Med. 2015;10:279–83.

70. Kolahian S, Fernandez IE, Eickelberg O, Hartl D. Immune mechanisms in pulmonary fibrosis. Am J Respir Cell Mol Biol. 2016;55:309–22.

71. Korthagen NM, van Moorsel CH, Zanen P, Ruven HJ, Grutters JC. Evaluation of circulating YKL-40

levels in idiopathic interstitial pneumonias. Lung. 2014;192:975–80.

72. Long X, He X, Ohshimo S, Griese M, Sarria R, Guzman J, Costabel U, Bonella F. Serum YKL-40 as predictor of outcome in hypersensitivity pneumonitis. Eur Respir J. 2017;49:1501924.

73. Hozumi H, Fujisawa T, Enomoto N, Nakashima R, Enomoto Y, Suzuki Y, Kono M, Karayama M, Furuhashi K, Murakami A, Inui N, Nakamura Y, Mimori T, Suda T. Clinical utility of YKL-40 in polymyositis/dermatomyositis-associated interstitial lung disease. J Rheumatol. 2017;44:1394–401.

74. Vaananen T, Lehtimaki L, Vuolteenaho K, Hamalainen M, Oksa P, Vierikko T, Jarvenpaa R, Uitti J, Kankaanranta H, Moilanen E. Glycoprotein YKL-40 levels in plasma are associated with fibrotic changes on HRCT in asbestos-exposed subjects. Mediat Inflamm. 2017;2017:1797512.

75. Korthagen NM, van Moorsel CH, Barlo NP, Ruven HJ, Kruit A, Heron M, van den Bosch JM, Grutters JC. Serum and BALF YKL-40 levels are predictors of survival in idiopathic pulmonary fibrosis. Respir Med. 2011;105:106–13.

76. Prasse A, Probst C, Bargagli E, Zissel G, Toews GB, Flaherty KR, Olschewski M, Rottoli P, Muller-Quernheim J. Serum CC-chemokine ligand 18 concentration predicts outcome in idiopathic pulmonary fibrosis. Am J Respir Crit Care Med. 2009;179:717–23.

77. Neighbors M, Cabanski CR, Ramalingam TR, Sheng XR, Tew GW, Gu C, Jia G, Peng K, Ray JM, Ley B, Wolters PJ, Collard HR, Arron JR. Prognostic and predictive biomarkers for patients with idiopathic pulmonary fibrosis treated with pirfenidone: post-hoc assessment of the CAPACITY and ASCEND trials. Lancet Respir Med. 2018;6:615–26.

78. Yang IV, Luna LG, Cotter J, Talbert J, Leach SM, Kidd R, Turner J, Kummer N, Kervitsky D, Brown KK, Boon K, Schwarz MI, Schwartz DA, Steele MP. The peripheral blood transcriptome identifies the presence and extent of disease in idiopathic pulmonary fibrosis. PLoS One. 2012;7:e37708.

79. Herazo-Maya JD, Noth I, Duncan SR, Kim S, Ma SF, Tseng GC, Feingold E, Juan-Guardela BM, Richards TJ, Lussier Y, Huang Y, Vij R, Lindell KO, Xue J, Gibson KF, Shapiro SD, Garcia JG, Kaminski N. Peripheral blood mononuclear cell gene expression profiles predict poor outcome in idiopathic pulmonary fibrosis. Sci Transl Med. 2013;5:205ra136.

80. Herazo-Maya JD, Sun J, Molyneaux PL, Li Q, Villalba JA, Tzouvelekis A, Lynn H, Juan-Guardela BM, Risquez C, Osorio JC, Yan X, Michel G, Aurelien N, Lindell KO, Klesen MJ, Moffatt MF, Cookson WO, Zhang Y, Garcia JGN, Noth I, Prasse A, Bar-Joseph Z, Gibson KF, Zhao H, Herzog EL, Rosas IO, Maher TM, Kaminski N. Validation of a 52-gene risk profile for outcome prediction in patients with idiopathic pulmonary fibrosis: an international, multicentre, cohort study. Lancet Respir Med. 2017;5:857–68.

Catherine A. Gao, John C. Huston,
Patricia Valda Toro, Samir Gautam,
and Charles S. Dela Cruz

Molecular Diagnostics— Recognition and Identification of the Pathogen

Illustrative Case (See Fig. 12.1)

A 45-year-old actively smoking male presents to the emergency department with a 3-day history of high fevers, cough productive of greenish sputum, and shortness of breath (SOB). In the emergency department, he is found to be hypoxemic and a portable chest X-ray shows a right lower lobe opacity read as infiltrate versus atelectasis. He is started on ceftriaxone and doxycycline per community-acquired pneumonia (CAP) guidelines and admitted to the medicine service. Five days into the hospitalization, the patient decompensates and ultimately requires intubation for

hypoxemic respiratory failure. Blood and sputum cultures are unrevealing. Urinary antigens for *Streptococcus pneumoniae* and *Legionella pneumophila* are negative. While in the intensive care unit, the patient continues to spike fevers. Blood cultures are obtained again but remain negative. The antimicrobial coverage is broadened to vancomycin and piperacillin-tazobactam. Eventually, the patient is extubated and transferred back to the general medical floor. He is eventually narrowed to amoxicillin/clavulanate. He is discharged to a short-term rehabilitation facility still requiring two liters of oxygen.

The Traditional Approach to Diagnosing Pneumonia: History, Physical Exam, and Basic Diagnostics

Confirming or refuting a suspected diagnosis of pneumonia has long depended on history-taking, physical examination, general laboratory studies,

---

These two authors contributed equally to this work and therefore the author list can be cited with either JH or CG as first author

---

C. A. Gao · J. C. Huston
Yale School of Medicine, Department of Internal Medicine, New Haven, CT, USA
e-mail: catherine.gao@yale.edu;
john.huston@yale.edu

P. V. Toro
Yale School of Medicine, New Haven, CT, USA
e-mail: patricia.valdatoro@yale.edu

S. Gautam
Yale School of Medicine, Department of Internal Medicine, Section of Pulmonary, Critical Care, and Sleep Medicine, New Haven, CT, USA
e-mail: samir.gautam@yale.edu

C. S. Dela Cruz (✉)
Yale School of Medicine, Department of Internal Medicine, Section of Pulmonary, Critical Care, and Sleep Medicine and Department of Microbial Pathogenesis, New Haven, CT, USA
e-mail: charles.delacruz@yale.edu

© Springer Nature Switzerland AG 2020
J. L. Gomez et al. (eds.), *Precision in Pulmonary, Critical Care, and Sleep Medicine*,
Respiratory Medicine, https://doi.org/10.1007/978-3-030-31507-8_12

Current Workup of Pneumonia

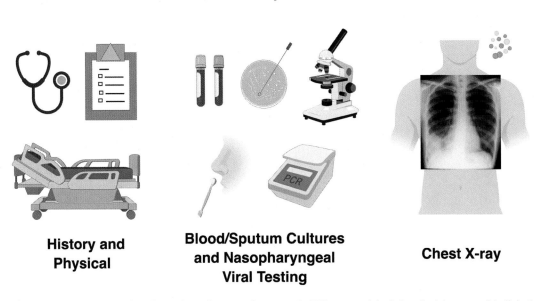

History and Physical **Blood/Sputum Cultures and Nasopharyngeal Viral Testing** **Chest X-ray**

Fig. 12.1 Current approach to the workup of suspected pneumonia. This approach includes obtaining a careful clinical history and physical exam, sputum and blood cultures, and chest X-ray

and basic radiologic studies including chest X-ray. A dichotomous approach aimed at defining both host and pathogen is generally taken. Important host-defining historical features include any degree of immunosuppression (e.g., neutropenia, chronic corticosteroid use, malignancy, liver or kidney disease, diabetes mellitus, immunosenescence), underlying structural lung disease (e.g., obstructive lung diseases, bronchiectasis), risk of aspiration (due to altered sensorium, bulbar muscle weakness, dysphagia, esophageal disorders), and relevant exposures (i.e., travel, sick contacts, animals). Regarding the pathogen, one probes the clinical history for susceptibilities and characteristic syndromes—for example, a background of chronic alcoholism or poorly treated HIV will point to aspiration pneumonia and opportunistic infections, respectively. The patient's clinical course is also closely observed in-house for clues to an etiology, for example, rapid response to empiric antibiotics indicating infection.

While these historical subtleties will provide important guidance for the seasoned, sophisticated clinician, simpler heuristics more often determine diagnostic decision-making. In the

case of pneumonia, the basic defining features include a radiographic infiltrate, systemic signs of infection (e.g., fever), and pulmonary symptoms of infection (e.g., productive cough, SOB, and occasionally pleuritic chest pain) [4]. Unfortunately, in practice, these historical features may be insufficient and potentially misleading as they may manifest in completely different disease processes, many of which do not require antibiotics. These include decompensated heart failure (SOB), pulmonary embolism (pleuritic chest pain), COPD exacerbation (SOB and cough), and even allergic rhinitis (fatigue, malaise, productive cough). Furthermore, studies have shown that history has poor interobserver reliability in the ability to record symptoms in patients with suspected pneumonia. For instance, the classic amalgam of fever, cough, tachycardia, and crackles has a sensitivity of less than 50% for the diagnosis of acute pneumonia, and no other constellation of historical and physical findings has performed better [5].

For the most part, microbiological diagnosis of bacterial pneumonia has remained unchanged since the 1800s, as we continue to rely on traditional sputum gram stain and culture. Its longevity, however, belies its relatively dismal diagnostic performance. This was starkly illustrated by a landmark study in 2015, which showed that in more than 60% of the cases, no bacterial or viral organism could be identified [6]. Equally poor results are seen in patients with ventilator-associated pneumonia, in whom only 50% of pathogens are identified [7]. In addition to poor sensitivity, traditional culture suffers from slow turn-around time, as they take on average 36–48 hours to result [8].

Chest radiography has long been considered essential in the diagnosis of pneumonia. However, the sensitivity of chest radiography for pneumonia is less than 50%, and the positive predictive value is only 30% [9]. Furthermore, chest X-rays are of variable quality and often difficult to interpret due to underlying cardiopulmonary disease, obesity, etc. Finally, initial studies may be falsely negative, due to a phenomenon known as "blos-soming infiltrate," which has been observed in up to 7% of patients in one study [10].

Given these many shortcomings of traditional diagnostics for pneumonia, the development of advanced tools is clearly needed. Excitingly, novel ways to diagnose pneumonia are rapidly emerging, with some already folded into practice. This section will cover these newer techniques, which run the technological gamut from protein biomarkers to whole genome sequencing and proteomic profiling.

Pathogen-Associated Biomarkers (See Table 12.1 **for Summary**)

An important component of the diagnostic armamentarium in pneumonia is a family of assays aimed at detecting bacterial antigens in bodily fluids (e.g., serum and urine). This approach is

Table 12.1 Summary of pathogen diagnostics

Test name	Test description	Sensitivity and specificity, approximate	Advantages and disadvantages	Availability	Selected references
Genomic profiling of pathogen					
RT- PCR	Real-time polymerase chain reaction to identify and quantify pathogen	Sensitivity 90% Specificity 100%	+ Simple and fast + Can quantify pathogen load + Allows identification of resistance genes − Inadequate sensitivity for lower respiratory samples	Commercially available	[3, 11–13]
Nucleic acid amplification test	Amplification of specific nucleic acids sequences followed by hybridization of probe		+ Fast diagnosis of TB (24–48 hours) + More sensitive than AFB smear + Works with low concentration samples + Fast test of drug resistance with high sensitivity and specificity − Less sensitive than culture		[19–25, 30]
Multiplex PCR	Amplification of many nucleic acid targets within one reaction		+ Allows diagnosis of multiple pathogens at once + Can quantify viral load − Lower sensitivity due to primer–primer interaction − May detect viruses not related to pathogenic process.	Commercially available	[13, 15, 19, 27]
Mass spectrometry for proteomic profiling					

(continued)

Table 12.1 (continued)

Test name	Test description	Sensitivity and specificity, approximate	Advantages and disadvantages	Availability	Selected references
MALDI-TOF MS	Mass spectrometry to identify bacterial organisms by their proteomic profile		+ Fast (minutes) + Low-cost per sample + Detects antibiotic resistance		[32–34]
Volatile organic compounds (VOCs)	Mass spectrometry to analyze VOCs in exhaled breath and diagnose pneumonia	Sensitivity 75% Specificity 73%	+ Noninvasive		[35–36]
Metataxonomics and metagenomics					
16S rRNA sequencing	Specific bacterial taxa are sequenced used primers to epitopes of highly conserved sequences of ribosomal RNA		+ Rapid identification of bacterial species + Provides quantification of pathogen abundance + Low-cost per sample − Resistance and virulence genes are not detected − Requires bronchial sample		[37–38]
Whole genome sequencing (WGS)	Wide net sequencing of sample		+ Includes resistance, virulence, and antimicrobial susceptibilities + Rapid detection of TB and drug resistance + Identification of mixed strains can help optimize therapies + Allows study of transmission patterns − May sequence colonizing nonpathogenic organism		[40–46]

already in widespread practice given its relatively low cost, high specificity, rapid processing times, and ready accessibility to samples. The principal disadvantage derives from the indirect detection of pathogen through an antigen rather than isolation of the organism, which is necessary for assessing antibiotic susceptibility [11, 12].

A common example is the assay for *S. pneumoniae* urinary antigen (the C-polysaccharide), which has a sensitivity and specificity of 72% and 96%, respectively, in patients with non-bacteremic pneumonia. Importantly, initiation of antibiotics does not impair test characteristics, as antigens remaining positive for at least 3 days after receiving appropriate therapy [13]. Another example is the urine immunoassay for detecting *Legionella pneu-*

mophilia serogroup 1, which causes between 50% and 70% of *Legionella* infections. This test has 80% sensitivity and greater than 99% specificity [14].

Genomic Profiling of Pathogen

Multiplex PCR

Polymerase Chain Reaction (RT-PCR) is a simple and rapid means of identifying bacterial and viral pathogens in the blood, sputum, and bronchoalveolar lavage (BAL) fluid in order identify causative organisms of pneumonia. Turnaround is typically on the scale of just a few hours.

Multiplex PCR allows for amplification of many nucleic acid targets within one reaction

[15], potentially enabling diagnosis of multiple pathogens simultaneously. There are numerous commercial multiplex PCR systems currently in use to diagnose pneumonia—mostly viral infection from nasopharyngeal sampling, but some bacterial pathogens as well. A downside to multiplex PCR is the potential for primer–primer interactions, which can interfere with amplification and decrease the sensitivity of the test; bead-array and microarrays are used to combat this issue [15]. A second issue is the risk of false positivity, which can stem either from the exquisite sensitivity of the test or from coincidental detection of organisms that are potentially pathogenic, but not producing disease in a given patient.

Multiplex PCR has changed our basic understanding of what causes pneumonia; in a landmark trial by the EPIC team, among more than 2000 patients with radiographic evidence of pneumonia, the majority of cases with a confirmed microbiological etiology were viral, and the most frequent pathogen was rhinovirus, accounting for 9% of cases [6, 16]. It should be noted, however, that the sampling site in this study was the nasopharynx, and therefore the recovered virus may simply represent a bystander and not the pathogen responsible for the lower respiratory tract infection (LRTI). Further complicating the interpretation of viral studies is that 15% of healthy individuals carry a respiratory tract pathogen at any given time [16].

Quantitative PCR

Recent studies have highlighted the prognostic importance of assessing pathogen load, which is enabled by real-time PCR (RT-PCR). For example, confirming an elevated *S. pneumoniae* DNA in the serum of patients with confirmed CAP was associated with a higher mortality, need for mechanical ventilation, and risk of shock [17]. Other studies have demonstrated a dose-dependent relationship, with higher bacterial DNA loads correlating with more severe disease [18].

PCR for Recognition of Genes Mediating Resistance or Virulence

In addition to defining the presence and quantity of pathogen, PCR can be used to identify genetic resistance determinants. The quintessential exam-

ple is identification of the mecA gene, which confers methicillin resistance to *Staphylococcus aureus* species, that is, methicillin-resistant *S. aureus* (MRSA). Specifically, the gene encodes for penicillin-binding protein 2a, which has a decreased affinity for beta-lactam antibiotics that renders almost the entire drug class obsolete, with the exception of late-generation cephalosporins [19, 20]. Multiple iterations of tests aimed at identifying MRSA have culminated in an effective multiplex assay that recognizes four pertinent genes in only 2–6 hours [21]. These include the SCCmec–orfX junction (which indicates the *Staphylococcus* genus), spa (which specifies *S. aureus*), mecA (the resistance gene), and mecC (a mecA homolog). Additional MRSA assays have been developed; as a class, they perform well with sensitivities greater than 90% and specificities approaching 100% [19].

PCR tests for virulence factors in common bacterial LRTI pathogens such as *S. pneumoniae* and *Moraxella catarrhalis* have been tested, but with mixed success, mainly due to the frequent colonization of these organisms in the upper respiratory tract [22]. For example, tests for the pneumolysin gene (a highly cytotoxic and inflammatory virulence factor for *S. pneumoniae*) in lower respiratory samples have shown inadequate sensitivity and specificity, and therefore have not been adopted into clinical practice [23].

PCR for Detection of Mycobacteria

An area of increasing interest is the rapid diagnosis of active *Mycobacterium tuberculosis* (MTb) infection. For decades, clinicians have relied on sputum acid-fast bacilli smears and culture, which have numerous drawbacks. First, the turnaround time is quite long—often taking months to result, resulting in delayed initiation of antimicrobials, and prolonged isolation of suspected patients. Second, sensitivity is quite poor, with detection rates estimated at 45–80% [24, 25]. Consequently, invasive testing may be necessary to make the diagnosis, including bronchoscopy and biopsy.

To address these issues, PCR assays are now being used in clinical practice. This technology can help diagnose pulmonary TB in 24–48 hours [26], and it has further utility in distinguishing between MTb and non-tuberculous mycobacteria on positive

AFB smears, with a positive predictive value of over 95%. Although still less sensitive than culture, the PCR test can detect MTb at a concentration of 1–10 organisms per milliliter [27–29]. This feature enables detection of MTb in patients with a negative AFB smear, with approximate 50–80% accuracy [30]. PCR tests can also detect resistance against drugs including rifampin or isoniazid with high sensitivity and specificity, can be completed in only 2 hours, and are highly sensitive and specific [31].

Mass Spectrometry for Proteomic Profiling

MALDI-TOF MS
Matrix-assisted laser desorption ionization time of flight mass spectrometry (MALDI-TOF MS) is a technique with the capacity to identify pathogens through recognition of unique proteomic profiles [32]. In contrast to traditional cultures, which take 36–48 hours to result, MALDI-TOF MS takes minutes, with a relatively low cost per sample [33]. In addition to pathogen identification, this methodology can also detect antibiotic resistance, for instance through recognition of specific proteins such as PBP2a in *S. aureus*, which indicates MRSA [34].

Volatile Organic Compounds
Another use of mass spectrometry is in the characterization of volatile organic compounds (VOCs)—so-called "breathomics," which has been hailed as a promising noninvasive method of sampling the respiratory tract [35]. Exhaled air contains numerous VOCs, including metabolites related to both host and pathogen. Select VOCs have been shown to be associated with pneumonia. As an example, one study identified 12 compounds that could correctly diagnose VAP with a sensitivity and specificity of 75% and 73% respectively [36], but concerns have been raised regarding the risk of bias in this and other early investigations.

Metataxonomics and Metagenomics

Whole genome sequencing (WGS) and 16S rRNA gene sequencing are high-output techniques that aim to comprehensively characterize the respiratory microbiome in a high-throughput manner.

16S rRNA sequencing depends on the use of nucleic acid primers against highly conserved sequences of ribosomal RNA. This allows identification of a bacterial species and some quantitative data on the relative abundance of the pathogen. Although rapid and relatively low in cost (per sample), it lacks the ability to detect genetic material outside of the ribosome, leaving resistance and virulence genes unrecognized.

A study using 16S rRNA sequencing on bronchial aspirates of mechanically ventilated patients with suspected VAP showed promising results. Compared to traditional bronchial aspirate cultures, 16S rRNA sequencing matched the culture result in 85% of cases, but time to identification was significantly shorter in the 16S group [37, 38], which is meaningful since early antibiotics (within 48 hours) are known to reduce mortality in patients with VAP [39].

Contrary to 16S, WGS fully sequences the respiratory microbiome, and as such can report on the presence of resistance and virulence genes [40, 41]. As discussed above, PCR-based assays have the capability to identify MTb and rifampin resistance in just 2 hours, but mutations outside of the probed sequence are not identified. WGS allows recognition of these, although the relative significance of such mutations may not be known [42, 43]. With time, this issue should be addressed with genome-wide association studies (GWAS), which aim to delineate a catalog of resistance loci [48–50]. This will serve as a reference for clinical samples and may help in creating models that predict future resistance to antimicrobials.

The granularity that WGS provides can also be used to trace transmission patterns of infection. This idea was exploited to track an outbreak of Human Adenovirus-7 (HAdV-7) causing ARDS at military training bases in Hubei Province, China. WGS helped identify a "super-spreader" who was not quarantined and had prolonged viral shedding [46]. Additionally, WGS can offer basic insight into the dysbiosis that often accompanies lung diseases such as chronic obstructive pulmonary disease (COPD). This is exemplified by a study examining rhinovirus-induced exacerbation, which demonstrated a significant rise in the overall bacterial burden [47].

One of the recognized weaknesses of WGS is target specificity. Though advanced post hoc processing methods allow for elimination of host genetic signal, there is no way to identify colonizing nonpathogenic or commensal organisms [44]. Additional disadvantages of meta-omics in general include the risk of contamination, inability to discriminate live from dead microbial DNA, and cost.

Molecular Diagnostics— Characterizing the Host Response

Host Response Biomarkers (See Table 12.2 **for Summary**)

In general, clinicians are alerted to infection by the host's inflammatory response to the pathogen. Observable manifestations of lung inflammation include classic systemic signs such as fever, local symptoms such as cough and purulent sputum, and radiographic evidence of neu-

Table 12.2 Summary of host response diagnostics

Test name	Test description	Sensitivity, specificity, odds ratio, hazard ratios, area under curve	Advantages, disadvantages	Availability	Selected references
C-reactive protein (CRP)	Early acute phase reactant synthesized in response to IL-6	Sensitivity: 60% Specificity 83%	+ Highly sensitive, elevated in Legionella as opposed to other biomarkers + Widely available, validated as point of care lab test − Nonspecific	Widespread; also available as point of care test	[51–55]
Procalcitonin	Prohormone of calcitonin; Elevates in response to PAMPs, DAMPs; Suppressed by type I IFN generated during viral infection	Sensitivity ranges from multiple studies: Averages approximately 74–87% Specificity approximately through numerous studies: 60–90%	+ Relatively widespread + More sensitive and specific in identifying bacterial infections + Not much affected by use of steroids + Validated in pneumonia, sepsis, shock + Beneficial in antimicrobial stewardship programs − Conflicting data (though mostly positive) in antibiotic algorithms − Elevated in renal disease and some non-specificity	Widespread and commonly available	[56–70]
Inflammatory cytokines (IL-6, IL-8, IL-10, among others)	Elevated in acute setting through a variety of pathways	Elevated levels of IL-6 and Il-10 correspond with risk of death with hazard ratio 20.5	+ Shown to predict mortality in hospitalized patients with CAP + Strong association with disease severity − Rapid rise/fall, on the order of hours	Available as send-out test but not commonly used in clinical care	[71–74]

(continued)

Table 12.2 (continued)

Test name	Test description	Sensitivity, specificity, odds ratio, hazard ratios, area under curve	Advantages, disadvantages	Availability	Selected references
Mid-regional pro-adrenomedullin (MR-proADM)	A member of the calcitonin peptide family, widely synthesized and elevated in acute infection	Sensitivity: 67–92% Specificity: 66–85%	+ Some studies have shown it to be superior compared with procalcitonin − Still not routinely used in clinical practice; not as much data as classic biomarkers	Not widely available yet	[81–82]
Pro-vasopressin (pro-VNP) Also called "copeptin" for C-terminal pro-vasopressin	Precursor to vasopressin, marker of stress, and fluid balance	Sensitivity 70% Specificity 85%	+ Promising data − Still not routinely used in clinical practice; not as much data as classic biomarkers	Not widely available yet	[79–80]
(Mid-regional) Pro-atrial natriuretic peptide (pro-ANP)	Family of natriuretic peptides, established for congestive heart disease but also elevated in high cardiac output, sympathetic stimulation, metabolism	To predict short-term death: sensitivity of 91%, specificity of 62%, positive predictive value of 10%, and negative predictive value of 99%	+ Promising data − Still not routinely used in clinical practice; not as much data as classic biomarkers	Not widely available yet	[77, 108]
Alveolar pentraxin 3 (PTX3)	An acute-phase mediator produced by lung cells	PTX3 levels ≥1 ng/ml in BAL fluid predicted pneumonia with sensitivity (92%), specificity (60%), and negative predictive value (95%)	+ Direct source—studied in BAL − Invasive sampling method	Not widely available yet	[84]

trophilic infiltrates. Inflammatory diagnostics have progressed immensely from simple leukocyte counts to serum biomarkers, such as C-reactive protein and procalcitonin, and more recently a wave of new biomarkers and genomic techniques. The sensitivity and specificity of these newer techniques vastly outstrips that of traditional pneumonia diagnostics; their implementation in clinical practice promises to improve not only diagnosis of infection, but also prediction of deterioration and tapering of therapy. These improvements should help to limit antibiotic overuse—one of the major unsolved problems in pneumonia.

C-reactive Protein

C-reactive protein (CRP) is an early acute phase reactant that is synthesized in the liver in response to IL-6 secreted by monocytes and macrophages. The "C" in its name derives from its reaction with the C-polysaccharide of *S. pneumoniae* as the first biomarker for pneumococcal pneumonia

[51, 52]. It is highly sensitive, but rather nonspecific as the level rises in most inflammatory conditions, and therefore must be used judiciously in the context of bacterial pneumonia. Interestingly, it is especially elevated in cases of *Legionella* infection compared with other biomarkers [53]. Given its widespread availability, it has been validated as a point-of-care (POC) lab test to guide antibiotic use in primary care [54], and levels have been correlated to disease severity and complications in community-acquired pneumonia [55]. Used with other inflammatory marker profiles, CRP may be used to pinpoint the time of infection: In patients who present within 3 days of disease onset, CRP was low, but in patients who present after more than 3 days of symptom onset, CRP levels rose significantly [56].

Procalcitonin

Procalcitonin is the prohormone of calcitonin, which is expressed mostly in the C-cells of the thyroid during health. In response to pathogen-associated molecular patterns (PAMPs), damage-associated molecular patterns (DAMPs), and inflammatory cytokines during infection, however, the expression of procalcitonin is upregulated in virtually every tissue and cell type [57]. Importantly, its expression is suppressed by type I interferons generated during viral infection, improving its specificity for bacterial etiologies. Serum levels elevate rapidly (within ~4 hours) and peak around 24–48 hours, making it an excellent early marker for infection [58]. Compared with CRP, it has been shown to be more sensitive and specific in identifying bacterial infections [59]. Also, unlike other infectious markers, its level is neither decreased (as is CRP) nor increased (as is white blood cell count) by the use of steroids [60]. An important drawback, however, is its lack of sensitivity for atypical infections such as *Legionella*, *Mycoplasma*, and *Chlamydophilia* [61].

First described as a biomarker for sepsis in 1993 [62], procalcitonin has since been validated repeatedly as not only a marker of bacterial infection, but also a correlate of severity in sepsis and

septic shock [63]. A meta-analysis of 21 studies including over 6000 patients showed that an elevated procalcitonin level was a risk factor for mortality (RR 4.38) [64]. A review of 1770 patients with CAP showed that procalcitonin levels had an approximately linear association with the need for invasive respiratory or vasopressor support; at levels >10 ng/mL, the risk was 22.4% compared to 4% in patients with procalcitonin <0.05 ng/mL [65].

Procalcitonin also serves as an important component of antimicrobial stewardship algorithms, helping to guide the decision to withhold antibiotics from low-risk patients and to abbreviate treatment courses in high-risk patients [66–68]. The latter is enabled by the progressive reduction in procalcitonin that accompanies successful treatment of infection; when its value drops to 80–90% (depending on the study) antibiotics can be stopped. Although numerous reports have shown the efficacy of procalcitonin-guided prescribing strategies in decreasing antibiotic usage, questions have lingered regarding safety. To address these questions, Schuetz et al. conducted a comprehensive meta-analysis, including studies across a variety of clinical settings including primary care, emergency departments, and the ICU. The study not only confirmed dramatic reductions in antibiotic exposure and safety, but in fact showed that procalcitonin-guided strategies *improve* clinical outcomes in terms of mortality and treatment failure [69].

Conflicting data, however, have been presented. Most prominently, a study in 1656 patients randomized to procalcitonin-guided versus usual antibiotic care in the emergency department failed to demonstrate even a reduction in antibiotic exposure [70]. These differences may have arisen due to heightened awareness of proper antibiotic prescribing practices and/or the relatively low acuity of the patients in the trial. Further studies will be necessary to clarify these issues.

Overall, procalcitonin has clear potential to aid in the diagnosis and management of pneumonia, but, like any biomarker, it has important limitations. These include its elevation in renal failure and relative nonspecificity for acute inflammation, including that related to cancer and tissue necrosis. Consequently, its usefulness will depend largely on the clinical setting (e.g., primary care vs. ICU) as well as the provider's knowledge of its biology and ability to integrate its significance within the larger clinical picture.

Cytokines

Inflammatory cytokines (IL-1, IL-6, IL-8, TNFα, among others) are significantly higher in patients with severe pneumonia than in those with milder disease, and can predict mortality in hospitalized patients with CAP [71]. For example, a 27-component panel was followed in 247 patients, with IL-6, IL-8, and MIP-1β showing a strong association with disease severity and adverse short-term outcome [72]. The levels rise and fall rapidly though, on the order of hours, and are usually highest at presentation [73]. A study of 1886 patients with CAP demonstrated an elevation of cytokine levels in 82% of patients, but the overall response was heterogeneous and no pattern clearly identified severe sepsis [74]. Though scientifically sensical, the optimal implementation of these cytokine panels in clinical practice remains unclear.

Newer Biomarkers

An array of novel biomarkers for CAP are now emerging, including pro-atrial natriuretic peptide (pro-ANP), C-terminal pro-vasopressin (copeptin or pro-VNP), mid-regional pro-adrenomedullin (MR-proADM), and others. These have shown advantages compared to CRP and PCT but have not yet been introduced into widespread clinical practice.

Pro-ANP is elevated in lower respiratory tract infections during CAP [75], and has the potential to predict both 30-day and 180-day mortality [76]. A study of 549 patients with mild CAP showed that a single pro-ANP measurement was more accurate than CRP and PCT in predicting need for admission [77]. Exciting data from the CAPNETZ network indicate that pro-ANP and

pro-VNP are significantly higher in fatal CAP and possess superior AUCs to those of WBC, CURB-65, CRP, and procalcitonin [78].

Copeptin has been shown likewise to be higher in patients with pneumonia before antibiotic treatment [79]; it also has been shown in a study of pediatric CAP to be significantly higher in pneumonia cases and non-survivors [80].

MR-proADM has been shown to be predictive of complications and mortality in patients with CAP in a meta-analysis of eight studies with 4119 patients [81]. A systematic review of 12 studies similarly found that elevated MR-proADM was highly associated with an increase in short term mortality (OR 6.8) and complications (OR 5.0) [82].

Alveolar pentraxin 3 (PTX3), an acute-phase mediator produced by lung cells, represents another promising biomarker for pneumonia. An examination of 82 intubated patients' BAL fluid showed that elevated PTX3 levels were able to identify bacterial pneumonia [83]. A subsequent nested case–control study found that a 2.56 ng/mL breakpoint had superb sensitivity and specificity for the diagnosis of VAP: 85% and 86%, respectively [84]. Finally, kallistatin, an anti-inflammatory kallikrein inhibitor, has been reported to be significantly consumed in severe CAP patients, and low levels early in admission are associated with increased mortality [85].

Genetics

It would be of great clinical value to have methods for predicting which patients will develop severe respiratory disease in response to a given pathogen and who will have milder courses, as at-risk patients can be given more prompt and aggressive care. A number of genetic analyses have been undertaken to address this need. Notable associations have been made with polymorphisms in pro-inflammatory factors such as TNF-α, IL-6, and lymphotoxin alpha (LTA) [86]. Additionally, several single nucleotide polymorphisms (SNPs) in immune-related genes have been shown to confer either resistance or susceptibility to Streptococcal infection; for instance, mutations in the toll-interleukin 1 receptor domain-containing adaptor protein (TIRAP) and the NF-kappaB pathway have been identified as protective [87].

Rautanen and the ESICM/ECCRN group evaluated over 2500 patients and found 11 loci that correlated significantly with 28-day survival in ICU patients with severe CAP [88]. They further found a SNP in the FER gene to be highly correlated with survival; mortality was 9.5% in patients with the CC genotype, 15.2% in the TC genotype patients, and 25.3% in the TT genotype patients [88]. A follow-up study looked at the FER polymorphism status in 441 patients with ARDS in the ICU, and again found that the TT genotype patients had higher mortality, with a 90-day hazard ratio of 4.62 [89].

Transcriptomics

In the past decade, significant efforts have been made to identify gene expression signatures that accurately identify host response to infection. With the increasing availability of transcriptomic analysis, it may soon be feasible to obtain expression profiles in high-risk patients to aid in the diagnosis and management of pneumonia.

Several groups have assembled gene expression microarrays to diagnose acute infections, with the specific goal of distinguishing viral versus bacterial pneumonia [90, 91]. In 2007, Ramilo and colleagues examined 131 peripheral blood samples and characterized 35 genes able to discriminate bacterial versus viral pneumonia with 95% accuracy [92]. Suarez et al. analyzed whole blood transcriptional data from 118 patients with lower respiratory tract infections and identified 3376 genes associated with bacterial infection and 2391 with viral infections. Using the K-nearest neighbors' algorithm, they identified a parsimonious ten-gene classifier that could distinguish between the two with 95% sensitivity and 92% specificity, greatly outperforming procalcitonin [93]. Scicluna's team looked at blood microarray analysis of critically ill patients with and without CAP and defined a 78-gene signature for CAP [94]. They narrowed this down to a ratio of the FAIM3 (fas apoptotic inhibitory

molecule 3) and PLAC8 (placenta specific 8) gene expression, leading to area under curve of 0.845, again outperforming procalcitonin [94].

Sweeney and Khatri have derived a set of seven genes that discriminate bacterial versus viral infections, which they validated in 30 independent cohorts [95]. Tsalik and his group looked at peripheral whole blood gene expression in 273 subjects with community onset respiratory infections, and used sparse logistic regression to develop classifiers for bacterial infections (71 probes) versus viral infections (33 probes) and noninfectious causes (26 probes); the overall accuracy was higher than that of procalcitonin and also three other published classifiers of bacterial versus viral infections [96].

While the foregoing studies require the use of multi-gene assays, Tang and colleagues recently used genomic analysis of 1071 patients to find a single gene capable of identifying viral infection, interferon alpha inducible protein 27 (IFI27) [97]. They demonstrated a considerable upregulation at the transcript level in patients with influenza as opposed to bacterial pneumonia, likely due to the specific activation of interferon signaling pathways downstream of pathogen recognition receptors selective for virus.

With regards to predicting host response to lung infections, there have been a number of recent advances. Meijas et al. looked at a cohort of infants hospitalized with RSV, HRV, and influenza and identified a score calculated from RSV transcriptional profiles that correlated with outcomes including length of hospitalization, duration of supplementation oxygen, and clinical disease severity score—an important example of the potential utility of transcriptomics in predicting the need for intensive care [98]. Banchereau et al. characterized whole blood transcriptional profiles of patients hospitalized with community-acquired *Staphylococcus aureus* infection and were able to generate a score they called molecular distance to health (MDTH), which correlated with elevated inflammatory markers, longer duration of hospitalization, and more severe disease [99].

A transcriptomic analysis of peripheral leukocytes from 265 ICU patients with sepsis from CAP found two distinct sepsis response signatures "SRS", which they categorized as "SRS1" and "SRS2". Over 3000 genes were noted to be differentially expressed between the groups, with 2260 downregulated in the SRS1 group. SRS1, which had lower expression of Toll-like receptor (TLR) signals, downregulation of human leukocyte antigen (HLA) class II genes, and decreased T-cell activation, was associated with a higher 14-day mortality than SRS2. They distilled out a set of just seven genes to classify patients into SRS1 or SRS2 [100]. Schaack et al. drew from over 900 microarray samples from public repositories from patients with sepsis and identified two clusters of patients according to global blood transcriptomes; these clusters exhibited expression of genes demonstrating a loss of monocyte and T-cell function, indicating a group of patients with higher immunosuppression that may need more aggressive care [101].

Metabolomics and Lipidomics

Metabolomics is an emerging area of investigation aimed at characterizing the cellular metabolic changes during infection [102]. Groups have found metabolic patterns specific to sepsis, some metabolites that potentially can identify severe versus less severe pneumonia, and certain metabolites that may predict poorer outcomes. For instance, To's group found that 13 lipid metabolites could discriminate between CAP and non-CAP cases with an AUC of >0.8, and that trihexosylceramide levels were higher in fatal cases [103]. A separate group used 1D 1H nuclear magnetic resonance (NMR) spectra to generate metabolic profiles from 15 patients with pneumonia; comparing the metabolic profiles using Orthogonal Partial Least Squares Discriminant Analysis (OPLS-DA) they were able to differentiate cases of VAP from those without [104]. Finally, Ning et al. analyzed 119 patients with CAP and found markedly different metabolic patterns as assessed by liquid chromatography-mass spectrometry (LC-MS) compared with control patients [105]. Sphinganine, p-Cresol sulfate, and DHEA-S were significantly lower, and in combination with lactate, this panel could dis-

criminate severe CAP from non-severe CAP with an impressive AUC of 0.911, better than the CURB-65, PSI, and APACHE II scores [105].

Sputum, Bronchoalveolar Lavage, and Exhaled Breath Sampling

Numerous studies have shown that the location of specimen sampling importantly influences diagnostic yield. While the most common tests are those tested in the serum, sputum and airway fluid (BAL, non-bronchoscopic BAL, tracheal aspirates) should also be evaluated. A study of BAL fluid from 47 patients found that median WBC count and neutrophil percentages were significantly higher in bacterial than viral pneumonia. Furthermore, BAL WBC count was an independent predictor of bacterial pneumonia, and when combined with procalcitonin or CRP, the composite reached a sensitivity of 95.8% and a specificity of 95.7% [106]. Importantly, the utility of BAL leukocytosis extends to immunocompromised patients as well, as demonstrated by a study of 107 patients with either hematological malignancy or solid organ transplant. This showed that BAL fluid neutrophil percentage had the highest AUC to predict bacterial infection; in contrast, neither the presence of infiltrates nor leukocyte count was helpful in diagnosing bacterial infection [107].

Interestingly, a discordant inflammatory response has been demonstrated in blood versus sputum in patients with severe CAP. Neutrophil respiratory burst was increased as expected in the blood, but significantly diminished in the lung, indicating either a local failure of inflammatory response or possibly an adaptive immunosuppression to protect lung tissue from immunopathology [108].

As discussed above, breathomics, or measurement of (VOCs) in exhaled breath, is a noninvasive means of sampling host metabolites. Promising early studies have shown discernable metabolomic changes in pneumonia due inflammation and oxidative stress [109]; further work will be necessary to understand the potential clinical utility of such methods.

Future Application of Technologies

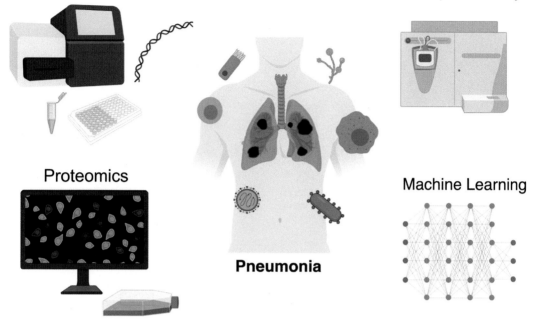

Genomics, Transcriptomics

Mass spectrometry

Proteomics

Machine Learning

Pneumonia

Fig. 12.2 Future application of technologies for the diagnosis and management of pneumonia. This approach may include whole genome sequencing, transcriptomics, proteomics, mass spectrometry, and other methods with the goal of improving precision in the treatment of patients with pneumonia

Conclusions

With ongoing advances in molecular and biochemical methods, we aim for an ever-greater level of diagnostic detail, with the ultimate goal of reliably diagnosing causative pathogens in pneumonia, as well as predicting decompensations, complications, and resolution. In addition to traditional clinical evaluation, we now employ powerful diagnostic tools to evaluate both host and pathogen including biomarkers and PCR; the advent of technologies such as mass spectroscopy and WGS promises further improvements in diagnostic clarity. In addition, the impressive (but potentially overwhelming) amount of data available through electronic medical records and multi-omics modalities including sequencing data may necessitate machine learning algorithms to further optimize pneumonia diagnosis and management.

Incorporating these techniques, we can re-envision the case presented at the outset of this chapter (see Fig. 12.2). The same 45-year-old patient presents with fever and cough. WGS is performed on a sputum sample and reveals influenza B infection with no bacterial superinfection. Antibiotics are withheld, and he initially improves on neuraminidase inhibitor therapy. However, 5 days later he has recurring fevers and worsening hypoxia. Analysis of his exhaled volatile compounds reveals a profile consistent with *S. aureus* pneumonia; mass spectrometry analysis of a sputum sample rapidly confirms *S. aureus* infection and further identifies mecA, indicating MRSA. Vancomycin is promptly added, and the team considers transferring him to a higher level

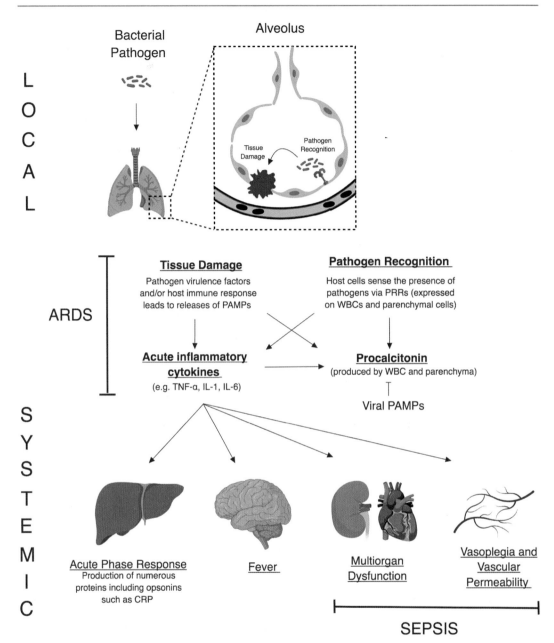

Fig. 12.3 A summary of local and systemic responses to lung infection. Using bacterial pneumonia as an example, pathogens access alveoli and trigger immune responses through the elaboration of pathogen associated molecular patterns (PAMPs), which activate pathogen recognition receptors (PRRs) and production of inflammatory cytokines. Pathogens also damage lung tissue directly, in some cases leading to acute respiratory distress syndrome (ARDS). In general, procalcitonin is secreted during bacterial and not viral infections. Bacterial lung infections can also result in systemic inflammation characterized by acute phase response and production of C-reactive protein (CRP), fever, multiorgan failure, vasoplegia, and vascular permeability that presents as sepsis

of care for closer monitoring. However, his pro-ANP and MR-pro-ADM are not elevated, and on-site transcriptomic analysis of peripheral leukocytes does not show an SRS1 pattern, reassuring the team that he is not a high risk for decompensating. He is safely sent to the general medicine floor, continues to improve, and is discharged home after his short hospitalization.

Several obstacles stand in the way of realizing this level of diagnostic precision and therapeutic sophistication, however. For instance, the costs associated with many of these tests are prohibitive, especially in smaller medical centers. Therefore, technological improvements will be necessary to decrease operating costs while clinical studies must be performed to identify those patients best suited for such advanced and more expensive diagnostics. Basic and translational studies are also needed to more fully elucidate the pathophysiology and natural history of pneumonia to inform future clinical studies and further explain existing data. Ultimately, a multidisciplinary approach involving clinical research, basic biology, chemical analysis, assay optimization, and computational science are needed to usher in an era where the potentially transformative technologies described above are used routinely in the diagnosis and management of pneumonia.

Key Point Summary (see Fig. 12.3)
- Traditional methods for the diagnosis and characterization of pulmonary infections are inadequate.
- The use of advanced molecular diagnostics such as newer biomarkers, multiplex PCR, mass spectrometry, metagenomics, and metataxonomics can improve clinical precision in the diagnosis of pneumonia.
- More studies involving biomarkers and multi-omics approaches are needed to help better characterize the host response to pulmonary infections.

- Incorporation of advanced tools for diagnostics and host response measurements will likely enable personalization of our management of pneumonia and improve outcomes.

References

1. Ferkol T, Schraufnagel D. The global burden of respiratory disease. Ann Am Thorac Soc. 2014;11(3):404–6.
2. Albaum MN, Hill LC, Murphy M, Li YH, Fuhrman CR, Britton CA, Kapoor WN, Fine MJ. Interobserver reliability of the chest radiograph in community-acquired pneumonia. PORT Investigators. Chest. 1996;110(2):343–50.
3. Kraus EM, et al. Antibiotic prescribing for acute lower respiratory tract infections (LRTI) – guideline adherence in the German primary care setting: an analysis of routine data. PLoS One. 2017;12(3):e0174584.
4. Mandell LA, et al. Infectious Diseases Society of America/American Thoracic Society consensus guidelines on the management of community-acquired pneumonia in adults. Clin Infect Dis. 2007;44(Suppl 2):S27–72.
5. Metlay JP. Does this patient have community-acquired pneumonia? Diagnosing pneumonia by history and physical examination. JAMA. 1997;278(17):1440–5.
6. Jain S, et al. Community-acquired pneumonia requiring hospitalization among U.S. adults. N Engl J Med. 2015;373(5):415–27.
7. Waters B, Muscedere J. A 2015 update on ventilator-associated pneumonia: new insights on its prevention, diagnosis, and treatment. Curr Infect Dis Rep. 2015;17(8):496.
8. Dixon P, et al. A systematic review of matrix-assisted laser desorption/ionisation time-of-flight mass spectrometry compared to routine microbiological methods for the time taken to identify microbial organisms from positive blood cultures. Eur J Clin Microbiol Infect Dis. 2015;34(5):863–76.
9. Self WH, et al. High discordance of chest x-ray and computed tomography for detection of pulmonary opacities in ED patients: implications for diagnosing pneumonia. Am J Emerg Med. 2013;31(2):401–5.
10. Basi SK, et al. Patients admitted to hospital with suspected pneumonia and normal chest radiographs: epidemiology, microbiology, and outcomes. Am J Med. 2004;117(5):305–11.
11. Andreo F, et al. Impact of rapid urine antigen tests to determine the etiology of community-acquired pneumonia in adults. Respir Med. 2006;100(5):884–91.
12. Sordé R, et al. Current and potential usefulness of pneumococcal urinary antigen detection in hospital-

ized patients with community-acquired pneumonia to guide antimicrobial therapy. Arch Intern Med. 2011;171(2):166–72.

13. Harris AM, et al. Influence of Antibiotics on the Detection of Bacteria by Culture-Based and Culture-Independent Diagnostic Tests in Patients Hospitalized With Community-Acquired Pneumonia. Open Forum Infect Dis. 2017;4(1):ofx014.

14. Dionne M, Hatchette T, Forward K. Clinical utility of a Legionella pneumophila urinary antigen test in a large university teaching hospital. Can J Infect Dis. 2003;14(2):85–8.

15. Poritz MA, et al. FilmArray, an automated nested multiplex PCR system for multi-pathogen detection: development and application to respiratory tract infection. PLoS One. 2011;6(10):e26047.

16. Jartti T, et al. Identification of respiratory viruses in asymptomatic subjects: asymptomatic respiratory viral infections. Pediatr Infect Dis J. 2008;27(12):1103–7.

17. Rello J, et al. Severity of pneumococcal pneumonia associated with genomic bacterial load. Chest. 2009;136(3):832–40.

18. Werno AM, Anderson TP, Murdoch DR. Association between pneumococcal load and disease severity in adults with pneumonia. J Med Microbiol. 2012;61(Pt 8):1129–35.

19. Patel PA, et al. Evaluation of multiple real-time PCR tests on nasal samples in a large MRSA surveillance program. Am J Clin Pathol. 2015;143(5):652–8.

20. Peacock SJ, Paterson GK. Mechanisms of methicillin resistance in *Staphylococcus aureus*. Annu Rev Biochem. 2015;84:577–601.

21. Carroll KC. Rapid diagnostics for methicillin-resistant *Staphylococcus aureus*. Mol Diagn Ther. 2008;12(1):15–24.

22. Kais M, et al. Quantitative detection of *Streptococcus pneumoniae*, Haemophilus influenzae, and Moraxella catarrhalis in lower respiratory tract samples by real-time PCR. Diagn Microbiol Infect Dis. 2006;55(3):169–78.

23. Abdeldaim G, et al. Is quantitative PCR for the pneumolysin (ply) gene useful for detection of pneumococcal lower respiratory tract infection? Clin Microbiol Infect. 2009;15(6):565–70.

24. Steingart KR, et al. Sputum processing methods to improve the sensitivity of smear microscopy for tuberculosis: a systematic review. Lancet Infect Dis. 2006;6(10):664–74.

25. Diagnostic Standards and Classification of Tuberculosis in Adults and Children. This official statement of the American Thoracic Society and the Centers for Disease Control and Prevention was adopted by the ATS Board of Directors, July 1999. This statement was endorsed by the Council of the Infectious Disease Society of America, September 1999. Am J Respir Crit Care Med. 2000;161(4 Pt 1):1376–95.

26. Marks SM, et al. The health-system benefits and cost-effectiveness of using *Mycobacterium tuberculosis* direct nucleic acid amplification testing to diagnose tuberculosis disease in the United States. Clin Infect Dis. 2013;57(4):532–42.

27. Lim TK, et al. Role of clinical judgment in the application of a nucleic acid amplification test for the rapid diagnosis of pulmonary tuberculosis. Chest. 2003;124(3):902–8.

28. Conaty SJ, et al. The interpretation of nucleic acid amplification tests for tuberculosis: do rapid tests change treatment decisions? J Infect. 2005;50(3):187–92.

29. Catanzaro A, et al. The role of clinical suspicion in evaluating a new diagnostic test for active tuberculosis: results of a multicenter prospective trial. JAMA. 2000;283(5):639–45.

30. Centers for Disease Control and Prevention (CDC). Updated guidelines for the use of nucleic acid amplification tests in the diagnosis of tuberculosis. JAMA. 2009;301(10):1014.

31. Centers for Disease, C. and Prevention. Availability of an assay for detecting *Mycobacterium tuberculosis*, including rifampin-resistant strains, and considerations for its use – United States, 2013. MMWR Morb Mortal Wkly Rep. 2013;62(41):821–7.

32. Vrioni G, et al. MALDI-TOF mass spectrometry technology for detecting biomarkers of antimicrobial resistance: current achievements and future perspectives. Ann Transl Med. 2018;6(12):240.

33. Angeletti S. Matrix assisted laser desorption time of flight mass spectrometry (MALDI-TOF MS) in clinical microbiology. J Microbiol Methods. 2017;138:20–9.

34. Jung JS, et al. Rapid detection of antibiotic resistance based on mass spectrometry and stable isotopes. Eur J Clin Microbiol Infect Dis. 2014;33(6):949–55.

35. van Oort PM, et al. The potential role of exhaled breath analysis in the diagnostic process of pneumonia-a systematic review. J Breath Res. 2018;12(2):024001.

36. Schnabel R, et al. Analysis of volatile organic compounds in exhaled breath to diagnose ventilator-associated pneumonia. Sci Rep. 2015;5:17179.

37. Toma I, et al. Single-molecule long-read 16S sequencing to characterize the lung microbiome from mechanically ventilated patients with suspected pneumonia. J Clin Microbiol. 2014;52(11):3913–21.

38. Conway Morris A, et al. 16S pan-bacterial PCR can accurately identify patients with ventilator-associated pneumonia. Thorax. 2017;72(11):1046–8.

39. Dupont H, et al. Impact of appropriateness of initial antibiotic therapy on the outcome of ventilator-associated pneumonia. Intensive Care Med. 2001;27(2):355–62.

40. Deng X, et al. Whole-genome sequencing for surveillance of invasive pneumococcal diseases in Ontario, Canada: rapid prediction of genotype, antibiotic resistance and characterization of emerging serotype 22F. Front Microbiol. 2016;7:2099.

41. Ellington MJ, et al. The role of whole genome sequencing in antimicrobial susceptibility testing of bacteria: report from the EUCAST Subcommittee. Clin Microbiol Infect. 2017;23(1):2–22.

42. Ocheretina O, et al. False-positive rifampin resistant results with Xpert MTB/RIF version 4 assay in clinical samples with a low bacterial load. Diagn Microbiol Infect Dis. 2016;85(1):53–5.

43. Doyle RM, et al. Direct whole-genome sequencing of sputum accurately identifies drug-resistant *mycobacterium tuberculosis* faster than MGIT culture sequencing. J Clin Microbiol. 2018;56(8):e00666–18.
44. Votintseva AA, et al. Same-day diagnostic and surveillance data for tuberculosis via whole-genome sequencing of direct respiratory samples. J Clin Microbiol. 2017;55(5):1285–98.
45. Cohen T, et al. Mixed-strain *mycobacterium tuberculosis* infections and the implications for tuberculosis treatment and control. Clin Microbiol Rev. 2012;25(4):708–19.
46. Qiu S, et al. Whole-genome sequencing for tracing the transmission link between two ARD outbreaks caused by a novel HAdV serotype 7 variant, China. Sci Rep. 2015;5(1):13617.
47. Molyneaux PL, et al. Outgrowth of the bacterial airway microbiome after rhinovirus exacerbation of chronic obstructive pulmonary disease. Am J Respir Crit Care Med. 2013;188(10):1224–31.
48. Coll F, et al. Genome-wide analysis of multi- and extensively drug-resistant *Mycobacterium tuberculosis*. Nat Genet. 2018;50(2):307–16.
49. Li Y, et al. Validation of β-lactam minimum inhibitory concentration predictions for pneumococcal isolates with newly encountered penicillin binding protein (PBP) sequences. BMC Genomics. 2017;18(1):621.
50. Nguyen M, et al. Developing an in silico minimum inhibitory concentration panel test for *Klebsiella pneumoniae*. Sci Rep. 2018;8(1):421.
51. Abernethy TJ, Avery OT. The occurrence during acute infections of a protein not normally present in the blood : i. Distribution of the reactive protein in patients' sera and the effect of calcium on the flocculation reaction with c polysaccharide of pneumococcus. J Exp Med. 1941;73(2):173–82.
52. Tillett WS, Francis T. Serological reactions in pneumonia with a non-protein somatic fraction of pneumococcus. J Exp Med. 1930;52(4):561–71.
53. García Vázquez E, et al. C-reactive protein levels in community-acquired pneumonia. Eur Respir J. 2003;21(4):702–5.
54. Aabenhus R, et al. Biomarkers as point-of-care tests to guide prescription of antibiotics in patients with acute respiratory infections in primary care. Cochrane Database Syst Rev. 2014;11:CD010130.
55. Hohenthal U, et al. Utility of C-reactive protein in assessing the disease severity and complications of community-acquired pneumonia. Clin Microbiol Infect. 2009;15(11):1026–32.
56. Méndez R, et al. Initial inflammatory profile in community-acquired pneumonia depends on time since onset of symptoms. Am J Respir Crit Care Med. 2018;198(3):370–8.
57. Müller B, et al. Ubiquitous expression of the calcitonin-I gene in multiple tissues in response to Sepsis1. J Clin Endocrinol Metab. 2001;86(1):396–404.
58. Meisner M. Update on procalcitonin measurements. Ann Lab Med. 2014;34(4):263–73.
59. Lee H. Procalcitonin as a biomarker of infectious diseases. Korean J Intern Med. 2013;28(3):285–91.
60. Reinhart K, et al. New approaches to sepsis: molecular diagnostics and biomarkers. Clin Microbiol Rev. 2012;25(4):609–34.
61. Jereb M, Kotar T. Usefulness of procalcitonin to differentiate typical from atypical community-acquired pneumonia. Wien Klin Wochenschr. 2006;118(5–6):170–4.
62. Assicot M, et al. High serum procalcitonin concentrations in patients with sepsis and infection. Lancet. 1993;341(8844):515–8.
63. Reinhart K, Meisner M. Biomarkers in the critically ill patient: procalcitonin. Crit Care Clin. 2011;27(2):253–63.
64. Liu D, et al. Prognostic value of procalcitonin in pneumonia: a systematic review and meta-analysis. Respirology. 2016;21(2):280–8.
65. Self WH, et al. Procalcitonin as an early marker of the need for invasive respiratory or vasopressor support in adults with community-acquired pneumonia. Chest. 2016;150(4):819–28.
66. Li H, et al. Meta-analysis and systematic review of procalcitonin-guided therapy in respiratory tract infections. Antimicrob Agents Chemother. 2011;55(12):5900–6.
67. Mueller B. Procalcitonin-guided antibiotic therapy and hospitalisation in patients with lower respiratory tract infections: the prohosp study. http://isrctn.org/, 2012.
68. Bouadma L, et al. Use of procalcitonin to reduce patients' exposure to antibiotics in intensive care units (PRORATA trial): a multicentre randomised controlled trial. Lancet. 2010;375(9713):463–74.
69. Schuetz P, et al. Effect of procalcitonin-guided antibiotic treatment on mortality in acute respiratory infections: a patient level meta-analysis. Lancet Infect Dis. 2018;18(1):95–107.
70. Huang DT, et al. Procalcitonin-guided use of antibiotics for lower respiratory tract infection. N Engl J Med. 2018;379(3):236–49.
71. Menendez R, et al. Biomarkers improve mortality prediction by prognostic scales in community-acquired pneumonia. Thorax. 2009;64(7):587–91.
72. Siljan WW, et al. Cytokine responses, microbial aetiology and short-term outcome in community-acquired pneumonia. Eur J Clin Investig. 2018;48(1):e12865.
73. Endeman H, et al. Systemic cytokine response in patients with community-acquired pneumonia. Eur Respir J. 2011;37(6):1431–8.
74. Kellum JA, et al. Understanding the inflammatory cytokine response in pneumonia and sepsis: results of the Genetic and Inflammatory Markers of Sepsis (GenIMS) Study. Arch Intern Med. 2007;167(15):1655–63.
75. Müller B, et al. Circulating levels of pro-atrial natriuretic peptide in lower respiratory tract infections. J Intern Med. 2006;260(6):568–76.
76. Vazquez M, et al. MR-pro-atrial natriuretic peptide (MR-proANP) predicts short- and long-term outcomes in respiratory tract infections: a prospective validation study. Int J Cardiol. 2012;156(1):16–23.
77. Claessens Y-E, et al. Accuracy of C-reactive protein, procalcitonin, and mid-regional pro-atrial natriuretic

peptide to guide site of care of community-acquired pneumonia. Intensive Care Med. 2010;36(5):799–809.

78. Welte T, Suttorp N, Marre R. CAPNETZ-community-acquired pneumonia competence network. Infection. 2004;32(4):234.

79. Krüger S, et al. C-terminal provasopressin (copeptin) in patients with community-acquired pneumonia–influence of antibiotic pre-treatment: results from the German competence network CAPNETZ. J Antimicrob Chemother. 2009;64(1):159–62.

80. Mohamed GB, et al. Predictive value of copeptin as a severity marker of community-acquired pneumonia. Electron Physician. 2017;9(7):4880–5.

81. Liu D, et al. Prognostic value of mid-regional pro-adrenomedullin (MR-proADM) in patients with community-acquired pneumonia: a systematic review and meta-analysis. BMC Infect Dis. 2016;16(1):232.

82. Cavallazzi R, et al. Midregional proadrenomedullin for prognosis in community-acquired pneumonia: a systematic review. Respir Med. 2014;108(11): 1569–80.

83. Mauri T, et al. Alveolar pentraxin 3 as an early marker of microbiologically confirmed pneumonia: a threshold-finding prospective observational study. Crit Care. 2014;18(5):562.

84. Bilgin H, et al. Sequential Measurements of Pentraxin 3 Serum Levels in Patients with Ventilator-Associated Pneumonia: A Nested Case-Control Study. Can J Infect Dis Med Microbiol. 2018;2018:4074169.

85. Lin W-C, et al. Plasma kallistatin levels in patients with severe community-acquired pneumonia. Crit Care. 2013;17(1):R27.

86. Chung LP, Waterer GW. Genetic predisposition to respiratory infection and sepsis. Crit Rev Clin Lab Sci. 2011;48(5–6):250–68.

87. Khor CC, et al. A Mal functional variant is associated with protection against invasive pneumococcal disease, bacteremia, malaria and tuberculosis. Nat Genet. 2007;39(4):523–8.

88. Rautanen A, et al. Genome-wide association study of survival from sepsis due to pneumonia: an observational cohort study. Lancet Respir Med. 2015;3(1):53–60.

89. Hinz J, et al. The FER rs4957796 TT genotype is associated with unfavorable 90-day survival in Caucasian patients with severe ARDS due to pneumonia. Sci Rep. 2017;7(1):9887.

90. Graf EH, et al. Unbiased detection of respiratory viruses by use of RNA sequencing-based metagenomics: a systematic comparison to a commercial PCR panel. J Clin Microbiol. 2016;54(4):1000–7.

91. Schlaberg R, et al. Viral pathogen detection by metagenomics and pan-viral group polymerase chain reaction in children with pneumonia lacking identifiable etiology. J Infect Dis. 2017;215(9):1407–15.

92. Ramilo O, et al. Gene expression patterns in blood leukocytes discriminate patients with acute infections. Blood. 2007;109(5):2066–77.

93. Suarez NM, et al. Superiority of transcriptional profiling over procalcitonin for distinguishing bacterial from viral lower respiratory tract infections in hospitalized adults. J Infect Dis. 2015;212(2):213–22.

94. Scicluna BP, et al. A molecular biomarker to diagnose community-acquired pneumonia on intensive care unit admission. Am J Respir Crit Care Med. 2015;192(7):826–35.

95. Sweeney TE, Wong HR, Khatri P. Robust classification of bacterial and viral infections via integrated host gene expression diagnostics. Sci Transl Med. 2016;8(346):346ra91.

96. Tsalik EL, et al. Host gene expression classifiers diagnose acute respiratory illness etiology. Sci Transl Med. 2016;8(322):322ra11.

97. Tang BM, et al. A novel immune biomarker discriminates between influenza and bacteria in patients with suspected respiratory infection. Eur Respir J. 2017;49(6):1602098.

98. Mejias A, et al. Whole blood gene expression profiles to assess pathogenesis and disease severity in infants with respiratory syncytial virus infection. PLoS Med. 2013;10(11):e1001549.

99. Banchereau R, et al. Host immune transcriptional profiles reflect the variability in clinical disease manifestations in patients with *Staphylococcus aureus* infections. PLoS One. 2012;7(4):e34390.

100. Davenport EE, et al. Genomic landscape of the individual host response and outcomes in sepsis: a prospective cohort study. Lancet Respir Med. 2016;4(4):259–71.

101. Schaack D, et al. The immunosuppressive face of sepsis early on intensive care unit-a large-scale microarray meta-analysis. PLoS One. 2018;13(6):e0198555.

102. Leoni D, Rello J. Severe community-acquired pneumonia: optimal management. Curr Opin Infect Dis. 2017;30(2):240–7.

103. To KK, et al. Lipid metabolites as potential diagnostic and prognostic biomarkers for acute community acquired pneumonia. Diagn Microbiol Infect Dis. 2016;85(2):249–54.

104. Antcliffe D, et al. Metabolic profiling in patients with pneumonia on intensive care. EBioMedicine. 2017;18:244–53.

105. Ning P, et al. Metabolic profiles in community-acquired pneumonia: developing assessment tools for disease severity. Crit Care. 2018;22(1):130.

106. Choi S-H, et al. Usefulness of cellular analysis of bronchoalveolar lavage fluid for predicting the etiology of pneumonia in critically ill patients. PLoS One. 2014;9(5):e97346.

107. Stolz D, et al. BAL neutrophils, serum procalcitonin, and C-reactive protein to predict bacterial infection in the immunocompromised host. Chest. 2007;132(2):504–14.

108. Fernandez-Botran R, et al. Contrasting inflammatory responses in severe and non-severe community-acquired pneumonia. Inflammation. 2014;37(4):1158–66.

109. Boots AW, et al. The versatile use of exhaled volatile organic compounds in human health and disease. J Breath Res. 2012;6(2):027108.

Biomarkers in Critical Care Illness: ARDS and Sepsis

13

Simon P. F. Lambden and Charlotte Summers

Introduction

The National Institutes for Health define a biomarker as 'a characteristic that is objectively measured and evaluated as an indicator of normal biological processes, pathogenic processes, or pharmacologic responses to a therapeutic intervention' [1]. The field of biomarker research across the breadth of medicine is considerable with a 2018 Pubmed search revealing more than 50,000 articles with 'biomarker' in the title. This work has led to the successful development of biomarkers across a range of clinical specialties and indications. Assays such as high-sensitivity troponin [2] and circulating d-dimer concentrations [3] are widely used to identify patients at low risk of acute coronary syndromes or deep vein thrombosis, respectively. In addition, the use of genetic biomarkers to determine likely therapeutic response has become the standard of care in breast [4] and haematological malignancies [5].

One of the key challenges in critical care medicine over the past few decades has been the syndromic nature of sepsis and acute respiratory distress syndrome. Understanding of the biological and pathogenic processes underlying these conditions is incomplete, and there are currently few efficacious pharmacotherapies, which has led to limited success in developing biomarkers that conform to the NIH definition above [6].

Identifying Biomarkers

Regardless of the proposed application, the identification of novel biomarkers is undertaken using one of two broad approaches. The traditional model involves target-based analysis of potential candidates. Based upon a specific hypothesis derived from either basic science or clinical observations, this approach typically explores the use of a single candidate as a biomarker for potential utility. These have, in the majority of cases, been circulating proteins or cytokines which have been implicated in the pathophysiology of the disease and isolated from the plasma.

In recent years, the advent of systems-based high-throughput technology has led to the development of '-omics' platforms that can undertake extensive unbiased screening and give detailed insights into the RNA (transcriptomic), DNA (genomic and epigenetic), protein (proteomic), and metabolic (metabolomic) status of the patient

S. P. F. Lambden
NIHR Clinical Lecturer in Intensive Care Medicine, Department of Medicine, University of Cambridge School of Clinical Medicine, Cambridge, UK
e-mail: spl48@cam.ac.uk

C. Summers (✉)
University Lecturer in Intensive Care Medicine, Department of Medicine, University of Cambridge School of Clinical Medicine, Cambridge, UK
e-mail: cs493@medschl.cam.ac.uk

© Springer Nature Switzerland AG 2020
J. L. Gomez et al. (eds.), *Precision in Pulmonary, Critical Care, and Sleep Medicine*, Respiratory Medicine, https://doi.org/10.1007/978-3-030-31507-8_13

using isolated cells or plasma. This allows a range of different potential targets to be identified and combined to offer greater sensitivity and specificity than that delivered by single candidates whilst still meeting the technical requirements of an effective biomarker. In practice, these approaches are often combined to narrow the range of targets and increase the face validity of a test.

Biomarkers may be employed in a range of roles to guide or support clinical decision-making in patients and could be employed to give insights into specific organ function or the patient as a whole. This chapter will categorise biomarkers as diagnostic, prognostic or theranostic. Diagnostic biomarkers could be employed to screen patients at risk and differentiate between the presence and absence of a disease or syndrome, which may facilitate early identification and initial management. A prognostic biomarker should determine the likely patient outcome and allow clinicians to stratify risk either on a population or personalised level. A further application of biomarkers is in the identification of patient populations suitable for a certain treatment and the measurement of the response to an intervention or therapy in a group known as theranostic biomarkers.

In this chapter the main features and roles of a high-quality biomarker will be explored and the technical approaches to their identification reviewed with accompanying discussion of potential candidates.

Defining Sepsis and Acute Respiratory Distress Syndrome

Sepsis is defined as life-threatening organ dysfunction caused by a dysregulated host response to infection [7]. Diagnosis is based on proven or clinical suspicion of infection combined with objective biological and physiological assessments. The challenge facing clinicians and researchers in this area is that in spite of recent revisions, the existing tools are neither entirely specific nor sensitive for diagnosing sepsis [8, 9]. In their 2015 study, Klouwenberg et al. [10] demonstrated using their previously validated tool for

analysis of the likelihood of sepsis [11] that in over 2500 patients admitted to the ICU and treated with antibiotics for infection, only 33% had a definite infection and 13% had a post hoc probability of infection of 'none'. Patients with a post hoc probability of 'none' had an increased risk of death, leading the group to suggest that harm may be associated with the incorrect diagnosis of sepsis. Even the definitive identification of infection is challenging with only around 30% of patients treated for sepsis developing positive blood cultures [12]. As a consequence of these issues, extensive work has been focused on identifying tools that facilitate identification of patients with, or at risk of, poor outcome from sepsis [13, 14]. To date however, only one biomarker (procalcitonin) appears in the surviving sepsis guidelines for use in the management of sepsis, with a weak recommendation for its use in the cessation of antimicrobial therapy [15].

First described in 1967 [16], the acute respiratory distress syndrome (ARDS) did not have a clear definition for more than 20 years. In 1994, following the formation of an international consensus panel, the terms ARDS and acute lung injury (ALI) were defined [17]. After a further consensus committee in 2013, the Berlin definition discarded the term ALI and described ARDS as 'an acute diffuse, inflammatory lung injury, leading to increased pulmonary vascular permeability, increased lung weight, and loss of aerated lung tissue … hypoxemia and bilateral radiographic opacities, associated with increased venous admixture, increased physiological dead space and decreased lung compliance' [18].

The Berlin definition of ARDS includes:

- Acute onset (onset or worsening over 1 week or less).
- Bilateral opacities consistent with pulmonary oedema must be present and may be detected on thoracic CT or chest radiograph.
- PaO_2/FiO_2 (P/F) ratio <300 mmHg with a minimum of 5 cm H_2O positive end expiratory pressure (PEEP) continuous positive airways pressure (CPAP).
- '…must not be fully explained by cardiac failure or fluid overload', in the physician's best

Table 13.1 ARDS is now categorised by the P/F ratio into three groups, which are associated with increasing mortality

ARDS severity	PaO$_2$/FiO$_2$	Mortality
Mild	200–300	27%
Moderate	100–200	32%
Severe	<100	45%

Table 13.2 Methods for identifying pathogenic microbes in sepsis

Diagnostic method	Time for pathogen identification
Microscopy	Morphology in minutes
Gram stain	General category in minutes
Culture and phenotypic biochemistry on/in artificial media (bacterial, mycobacterial, fungal)	Days to weeks
In vitro antimicrobial susceptibility	Days to weeks
Acute and convalescent antibody	Weeks
Monoclonal antibodies	Hours
Antigen detection	Minutes to hours
Real-time polymerase chain reaction for microorganisms and drug resistance genes	One to several hours
Mass spectrometry	Seconds to minutes, after growth on/in media

Adapted from Caliendo et al. [19]

estimation using available information – an 'objective assessment' (e.g. echocardiogram) should be performed in most cases if there is no clear cause such as trauma or sepsis [18].

ARDS is now categorised by the P/F ratio into three groups, which are associated with increasing mortality (Table 13.1):

Diagnostic Biomarkers in Sepsis

The detection of an infectious pathogen is at the heart of the diagnosis and management of patients with sepsis, and extensive work has been done to improve our ability to isolate pathogenic species early to facilitate rapid and focused antimicrobial therapy. The conduct of this work is beyond the scope of this chapter although several methods have been validated as possible tools for the rapid recognition of infection (Table 13.2), and these may become more prevalent as the technology becomes more widely available [19]. There is, however, an important distinction between identification of a potential pathogen, confirming it as the cause of infection and recognising the presence of the sepsis syndrome.

Biomarkers in Existing Definitions of Sepsis

The use of biomarkers in the identification of sepsis is well established, with white cell count forming part of the systemic inflammatory response syndrome (SIRS) criteria that were originally proposed in 1992 and went on, in conjunction with the presence of confirmed or presumed infection, to constitute the diagnostic criteria for sepsis [20], which became a cornerstone of critical care research and clinical practice. Some concerns were identified with their use however, including poor construct validity [21], the of lack of sensitivity and specificity [22] and the heterogeneity of population that was identified by these criteria, making comparison of studies in sepsis outcomes difficult to interpret [23]. The definition of sepsis remained unchanged until 2016, when a new definition and set of diagnostic criteria were developed and presented in the Third International Consensus on Septic Shock in an attempt to address some of these issues [7].

The revised definitions removed the SIRS criteria and replaced them with 'an increase in the Sequential [Sepsis-related] Organ Failure Assessment (SOFA) score of two points or more'. The SOFA score (Table 13.3) was developed based on expert opinion and contains six domains each scored from zero to four. The six organ-specific domains use clinical and laboratory data to quantify the severity of organ dysfunction or failure. An increase in the SOFA score is associated with increasing risk of death [24] and was the most widely used sepsis-specific scoring system at the time of the development of the

Table 13.3 The SOFA score

Score	0	1	2	3	4
Respiration: PaO_2/ FIO_2, mm Hg (kPa)	≥400 (53.3)	<400 (53.3)	<300 (40)	<200 (26.7) with respiratory support	<100 (13.3) with respiratory support
Coagulation: platelets, ×10³/μL	≥150	<150	<100	<50	<20
Liver (bilirubin, mg/ dL [μmol/L])	<1.2 (20)	1.2–1.9 (20–32)	2.0–5.9 (33–101)	6.0–11.9 (102–204)	>12.0 (204)
Cardiovascular	MAP ≥70 mm Hg	MAP <70 mm Hg	Dopamine <5 or dobutamine (any dose)	Dopamine 5.1–15 or epinephrine ≤0.1 or norepinephrine ≤0.1	Dopamine >15 or epinephrine >0.1 or norepinephrine >0.1
Central nervous system (Glasgow Coma Scale score	15	13–14	10–12	6–9	<6
Renal: creatinine, mg/ dL (μmol/L), or urine output, mL/day	<1.2 (110)	1.2–1.9 (110– 170)	2.0–3.4 (171–299)	3.5–4.9 (300–440) <500	>5.0 (440) <200

Adapted from Singer et al. [7]

guidelines. The increase of two or more points in the SOFA score was associated with a 10% mortality in patients with presumed infection and the revised definition proved superior to the SIRS criteria in terms of sensitivity and specificity in retrospective interrogation of a large data set (0.74; 95% CI, 0.73–0.76 vs. 0.64; 95% CI, 0.62–0.66, respectively) [7].

Whilst the revised guidelines offered improved validity, they acknowledged that the new criteria were not perfect and that there was no biomarker available that could reliably detect sepsis. The authors proposed the use of these guidelines to improve identification of patients with sepsis whilst recommending continued work to better define the sepsis syndrome. A range of candidate biomarkers for the diagnosis of sepsis have been proposed as tools to differentiate the dysregulated response to infection from other clinical conditions that can present with sepsis-like features.

Hypothesis-Based Candidates

Over 30 years of study, numerous pathways have been implicated in the pathophysiology of sepsis. The selection of a potential biomarker based upon its role in the development of the target disease or syndrome has a high degree of face validity and is an appealing approach to biomarker

discovery. It has been used successfully in other areas of medicine and extensive work has been undertaken using this strategy.

The best evaluated biomarker for the diagnosis of sepsis is procalcitonin (PCT). PCT has been explored as a potential diagnostic biomarker and as guide to antimicrobial cessation, an application which is considered in a subsequent section. PCT is a 116 peptide amino acid that is encoded by the *CALC-1* gene [25]. Normally only expressed in neuroendocrine tissues, in the presence of bacterial infection *CALC-1* is expressed throughout the body and the synthesis of PCT increases substantially. With a half-life of more than 25 hours, a positive PCT test result associated with clinical features of inflammation has been proposed as a diagnostic tool for sepsis. Of 30 studies included in their analysis, a review of the use of PCT to differentiate between sepsis and infectious inflammation demonstrated an area under the receiver operator characteristic (ROC) curve of 0.85 (95% CI 0·81–0·88) [26], suggesting that PCT was a potentially useful adjunct in making the diagnosis. One of the key limiting factors in interpreting the potential clinical use of PCT is the threshold at which the test is considered positive. A range between 0.1 and 5 ng/ml or a relative change from baseline levels has been considered positive with differences in sensitivity and specificity reported based on the threshold selected. In addition, PCT expression is not unique to infection with elevated levels seen in a range of acute conditions including trauma [27], pancreatitis [28], cardiogenic shock [29], renal failure [30], and following surgery [31], which may limit its application as a diagnostic biomarker, although the use of differing thresholds may still offer promise in the identification of infection in these populations.

In addition to PCT, a large number of hypothesis-based candidates have been assessed in one or more clinical populations with sepsis. In their detailed review in 2010, Pierrakos and Vincent [14] identified more than 3000 studies exploring 178 biomarker candidates. Of the 34 that had been specifically examined as diagnostic biomarkers, several had been shown to display a greater than 90% of sensitivity and specificity in neonates and paediatric sepsis. Of those examined in adults, only one delivered a similar performance, the degree of CD64 expression on circulating neutrophils assessed using flow cytometry. In those patients with a CD64 expression above a defined threshold, the sensitivity (96%) and specificity (95%) of this test delivered an area under the ROC of 0.97 in a group of 50 patients with blood culture positive for sepsis compared to patients without positive blood cultures [32].

Of other potential candidates considered for use as diagnostic tools, C reactive protein (CRP) is the most widely employed in clinical practice. Initially discovered in the context of acute infection with streptococcus and later with other microbes, CRP is an acute phase protein that is elevated in a range of inflammatory disorders including burns, trauma, and following surgery. As such its sensitivity and specificity for the diagnosis of sepsis is limited [33]. A similar challenge has been faced by efforts to validate other cytokines as diagnostic biomarkers such as tumour necrosis factor-α (TNF-α), interleukin-6 and interleukin-1β (IL-6 and IL-1β). Biomarkers such as these were identified as important mediators of the innate immune response and have been widely demonstrated to play important roles in the pathophysiology of sepsis. The value of these markers as diagnostics has been shown to be limited however, because these pathways are activated by a diverse range of stimuli and also many of these

cytokines have a short half-life which may explain the variability in plasma concentrations seen in sepsis and control populations [34].

Other candidates include presepsin, formed by the solubilisation of the shed CD14/LPS complex [35] and include soluble triggering receptor expressed on myeloid cells-1 (sTREM-1) [36, 37]. In a range of small studies undertaken subsequently, it has been demonstrated that biomarkers have shown adequate sensitivity and specificity in the diagnosis of infection-related inflammation but without significant advantage over existing clinical and biochemical tools, with an area under the ROC curve ranging between 0.75 and 0.9 in differentiating infectious and non-infectious inflammation [38].

MicroRNAs

MicroRNAs (miRNAs) have become an area of considerable interest to all branches of medicine in recent years. They are small RNAs in the region of 20–25 nucleotides in length that do not code for proteins but regulate gene expression. miRNAs may cause increased or reduced translation of a gene target and play a role in the regulation of as much as 60% of the genes that code for proteins [39]. Because of this extensive role, numerous miRNAs have been implicated in the pathophysiology of sepsis [40] and have also been considered as candidate biomarkers for the diagnosis or prognosis of the syndrome. In a small study of a patients with severe non-infective SIRS or severe sepsis, of the 116 miRNAs detected in plasma, a panel of six (miR-30d-5p, miR-30a-5p, miR-192-5p, miR-26a-5p, miR-23a-5p, miR-191-5p) were considered to be potential candidates. All were associated with significant differences in expression between the two groups of patients, and when considered in combination, they offered an AUC of 0.917 for the diagnosis of sepsis [41]. In a subsequent study, levels of miRNA displayed some correlation between illness severity described by the SOFA score in patients with non-infective systemic inflammation; however, none of them showed a significant correlation in patients with sepsis [42]. Further limitations of miRNA-based methods have included significant inter-study and inter-assay variability which has limited the potential utility of this approach, although considerable development of methodology continues which may improve the reliability of studies in this area [43].

Transcriptomics

RNA is the key intermediary between the information storage of the genome and is the key driver of protein synthesis. Transcriptomics describes the analysis of a snapshot of patients' RNA expression and approaches typically involve the isolation of RNA from a cellular source followed by global analysis or interrogation of a specific selection of candidates. This approach has appeal because the transcriptional response to critical illness is extensive and describes those pathways that are activated and inhibited by the stressor, meaning that potential candidates can be analysed individually or in combination.

The transcriptomic tool Septicyte™ was recently approved for use by the Food and Drug Administration as a diagnostic tool for the differentiation of sepsis from systemic inflammation on the ICU and is based on the expression of RNA of four genes – *CEACAM4, LAMP1, PLA2G7,* and *PLAC8* [44]. In prospective evaluation in a heterogeneous group of patients from the USA and Europe, Septicyte offered an AUROC of between 0.82 and 0.89 which was independent of demographic factors and the addition on clinical variables or PCT [45].

In an analysis of publicly available data sets, Sweeney et al. [46] developed the infection z score using an unbiased analytical approach. The z score offered a different panel of 11 transcriptomic markers in peripheral blood that differentiated between infection- and non-infection-related systemic inflammation. Use of the panel to identify sepsis gave an AUROC of 0.87 in the discovery set and 0.83 in the validation cohort which was derived using isolated neutrophils and was independent of the nature of the infective organism.

In their analysis of transcriptomic biomarkers from critically ill patients as a potential diagnostic platform, Bauer et al. [47] considered the dys-regulated nature of the immune response in sepsis and identified a panel of 7 RNA targets, three of which were upregulated (*TLR5, CD59, CLU*) and four of which were downregulated (*FGL2, IL7R, HLA-DPA1* and *CPVL*). Using this panel and data sets from German and Greek populations, the group were able to demonstrate an AUROC of 0.812. They also demonstrated that the process could be effectively transferred to a RT-PCR platform to improve potential clinical utility by providing a gene expression score that displayed differentiation between those with either proven or suspected infection and those without. A further example of the use of transcriptomic platforms in the diagnosis of sepsis comes from the *FAIM3/PLAC8* ratio, derived from a 78 gene expression panel and originally validated as a tool to diagnose community-acquired pneumonia in patients admitted to ICU [48]. The AUC of 0.845 they observed in their study was recapitulated in a follow-up validation of multiple cohorts in which the tool offered similar performance in a range of diseases and time points [49].

Metabolomics

Metabolomics interrogates the cellular 'fingerprint' that is the product of the functional activity of the cell and as such has appeal in critical illness as a tool to understand the narrative course of a dynamic disease process in patients.

Most commonly interrogated using mass spectrometry techniques, metabolomic approaches offer an attractive potential platform for the differentiation of patients with the sepsis syndrome from those with inflammation without infection. A range of studies have shown that metabolites associated with energy metabolism show consistent directional changes in a range of populations with infection [50]. In a study of six classes of analyte totalling more than 180 metabolites from 143 patients, Schmerler et al. found two candidates (acylcarnitine C10:1 and glycerophospholipid PCaaC32:0) that offered an AUC of 0.831 and 0.855 individually and 0.886 in combination [51]. In a retrospective study of metabolomic candidates, a regression model combining two analytes (the sphingolipid SM C22:3 and the glycerophospholipid lysoPCaC24:0) offered an AUC of 0.90 and also offered some ability to differentiate between the sources of infection [52].

Prognostic Biomarkers in Sepsis and ARDS

Survival Prognostication in Sepsis and ARDS

Sepsis is a syndrome that is associated with a mortality of more than 10% and septic shock with a mortality of at least 30% [7], and ARDS is associated with a mortality of 35–50% depending on severity [17, 18]. Identifying one or more biomarkers that would allow clinicians to prognosticate survival with a high degree of certainty is appealing as it would potentially facilitate improved end-of-life care for those who are not going to survive and efficient resource allocation in those whose clinical course may be modifiable. There has been a wealth of research with this end in mind, and many hypothesis-based biomarkers have been suggested to provide some degree of prognostication or association with illness severity. These candidates may be divided into a number of categories including cytokines, cell surface receptors, coagulation proteins, vasculature derived, and circulating proteins, as well as physiological measurements. An exhaustive review of these is not within the purview of this chapter; however, here we highlight some exemplars. Whilst many of these candidates have some value in determining those populations of patients with the greatest risk of death or highest severity of illness, none can offer individual prognostication, making their utility limited.

With the development of transcriptomic profiling, new observations have been made in studies of patients with sepsis. In particular, it has been shown that patients with the same or similar clinical presentations can have extensive differences in their transcriptomic profiles and that they can be divided into distinct phenotypic groups which are associated with prognosis. In their study of more than 250 patients with community-acquired pneumonia and organ dysfunction admitted to intensive care units in the UK, Davenport et al. [53]

used peripheral blood leukocyte transcriptomics to determine the expression profiles of these cells and associate them with outcome. They identified two groups, SRS1 found in 41% of the patients and expressing an immunosuppression pattern compared to the second group (SRS2). This immunosuppression phenotype was associated with a significantly increased hazard ratio for death compared to the SRS2 patients that could be identified by a panel of seven genes (*DYRK2, CCNB1IP1, TDRD9, ZAP70, ARL14EP, MDC1,* and *ADGRE3*). Of note, the group made the observation that clinical scoring systems, the timing of sample collection and expression of common pro-inflammatory activators such as IL-1, IL-6, or TNF did not predict membership of the SRS1 population.

Proteomic approaches show promise in identifying the presence [54] or nature [55] of an infectious insult; however, issues with reproducibility have meant that isolated proteomic approaches have proven limited. In one small study that targeted plasma glycopeptides in an effort to eliminate signal noise produced by more abundant proteins, the team identified 54 proteins unique to survivors and 43 unique to non-survivors of a total of 234. These were mapped onto a series of pathways which were associated with outcome [56].

In a combined protein and transcriptomic analysis, the PERSEVERE [57] and updated PERSEVERE XP [58] platforms were developed for prediction of survival status in paediatric sepsis. This approach used a selection of potential candidates based on previous genome-wide studies and predictive modelling. The PERSEVERE XP has shown a high degree of differentiation between survivors and non-survivors with an area under the ROC curve of 0.90 in the derivation and 0.96 in the test cohort. In adults, the group took a similar approach and developed a decision tree with five biomarkers (granzyme B, heat shock protein 70 kDa 1B, CCL3, IL-8, IL-1a, and CCL4) which had some crossover with the paediatric model, as well as serum lactate and the presence of chronic disease to quantify risk [59]. This tool had a high degree of sensitivity, although specificity was poor leading to an AUROC of 0.784.

In ARDS, a different approach has led to a similar observation that in patients who were included in randomised controlled trials of ARDS therapies, two distinct phenotypes of patients could be identified based on a range of clinical, biochemical and biomarkers in combination. In their study, Calfee et al. [60] identified a cohort of patients characterised by higher expression of pro-inflammatory biomarkers, vasopressor use, and the presence of sepsis, which was associated with significantly higher mortality and critical care utilisation. There was also a difference between these groups in response to positive end expiratory pressure suggesting that heterogeneous treatment responses within a study population may obscure a clinically relevant benefit in some patients, an observation which may provoke change in patient selection for studies of this kind.

Metabolomics approaches have also offered some candidate prognostic biomarkers in sepsis. In a study that used data from two independent cohorts, 12 metabolite profiles were selected based on previous studies or pilot data, combined with a series of clinical features (age, mean arterial pressure, haematocrit, and temperature). This approach was associated with sensitivity and specificity consistent with an AUC of 0.73–0.85 for the prediction of survival [61]. Further work in the same patients identified 31 metabolites that were different in sepsis survivors and non-survivors from two different patient cohorts. They also used a Bayesian approach to develop a metabolomic network of seven metabolites associated with death that offered an AUC of 0.74 and 0.91 [62].

A defining feature of ARDS is the presence of non-cardiogenic pulmonary oedema fluid within the alveolar space, which accumulates due to increased permeability of the alveolar–capillary barrier. Transpulmonary thermodilution techniques provide an estimation of extravascular lung water (EVLW) [63] and pulmonary blood volume. The ratio between these two parameters, called pulmonary vascular permeability index (PVPI), is thought to reflect the permeability of the alveolocapillary barrier [64]. A thermistor placed into a femoral arterial catheter measures the downstream temperature changes induced by the injection of a bolus of cold saline solution into the superior vena cava and calculates cardiac output from the thermodilution curve using the

Stewart–Hamilton algorithm, as well as the mean transit time and exponential downslope time of the transpulmonary thermodilution curve. The product of cardiac output and mean transit time is the intrathoracic thermal volume. The product of cardiac output and exponential downslope time is the pulmonary thermal volume [65]. The EVLW value is deducted from the difference between the intrathoracic thermal volume and the estimated intrathoracic blood volume. The pulmonary blood volume is deducted from the difference between the pulmonary thermal volume and the EVLW.

In ARDS, it has been repeatedly observed that high values of EVLW indexed to predicted body weight (EVLWI) are significantly associated with mortality [66–71] and further that daily changes in EVLWI may be associated with survival [68, 69]. EVLWI has also been shown to be a good predictor of mortality [67–70]. PVPI has also been shown to be related to the prognosis of patients with ARDS [67, 71] and to predict mortality in an independent manner [67]. PVPI and EVLWI predict mortality in an independent manner, suggesting that they may indicate a different pathophysiological aspect of ARDS. Whilst PVPI appears to characterise the degree of impairment of the alveolocapillary barrier, EVLWI may indicate the severity of the pulmonary leak resulting from this injury. EVLWI has been successfully used in clinical trials of pharmacotherapy in patients with ARDS [72, 73].

Biomarkers in Survivors of Critical Illness

In addition to survival, there is burgeoning recognition that survivors of critical illness are at significantly increased risk of long-term complications including biological, physical, and psychological issues that extend beyond discharge from hospital and often for prolonged periods [74]. Prognostic biomarkers in critical illness could be employed to identify those likely to survive their admission to hospital, but also to determine the population at risk of specific complications arising from the syndrome. These tools could allow clinicians to focus interventions and follow-up on those patients most at risk. An example of this strategy was seen in the study by Hughes et al. which looked at the presence of persistent cognitive impairment in more than 400 survivors of critical illness [75]. The group showed that higher circulating levels of biomarkers of brain injury and endothelial dysfunction (S100B and E-selectin, respectively) measured within 72 hours of ICU admission was associated with cognitive dysfunction at 3 and 12 months.

Theranostic Biomarkers in Sepsis and ARDS

Theranostic approaches describes the use of one or more biomarkers to identify patients who may benefit from specific treatments. This strategy is well established in a number of fields of medicine, with examples including elevated HER2 receptor expression in the therapeutic treatment of breast cancer with trastuzumab (Herceptin™) [76] and the presence of gain or loss of function polymorphisms of the *CYP2C19* gene which determine the effectiveness of clopidogrel as an anti-platelet therapy [77]. Theranostic biomarkers can be employed in a range of roles including the selection of the optimum treatment option or driving the initiation or cessation of a specific intervention. In critical care, a number of different approaches have been validated as potential candidates ranging from plasma cytokines through to genomic strategies.

An early effort to use biomarkers as theranostics came in 2001 when Reinhart *et al.* trialled anti-TNF-α monoclonal antibody therapy in a population of septic shock patients who had a serum IL-6 concentration >1000 pg/mL using a point-of-care test undertaken prior to randomisation [78]. The study showed the feasibility of large-scale studies using biomarkers to enrich study populations in clinical trials of potential therapies. In a subsequent randomised controlled trial of the same agent, patients with an elevated IL-6 experienced a modest survival benefit from the therapy, whereas no benefit was seen in the unenriched population [79].

Of theranostic candidates, the best-evaluated hypothesis-based approach is the use of PCT, not as a diagnostic biomarker, but to provide insight into the appropriate time to initiate or stop antimicrobial therapy in patients with infection. A number of clinical trials have tested the impact of PCT testing on duration of antimicrobial therapy in patients with sepsis or septic shock. Bloos et al. [80] and de Jong et el. [81] have demonstrated significant reductions in the duration of antimicrobial therapy without apparent increases in treatment failures. Meta-analysis of randomised trials in this area suggests a potential benefit [82] leading to PCT being recommended for this indication in some national guidelines [83]. However, as with diagnostics, the threshold at which treatment is stopped is an important consideration and may impact on efficacy [84]. In addition, the application of these tests in normal clinical practice may be less effective than that seen in studies, with an observational study of more than 20,000 patients reporting that in the 18% of patients in whom PCT was measured, there was no change in duration of antimicrobial therapy or other outcomes [85]. As a consequence of these data and the challenge of controlling for the prompting effect seen in trials of this kind [86], the 2016 iteration of the Surviving Sepsis guidelines offers only a weak recommendation for PCT use in patients who had previously displayed features of sepsis in whom there is limited clinical evidence of infection [15].

A more recent example of theranostics is the work by Calfee et al. [87], where retrospective analysis of the HARP2 clinical trial of statin therapy in acute respiratory distress syndrome identified two subtypes of ARDS with differential responses to therapy: hyper- and hypoinflammatory phenotypes similar to those identified in earlier work [60]. Patients with the hyperinflammatory subphenotype treated with simvastatin had significantly higher 28-day survival than those given placebo, with a similar pattern observed for 90-day survival. No benefit of statins was seen in the hypoinflammatory subphenotype. Whilst these findings need prospective validation, they support the idea that not all patients have similar responses to therapy and that identification of subpopulations who derive benefit (or harm) from a given intervention is an important aim.

Pharmacogenomics holds considerable promise for the identification of patients who may benefit from specific treatments. Identifying those patients with polymorphisms that place them at increased risk and modulating the specific pathway may offer personalised treatment strategies that can overcome the heterogeneity of response seen in clinical trials of the wider sepsis population.

A potential candidate for a pharmacogenomic approach is expression of polymorphisms of the *PCSK9* gene. Already well established as a potential treatment for hypercholesterolaemia [88], Walley et al. [89] demonstrated in patients with septic shock that the expression of loss or gain of function polymorphisms of *PCSK9* was associated with significant alterations in mortality. They also showed that pharmacological inhibition of *PCSK9* may be a therapeutic option in sepsis. Other candidates include vasopressors, where changes in the response to specific vasoactive therapies such as catecholamines, vasopressin, or angiotensin II [90] could be governed by receptor polymorphisms which may in turn make one therapy preferable over another. Caution should be expressed in this area as polymorphisms do not account for all the apparent variability in response and subsequent failure of therapies. In a study that may offer a model for future trials in this area, the impact of four polymorphisms on the response to activated protein C therapy was explored in 639 patients, compared to more than 1500 matched controls. Of the four single nucleotide polymorphisms (SNPs) identified through high-throughput screens, the group used two 'improved response polymorphism (IRP)' groups each containing two of the target SNPs [91]. No impact of the presence of these proposed IRPs was seen in the response to activated protein C therapy.

Evaluation of the response to therapy may also be guided in the future by platform-based approaches such as metabolomics. In an exploratory analysis of samples from a pilot randomised controlled trial of L-carnitine therapy in sepsis [92], the authors identified a responder and non-responder population based on their metabolomic profiles after initiation of treatment, with responders appearing to have better outcomes when treated with L-carnitine [93]. The authors suggested that this was a potential approach to subsequent trial design and patient selection for studies in critical illness.

Conclusions

A major effort has been invested in the identification of biomarkers that can assist clinicians in the diagnosis, prognostication or selection of therapeutic options for patients with sepsis or ARDS. To date, the uptake of these approaches has been limited to a few biomarkers in selected cases, and even then penetration into the real-world clinical environment has been incomplete. There are a number of reasons for this which must be considered as we move forward with development and validation of candidates in this area.

The challenge of a syndrome: Both sepsis and ARDS are not in themselves diseases; they exist on a spectrum with mild features at one end and catastrophic organ failure at the other. The heterogeneity of the syndromes makes developing a test to confirm their presence challenging as the presence of the syndrome or the risk of death increase as the patient progresses along the spectrum of illness. This is true both of conventional diagnostic definitions and of efforts to develop tests to confirm their presence.

Construct validity: In a number of cases, across all of the proposed platforms, there is considerable variability between the biomarkers/profiles identified. This remains the case even in similar populations and raises the question of how translatable to clinical practice the biomarkers are. This concern is confirmed when 'real-world' assessments of these tools are undertaken. In these studies, the performance of candidates is rarely as good as in controlled study conditions. Larger sample, prospective studies are necessary to increase the confidence that a target may be worthy of consideration in a real-world setting.

Analytic complexity: In order for a biomarker or platform to be valuable, it must fulfil the criteria that are laid out in this chapter for the ideal biomarker. Without rapid turnaround, ease of use, and economic methods, clinicians will not be able to build a case for their use. Before companies will invest in simplifying methods to facilitate this approach however, a highly robust target must be found to justify their investment.

Precision approaches: In the face of a large body of evidence that delays in appropriate treatment are associated with significantly increased mortality, a biomarker that has even a modest false-negative rate would be associated with potentially significant harm. In contrast, the negative impacts of excessive antimicrobial therapy are also well documented so a test that provides a false positive and provokes an unnecessary intervention may also cause concern. Therefore, given the clinical uncertainty associated with the diagnosis of sepsis, a biomarker or platform must offer more precision than is currently available before clinicians will accept their routine use.

The future of biomarker selection and identification may lie in combinations of approaches including the use of combination platforms which use candidate DNA, RNA, proteins, and metabolites to improve the personalisation of biomarker results. This, in combination with large databases and sample libraries, will facilitate greater success in the next generation of diagnostic, prognostic, and theranostic tests in sepsis or ARDS.

References

1. Group BDW. Biomarkers and surrogate endpoints: preferred definitions and conceptual framework. Clin Pharmacol Ther. 2001;69:89–95.
2. Garg P, Morris P, Fazlanie AL, Vijayan S, Dancso B, Dastidar AG, Plein S, Mueller C, Haaf P. Cardiac biomarkers of acute coronary syndrome: from history to high-sensitivity cardiac troponin. Intern Emerg Med. 2017;12:147–55.
3. Riley RS, Gilbert AR, Dalton JB, Pai S, McPherson RA. Widely used types and clinical applications of D-dimer assay. Lab Med. 2016;47:90–102.
4. Duffy MJ, Harbeck N, Nap M, Molina R, Nicolini A, Senkus E, Cardoso F. Clinical use of biomarkers in breast cancer. Updated guidelines from the European Group on Tumor Markers (EGTM). Eur J Cancer. 2017;75:284–98.
5. Hussaini M. Biomarkers in hematological malignancies: a review of molecular testing in hematopathology. Cancer Control. 2015;22:158–66.
6. Shankar-Hari M, Summers C, Baillie JK. In pursuit of precision medicine in the critically ill. In: Vincent J-L, editor. Annual update in intensive care medicine. Switzerland: Springer International Publishing; 2018.
7. Singer M, Deutschman CS, Seymour C, Shankar-Hari M, Annane D, Bauer M, Bellomo R. The third international consensus definitions for sepsis and septic shock (sepsis-3). JAMA. 2016;315:801–10.
8. Finkelsztein EJ, Jones DS, Ma KC, Pabón MA, Delgado T, Nakahira K, Arbo JE, Berlin DA, Schenck EJ, Choi AMK, et al. Comparison of qSOFA and SIRS for predicting adverse outcomes of patients with suspicion of sepsis outside the intensive care unit. Crit Care. 2017;21:73.
9. Seymour CW, Liu VX, Iwashyna TJ, Brunkhorst FM, Rea TD, Scherag A, Rubenfeld G, Kahn JM, Shankar-Hari M, Singer M. Assessment of clinical criteria for sepsis for the third international consensus definitions for sepsis and septic shock (Sepsis-3). JAMA. 2016;315:762–74.
10. Klein Klouwenberg PMC, Cremer OL, van Vught LA, Ong DSY, Frencken JF, Schultz MJ, Bonten MJ, van der Poll T. Likelihood of infection in patients with presumed sepsis at the time of intensive care unit admission: a cohort study. Crit Care. 2015;19:319.
11. Klein Klouwenberg PM, Ong DS, Bos LD, de Beer FM, van Hooijdonk RT, Huson MA, Straat M, van Vught LA, Wieske L, Horn J, et al. Interobserver agreement of Centers for Disease Control and Prevention criteria for classifying infections in critically ill patients. Crit Care Med. 2013;41:2373–8.
12. Minderhoud TC, Spruyt C, Huisman S, Oskam E, Schuit SCE, Levin MD. Microbiological outcomes and antibiotic overuse in Emergency Department patients with suspected sepsis. Netherlands J Med. 2017;75:196–203.
13. Van Engelen TSR, Wiersinga WJ, Scicluna BP, van der Poll T. Biomarkers in Sepsis. Critical Care Clin. 2018;34:139–52.
14. Pierrakos C, Vincent JL. Sepsis biomarkers: a review. Crit Care. 2010;14:R15.
15. Rhodes A, Evans LE, Alhazzani W, Levy MM, Antonelli M, Ferrer R, Kumar A, Sevransky JE, Sprung CL, Nunnally ME, et al. Surviving Sepsis Campaign: international guidelines for management of sepsis and septic shock: 2016. Intensive Care Med. 2017;43:304–77.
16. Ashbaugh DG, Bigelow DB, Petty TL, Levine BE. Acute respiratory distress in adults. Lancet. 1967;2:319–23.
17. Bernard GR, Artigas A, Brigham KL, Carlet J, Falke K, Hudson L, Lamy M, Legall JR, Morris A, Spragg R. The American-European Consensus Conference on ARDS. Definitions, mechanisms, relevant outcomes, and clinical trial coordination. Am J Respir Crit Care Med. 1994;149:818–24.
18. Ranieri VM, Rubenfeld GD, Thompson BT, Ferguson ND, Caldwell E, Fan E, Camporota L, Slutsky AS. Acute respiratory distress syndrome: the Berlin Definition. JAMA. 2012;307:2526–33.
19. Caliendo AM, Gilbert DN, Ginocchio CC, Hanson KE, May L, Quinn TC, Tenover FC, Alland D, Blaschke AJ, Bonomo RA, et al. Better tests, better care: improved diagnostics for infectious diseases. Clinical Infect Dis. 2013;57(Suppl 3):S139–70.
20. American College of Chest Physicians/Society of Critical Care Medicine Consensus Conference: definitions for sepsis and organ failure and guidelines for the use of innovative therapies in sepsis. Crit Care Med. 1992;20:864–74.
21. Shankar-Hari M, Bertolini G, Brunkhorst FM, Bellomo R, Annane D, Deutschman CS, Singer

M. Judging quality of current septic shock definitions and criteria. Crit Care. 2015;19:1–5.

22. Churpek MM, Snyder A, Han X, Sokol S, Pettit N, Howell MD, Edelson DP. Quick sepsis-related organ failure assessment, systemic inflammatory response syndrome, and early warning scores for detecting clinical deterioration in infected patients outside the intensive care unit. Am J Respir Crit Care Med. 2017;195:906–11.

23. Shankar-Hari M, Deutschman CS, Singer M. Do we need a new definition of sepsis? Intensive Care Med. 2015;41:909–11.

24. Vincent JL, de Mendonca A, Cantraine F, Moreno R, Takala J, Suter PM, Sprung CL, Colardyn F, Blecher S. Use of the SOFA score to assess the incidence of organ dysfunction/failure in intensive care units: results of a multicenter, prospective study. Working group on "sepsis-related problems" of the European Society of Intensive Care Medicine. Crit Care Med. 1998;26:1793–800.

25. Jin M, Khan AI. Procalcitonin: uses in the clinical laboratory for the diagnosis of sepsis. Lab Med. 2010;41:173–7.

26. Wacker C, Prkno A, Brunkhorst FM, Schlattmann P. Procalcitonin as a diagnostic marker for sepsis: a systematic review and meta-analysis. Lancet Infect Dis. 2013;13:426–35.

27. Meisner M, Adina H, Schmidt J. Correlation of procalcitonin and C-reactive protein to inflammation, complications, and outcome during the intensive care unit course of multiple-trauma patients. Crit Care. 2006;10:R1.

28. Rau B, Steinbach G, Baumgart K, Gansauge F, Grunert A, Beger HG. The clinical value of procalcitonin in the prediction of infected necrosis in acute pancreatitis. Intensive Care Med. 2000;26(Suppl 2):S159–64.

29. Geppert A, Steiner A, Delle-Karth G, Heinz G, Huber K. Usefulness of procalcitonin for diagnosing complicating sepsis in patients with cardiogenic shock. Intensive Care Med. 2003;29:1384–9.

30. Sabat R, Hoflich C, Docke WD, Oppert M, Kern F, Windrich B, Rosenberger C, Kaden J, Volk HD, Reinke P. Massive elevation of procalcitonin plasma levels in the absence of infection in kidney transplant patients treated with pan-T-cell antibodies. Intensive Care Med. 2001;27:987–91.

31. Syvanen J, Peltola V, Pajulo O, Ruuskanen O, Mertsola J, Helenius I. Normal behavior of plasma procalcitonin in adolescents undergoing surgery for scoliosis. Scand J Surgery. 2014;103:60–5.

32. Cardelli P, Ferraironi M, Amodeo R, Tabacco F, De Blasi RA, Nicoletti M, Sessa R, Petrucca A, Costante A, Cipriani P. Evaluation of neutrophil CD64 expression and procalcitonin as useful markers in early diagnosis of sepsis. Int J Immunopathol Pharmacol. 2008;21:43–9.

33. Vincent JL, Donadello K, Schmit X. Biomarkers in the critically ill patient: C-reactive protein. Crit Care Clin. 2011;27:241–51.

34. Pinsky MR, Vincent J-L, Deviere J, Alegre M, Kahn RJ, Dupont E. Serum cytokine levels in human septic shock: relation to multiple-system organ failure and mortality. Chest. 1993;103:565–75.

35. Limongi D, D'Agostini C, Ciotti M. New sepsis biomarkers. Asian Pac J Trop Biomed. 2016;6:516–9.

36. Brenner T, Uhle F, Fleming T, Wieland M, Schmoch T, Schmitt F, Schmidt K, Zivkovic AR, Bruckner T, Weigand MA, et al. Soluble TREM-1 as a diagnostic and prognostic biomarker in patients with septic shock: an observational clinical study. Biomarkers. 2017;22:63–9.

37. Aksaray S, Alagoz P, Inan A, Cevan S, Ozgultekin A. Diagnostic value of sTREM-1 and procalcitonin levels in the early diagnosis of sepsis. North Clin Istanb. 2016;3:175–82.

38. Chenevier-Gobeaux C, Borderie D, Weiss N, Mallet-Coste T, Claessens Y-E. Presepsin (sCD14-ST), an innate immune response marker in sepsis. Clin Chim Acta. 2015;450:97–103.

39. Friedman RC, Farh KK, Burge CB, Bartel DP. Most mammalian mRNAs are conserved targets of microRNAs. Genome Res. 2009;19:92–105.

40. Benz F, Roy S, Trautwein C, Roderburg C, Luedde T. Circulating MicroRNAs as biomarkers for sepsis. Int J Mol Sci. 2016;17:78.

41. Caserta S, Kern F, Cohen J, Drage S, Newbury SF, Llewelyn MJ. Circulating plasma microRNAs can differentiate human sepsis and systemic inflammatory response syndrome (SIRS). Sci Rep. 2016;6:28006.

42. Caserta S, Mengozzi M, Kern F, Newbury SF, Ghezzi P, Llewelyn MJ. Severity of systemic inflammatory response syndrome affects the blood levels of circulating inflammatory-relevant microRNAs. Front Immunol. 2018;8:1977.

43. Buschmann D, Kirchner B, Hermann S, Märte M, Wurmser C, Brandes F, Kotschote S, Bonin M, Steinlein OK, Pfaffl MW, et al. Evaluation of serum extracellular vesicle isolation methods for profiling miRNAs by next-generation sequencing. J Extracellular Vesicles. 2018;7:1481321.

44. McHugh L, Seldon TA, Brandon RA, Kirk JT, Rapisarda A, Sutherland AJ, Presneill JJ, Venter DJ, Lipman J, Thomas MR, et al. A molecular host response assay to discriminate between sepsis and infection-negative systemic inflammation in critically ill patients: discovery and validation in independent cohorts. PLoS Med. 2015;12:e1001916.

45. Miller RR 3rd, Lopansri BK, Burke JP, Levy M, Opal S, Rothman RE, D'Alessio FR, Sidhaye VK, Aggarwal NR, Balk R, et al. Validation of a host response assay, Septicyte™ LAB, for discriminating sepsis from SIRS in the ICU. Am J Respir Crit Care Med. 2018;198:903–13.

46. Sweeney TE, Shidham A, Wong HR, Khatri P. A comprehensive time-course–based multicohort analysis of sepsis and sterile inflammation reveals a robust diagnostic gene set. Sci Transl Med. 2015;7:287ra71.

47. Bauer M, Giamarellos-Bourboulis EJ, Kortgen A, Möller E, Felsmann K, Cavaillon JM, Guntinas-Lichius O, Rutschmann O, Ruryk A, Kohl M, et al. A transcriptomic biomarker to quantify systemic inflam-

mation in sepsis: a prospective multicenter phase II diagnostic study. EBioMedicine. 2016;6:114–25.

48. Scicluna BP, Klein Klouwenberg PM, van Vught LA, Wiewel MA, Ong DS, Zwinderman AH, Franitza M, Toliat MR, Nurnberg P, Hoogendijk AJ, et al. A molecular biomarker to diagnose community-acquired pneumonia on intensive care unit admission. Am J Respir Crit Care Med. 2015;192:826–35.

49. Sweeney TE, Khatri P. Comprehensive validation of the FAIM3:PLAC8 ratio in time-matched public gene expression data. Am J Respir Crit Care Med. 2015;192:1260–1.

50. Eckerle M, Ambroggio L, Puskarich MA, Winston B, Jones AE, Standiford TJ, Stringer KA. Metabolomics as a driver in advancing precision medicine in sepsis. Pharmacotherapy. 2017;37:1023–32.

51. Schmerler D, Neugebauer S, Ludewig K, Bremer-Streck S, Brunkhorst FM, Kiehntopf M. Targeted metabolomics for discrimination of systemic inflammatory disorders in critically ill patients. J Lipid Res. 2012;53:1369–75.

52. Neugebauer S, Giamarellos-Bourboulis EJ, Pelekanou A, Marioli A, Baziaka F, Tsangaris I, Bauer M, Kiehntopf M. Metabolite profiles in sepsis: developing prognostic tools based on the type of infection. Crit Care Med. 2016;44:1649–62.

53. Davenport EE, Burnham KL, Radhakrishnan J, Humburg P, Hutton P, Mills TC, Rautanen A, Gordon AC, Garrard C, Hill AVS, et al. Genomic landscape of the individual host response and outcomes in sepsis: a prospective cohort study. Lancet Respir Med. 2016;4:259–71.

54. Joenvaara S, Saraswat M, Kuusela P, Saraswat S, Agarwal R, Kaartinen J, Järvinen A, Renkonen R. Quantitative N-glycoproteomics reveals altered glycosylation levels of various plasma proteins in bloodstream infected patients. PLoS One. 2018;13:e0195006.

55. Oved K, Cohen A, Boico O, Navon R, Friedman T, Etshtein L, Kriger O, Bamberger E, Fonar Y, Yacobov R, et al. A novel host-proteome signature for distinguishing between acute bacterial and viral infections. PLoS One. 2015;10:e0120012.

56. DeCoux A, Tian Y, DeLeon-Pennell KY, Nguyen NT, de Castro Brás LE, Flynn ER, Cannon PL, Griswold ME, Jin Y-F, Puskarich MA, et al. Plasma glycoproteomics reveals sepsis outcomes linked to distinct proteins in common pathways. Crit Care Med. 2015;43:2049–58.

57. Wong HR, Salisbury S, Xiao Q, Cvijanovich NZ, Hall M, Allen GL, Thomas NJ, Freishtat RJ, Anas N, Meyer K, et al. The pediatric sepsis biomarker risk model. Crit Care. 2012;16:R174.

58. Wong HR, Cvijanovich NZ, Anas N, Allen GL, Thomas NJ, Bigham MT, Weiss SL, Fitzgerald JC, Checchia PA, Meyer K, et al. Improved risk stratification in pediatric septic shock using both protein and mRNA biomarkers. PERSEVERE-XP. Am J Respir Crit Care Med. 2017;196:494–501.

59. Wong HR, Lindsell CJ, Pettilä V, Meyer NJ, Thair SA, Karlsson S, Russell JA, Fjell CD, Boyd JH, Ruokonen E, et al. A multibiomarker-based outcome risk stratification model for adult septic shock. Crit Care Med. 2014;42:781–9.

60. Calfee CS, Delucchi K, Parsons PE, Thompson BT, Ware LB, Matthay MA. Subphenotypes in acute respiratory distress syndrome: latent class analysis of data from two randomized controlled trials. Lancet Respir Med. 2014;2:611–20.

61. Langley RJ, Tsalik EL, Velkinburgh JCV, Glickman SW, Rice BJ, Wang C, Chen B, Carin L, Suarez A, Mohney RP, et al. An integrated clinico-metabolomic model improves prediction of death in sepsis. Sci Transl Med. 2013;5:195ra195.

62. Rogers AJ, McGeachie M, Baron RM, Gazourian L, Haspel JA, Nakahira K, Fredenburgh LE, Hunninghake GM, Raby BA, Matthay MA, et al. Metabolomic derangements are associated with mortality in critically ill adult patients. PLoS One. 2014;9:e87538.

63. Sakka SG, Ruhl CC, Pfeiffer UJ, Beale R, McLuckie A, Reinhart K, Meier-Hellmann A. Assessment of cardiac preload and extravascular lung water by single transpulmonary thermodilution. Intensive Care Med. 2000;26:180–7.

64. Katzenelson R, Perel A, Berkenstadt H, Preisman S, Kogan S, Sternik L, Segal E. Accuracy of transpulmonary thermodilution versus gravimetric measurement of extravascular lung water. Crit Care Med. 2004;32:1550–4.

65. Newman EV, Merrell M, Genecin A, Monge C, Milnor WR, McKeever WP. The dye dilution method for describing the central circulation. An analysis of factors shaping the time-concentration curves. Circulation. 1951;4:735–46.

66. Cordemans C, De Laet I, Van Regenmortel N, Schoonheydt K, Dits H, Huber W, Malbrain MLNG. Fluid management in critically ill patients: the role of extravascular lung water, abdominal hypertension, capillary leak, and fluid balance. Ann Intensive Care. 2012;2:S1.

67. Jozwiak M, Silva S, Persichini R, Anguel N, Osman D, Richard C, Teboul JL, Monnet X. Extravascular lung water is an independent prognostic factor in patients with acute respiratory distress syndrome. Crit Care Med. 2013;41:472–80.

68. Brown LM, Calfee CS, Howard JP, Craig TR, Matthay MA, McAuley DF. Comparison of thermodilution measured extravascular lung water with chest radiographic assessment of pulmonary oedema in patients with acute lung injury. Ann Intensive Care. 2013;3:25.

69. Phillips CR, Chesnutt MS, Smith SM. Extravascular lung water in sepsis-associated acute respiratory distress syndrome: indexing with predicted body weight improves correlation with severity of illness and survival. Crit Care Med. 2008;36:69–73.

70. Craig TR, Duffy MJ, Shyamsundar M, McDowell C, McLaughlin B, Elborn JS, McAuley DF. Extravascular lung water indexed to predicted body weight is a novel predictor of intensive care unit mortality in patients with acute lung injury. Crit Care Med. 2010;38:114–20.

71. Kuzkov VV, Kirov MY, Sovershaev MA, Kuklin VN, Suborov EV, Waerhaug K, Bjertnaes LJ. Extravascular lung water determined with single transpulmonary thermodilution correlates with the severity of sepsis-induced acute lung injury. Crit Care Med. 2006;34:1647–53.

72. Craig TR, Duffy MJ, Shyamsundar M, McDowell C, O'Kane CM, Elborn JS, McAuley DF. A randomized clinical trial of hydroxymethylglutaryl- coenzyme a reductase inhibition for acute lung injury (The HARP Study). Am J Respir Crit Care Med. 2011;183:620–6.

73. Perkins GD, McAuley DF, Thickett DR, Gao F. The beta-agonist lung injury trial (BALTI): a randomized placebo-controlled clinical trial. Am J Respir Crit Care Med. 2006;173:281–7.

74. Prescott HC, Costa DK. Improving long-term outcomes after sepsis. Crit Care Clinics. 2018;34:175–88.

75. Hughes CG, Patel MB, Brummel NE, Thompson JL, McNeil JB, Pandharipande PP, Jackson JC, Chandrasekhar R, Ware LB, Ely EW, et al. Relationships between markers of neurologic and endothelial injury during critical illness and long-term cognitive impairment and disability. Intensive Care Med. 2018;44:345–55.

76. Mitri Z, Constantine T, O'Regan R. The HER2 receptor in breast cancer: pathophysiology, clinical use, and new advances in therapy. Chemother Res Pract. 2012;2012:743193.

77. Mirabbasi SA, Khalighi K, Wu Y, Walker S, Khalighi B, Fan W, Kodali A, Cheng G. CYP2C19 genetic variation and individualized clopidogrel prescription in a cardiology clinic. J Community Hosp Intern Med Perspect. 2017;7:151–6.

78. Reinhart K, Menges T, Gardlund B, Harm Zwaveling J, Smithes M, Vincent J-L, Maria Tellado J, Salgado-Remigio A, Zimlichman R, Withington S, et al. Randomized, placebo-controlled trial of the antitumor necrosis factor antibody fragment afelimomab in hyperinflammatory response during severe sepsis: The RAMSES Study. Crit Care Med. 2001;29:765–9.

79. Panacek EA, Marshall JC, Albertson TE, Johnson DH, Johnson S, MacArthur RD, Miller M, Barchuk WT, Fischkoff S, Kaul M, et al. Efficacy and safety of the monoclonal anti-tumor necrosis factor antibody F(ab')2 fragment afelimomab in patients with severe sepsis and elevated interleukin-6 levels. Crit Care Med. 2004;32:2173–82.

80. Bloos F, Trips E, Nierhaus A, et al. Effect of sodium selenite administration and procalcitonin-guided therapy on mortality in patients with severe sepsis or septic shock: a randomized clinical trial. JAMA Intern Med. 2016;176:1266–76.

81. de Jong E, van Oers JA, Beishuizen A, Vos P, Vermeijden WJ, Haas LE, Loef BG, Dormans T, van Melsen GC, Kluiters YC, et al. Efficacy and safety of procalcitonin guidance in reducing the duration of antibiotic treatment in critically ill patients: a randomised, controlled, open-label trial. Lancet Infect Dis. 2016;16:819–27.

82. Kopterides P, Siempos II, Tsangaris I, Tsantes A, Armaganidis A. Procalcitonin-guided algorithms of antibiotic therapy in the intensive care unit: a systematic review and meta-analysis of randomized controlled trials. Crit Care Med. 2010;38:2229–41.

83. Barlam TF, Cosgrove SE, Abbo LM, MacDougall C, Schuetz AN, Septimus EJ, Srinivasan A, Dellit TH, Falck-Ytter YT, Fishman NO, et al. Implementing an antibiotic stewardship program: guidelines by the Infectious Diseases Society of America and the Society for Healthcare Epidemiology of America. Clin Infect Dis. 2016;62:e51–77.

84. Shehabi Y, Sterba M, Garrett PM, Rachakonda KS, Stephens D, Harrigan P, Walker A, Bailey MJ, Johnson B, Millis D, et al. Procalcitonin Algorithm in critically ill adults with undifferentiated infection or suspected sepsis. A randomized controlled trial. Am J Respir Crit Care Med. 2014;190:1102–10.

85. Chu DC, Mehta AB, Walkey AJ. Practice patterns and outcomes associated with procalcitonin use in critically ill patients with sepsis. Clin Infect Dis. 2017;64:1509–15.

86. Weiss CH, Persell SD, Wunderink RG, Baker DW. Empiric antibiotic, mechanical ventilation, and central venous catheter duration as potential factors mediating the effect of a checklist prompting intervention on mortality: an exploratory analysis. BMC Health Services Res. 2012;12:198.

87. Calfee CS, Delucchi KL, Sinha P, Matthay MA, Hackett J, Shankar-Hari M, McDowell C, Laffey JG, O'Kane CM, McAuley DF. Acute respiratory distress syndrome subphenotypes and differential response to simvastatin: secondary analysis of a randomised controlled trial. Lancet Respir Med. 2018;6:691–8.

88. McGettigan P, Ferner RE. PCSK9 inhibitors for hypercholesterolaemia. BMJ. 2017;356:j188.

89. Walley KR, Thain KR, Russell JA, Reilly MP, Meyer NJ, Ferguson JF, Christie JD, Nakada T-A, Fjell CD, Thair SA, et al. PCSK9 is a critical regulator of the innate immune response and septic shock outcome. Sci Transl Med. 2014;6:258ra143.

90. Russell JA. Genomics and pharmacogenomics of sepsis: so close and yet so far. Crit Care. 2016;20:185.

91. Annane D, Mira JP, Ware LB, Gordon AC, Hinds CJ, Christiani DC, Sevransky J, Barnes K, Buchman TG, Heagerty PJ, et al. Pharmacogenomic biomarkers do not predict response to drotrecogin alfa in patients with severe sepsis. Ann Intensive Care. 2018;8:16.

92. Puskarich MA, Kline JA, Krabill V, Claremont H, Jones AE. Preliminary safety and efficacy of L-carnitine infusion for the treatment of vasopressor-dependent septic shock: a randomized control trial. JPEN. 2014;38:736–43.

93. Puskarich MA, Finkel MA, Karnovsky A, Jones AE, Trexel J, Harris BN, Stringer KA. Pharmacometabolomics of L-carnitine treatment response phenotypes in patients with septic shock. Ann Am Thorac Soc. 2015;12:46–56.

Part IV

Precise Phenotyping

Lessons for Precision Medicine from Lung Cancer

Brett C. Bade, Finbar T. Foley, and Lynn T. Tanoue

Key Points
- Assessment of patients with lung cancer should be standardized and structured, with each individual assessment being *unique* and *uniquely* informing optimal personalized treatment.
- Advances in the understanding of the biology of lung cancer have facilitated precise risk assessment tools, safer and more efficient diagnostic algorithms, and individualization of treatment.
- Priorities in precision lung cancer care include individualized assessment of the patient's stage of disease, physiology and ability to undergo diagnostic procedures and treatment, characterization of the individual tumor, and an understanding of the patient's personal goals and preferences, supported by a comprehensive current knowledge of the biology of neoplasia.
- The increasingly broader array of precision therapies mandates that histologic evaluation be performed to the level of tumor-specific molecular and immunologic characteristics.

Introduction

Precision medicine, defined by Collins and Varmus as "prevention and treatment strategies that take individual variability into account," has been the long-standing paradigm for evaluation and management of patients with lung cancer [1]. The approach to optimizing care for an individual with lung cancer has its original foundation in anatomic staging. Impressive progress in personalized evaluation and care has been achieved over the last several decades by scientific advances in our understanding of cancer pathobiology. These findings, in turn, have led to breakthroughs in treatment informed by more precise knowledge of the molecular processes that drive neoplasia.

The global burden of lung cancer morbidity and mortality is enormous. Lung cancer is the leading cause of cancer death in the world; in 2015, the World Health Organization (WHO) estimated that lung cancer caused 1.69 million deaths worldwide [2]. Moreover, lung cancer burden is on the rise. In WHO low-income coun-

B. C. Bade (✉) · F. T. Foley · L. T. Tanoue
Section of Pulmonary, Critical Care, and Sleep Medicine, Department of Internal Medicine, Yale School of Medicine, New Haven, CT, USA
e-mail: brett.bade@yale.edu; finbar.foley@yale.edu; lynn.tanoue@yale.edu

© Springer Nature Switzerland AG 2020
J. L. Gomez et al. (eds.), *Precision in Pulmonary, Critical Care, and Sleep Medicine*, Respiratory Medicine, https://doi.org/10.1007/978-3-030-31507-8_14

tries, the most common cause of death is lower respiratory infections [3]. By contrast, cancer of the trachea and bronchus is the fourth leading cause of mortality in WHO high-income countries, leading to more deaths than either lower respiratory infections or chronic obstructive pulmonary disease (COPD) [3]. We have witnessed that economic development is accompanied by a changing disease spectrum. It seems unfortunately inevitable that lung cancer is destined to become an even greater cause of mortality worldwide.

Lung cancer is not a single entity. Among all cancers, lung cancers are among the most highly mutated, consistent with the wide array of known associated carcinogenic factors [4]. However, we recognize that this paradigm is not true for all lung cancers; it is increasingly clear that the neoplastic process is driven in some tumors by mutations or alterations in single genes. The multistep process of genetic and epigenetic alterations that results in lung neoplasia generates clinical, biologic, histologic, and molecular heterogeneity. Recognizing this heterogeneity, an individualized approach is clearly necessary; one size will not fit all. Personalizing evaluation of the individual requires an understanding of the characteristics of his/her specific lung cancer. Importantly, treatment decisions must take into consideration all other aspects of his/her individual health as a whole human organism. A population health approach reminds us that genetics is only part of the story. Lung cancer is a prime example of disease where other determinants of health, including behavioral patterns, environmental exposures, social circumstances, and interaction with the medical system, play clear and critical roles in disease development, presentation, treatment, and outcomes [5].

To provide an understanding of how precision medicine has become the standard approach for lung cancer diagnosis and care, we feel it is useful to reflect on the advances made over the past decade. Let us consider the following patient with lung cancer in 2008; we will return to this patient later and reconsider his case in 2019.

PM is a 67-year-old male former smoker who presented with several months of persistent cough and worsening dyspnea. A chest radiograph demonstrated a right lower lobe abnormality; chest CT confirmed a 3.5-cm right lower lobe mass and enlarged right hilar and subcarinal lymph nodes, without abnormalities in the liver, adrenal glands, or bones. Bronchoscopic biopsy of the mass demonstrated non-small cell lung cancer. PET imaging showed intense fluorodeoxyglucose (FDG) uptake in the mass and multiple mediastinal and hilar lymph nodes; brain MRI demonstrated an enhancing right parietal lesion. The clinical stage was T2N2M1 (stage IV). PM received chemotherapy with cisplatin, gemcitabine and bevacizumab, and whole brain radiation. His treatment course was complicated by anorexia, fatigue, and one episode of pneumonia-related sepsis requiring hospitalization. Five months later, follow-up imaging demonstrated new liver abnormalities consistent with metastases. PM underwent second-line chemotherapy with pemetrexed but without response. His overall status continued to decline; chemotherapy was discontinued, and he was referred for palliative care.

PM's course followed the standard of care guidelines for patients with stage IV non-small cell lung cancer (NSCLC) in 2008 as outlined by the National Comprehensive Cancer Network (NCCN) (Fig. 14.1a). The three lessons in precision medicine for lung cancer care presented below will demonstrate the evolution of personalized lung cancer care over the past decade and articulate current recommendations. Lesson #1 will highlight milestones in our understanding of lung cancer and the subsequent "tools" that followed. Lesson #2 will explain how our tools enable individualized diagnostic evaluations and patient assessments. Lesson #3 will consider the impact of patient preferences and goals, and consider how PM's course of diagnosis and treatment has changed in 2019. These lessons inform an individualized approach for the evaluation and care of the patient with lung cancer. We offer them as a paradigm for a precision approach that may be applied to many other diseases.

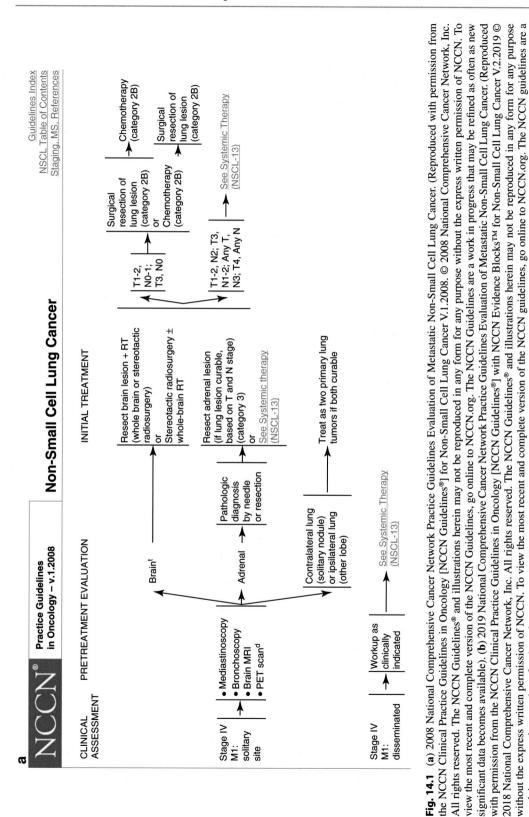

Fig. 14.1 (**a**) 2008 National Comprehensive Cancer Network Practice Guidelines Evaluation of Metastatic Non-Small Cell Lung Cancer. (Reproduced with permission from the NCCN Clinical Practice Guidelines in Oncology [NCCN Guidelines®] for Non-Small Cell Lung Cancer V.1.2008. © 2008 National Comprehensive Cancer Network, Inc. All rights reserved. The NCCN Guidelines® and illustrations herein may not be reproduced in any form for any purpose without the express written permission of NCCN. To view the most recent and complete version of the NCCN Guidelines, go online to NCCN.org. The NCCN Guidelines are a work in progress that may be refined as often as new significant data becomes available). (**b**) 2019 National Comprehensive Cancer Network Practice Guidelines Evaluation of Metastatic Non-Small Cell Lung Cancer. (Reproduced with permission from the NCCN Clinical Practice Guidelines in Oncology [NCCN Guidelines®] with NCCN Evidence Blocks™ for Non-Small Cell Lung Cancer V.2.2019 © 2018 National Comprehensive Cancer Network, Inc. All rights reserved. The NCCN Guidelines® and illustrations herein may not be reproduced in any form for any purpose without the express written permission of NCCN. To view the most recent and complete version of the NCCN guidelines, go online to NCCN.org. The NCCN guidelines are a work in progress that may be refined as often as new significant data becomes available)

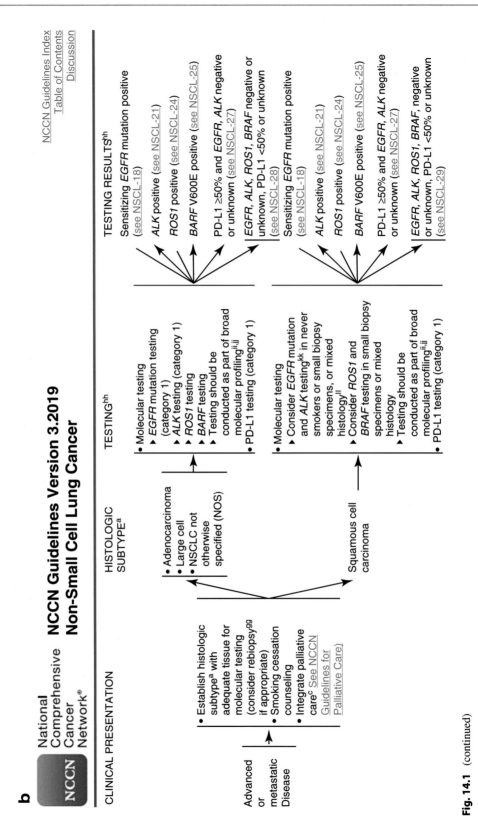

Fig. 14.1 (continued)

Lesson #1: Precision Medicine Is an Iterative Process: Better Disease Understanding Facilitates Better Individualized Assessment

Precision medicine in lung cancer has been an iterative process over the past half century spanning multiple areas, including individualized risk assessment, more specific tissue characterization, refinements in staging techniques, and better treatments. Advances in our understanding of the biology of neoplasia have informed the development of additional tools that improve evaluation and management. Some of the most exciting advances are targeted and immunologic therapies, where a drug is developed based on specific knowledge of molecular abnormalities or immunologic pathways important to the neoplastic process. These treatment opportunities are the culmination of years of scientific progress in the field. In this lesson, we will review several advances in our understanding of lung cancer biology as well as the relevant tools that are improving and personalizing lung cancer care. Figure 14.2 provides a timeline for several of the discoveries that will be discussed. How those tools are utilized in individualized assessments will be further described in Lessons #2 and #3. Since most advances have been made in NSCLC, we will focus on this group, which includes >80% of all lung cancer patients [6].

Lung Cancer Is a Heterogeneous Disease

In a 1964 report by the Surgeon General on the consequences of smoking on health, tobacco smoking was identified as a cause of lung cancer in men and a probable cause of lung cancer in women [7]. Those early findings contributed to general stereotypes about lung cancer that persist, including that lung cancer is predominately seen in older male smokers, and prognosis is very poor. Several recent trends have demonstrated the clinical heterogeneity of lung cancer. First, we now recognize that 10–25% of patients who develop lung cancer are never-smokers [8, 9].

Second, more recent Surveillance, Epidemiology, and End Results (SEER) data demonstrate that lung cancer incidence and mortality rates by gender are converging (Fig. 14.3) [6], with recent work by Jemal and colleagues showing that lung cancer incidence rates are now *higher* in young non-Hispanic white and Hispanic women compared to young men [10]. Finally, though lung cancer has lower 5-year survival (18.6%) than most other solid tumors [11], there is growing recognition that lung cancer can be indolent. We are increasingly aware of slow-growing lesions along the spectrum of adenocarcinoma (e.g., atypical adenomatous hyperplasia, adenocarcinoma in situ, minimally invasive adenocarcinoma), which may remain stable for many years [12]. How do we explain the changing trends in lung cancer, development of the same disease in very different populations, and unique clinical courses? Improved understanding of risk factors and pathobiology of lung cancer are helping us begin to answer these questions.

An individual's risk of developing lung cancer is multifactorial. Tobacco use remains the predominant risk factor and is implicated in 80–90% of lung cancers [13]. However, many non-tobacco risk factors have been identified and contribute to lung cancer in diverse populations. For example, age, exposures to inhaled carcinogens other than tobacco, chronic lung injury/inflammation (e.g., chronic lung diseases), inherited or genetic factors, diet, and physical activity level (particularly in former smokers) all contribute to risk [14–16].

A more comprehensive understanding of risk factors has led to the development of tools designed to assess risk of developing lung cancer in specific populations. One of the earliest models was developed by Bach and colleagues in 18,172 subjects participating in a multicenter, randomized, controlled study evaluating the potential benefit of supplementation with beta-carotene and vitamin A in a population at increased risk of lung cancer [17, 18]. Patient characteristics including age, sex, asbestos exposure, and smoking history were included in the model. Two interesting findings from this study are important in understanding the utility of models in risk assessment. First, even among smok-

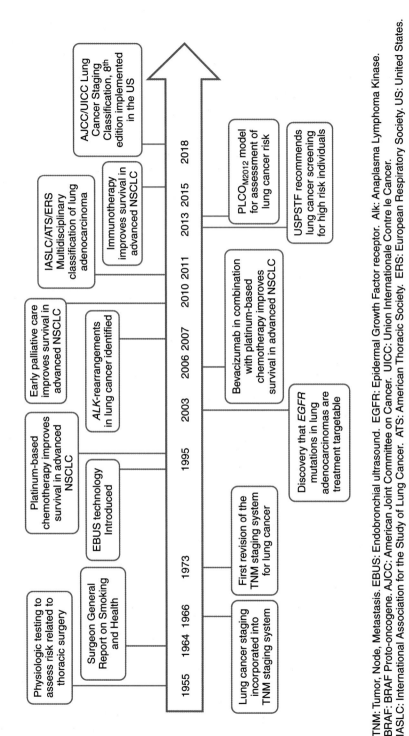

TNM: Tumor, Node, Metastasis. EBUS: Endobronchial ultrasound. EGFR: Epidermal Growth Factor receptor. Alk: Anaplasma Lymphoma Kinase. BRAF: BRAF Proto-oncogene. AJCC: American Joint Committee on Cancer. UICC: Union Internationale Contre le Cancer. IASLC: International Association for the Study of Lung Cancer. ATS: American Thoracic Society. ERS: European Respiratory Society. US: United States.

Fig. 14.2 Advances in personalized therapy for non-small cell lung cancer (NSCLC)

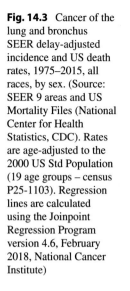

Fig. 14.3 Cancer of the lung and bronchus SEER delay-adjusted incidence and US death rates, 1975–2015, all races, by sex. (Source: SEER 9 areas and US Mortality Files (National Center for Health Statistics, CDC). Rates are age-adjusted to the 2000 US Std Population (19 age groups – census P25-1103). Regression lines are calculated using the Joinpoint Regression Program version 4.6, February 2018, National Cancer Institute)

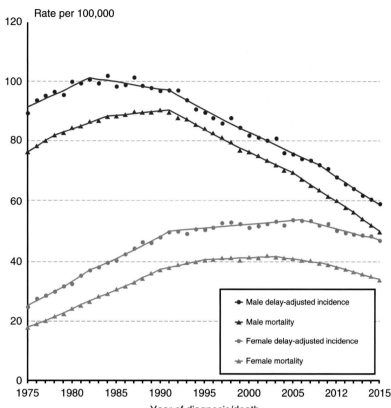

ers, the risk of lung cancer development is widely variable. This finding suggests that individual genetic factors or other exposures lead to differential risk of developing lung cancer. Second, the majority of lung cancers develop in the highest-risk patients. In the Bach model, approximately 50% of lung cancers developed in the quartile of patients with the highest model-predicted risk [17]. More recent risk assessment models have become more complex and include more patient-level factors. One of the most robust models is the PLCO$_{M2012}$ [19], which was developed and validated in current or former smokers participating in the Prostate, Lung, Colorectal, and Ovarian (PLCO) cancer screening trial and the National Lung Screening Trial (NLST) [20, 21]. Table 14.1 shows the patient-level components in the model. There is ongoing debate as to the role of PLCO$_{M2012}$ or other lung cancer risk assessment tools in identifying patients at sufficiently high risk to be considered candidates for lung cancer

Table 14.1 PLCO$_{M2012}$ model for lung cancer risk assessment: Patient-level components

Components of PLCO$_{M2012}$
Age
Race
Education
Body mass index
Chronic obstructive pulmonary disease
Personal history of cancer
Family history of lung cancer
Smoking status (current vs. former)
Smoking intensity
Duration of smoking
Smoking quit time

screening, compared to the current practice of identification based solely on age and smoking history. We will address this topic further in Lesson #2.

A better understanding of lung cancer genetics has also helped explain the clinical heterogeneity that is widely described in lung cancer. Lung cancer development in younger, nonsmoking women as well as older, heavily smoking men suggests distinct and different biologic processes in the two groups. We now recognize that classic lung cancer is the result of multiple sequential mutations that generally occur in association with tobacco use and chronic lung injury and result in uncontrolled cell growth. In contrast, several individual "driver" mutations and gene rearrangements have been identified that are typically not associated with tobacco use. Epidermal growth factor receptor (*EGFR*) mutations were the earliest described of these, with *EGFR* mutations identified more frequently in never-smokers [8], females [22, 23], and Asian patients [24]. Anaplastic lymphoma kinase (*ALK*) rearrangements, rat osteosarcoma (*ROS1*) rearrangements, and B-Raf proto-oncogene (*BRAF*) mutations are other examples of molecular alterations associated with lung cancer. These mutations and rearrangements also tend to follow patient clinical patterns. *ALK*-rearranged tumors are more likely in never/light smokers [25]. Compared to patients with *EGFR* mutations, patients with *ALK* rearrangements are younger and more likely to be men. *ROS-1* rearrangement is also more frequently seen in younger, never-smokers [26]. In contrast, Kirsten Ras (*KRAS*) oncogene and *BRAF* mutations are found more frequently in current or former smokers [15, 27]. The critical importance of identification of such driver mutations is that they identify individual tumors that are potentially therapeutically targetable. The development of targeted treatments now mandates that molecular information be incorporated in diagnostic and treatment algorithms for metastatic NSCLC (Fig. 14.1b) [28]. Additional details about lung cancer genetics and the mechanisms of neoplasia resulting from driver mutations are described in Chap. 7 (Genetics of Lung Cancer).

As effective targeted treatment options for several driver mutations have become available, specific identification of these mutations is important. Today, multiple commercial testing options are available to identify these mutations, including real-time polymerase chain reaction,

Sanger sequencing, next-generation sequencing (allowing identification of multiple commonly mutated genes) [29], and others [28]. Such technologies have made identification of multiple molecular alterations easily accessible to the clinician. We will further discuss mutation testing and molecular evaluation in lung cancer diagnosis in Lesson #2.

Determining the Extent of Disease Predicts Outcome

One of the simplest but most important principles in lung cancer is that accurate assessment of extent of disease (i.e., staging) is associated with better lung cancer outcome. Furthermore, extent of disease is the major determinant of treatment [30]. The most updated staging tool is the Eighth Edition Lung Cancer Stage Classification, a monumental work performed by the International Association for the Study of Lung Cancer (IASLC) involving 94,708 lung cancer patients from 16 countries (Table 14.2) [31]. Fundamentally, stages of cancer are defined by differences in survival; patients with tumors of different combinations of T (tumor), N (nodal), and M (metastasis) descriptors will be grouped together in a single stage if they share similar survival (Fig. 14.4). Sixty-four stage groupings currently result from combinations of T, N, and M, compared to 32 and 48 stage groupings in the sixth and seventh staging classifications, respectively. This highlights the effort to "split" (as opposed to "lump") individual patients into more specific groups for the purposes of more precise treatment as well as identifying eligibility for focused clinical trial participation. Farjah and colleagues showed that multimodality (i.e., computed tomography [CT], positron emission tomography [PET], and invasive mediastinal staging) as compared to single modality staging was associated with better survival, and use of more modalities was associated with lower risk of death [32]. Vokes and colleagues reported longer overall survival and progression-free survival in patients with stage III NSCLC who received PET imaging than those who did not [33]. The

Table 14.2 Eighth Edition Lung Cancer Staging Classification: Definitions for T, N, and M descriptors

T (primary tumor)		Label
T0	No primary tumor	
Tis	Carcinoma in situ (squamous or adenocarcinoma)	Tis
T1	Tumor ≤3 cm	
T1a(mi)	Minimally invasive adenocarcinoma	T1a*(mi)*
T1a	Superficial spreading tumor in central airways[a]	T1a *ss*
T1a	Tumor ≤1 cm	T1a *≤1*
T1b	Tumor >1 but ≤2 cm	T1b *>1–2*
T1c	Tumor >2 but ≤3 cm	T1c *>2–3*
T2	Tumor >3 but ≤5 cm or tumor involving:	
	Visceral pleura[b]	T2 *Visc Pl*
	Main bronchus (not carina), atelectasis to hilum[b]	T2 *Centr*
T2a	Tumor >3 but ≤4 cm	T2a *>3–4*
T2b	Tumor >4 but ≤5 cm	T2b *>4–5*
T3	Tumor >5 but ≤7 cm	T3 *>5–7*
	Or invading chest wall, pericardium, phrenic nerve	T3*Inv*
	Or separate tumor nodule(s) in the same lobe	T3 *Satell*
T4	Tumor >7 cm	T4 *>7*
	Or tumor invading: mediastinum, diaphragm, heart, great vessels, recurrent laryngeal nerve, carina, trachea, esophagus, spine	T4 *Inv*
	Or tumor nodule(s) in a different ipsilateral lobe	T4 *Ipsi Nod*
N (regional lymph nodes)		
N0	No regional node metastasis	
N1	Metastasis in ipsilateral pulmonary or hilar nodes	
N2	Metastasis in ipsilateral mediastinal/subcarinal nodes	
N3	Metastasis in contralateral mediastinal/hilar, or supraclavicular nodes	
M (distant metastasis)		
M0	No distant metastasis	
M1a	Malignant pleural/pericardial effusion[c] or pleural/pericardial nodules	M1a *Pl Dissem*
	Or separate tumor nodule(s) in a contralateral lobe	M1a *Contr Nod*
M1b	Single extrathoracic metastasis	M1b *Single*
M1c	Multiple extrathoracic metastases (1 or >1 organ)	M1c *Multi*

Reprinted from Detterbeck et al. [98] with permission from Elsevier

TX, NX: T or N status not able to be assessed

[a]Superficial spreading tumor of any size but confined to the tracheal or bronchial wall

[b]Such tumors are classified as T2a if >3 ≤ 4 cm, T2b if >4 ≤ 5 cm

[c]Pleural effusions are excluded that are cytologically negative, non-bloody, transudative, and clinically judged not to be due to cancer

benefit of accurate staging is likely related to avoiding stage-inappropriate therapy. For example, treating widely metastatic lung cancer with a local approach (surgery or radiation) due to not recognizing disease outside the chest is unlikely to be curative, may subject the patient to an unnecessary procedure, and potentially results in delivery of the wrong therapies.

The multimodality tools used in the study by Farjah and colleagues – chest CT, functional imaging (PET), and needle-based invasive mediastinal staging techniques – represent significant technological and procedural advancements in lung cancer diagnostic and staging tools. Chest CT has the highest anatomic accuracy in measuring the size of a lung cancer, determining its location within the lungs, and identifying any enlarged lymph nodes or involvement of local structures (e.g., rib, mediastinal structures, or chest wall). Compared to CT alone, PET imaging has addi-

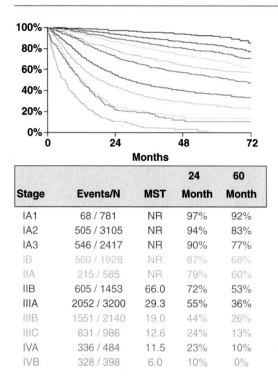

Stage	Events/N	MST	24 Month	60 Month
IA1	68 / 781	NR	97%	92%
IA2	505 / 3105	NR	94%	83%
IA3	546 / 2417	NR	90%	77%
IB	560 / 1928	NR	87%	68%
IIA	215 / 585	NR	79%	60%
IIB	605 / 1453	66.0	72%	53%
IIIA	2052 / 3200	29.3	55%	36%
IIIB	1551 / 2140	19.0	44%	26%
IIIC	831 / 986	12.6	24%	13%
IVA	336 / 484	11.5	23%	10%
IVB	328 / 398	6.0	10%	0%

Fig. 14.4 Overall survival by clinical stage according to the eighth edition using the entire database available for the eighth edition. MST, mean survival time. Survival is weighted by type of database submission: registry vs other. (Reprinted from Goldstraw et al. [31] with permission from Elsevier)

tional advantages, including identification of metabolic activity in the pulmonary lesion, mediastinal or hilar lymph nodes, or extrathoracic sites [30]. Several studies have shown that use of PET imaging can reduce the number of noncurative lung cancer surgeries [34] and more accurately identifies patients with N2 (mediastinal) or N3 (supraclavicular or contralateral mediastinal) nodal disease [35, 36]. It is important to note that tissue confirmation of sites identified as abnormal on PET scanning should be pursued, as inflammation or infection may also be metabolically active and misinterpreted as malignant. Finally, endoscopic needle-based techniques (endobronchial ultrasound [EBUS] and endoscopic ultrasound [EUS]) have been shown to accurately confirm or exclude nodal metastasis less invasively than surgical procedures in patients with abnormal radiographic findings [37]. Each of these tools allows clinicians to more precisely define disease stage, so that stage-appropriate treatment can be considered.

A Patient's Functional Status Influences Outcome

Advances in lung cancer diagnosis and treatment have not been limited to better diagnostic and staging techniques. Another step in precision lung cancer care has been the recognition that a given patient's physiology also influences outcome and should factor into decisions about treatment approach. We clinically observe that some patients may not have the physiologic reserve to tolerate surgical resection, even if that might generally be the approach with the best oncologic outcome. We also know that more extensive resections have consequences; for example, operative mortality is higher with pneumonectomy compared to lobectomy [38, 39]. Tools to estimate pre- and posttreatment functional and physiologic capacity include performance status, pulmonary function testing, and cardiopulmonary exercise testing.

Measures of individual performance status help predict lung cancer outcomes. The Eastern Cooperative Oncology Group (ECOG) performance status score is based on simple assessment of a patient's overall functional status (Table 14.3) and is widely accepted as a powerful predictor of outcomes [40]. The ECOG performance status predicts an individual patient's ability to tolerate treatment and influences his/her eligibility for participation in clinical trials. For patients with advanced stage disease, performance status can help determine which patients may be at increased risk for complications of systemic therapy. For example, in patients with metastatic NSCLC and PD-L1 expression <50%, no contraindications to immunotherapy, no targetable mutations, and an ECOG performance status of 0–1, the current NCCN guidelines recommend treatment with combination immunotherapy and chemotherapy [28]. For the same group of patients with ECOG performance status 3–4, best supportive care is recommended [28]. Of note, targeted therapies are associated with less severe side effect profiles and are generally offered to patients with ECOG PS 0–4. Determination of an individual patient's performance status is a standard consideration for undergoing any therapy, particularly systemic therapies such as chemotherapy.

Table 14.3 Eastern Cooperative Oncology Group performance status. Developed by the Eastern Cooperative Oncology Group, Robert L. Comis, MD, Group Chair[a]

Grade	ECOG performance status
0	Fully active, able to carry on all pre-disease performance without restriction
1	Restricted in physically strenuous activity but ambulatory and able to carry out work of a light or sedentary nature, e.g., light housework, office work
2	Ambulatory and capable of all self-care but unable to carry out any work activities; up and about more than 50% of waking hours
3	Capable of only limited self-care; confined to bed or chair more than 50% of waking hours
4	Completely disabled; cannot carry on any self-care; totally confined to bed or chair
5	Dead

[a]Oken et al. [99]

Physiologic testing can include pulmonary function testing (PFTs) and cardiopulmonary exercise testing (CPET). PFTs measure volume and flow of air and diffusion capacity (DLCO); CPET measures maximal oxygen consumption (VO2max) as well as cardiac or ventilatory limitation to exercise. Ventilation/perfusion scanning is typically obtained to determine the relative contribution of each lung or lung zones and helps predict postoperative function. Bolliger and colleagues reported that predicted postoperative VO2max correlated with operative morbidity and mortality in patients undergoing lung resections; in their series, 100% mortality was observed in those patients with an estimated postoperative VO2max <10 mL/kg/min [41]. Multiple studies have demonstrated that patients with better functional and physiologic capacities have better clinical outcomes. Conversely, patients with worse functional and physiologic status are at increased risk of postoperative complications, lower survival, and death if treated with more aggressive surgical resection [42, 43]. Estimated postoperative physiologic capacity is standard of care for patients being considered for surgical resection. The American College of Chest Physicians (ACCP) lung cancer guidelines offer an algorithm for physiologic assessment using simple exercise testing (i.e., walk testing or stair climbing) or CPET to estimate postoperative physiologic function [44].

Lesson #2: Tools for Individualized Assessments: Lung Cancer Risk, Diagnosis, and Staging

In Lesson #1, we identified several important advances in our understanding of lung cancer and described tools that have been developed to improve evaluation and management. In Lesson #2, we will consider how those tools are utilized to individualize lung cancer risk assessment, diagnosis, staging, and tumor tissue analysis.

Lung Cancer Screening

Lung cancer screening gives us an opportunity to understand how risk assessment for NSCLC is becoming more individualized and how that knowledge can be practically implemented. In 2011, the National Lung Screening Trial (NLST) showed that annual screening with low-dose CT (LDCT) improved overall and lung cancer-associated mortality in asymptomatic patients at high risk for lung cancer [21]. "High risk" in NLST was defined by two patient-level factors: age (55–74 years) and smoking status (≥30 pack-year smoking history in current smokers or former smokers quitting within the last 15 years). Based on NLST findings and a separate modeling study performed by the Cancer Intervention and Surveillance Modeling Network for Healthcare Research and Quality (CISNET) [45], the United States Preventive Services Task Force (USPSTF) endorsed lung cancer screening for individuals ages 55–80 who are either currently smoking or have quit within the previous 15 years and have accumulated ≥30 pack-years of smoking [45, 46].

Subsequent evaluation of NLST demonstrated a similar pattern to that discovered from the Bach risk assessment model: The most benefit from screening is obtained by the highest-risk patients. Kovalchik and colleagues assigned patients in NLST into quintiles of risk for developing lung cancer based on a risk prediction model developed in an NLST study subpopulation and validated in the PLCO cancer screening trial population [47]. Most (88%) of the screening-averted deaths from lung cancer were identified in the three highest-risk quintiles. Furthermore, the incidence of false-positive findings was lower in the higher-risk groups [47]. The number needed to screen (NNS) to prevent one lung cancer death in the highest-risk quintile was 161, compared to 320 in the overall NLST population [21, 47]. Caverly and colleagues performed a similar analysis in the Veterans Affairs (VA) Lung Cancer Screening Demonstration Project [48]. Again, the highest-risk quintiles had more lung cancers identified and a lower NNS. These findings suggest that individualized patient assessments for lung cancer screening may maximize the number of lung cancer deaths averted and minimize false-positive findings.

Compared to the NLST inclusion criteria, individualized risk assessment models incorporating more patient-level factors may increase the accuracy of identifying patients who would benefit from lung cancer screening. Tammemagi and colleagues compared application of the $PLCO_{M2012}$ model to NLST criteria and observed that $PLCO_{M2012}$ had higher sensitivity (83.0% vs. 71.1%, $p < 0.001$) and positive predictive value (4.0% vs. 3.4%, $p = 0.01$) with similar specificity (62.9% vs. 62.7%, $p = 0.54$) [19]. Katki and colleagues similarly developed and validated risk models for lung cancer incidence and death using patients from the PLCO and NLST trials as well as the National Health Interview Survey (NHIS) [49]. Using their model, the NNS to avert one lung cancer death for the highest-risk group was 162 [49]. These studies suggest that predictive models may be more efficient in identifying individuals who will benefit from lung cancer screening than the USPSTF criteria. Moreover, the models identify some patients who do not meet the USPSTF criteria but have high enough risk to benefit from screening [50]. In a recent update to the CHEST Guidelines for lung cancer screening, a $PLCO_{M2012}$-calculated risk of 1.51% over 6 years was proposed as a potential threshold for defining patients at high enough risk for lung cancer to consider screening [51]. It is important to note that routine lung cancer screening in patients who do not meet USPSTF criteria is *not* recommended, as there is no evidence demonstrating benefit. However, studies to address alternative screening criteria will be difficult to achieve as they require long duration of follow-up and are extremely costly; the guidelines acknowledge this dilemma [51]. Available models do give us the opportunity to individualize risk assessment, and decisions about screening still will remain at the discretion of shared decision-making between a physician and an individual patient.

Anatomic Staging

Personalized medicine for lung cancer has its foundations in anatomic staging, which has been the cornerstone of individualization of evaluation and treatment since Mountain's seminal first revision of the lung cancer staging system in 1973 [52]. Clinical staging is based on all information available short of a complete surgical specimen. Every patient should receive T, N, M designations for clinical stage. Complete pathologic staging should be performed for every patient undergoing surgical resection with intent to cure. In 2019, precise understanding of an individual tumor additionally requires histologic classification (i.e., adenocarcinoma, squamous cell carcinoma, small cell carcinoma) and subclassification when possible. Pathologic information is now routinely further augmented by description of individual tumor molecular and biochemical characteristics. Precise staging ensures that a patient's individual treatment is accurately based on stage and tumor factors, maximizing possible benefit and minimizing risk of treatment-related complications. Personalization of care is further informed by a global assessment of patient performance and physiologic status (see Lesson #1). Of note, though presented separately here, evaluation for diagnosis, staging, and patient values (see Lesson #3) are performed concurrently in clinical practice. In this section, we will highlight how imaging and procedures for NSCLC staging have become more precise over time. For a full review of staging approaches and procedures, we refer the reader to the ACCP and NCCN guidelines on lung cancer diagnosis and treatment [28, 53].

The benefit of accurate staging was discussed in Lesson #1. As already stated, staging evaluations are standardized but individualized using the above-mentioned tools. The goal of lung cancer staging is to identify all sites of disease and ideally to pathologically confirm the site of highest disease stage. Importantly, the least invasive test for the site of highest disease should be utilized [30, 54]. The goal of the clinician is to determine the "right" test for an individual patient. In general, the ACCP and NCCN lung cancer guidelines recommend that all patients with known or suspected lung cancer undergo history, physical, chest CT (including liver/adrenal glands), and lab testing (blood counts and basic metabolic profile) [28, 55]. Further evaluation, including histologic confirmation of disease, should be directed by the results of the baseline assessment and informed by individual patient characteristics.

Most patients suspected of having lung cancer undergo CT and PET imaging. There are several noteworthy examples where the extent of imaging should be individually tailored. First, patients with less aggressive or very early disease may not require PET imaging. Specifically, (1) patients with pure ground glass opacities without other abnormalities on CT and (2) patients with peripheral stage IA tumors do not require PET imaging [30]. In both cases, the likelihood of identifying more advanced disease with additional imaging is low and the likelihood that abnormal findings are false positives is high. In contrast, patients with abnormal baseline clinical evaluations should undergo PET imaging to evaluate for distant disease in addition to focused evaluation of any suspicious site. The choice of imaging for a focal suspicious site should be directed by the best imaging modality for that site. For example, dedicated brain imaging is recommended for a patient with a focal neurologic abnormality on physical exam, with contrast-enhanced brain MRI the preferred diagnostic test. Similarly, abnormal CT or PET findings in the liver or adrenal glands may be best assessed by MRI of these areas. Finally, dedicated brain imaging is recommended in all patients with stage III or IV lung cancer even in the absence of focal findings, as the likelihood of identifying asymptomatic brain metastasis is much higher with advanced stage

disease [30]. The complexity of imaging recommendations for patients with NSCLC reinforces the importance of individualization of the evaluative process.

Lung cancer cannot (yet) be diagnosed without tissue acquisition and pathologic confirmation. Among the major advances in lung cancer care, the development of minimally invasive procedures has preserved or improved accuracy of diagnosis and staging with less risk to patients. Endoscopy allows tissue acquisition that, in many cases, avoids a surgery. Notably, endoscopic needle-based techniques for mediastinal, hilar, paraesophageal, and even adrenal lymph node sampling are now the preferred first tests for patients with radiographic abnormalities suggestive of disease involvement [30]. Needle-based techniques utilize endobronchial ultrasound (EBUS) in the bronchial tree or endoscopic ultrasound (EUS) in the gastrointestinal tract. Both procedures are associated with high diagnostic yields due to real-time visualization of the needle entering the biopsy target. Ultrasound-guided needle-based techniques have been associated with high diagnostic sensitivity and with reduction in more invasive surgical procedures. For example, Annema and colleagues demonstrated a reduction in the number of unnecessary thoracotomies by implementing a staging strategy preferentially using EUS/EBUS as the initial approach, followed by surgical staging only if the needle-based approach was nondiagnostic [37].

For diagnosis of peripheral pulmonary lesions, the choice of the "right" biopsy technique for a given patient must be individualized. CT-guided biopsy has high yield for peripheral lesions but with a high rate of pneumothorax; bronchoscopic biopsy may have more variable yield, but has a lower rate of pneumothorax [54]. A meta-analysis of patients undergoing bronchoscopic biopsies for peripheral pulmonary nodules reported 70% pooled yield [56], whereas a multicenter study estimated yield between 39% and 64%, with higher yield associated with non-upper lobe larger lesions and tobacco use [57]. Technologies are developing to optimize yield, including "thin" bronchoscopes facilitating access to more distal airways and image guidance with radial ultrasound and electromagnetic navigation. Presently, the discussion regarding the "right" biopsy technique must include consideration of the degree of invasiveness, the anticipated yield, potential complications, and the patient's ability to tolerate the procedure.

The future of staging procedures for lung cancer will include even less invasive diagnostic testing to diagnose lung cancer or lung cancer recurrence. Specifically, "liquid" biopsies hold the promise of a lung cancer diagnosis through examination of blood or plasma as opposed to tissue. Liquid biopsies of peripheral blood can detect circulating tumor cells, tumor DNA or RNA, or tumor proteins [58]. At present, liquid biopsies can be used in clinical practice for detection of driver mutations [59]. As the technology improves, it is likely these noninvasive evaluations will play increasingly important roles in lung cancer diagnosis.

Tumor Tissue Evaluation

The complexity of accurate pathologic diagnosis for patients with NSCLC further highlights how precision medicine has become the routine approach. Figure 14.1a, b demonstrate the 2008 and 2019 NCCN guidelines for treatment of stage IV NSCLC, respectively. Clinical staging gets us to the beginning of both these algorithms, and the individual patient's global status will inform final decisions about treatment. What is immediately evident is that over the 10 years between these guidelines, a precision landscape for lung cancer evaluation and treatment has dramatically evolved, based on important advances in our ability to characterize individual tumors. Pathologic diagnosis is defined by the 2015 WHO Classification of Lung Tumors [60]. Increasingly, molecular and biochemical evaluation are routinely performed for NSCLC and are essential components of the tissue evaluation for advanced stage disease. Though a complete discussion is beyond the scope of this chapter, Reck and Rabe provide a helpful diagnostic pathologic algorithm for advanced NSCLC (Fig. 14.5). In general, more advanced lung cancers require more exten-

sive tissue evaluation, with particular focus on molecular testing.

Three important precision aspects of tissue diagnosis should be considered: histology, molecular testing, and immunologic status. With regard to histology, "NSCLC" as a final pathologic diagnosis is no longer acceptable. In the 2008 NCCN guidelines for metastatic NSCLC (Fig. 14.1a), determination of NSCLC (regardless of histology) and stage was considered sufficient evaluation to guide treatment. In contrast, the 2019 NCCN guidelines (Fig. 14.1b) mandate specific histology determination (i.e., squamous cell carcinoma, adenocarcinoma, large cell, or NSCLC not otherwise specified [NOS]); more precise histologic categorization enables prioritization of molecular/immunologic testing (see below), which is necessary for treatment decisions. The 2019 guidelines assume that distinguishing squamous cell carcinoma from non-squamous cell carcinoma (i.e., adenocarcinoma or large cell carcinoma) will occur. The overarching reason for separating these entities is the increasing evidence base that they are fundamentally different and will demonstrate distinct outcomes to treatments. For example, *EGFR* mutations, *ALK* and *ROS1* rearrangements, and *BRAF* mutations are more frequently seen in non-squamous NSCLC [60]. Pemetrexed is effective in non-squamous NSCLC but not in squamous cell carcinoma [61, 62]. Bevacizumab, a monoclonal antibody targeting vascular endothelial growth factor (VEGF), is contraindicated in patients with squamous cell carcinoma due to risk of hemorrhage and/or hemoptysis [60, 63]. Numerous such examples compel pathologists to make this first, critical distinction in major histologic type. A much more granular analysis of the broad category of NSCLC is now required to facilitate appropriate treatment, particularly for metastatic disease.

Molecular testing of individual tumors is now a requirement for patients with advanced stage disease. The discovery that inhibitors of *EGFR* could result in dramatic benefit for patients with metastatic *EGFR*-mutant adenocarcinoma was an enormous leap forward in precision medicine for lung cancer [64, 65]. As mentioned in Lesson

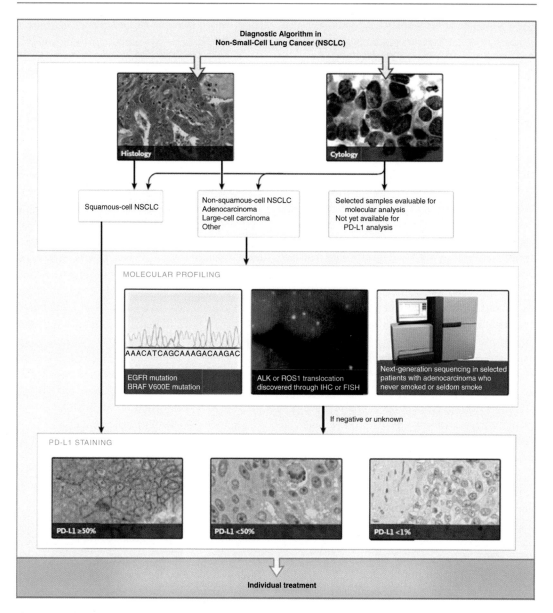

Fig. 14.5 Diagnostic algorithm in non-small cell lung cancer (NSCLC). The upper portion of the algorithm shows the morphologic classification of NSCLC based on histology (hematoxylin and eosin) and cytologic (Giemsa) evaluation. The middle portion of the algorithm shows the molecular analysis for the key treatable oncogenic alterations: *EGFR* and *BRAF* V600E mutations and *ALK* and *ROS1* translocations, as well as additional molecular analyses in selected patients. The lower portion of the algorithm shows the assessment of programmed death ligand 1 (PD-L1) expression by means of immunohistochemical staining. FISH denotes fluorescence in situ hybridization and IHC analysis. (Reproduced from Reck and Rabe [9] with permission from the Massachusetts Medical Society)

#1, *EGFR* mutations, *ALK* and *ROS1* rearrangements, and *BRAF* mutations are all potentially targetable; testing for these abnormalities is recommended for all non-squamous NSCLCs (Fig. 14.5). Targetable alterations are infrequently identified in squamous cell carcinoma; for example, <5% of squamous cell carcinomas will demonstrate *EGFR* mutations [66]. In metastatic squamous cell carcinoma, NCCN guidelines recommend consideration of *EGFR* and

ALK testing in never-smokers, when biopsy specimens are small, or with mixed histology; *ROS1* and *BRAF* testing for metastatic squamous cell carcinoma should be considered with small biopsy specimens or mixed histology (Fig. 14.1b). In contrast, testing for targetable mutations is recommended for all non-squamous tumors. Testing of small biopsy samples is discussed due to the potential for incomplete sampling and histologic uncertainty [28, 67]. It should be noted that molecular testing is not currently recommended for nonmetastatic lung cancers because optimal treatment for those patients is achieved predominantly with local therapy; in these cases, molecular testing would add little other than cost to treatment decisions.

Lastly, determining the immunologic status of a tumor is yet another important determinant of personalized treatment. The role of the immune system in neoplasia has long been appreciated, and the recent development of successful immunotherapies for lung cancer is dramatically and rapidly changing our therapeutic approach. Agents targeting checkpoint inhibition have been rapidly integrated into advanced stage lung cancer treatment. Immunologic tumor evaluation specifically relates to tumor expression of programmed death ligand 1 (PD-L1). PD-L1 on the surface of the tumor cell binds the programmed death-1 (PD-1) receptor on T-cells, resulting in downregulation of T-cell activity and tumor evasion of immune system detection [68]. Agents that block the interaction of tumor PD-L1 and host PD-1 prevent the tumor from escaping immune surveillance. Nivolumab and pembrolizumab (antibodies targeting the PD-1 receptor on T-cells) were two of the first such immunotherapies. In 2016, Reck and colleagues showed that advanced squamous and non-squamous NSCLC with tumor PD-L1 expression ≥50% had improved progression-free survival and overall survival when treated with pembrolizumab, compared to standard platinum-based chemotherapy [69]. Tumor PD-L1 testing is now recommended by NCCN for all metastatic NSCLCs.

As we consider the future role of molecular and immunologic testing for lung cancer, three trends should be highlighted. First, recent studies have shown clinical improvements in stage III and IV NSCLC with immunotherapy independent of tumor PD-L1 status [70–72]. Therefore, PD-L1 may not be the ideal biomarker on which to base decisions about immunotherapy, and other biomarkers will likely be considered [73]. Higher tumor mutational burden may be a poor prognostic marker in NSCLC [74], but it is associated with a higher likelihood of response to immunotherapy and is being studied as another possible biomarker [75]. Second, since current trials are studying immunotherapies in conjunction with chemotherapy and surgery in the setting of nonmetastatic disease [71, 76], it seems likely that immunotherapy use will be extended to earlier stages. Third, genomic evaluation now makes it clear that the majority of adenocarcinomas have potentially targetable driver mutations. Since only a few of these are currently actionable with available therapies, broad-based genomic sequencing as compared to focused *EGFR* and *ALK* testing may not be of current benefit [77]. Nonetheless, identification of those potential targets opens a wide spectrum of possible new precision therapies for lung cancer.

Lesson #3: From Individualization to Personalization – The Patient as Stakeholder

Lessons #1 and #2 have highlighted significant advances in our understanding of lung cancer biology, identified the resultant assessment tools, and outlined how lung cancer risk assessment, diagnosis, and tissue evaluation have become much more individualized, with the result being better personalized treatment with better outcome. We have conceptualized "precision medicine" primarily as "personalized medicine," utilizing data specific to the patient including lung cancer risk modeling, individual staging, and more precise understanding of tumor pathology within the context of a given patient's comorbidities and functional status. These data permit providers to present a plan of care specific to that patient. However, we have not yet included the patient's own preferences into the decision-making process. This final lesson will emphasize the importance of utilizing data at the level of the individual to make personalized treatment decisions.

A Precise Approach: From Individualized to Personalized

Once the patient's preferences are considered, "individualized medicine" may become "personalized medicine," in which the patient's values factor into the ultimate treatment plan. In their evaluation of nationwide healthcare differences, the Dartmouth Atlas Project recognized various categories of medical services, including "effective care" and "preference sensitive care" [78]. "Effective care" describes a service wherein the weight of theory and evidence supports efficacy, and excepting unusual circumstances this service should be provided to all qualifying patients [78]. An example of effective care would be the use of *EGFR* tyrosine kinase inhibitors as first-line therapy. For patients with advanced stage NSCLC and susceptible *EGFR* mutations, higher response rate, longer progression-free survival, and improved quality of life measures favor *EGFR* inhibitors such that they should be offered first line in virtually all cases, as opposed to treatment with cytotoxic chemotherapy [79]. Another example of effective care would be early palliative care intervention for patients with metastatic NSCLC. Temel and colleagues reported that, compared to standard of care, early palliative care resulted in better quality of life, fewer depressive symptoms, and longer median survival, with survival benefits comparable to medical treatment with chemotherapy [80]. Routine early integration of palliative care into lung cancer care is now recommended as standard practice [81], ensuring that there is a consistent focus on patient symptoms and values.

"Preference sensitive care" refers to medical services in which valid alternative treatment strategies exist, and the choice of treatment involves balancing risks and benefits [78]. The choice of the second agent in platinum-based doublet chemotherapy for advanced stage NSCLC is an example of such clinical equipoise. Prior work has shown that there is no significant difference in response rates or overall survival whether the second agent is gemcitabine, docetaxel, or paclitaxel [82]. Patients may have treatment preferences based on factors such as toxicity, convenience, and cost [83], with priorities varying significantly between patients. For example, one survey noted that, for female patients, concerns relating to infection risk or hair loss may be more prominent than for male patients [84].

Shared Decision-Making

The practice of "shared decision-making" (SDM) has been defined as "an approach where clinicians and patients share the best available evidence when faced with the task of making decisions, and where patients are supported to consider options, to achieve informed preferences" [85]. In SDM, clinicians present the risks and benefits associated with different options, and patients weigh in with their own values and preferences [85]. Having an honest and open-ended discussion early in the evaluation process ensures that patient and treatment goals are aligned. A review by Geerse and colleagues suggests that shared decision-making may be associated with improved emotional outcomes in patients with lung cancer [86]. Specific mechanisms for enhancing SDM include decision-aid tools (such as pamphlets or videos) designed to help patients make choices among healthcare options. A Cochrane review by Stacey and colleagues reported that use of decision aids increases patient knowledge and risk perception, enhances participation in decisions, and increases satisfaction with decisions, with no adverse effects on outcomes [87]. We will review the importance of shared decision-making in lung cancer screening and early-stage lung cancer management.

The role of SDM in lung cancer is perhaps most evident in the lung cancer screening process. The USPSTF recommends (and the Centers for Medicare and Medicaid Services mandate) a counseling and SDM visit for lung cancer screening; the visit includes a determination of lung cancer screening eligibility, SDM with one or more decision aids, and smoking cessation counseling [88]. The SDM visit was specifically included by USPSTF because of the complexity of lung cancer screening, including the potential for both benefit and harm, and the importance of patient participation in deciding whether to screen. For example, the benefits of lung cancer screening have only been established in a select population, and there is additive benefit to smoking cessation [89]. Further, lung cancer screening entails potential harms, including false-positive results, incidental findings, subsequent diagnostic procedures, and anxiety. Lung cancer screening may also result in overdiagnosis, defined as detection of a cancer that would not in the future have resulted in clinically significant disease [90]. As noted in Lesson #1, in NLST the number needed to screen was 320 [21]; thus, the majority of patients do not obtain benefit from lung cancer screening, though all are exposed to the harms. One means of facilitating SDM involves performance of screening at specialized centers with substantial expertise, access to enhanced resources, and dedicated knowledgeable providers. Mazzone and colleagues demonstrated that a centralized counseling and decision-making visit is feasible and improves knowledge surrounding lung cancer screening [91]. With this knowledge, patients have a greater chance of making decisions that best reflect their goals.

Management of early-stage lung cancer provides another opportunity for personalization of care through shared decision-making. In Lesson #1, we reviewed the impact of a patient's functional status on surgical decisions. The ability to tolerate more extensive resection is important because lobectomy with mediastinal dissection or systematic lymph node sampling for stage I cancer is considered standard of care. Alternatives to lobectomy include sublobar resection or stereotactic ablative radiotherapy (SABR; also known as stereotactic body radiation therapy [SBRT]). Oncologic outcomes with lobectomy are superior to sublobar resection [92, 93], and current evidence does not support the use of SABR in patients who are suitable candidates for

lobectomy [94, 95]. There is greater equipoise, however, when comparing sublobar resection (segmentectomy or wedge resection) against SABR in patients who are unable or unwilling to undergo full lobectomy. There are no large, randomized, head-to-head comparative studies, but there are significant data demonstrating the efficacy of SABR in medically inoperable patients with early stage peripheral cancers. For example, Timmerman and colleagues demonstrated that, in a group of 55 patients with medically inoperable stage I NSCLC treated with SABR and followed for a median of 3 years, tumor control rate was 97.6%, 3-year tumor and lobe control rate was 90.6%, and median overall survival was 4 years [96]. These 3-year outcomes are similar to those observed with sublobar resection, suggesting that SABR is a reasonable alternative for high-risk surgical patients who cannot undergo lobectomy [97]. If a patient with an early stage NSCLC is not a candidate for lobectomy, whether due to poor functional status (unacceptable risk of complications) or patient preference (desire to avoid surgical interventions or minimize perioperative complications), the discussion can then proceed toward a shared decision-making process outlining the relative risks and benefits of more limited surgical intervention versus radiation therapy. While it is important to maximize the chance for survival, this needs to be balanced against the patient's goals and the physician's concern for quality of life.

Ultimately, personalization of treatment must include the patient's preferences, which may only be known if we remember to ask. A multitude of decision points will be encountered in every lung cancer case. Standardized evaluation to guide decision-making is necessary to prevent undue variation and ensure thoroughness and efficiency. Precise staging and tissue evaluation represent critical points in the evaluation pathway informing treatment, and we can now characterize neoplasms at the level of single mutations or cell surface ligands to determine optimal treatments. However, we need to remember that the patient is not defined by their tumor. Rather, each patient is a whole human person, who should be fully engaged and participating in decision-making relating to their care. Shared decision-making allows us to use the tools of precision medicine to provide personalized care concordant with patient goals and values.

Conclusion

The evolution of diagnosis, evaluation, and treatment of lung cancer is an ideal model for understanding precision medicine and the personalization of care. Lung cancer research extends from large-scale studies providing insight into the epidemiology of lung cancer, permitting earlier identification and intervention, to molecular evaluation of single tumors. We have gained enormous insight into the heterogeneity of lung cancer and a profound appreciation that more precise understanding of genetic and biochemical differences informed by the backdrop of behavioral and social characteristics should guide individualized decisions relating to screening, staging, and treatment for a given patient. The old, nihilistic perception of lung cancer as a uniformly morbid disease with limited treatment options should be firmly rejected.

We can now return to our patient PM and compare his experience from 2008 as described above with what he would experience today, based on the remarkable advances made in the field of lung cancer over the past decade. This comparison highlights multiple ways in which scientific discoveries have been implemented into patient care, with emphasis on an individualized approach.

PM is a 65-year-old male current smoker with moderate COPD, who presented for routine health evaluation. His primary care physician initiated a discussion about lung cancer risk, as PM met USPSTF criteria for screening. PM was counseled about smoking cessation, and after a shared decision-making discussion, he elected to undergo screening low-dose chest CT (LDCT). The LDCT identified a solid 2.1-cm right upper lobe (RUL) nodule, without hilar or mediastinal adenopathy. PET-CT showed intense FDG uptake only in the nodule. EBUS biopsy of the nodule confirmed squamous cell carcinoma; biopsies of

right hilar and mediastinal nodes were negative. The clinical stage was T1cN0M0. PM had comprehensive physiologic evaluation, which demonstrated adequate predicted postoperative function. He underwent RUL lobectomy; pathologic stage was pT1cN0M0 (stage IA3). PM successfully quit smoking and was followed for several years without evidence of disease recurrence, but was then lost to follow-up. Ten years after the original LDCT, PM presented with several months of worsening cough and dyspnea. A chest radiograph demonstrated a right lower lobe abnormality; chest CT confirmed a 3.5-cm right lower lobe mass and enlarged right hilar and subcarinal lymph nodes, without abnormalities in the liver, adrenal glands, or bones. PET imaging showed intense FDG uptake in the mass and in mediastinal and hilar lymph nodes; brain MRI demonstrated two enhancing 1.0-cm lesions in the right parietal and temporal regions. Bronchoscopy with EBUS confirmed adenocarcinoma in the RLL mass as well as in multiple mediastinal nodes. The clinical stage was T2aN2M1c (stage IVB). Molecular testing was negative for *EGFR* or *BRAF* mutations or *ALK* or *ROS1* rearrangements; tumor PD-L1 was >50%. PM indicated that, at his age of 75 and with other health conditions, he wanted treatment that would balance survival benefit while limiting adverse reactions. After discussions with his multidisciplinary team, PM started immunotherapy with pembrolizumab, underwent stereotactic radiosurgery for the brain metastasis, and initiated care with the palliative medicine service. PM tolerated immunotherapy well with measurable response to treatment. However, follow-up imaging 18 months later demonstrated new liver abnormalities consistent with metastases. He was presented with the option of systemic chemotherapy, but after discussion of benefits and risks, elected to discontinue active treatment and focus with his primary care and palliative medicine teams on quality of life.

In the words of Sir William Osler, "The good physician treats the disease; the great physician treats the patient who has the disease." The advances of precision medicine in lung cancer increase the frequency with which cure can be obtained and permit greater flexibility in promoting survival while balancing individual goals relating to aggressiveness of care and potential toxicities. While specific tools, treatments, and guidelines presented today will inevitably become obsolete, the general approach to precision medicine that guides future research will remain durable. Through studying disease at the most fundamental molecular level to the broadest population-based level, we aim to predict those at greatest risk, take steps to attenuate that risk, identify cases sooner, rigorously define an individual's unique disease, and apply individualized therapies with greater efficacy and lower morbidity. Patient assessments should be standardized and structured, but each individual assessment will be *unique* and will *uniquely* inform optimal personalized treatment.

References

1. Collins FS, Varmus H. A new initiative on precision medicine. N Engl J Med. 2015;372(9):793–5.
2. World Health Organization. Cancer 2018. Available from: http://www.who.int/en/news-room/fact-sheets/detail/cancer. Accessed 27 Aug 2018.
3. World Health Organization. The top 10 causes of death 2018. Available from: http://www.who.int/mediacentre/factsheets/fs310/en/index1.html. Accessed 27 Aug 2018.
4. Chalmers ZR, Connelly CF, Fabrizio D, Gay L, Ali SM, Ennis R, et al. Analysis of 100,000 human cancer genomes reveals the landscape of tumor mutational burden. Genome Med. 2017;9(1):34.
5. Schroeder SA. Shattuck Lecture. We can do better–improving the health of the American people. N Engl J Med. 2007;357(12):1221–8.
6. Noone AM, Howlader N, Krapcho M, Miller D, Brest A, Yu M, Ruhl J, Tatalovich Z, Mariotto A, Lewis DR, Chen HS, Feuer EJ, Cronin KA, editors. SEER cancer statistics review, 1957–2015. Bethesda: National Cancer Institute; 2015.
7. Centers for Disease Control and Prevention. History of the surgeon general's reports on smoking health 2018. Available from: https://www.cdc.gov/tobacco/data_statistics/sgr/history/index.htm. Accessed 28 Aug 2018.
8. Subramanian J, Govindan R. Lung cancer in never smokers: a review. J Clin Oncol. 2007;25(5):561–70.
9. Reck M, Rabe KF. Precision diagnosis and treatment for advanced non-small-cell lung cancer. N Engl J Med. 2017;377(9):849–61.
10. Jemal A, Miller KD, Ma J, Siegel RL, Fedewa SA, Islami F, et al. Higher lung cancer incidence in young women than young men in the United States. N Engl J Med. 2018;378(21):1999–2009.
11. National Cancer Institute Surveillance, Epidemiology, and End Results Program. Cancer stat facts: lung and bronchus cancer. Available from: https://seer.cancer.gov/statfacts/html/lungb.html. Accessed 28 Aug 2018.
12. Detterbeck FC. Achieving clarity about lung cancer and opacities. Chest. 2017;151(2):252–4.
13. Centers for Disease Control and Prevention. What are the risk factors for lung cancer 2018. Available from: https://www.cdc.gov/cancer/lung/basic_info/risk_factors.htm. Accessed 28 Aug 2018.
14. MacMahon H, Naidich DP, Goo JM, Lee KS, Leung ANC, Mayo JR, et al. Guidelines for management of incidental pulmonary nodules detected on CT images: from the Fleischner Society 2017. Radiology. 2017;284(1):228–43.
15. Dela Cruz CS, Tanoue LT, Matthay RA. Lung cancer: epidemiology, etiology, and prevention. Clin Chest Med. 2011;32(4):605–44.
16. Moore SC, Lee IM, Weiderpass E, Campbell PT, Sampson JN, Kitahara CM, et al. Association of leisure-time physical activity with risk of 26 types of cancer in 1.44 million adults. JAMA Intern Med. 2016;176(6):816–25.
17. Bach PB, Kattan MW, Thornquist MD, Kris MG, Tate RC, Barnett MJ, et al. Variations in lung cancer risk among smokers. J Natl Cancer Inst. 2003;95(6):470–8.
18. Omenn GS, Goodman G, Thornquist M, Grizzle J, Rosenstock L, Barnhart S, et al. The beta-carotene and retinol efficacy trial (CARET) for chemoprevention of lung cancer in high risk populations: smokers and asbestos-exposed workers. Cancer Res. 1994;54(7 Suppl):2038s–43s.
19. Tammemagi MC, Katki HA, Hocking WG, Church TR, Caporaso N, Kvale PA, et al. Selection criteria for lung-cancer screening. N Engl J Med. 2013;368(8):728–36.
20. Tammemagi CM, Pinsky PF, Caporaso NE, Kvale PA, Hocking WG, Church TR, et al. Lung cancer risk prediction: prostate, lung, colorectal and ovarian cancer screening trial models and validation. J Natl Cancer Inst. 2011;103(13):1058–68.
21. National Lung Screening Trial Research Team, Aberle DR, Adams AM, Berg CD, Black WC, Clapp JD, et al. Reduced lung-cancer mortality with low-dose computed tomographic screening. N Engl J Med. 2011;365(5):395–409.
22. Rosell R, Moran T, Queralt C, Porta R, Cardenal F, Camps C, et al. Screening for epidermal growth factor receptor mutations in lung cancer. N Engl J Med. 2009;361(10):958–67.
23. Ou SH. Lung cancer in never-smokers. Does smoking history matter in the era of molecular diagnostics and targeted therapy? J Clin Pathol. 2013;66(10):839–46.
24. Shi Y, Au JS, Thongprasert S, Srinivasan S, Tsai CM, Khoa MT, et al. A prospective, molecular epidemiology study of EGFR mutations in Asian patients with advanced non-small-cell lung cancer of adeno-

carcinoma histology (PIONEER). J Thorac Oncol. 2014;9(2):154–62.

25. Shaw AT, Yeap BY, Mino-Kenudson M, Digumarthy SR, Costa DB, Heist RS, et al. Clinical features and outcome of patients with non-small-cell lung cancer who harbor EML4-ALK. J Clin Oncol. 2009;27(26):4247–53.

26. Bergethon K, Shaw AT, Ou SH, Katayama R, Lovly CM, McDonald NT, et al. ROS1 rearrangements define a unique molecular class of lung cancers. J Clin Oncol. 2012;30(8):863–70.

27. Paik PK, Arcila ME, Fara M, Sima CS, Miller VA, Kris MG, et al. Clinical characteristics of patients with lung adenocarcinomas harboring BRAF mutations. J Clin Oncol. 2011;29(15):2046–51.

28. National Comprehensive Cancer Network. NCCN Clinical Practice Guidelines in Oncology. Non-Small Cell Lung Cancer, Version 3.2019 – January 18, 2019: National Comprehensive Cancer Network; 2019 [11 February 2019]. Available from: https://www.nccn.org/professionals/physician_gls/pdf/nscl.pdf. Referenced with permission from the NCCN Guidelines® for Non-Small Cell Lung Cancer V.6.2018 © National Comprehensive Cancer Network, Inc. 2018. All rights reserved. Accessed 17 Aug 2018. Available online at www.NCCN.org. NCCN makes no warranties of any kind whatsoever regarding their content, use or application and disclaims any responsibility for their application or use in any way.

29. Hagemann IS, Devarakonda S, Lockwood CM, Spencer DH, Guebert K, Bredemeyer AJ, et al. Clinical next-generation sequencing in patients with non-small cell lung cancer. Cancer. 2015;121(4):631–9.

30. Silvestri GA, Gonzalez AV, Jantz MA, Margolis ML, Gould MK, Tanoue LT, et al. Methods for staging non-small cell lung cancer: Diagnosis and management of lung cancer, 3rd ed: American College of Chest Physicians evidence-based clinical practice guidelines. Chest. 2013;143(5 Suppl):e211S–e50S.

31. Goldstraw P, Chansky K, Crowley J, Rami-Porta R, Asamura H, Eberhardt WE, et al. The IASLC lung cancer staging project: proposals for revision of the TNM stage groupings in the forthcoming (eighth) edition of the TNM classification for lung cancer. J Thorac Oncol. 2016;11(1):39–51.

32. Farjah F, Flum DR, Ramsey SD, Heagerty PJ, Symons RG, Wood DE. Multi-modality mediastinal staging for lung cancer among medicare beneficiaries. J Thorac Oncol. 2009;4(3):355–63.

33. Vokes EE, Govindan R, Iscoe N, Hossain AM, San Antonio B, Chouaki N, et al. The impact of staging by positron-emission tomography on overall survival and progression-free survival in patients with locally advanced NSCLC. J Thorac Oncol. 2018;13(8):1183–8.

34. Fischer B, Lassen U, Mortensen J, Larsen S, Loft A, Bertelsen A, et al. Preoperative staging of lung cancer with combined PET-CT. N Engl J Med. 2009;361(1):32–9.

35. Viney RC, Boyer MJ, King MT, Kenny PM, Pollicino CA, McLean JM, et al. Randomized controlled trial of the role of positron emission tomography in the management of stage I and II non-small-cell lung cancer. J Clin Oncol. 2004;22(12):2357–62.

36. van Tinteren H, Hoekstra OS, Smit EF, van den Bergh JH, Schreurs AJ, Stallaert RA, et al. Effectiveness of positron emission tomography in the preoperative assessment of patients with suspected non-small-cell lung cancer: the PLUS multicentre randomised trial. Lancet. 2002;359(9315):1388–93.

37. Annema JT, van Meerbeeck JP, Rintoul RC, Dooms C, Deschepper E, Dekkers OM, et al. Mediastinoscopy vs endosonography for mediastinal nodal staging of lung cancer: a randomized trial. JAMA. 2010;304(20):2245–52.

38. Boffa DJ, Allen MS, Grab JD, Gaissert HA, Harpole DH, Wright CD. Data from The Society of Thoracic Surgeons General Thoracic Surgery database: the surgical management of primary lung tumors. J Thorac Cardiovasc Surg. 2008;135(2):247–54.

39. Seder CW, Wright CD, Chang AC, Han JM, McDonald D, Kozower BD. The society of thoracic surgeons general thoracic surgery database update on outcomes and quality. Ann Thorac Surg. 2016;101(5):1646–54.

40. Finkelstein DM, Ettinger DS, Ruckdeschel JC. Long-term survivors in metastatic non-small-cell lung cancer: an Eastern Cooperative Oncology Group Study. J Clin Oncol. 1986;4(5):702–9.

41. Bolliger CT, Wyser C, Roser H, Soler M, Perruchoud AP. Lung scanning and exercise testing for the prediction of postoperative performance in lung resection candidates at increased risk for complications. Chest. 1995;108(2):341–8.

42. Alam N, Park BJ, Wilton A, Seshan VE, Bains MS, Downey RJ, et al. Incidence and risk factors for lung injury after lung cancer resection. Ann Thorac Surg. 2007;84(4):1085–91; discussion 91.

43. Ferguson MK, Dignam JJ, Siddique J, Vigneswaran WT, Celauro AD. Diffusing capacity predicts long-term survival after lung resection for cancer. Eur J Cardiothorac Surg. 2012;41(5):e81–6.

44. Brunelli A, Kim AW, Berger KI, Addrizzo-Harris DJ. Physiologic evaluation of the patient with lung cancer being considered for resectional surgery: diagnosis and management of lung cancer, 3rd ed: American College of Chest Physicians evidence-based clinical practice guidelines. Chest. 2013;143(5 Suppl):e166S–e90S.

45. de Koning HJ, Meza R, Plevritis SK, ten Haaf K, Munshi VN, Jeon J, et al. Benefits and harms of computed tomography lung cancer screening strategies: a comparative modeling study for the U.S. Preventive Services Task Force. Ann Intern Med. 2014;160(5):311–20.

46. Moyer VA, Force USPST. Screening for lung cancer: U.S. Preventive Services Task Force recommendation statement. Ann Intern Med. 2014;160(5):330-8.

47. Kovalchik SA, Tammemagi M, Berg CD, Caporaso NE, Riley TL, Korch M, et al. Targeting of low-dose CT screening according to the risk of lung-cancer death. N Engl J Med. 2013;369(3):245–54.

48. Caverly TJ, Fagerlin A, Wiener RS, Slatore CG, Tanner NT, Yun S, et al. Comparison of observed harms and expected mortality benefit for persons in the veterans health affairs lung cancer screening demonstration project. JAMA Intern Med. 2018;178(3):426–8.

49. Katki HA, Kovalchik SA, Berg CD, Cheung LC, Chaturvedi AK. Development and validation of risk models to select ever-smokers for CT lung Cancer screening. JAMA. 2016;315(21):2300–11.

50. Tammemagi MC. Selecting lung cancer screenees using risk prediction models-where do we go from here. Transl Lung Cancer Res. 2018;7(3):243–53.

51. Mazzone PJ, Silvestri GA, Patel S, Kanne JP, Kinsinger LS, Wiener RS, et al. Screening for lung cancer: CHEST guideline and expert panel report. Chest. 2018;153(4):954–85.

52. Mountain CF, Carr DT, Anderson WA. A system for the clinical staging of lung cancer. Am J Roentgenol Radium Ther Nucl Med. 1974;120(1):130–8.

53. Detterbeck FC, Lewis SZ, Diekemper R, Addrizzo-Harris D, Alberts WM. Executive summary: diagnosis and management of lung cancer, 3rd ed: American College of Chest Physicians evidence-based clinical practice guidelines. Chest. 2013;143(5 Suppl):7S–37S.

54. Rivera MP, Mehta AC, Wahidi MM. Establishing the diagnosis of lung cancer: diagnosis and management of lung cancer, 3rd ed: American College of Chest Physicians evidence-based clinical practice guidelines. Chest. 2013;143(5 Suppl):e142S–e65S.

55. Ost DE, Jim Yeung SC, Tanoue LT, Gould MK. Clinical and organizational factors in the initial evaluation of patients with lung cancer: diagnosis and management of lung cancer, 3rd ed: American College of Chest Physicians evidence-based clinical practice guidelines. Chest. 2013;143(5 Suppl):e121S–e41S.

56. Wang Memoli JS, Nietert PJ, Silvestri GA. Meta-analysis of guided bronchoscopy for the evaluation of the pulmonary nodule. Chest. 2012;142(2):385–93.

57. Ost DE, Ernst A, Lei X, Kovitz KL, Benzaquen S, Diaz-Mendoza J, et al. Diagnostic yield and complications of bronchoscopy for peripheral lung lesions. Results of the AQuIRE Registry. Am J Respir Crit Care Med. 2016;193(1):68–77.

58. Hofman P. Liquid biopsy for early detection of lung cancer. Curr Opin Oncol. 2017;29(1):73–8.

59. Rolfo C, Mack PC, Scagliotti GV, Baas P, Barlesi F, Bivona TG, et al. Liquid biopsy for advanced non-small cell lung Cancer (NSCLC): a statement paper from the IASLC. J Thorac Oncol. 2018;13:1248.

60. Travis WD, Brambilla E, Nicholson AG, Yatabe Y, Austin JHM, Beasley MB, et al. The 2015 World Health Organization classification of lung tumors: impact of genetic, clinical and radiologic advances since the 2004 classification. J Thorac Oncol. 2015;10(9):1243–60.

61. Scagliotti G, Hanna N, Fossella F, Sugarman K, Blatter J, Peterson P, et al. The differential efficacy of pemetrexed according to NSCLC histology: a review of two Phase III studies. Oncologist. 2009;14(3):253–63.

62. Al-Saleh K, Quinton C, Ellis PM. Role of pemetrexed in advanced non-small-cell lung cancer: meta-analysis of randomized controlled trials, with histology subgroup analysis. Curr Oncol. 2012;19(1):e9–e15.

63. Lauro S, Onesti CE, Righini R, Marchetti P. The use of bevacizumab in non-small cell lung cancer: an update. Anticancer Res. 2014;34(4):1537–45.

64. Paez JG, Janne PA, Lee JC, Tracy S, Greulich H, Gabriel S, et al. EGFR mutations in lung cancer: correlation with clinical response to gefitinib therapy. Science. 2004;304(5676):1497–500.

65. Lynch TJ, Bell DW, Sordella R, Gurubhagavatula S, Okimoto RA, Brannigan BW, et al. Activating mutations in the epidermal growth factor receptor underlying responsiveness of non-small-cell lung cancer to gefitinib. N Engl J Med. 2004;350(21):2129–39.

66. Perez-Moreno P, Brambilla E, Thomas R, Soria JC. Squamous cell carcinoma of the lung: molecular subtypes and therapeutic opportunities. Clin Cancer Res. 2012;18(9):2443–51.

67. Paik PK, Varghese AM, Sima CS, Moreira AL, Ladanyi M, Kris MG, et al. Response to erlotinib in patients with EGFR mutant advanced non-small cell lung cancers with a squamous or squamous-like component. Mol Cancer Ther. 2012;11(11):2535–40.

68. Carbone DP, Gandara DR, Antonia SJ, Zielinski C, Paz-Ares L. Non-small-cell lung cancer: role of the immune system and potential for immunotherapy. J Thorac Oncol. 2015;10(7):974–84.

69. Reck M, Rodriguez-Abreu D, Robinson AG, Hui R, Csoszi T, Fulop A, et al. Pembrolizumab versus chemotherapy for PD-L1-positive non-small-cell lung cancer. N Engl J Med. 2016;375(19):1823–33.

70. Antonia SJ, Villegas A, Daniel D, Vicente D, Murakami S, Hui R, et al. Durvalumab after chemoradiotherapy in stage III non-small-cell lung cancer. N Engl J Med. 2017;377(20):1919–29.

71. Gandhi L, Rodriguez-Abreu D, Gadgeel S, Esteban E, Felip E, De Angelis F, et al. Pembrolizumab plus chemotherapy in metastatic non-small-cell lung cancer. N Engl J Med. 2018;378(22):2078–92.

72. Paz-Ares L, Luft A, Vicente D, Tafreshi A, Gumus M, Mazieres J, et al. Pembrolizumab plus chemotherapy for squamous non-small-cell lung cancer. N Engl J Med. 2018;379(21):2040–51.

73. Beattie J, Yarmus L, Wahidi M, Rivera MP, Gilbert C, Maldonado F, et al. The immune landscape of non-small-cell lung cancer. Utility of cytologic and histologic samples obtained through minimally invasive pulmonary procedures. Am J Respir Crit Care Med. 2018;198(1):24–38.

74. Owada-Ozaki Y, Muto S, Takagi H, Inoue T, Watanabe Y, Fukuhara M, et al. Prognostic impact of tumor mutation burden in patients with completely resected non-small cell lung cancer: brief report. J Thorac Oncol. 2018;13(8):1217–21.

75. Hellmann MD, Ciuleanu TE, Pluzanski A, Lee JS, Otterson GA, Audigier-Valette C, et al. Nivolumab

plus ipilimumab in lung cancer with a high tumor mutational burden. N Engl J Med. 2018;378(22):2093–104.

76. Forde PM, Chaft JE, Smith KN, Anagnostou V, Cottrell TR, Hellmann MD, et al. Neoadjuvant PD-1 blockade in resectable lung cancer. N Engl J Med. 2018;378(21):1976–86.

77. Presley CJ, Tang DW, Soulos PR, Chiang AC, Longtine JA, Adelson KB, et al. Association of broad-based genomic sequencing with survival among patients with advanced non-small cell lung cancer in the community oncology setting. JAMA. 2018;320(5):469–77.

78. Wennberg JE, Fisher ES, Skinner JS. Geography and the debate over Medicare reform. Health Aff (Millwood). 2002;Suppl Web Exclusives:W96–114.

79. Langer CJ. Epidermal growth factor receptor inhibition in mutation-positive non-small-cell lung cancer: is afatinib better or simply newer? J Clin Oncol. 2013;31(27):3303–6.

80. Temel JS, Greer JA, Muzikansky A, Gallagher ER, Admane S, Jackson VA, et al. Early palliative care for patients with metastatic non-small-cell lung cancer. N Engl J Med. 2010;363(8):733–42.

81. Ferrell BR, Temel JS, Temin S, Alesi ER, Balboni TA, Basch EM, et al. Integration of palliative care into standard oncology care: American Society of Clinical Oncology Clinical Practice Guideline Update. J Clin Oncol. 2017;35(1):96–112.

82. Schiller JH, Harrington D, Belani CP, Langer C, Sandler A, Krook J, et al. Comparison of four chemotherapy regimens for advanced non-small-cell lung cancer. N Engl J Med. 2002;346(2):92–8.

83. Goffin J, Lacchetti C, Ellis PM, Ung YC, Evans WK, Lung Cancer Disease Site Group of Cancer Care Ontario's Program in Evidence-Based C. First-line systemic chemotherapy in the treatment of advanced non-small cell lung cancer: a systematic review. J Thorac Oncol. 2010;5(2):260–74.

84. Dubey S, Brown RL, Esmond SL, Bowers BJ, Healy JM, Schiller JH. Patient preferences in choosing chemotherapy regimens for advanced non-small cell lung cancer. J Support Oncol. 2005;3(2):149–54.

85. Barry MJ, Edgman-Levitan S. Shared decision making–pinnacle of patient-centered care. N Engl J Med. 2012;366(9):780–1.

86. Geerse OP, Stegmann ME, Kerstjens HAM, Hiltermann TJN, Bakitas M, Zimmermann C, et al. Effects of shared decision making on distress and health care utilization among patients with lung cancer: a systematic review. J Pain Symptom Manag. 2018;56:975.

87. Stacey D, Legare F, Lewis K, Barry MJ, Bennett CL, Eden KB, et al. Decision aids for people facing health treatment or screening decisions. Cochrane Database Syst Rev. 2017;4:CD001431.

88. Centers for Medicare and Medicaid Services. Decision memo for screening for lung cancer with low dose computed tomography (LDCT) (CAG-00439N). Available from: https://www.cms.gov/medicare-coverage-database/details/nca-decision-memo.aspx?NCAId=274.

89. Tanner NT, Kanodra NM, Gebregziabher M, Payne E, Halbert CH, Warren GW, et al. The association between smoking abstinence and mortality in the National Lung Screening Trial. Am J Respir Crit Care Med. 2016;193(5):534–41.

90. Patz EF Jr, Pinsky P, Gatsonis C, Sicks JD, Kramer BS, Tammemagi MC, et al. Overdiagnosis in low-dose computed tomography screening for lung cancer. JAMA Intern Med. 2014;174(2):269–74.

91. Mazzone PJ, Tenenbaum A, Seeley M, Petersen H, Lyon C, Han X, et al. Impact of a lung cancer screening counseling and shared decision-making visit. Chest. 2017;151(3):572–8.

92. Dai C, Shen J, Ren Y, Zhong S, Zheng H, He J, et al. Choice of surgical procedure for patients with non-small-cell lung cancer </= 1 cm or > 1–2 cm among lobectomy, segmentectomy, and wedge resection: a population-based study. J Clin Oncol. 2016;34(26):3175–82.

93. Ginsberg RJ, Rubinstein L. The comparison of limited resection to lobectomy for T1N0 non-small cell lung cancer. LCSG 821. Chest. 1994;106(6 Suppl):318S–9S.

94. Bryant AK, Mundt RC, Sandhu AP, Urbanic JJ, Sharabi AB, Gupta S, et al. Stereotactic body radiation therapy versus surgery for early lung cancer among US veterans. Ann Thorac Surg. 2018;105(2):425–31.

95. Cao C, Wang D, Chung C, Tian D, Rimner A, Huang J, et al. A systematic review and meta-analysis of stereotactic body radiation therapy versus surgery for patients with non-small cell lung cancer. J Thorac Cardiovasc Surg. 2019;157(1):362–73.e8.

96. Timmerman R, Paulus R, Galvin J, Michalski J, Straube W, Bradley J, et al. Stereotactic body radiation therapy for inoperable early stage lung cancer. JAMA. 2010;303(11):1070–6.

97. Grills IS, Mangona VS, Welsh R, Chmielewski G, McInerney E, Martin S, et al. Outcomes after stereotactic lung radiotherapy or wedge resection for stage I non-small-cell lung cancer. J Clin Oncol. 2010;28(6):928–35.

98. Detterbeck FC, Boffa DJ, Kim AW, Tanoue LT. The eighth edition lung cancer stage classification. Chest. 2017;151(1):193–203.

99. Oken M, Creech R, Tormey D, et al. Toxicity and response criteria of the Eastern Cooperative Oncology Group. Am J Clin Oncol. 1982;5:649–55.

COPD Phenotyping

Emmet O'Brien, Frank C. Sciurba, and Jessica Bon

Abbreviations

AATD	Alpha-1 antitrypsin deficiency
ACO	Asthma COPD overlap
COPD	Chronic obstructive pulmonary disease
CRP	C reactive protein
CT	Computerized tomography
DLCO	Diffusion capacity for carbon monoxide
FEV1	Forced expiratory volume in 1 second
FFMI	Fat free mass index
FVC	Forced vital capacity in 1 second
GERD	Gastroesophageal reflux disease
GOLD	Global initiative for obstructive lung disease
HU	Hounsfield unit
ICS	Inhaled corticosteroid
IL-5	Interleukin-5
LABA	Long-acting beta agonist
LAMA	Long-acting muscarinic antagonist
mMRC	Modified Medical Research Council (Dyspnea Score)
PD15	HU value at the 15th percentile of the HU value histogram of lung voxels
PRISm	Preserved ratio impaired spirometry
RV	Residual volume
SPD	Surfactant protein D
sRAGE	Soluble advanced glycosylation end products
TLC	Total lung capacity

E. O'Brien
Department of Medicine, Beaumont Hospital, Dublin, Ireland

F. C. Sciurba
Department of Medicine, Beaumont Hospital, Dublin, Ireland

Division of Pulmonary, Allergy and Critical Care Medicine, Department of Medicine, University of Pittsburgh, Pittsburgh, PA, USA
e-mail: sciurbafc@upmc.edu

J. Bon (✉)
Division of Pulmonary, Allergy and Critical Care Medicine, Department of Medicine, University of Pittsburgh, Pittsburgh, PA, USA
e-mail: bonjm@upmc.edu

General Considerations for Prevention, Diagnosis, and Treatment of Chronic Obstructive Pulmonary Disease

Chronic obstructive pulmonary disease (COPD), while defined as incompletely reversible obstruction to expiratory airflow, is in reality a complex and heterogeneous constellation of mechanisms and multisystem clinical features. COPD is a major healthcare burden and a leading cause of death worldwide. Inhalational exposure to noxious gases, notably tobacco and environmental smoke, has a causal relationship for the development of COPD [1]. Critically, improvements in air quality and smoking cessation improve the

© Springer Nature Switzerland AG 2020
J. L. Gomez et al. (eds.), *Precision in Pulmonary, Critical Care, and Sleep Medicine*,
Respiratory Medicine, https://doi.org/10.1007/978-3-030-31507-8_15

burden of symptoms and halt the progressive decline in parameters of lung function in those susceptible to COPD [2].

The foundation of the term COPD arose in the 1960s through a concerted effort to physiologically define the clinically overlapping conditions of chronic bronchitis, emphysema, and asthma using forced spirometric maneuvers [3]. These classic COPD phenotypes were recognized over a century earlier to share similar origins despite being pathologically distinct [4]. Persistent obstruction on post bronchodilator spirometry is the cornerstone for establishing the diagnosis of COPD. Bronchodilator reversibility, initially adopted as a distinguishing characteristic between COPD and bronchial asthma, is now recognized as prevalent among patients with both COPD and asthma and can be diminished or absent in patients with severe asthma [5, 6]. Further, bronchodilator reversibility is a poor predictor of clinical and functional outcomes, such as exacerbation frequency, exercise capacity, and patient-reported health status. The availability of advanced pulmonary diagnostics has enhanced the more precise delineation of COPD phenotypes beyond basic spirometric airflow obstruction and symptomatology through the use of body plethysmography to define lung volume compartments and hyperinflation, lung imaging for the quantification and distribution of parenchymal emphysema and airway dimensions, and blood testing to screen for genetic risk factors such as alpha-1 antitrypsin deficiency (AATD) and other cellular and protein biomarkers of disease activity.

There remains a strong impetus to better characterize individual patients at risk of COPD incidence and progression so that we may develop novel therapies to alleviate suffering, improve survival, and, ultimately, reverse the course of this devastating illness. Our current understanding of clinical phenotypes in COPD reveal a mixture of disease endotypes that remain loosely classified by symptom burden, pulmonary function testing, and radiographic characteristics (Table 15.1). A key unanswered question in the field is why certain disease traits or phenotypes of COPD emerge among smokers while others with similar exposure history remain unaffected. The recognition of AATD as a key genetic determinant of emphysema by Laurell and Eriksson was a critical milestone, promulgating our current understanding of the role of protease: Anti-protease balance in the pathobiology of COPD and leading to the development of a disease-specific treatment for affected individuals [7]. Other host attributes that lead to COPD, in particular genetic susceptibility factors and early life disadvantage, are areas of interest being addressed within several large international prospective studies [8, 9].

The heterogeneous nature of COPD highlights the importance of precision phenotyping in clinical trials whereby patient selection permits benefits from therapeutic intervention to be relevant and applicable to the target population [5, 10]. Several randomized controlled trials have revealed clinically significant benefits in certain COPD phenotypes through subgroup analyses of secondary endpoints, for example, roflumilast has been shown to improve parameters of lung

Table 15.1 Common COPD clinical phenotypes

	PRISm	ACO	Low symptom burden	Hyperinflated	Frequent exacerbator
Active smoker	+	−	−	+/−	+
Pack year smoking history	Low	Low	Low	High	High
Airflow obstruction (FEV1/FVC <0.7)	−	+	+	+	+
Bronchial hyper-responsiveness	−	+	−	+/−	+
Exacerbations	+	+	−	+/−	+
Dyspnea	+	+	−	+	+/−
Emphysema	+/−	−	+/−	+	+/−
Oxygen use	−	−	−	+/−	+/−
Comorbid illness	+	+	+/−	+	+

function and reduce exacerbation frequency in symptomatic patients with moderate to severe COPD and prior history of exacerbation [11]. In this new era of personalized medicine, such complex and detailed phenotyping is not only feasible but can be integrated into clinical decision-making and applied in clinical practice.

Current COPD Management

Smoking cessation is central to halting disease progression, improving symptom burden, and reducing healthcare utilization in COPD while the prevailing therapeutic paradigm includes bronchodilation, suppression of airway inflammation, and minimizing the impact of respiratory failure. The Global Initiative for Obstructive Lung Disease (GOLD) has developed guidelines to classify and direct treatment for COPD internationally [6]. Current GOLD guidelines have evolved to emphasize pulmonary exacerbation history and symptom burden over the degree of airflow limitation to guide therapy by ABCD class [12]. Short-acting bronchodilators are recommended as reliever therapy for all symptomatic patients with COPD, while long-acting beta agonists (LABA) or muscarinic antagonists (LAMA) alone or in combination are recommended as an initial approach, as maintenance therapy. Exacerbation-prone patients may benefit from the addition of inhaled corticosteroids (ICS) with respect to exacerbation frequency and quality of life while ICS can be safely withdrawn in others, thereby limiting associated short- and long-term adverse events such as pneumonia and osteopenia [13]. "Precision" targeting of patients with persistent exacerbations despite optimal maintenance inhaler therapy may include the addition of a macrolide antibiotic, if not currently smoking, or a phosphodiesterase inhibitor type-4 inhibitor, such as roflumilast, in more severe patients with a chronic bronchitic phenotype. Long-term oxygen therapy is associated with improved survival in patients with resting hypoxemia (SpO2 <89%, or <90% in the presence of cor pulmonale) [14, 15]; however that benefit does not extend to patients with moderately low arterial oxygen at rest (SpO$_2$ 89–93%) and desaturation only with exertion [16].

A desirable goal to lower treatment burden and associated healthcare costs would be through the precision delivery of therapies to patients with COPD phenotypes that derive clinically significant benefits while avoiding indiscriminate use for those who do not. Non-pharmacological interventions in COPD, such as pulmonary rehabilitation, are invariably underutilized [17] though proven to improve exercise capacity and quality of life in patients with stable COPD or following an acute exacerbation [18, 19]. Much debate still exists regarding exacerbation-prone symptomatic individuals without airflow obstruction as they fall outside current COPD classification criteria and lack evidence-based treatment options [20–22].

General Principles of Novel Concepts with Relevance for Precision Medicine

Identification of relevant COPD phenotypes has shifted from the historic narrative of descriptive physiological manifestations, such as "pink puffers" and "blue bloaters" in the context of hypoxic respiratory failure, to more tangible predictors of clinical response (Table 15.2).

Bronchial Hyper-responsiveness

Bronchial hyper-responsiveness is reportedly highly prevalent in smokers, more common in females, and related to lower baseline lung function [23]. The presence of bronchial hyper-responsiveness has underlying biological relevance in COPD as it is associated with physiologic air trapping, airway inflammation, peripheral eosinophilia, accelerated decline in lung function, and mortality [24–26]. In the absence of a clear delineation in diagnostic parameters, together with shared phenotypic similarities between asthma and of bronchial hyper-responsiveness in COPD, the term asthma–COPD overlap (ACO) has arisen to assuage the clinical dilemma of differentiating this patient population [27]. Applying the expanding arsenal of precision asthma therapeutics to patients with ACO is enticing; however, in the

Table 15.2 Tools for precision COPD phenotyping

Clinical tools		
Clinical history	Exacerbations	
	Hospitalization	
Clinical severity scoring	COPD assessment test	
	Modified Medical Research Council (mMRC) Dyspnea Scale	
	Six minute walk test	
Pulmonary function testing	Spirometry	
	Lung volumes	
	DLCO	
	Impulse oscillometry	
Radiographic	Emphysema distribution	
	Emphysema quantitative analysis	
	Fissure integrity	
Biomarkers	Fibrinogen	
	Blood eosinophilia	
Genetic	Plasma AAT level	
	AAT phenotyping/genotyping	
Comorbidities	Cardiovascular disease	Neurocognitive decline
	Lung cancer	GERD
	Anxiety	Osteoporosis
	Depression	Skeletal muscle atrophy
Research tools		
Clinical history	St. George's Respiratory Questionnaire	
Genetic	Epigenetics	
	Whole-genome sequencing	
	Telomere length	
Biomarkers	Markers of inflammation	Auto-immunity
	Proteomics	
	Metabolomics	
Radiographic	Parametric response mapping	
Microbiome	16S ribosomal RNA sequencing	
	Shotgun metagenomics	

absence of international societal guidelines or endorsement, standardized definition, and discernable evidence base it remains premature [28]. Further, other elements of traditional asthma such as bronchodilator reversibility, a history of allergies or childhood asthma, and blood eosinophil levels are only modestly correlated in COPD.

Exacerbations

Pulmonary exacerbation frequency is associated with the severity of airflow limitation and spirometric GOLD stage; however, it is now recog-

nized that the most important predictor is an individual's own history of exacerbations [29]. In the clinical context, moderate and severe pulmonary exacerbations are a key driver for resource utilization and healthcare cost [30]. Identifying exacerbation-prone COPD phenotypes that may benefit from targeted preventative therapies, such as roflumilast, and the institution of early treatment strategies that may diminish symptom burden, treatment failure, length of hospital stay, and hospital readmission is desirable [31]. As an important healthcare metric, minimizing pulmonary exacerbation frequency now influences clinical trial design, drug development, and the goals of COPD therapy [32–36]. A limitation in using exacerbation frequency to define treatment is that the phenotype is only modesty reproduced from year to year [37].

Comorbidities

Comorbidities contribute to the clinical phenotype in COPD and are highly prevalent, linked to poorer health outcomes, increased healthcare utilization, and contribute significantly to all-cause mortality [38]. It is difficult to extricate illnesses, such as cardiovascular disease, lung cancer, and osteoporosis, as comorbid rather than nonpulmonary sequelae of COPD (Fig. 15.1) [39]. Complications of chronic hypoxia, such as cor pulmonale, are important to recognize in end-stage disease and to differentiate from primary cardiac etiologies [40]. Anxiety and depression are strongly associated with phenotypes of severe COPD and contribute to perceptions of well-being, social isolation, and correlate with mortality [41, 42]. Initially described as "pulmonary cachexia" [43], skeletal muscle atrophy is an important clinical phenotype in COPD that is characterized by altered muscle structure, sarcopenia, and impaired exercise capacity [44–46]. A strong association exists between declining respiratory function and oxidative shift in peripheral muscle fibers in moderate and severe COPD [47]. These alterations in muscle fiber type, in conjunction with decreased physical activity, result in reduced thigh cross-sectional area and quadriceps

Pulmonary morbidity

Systemic comorbidities

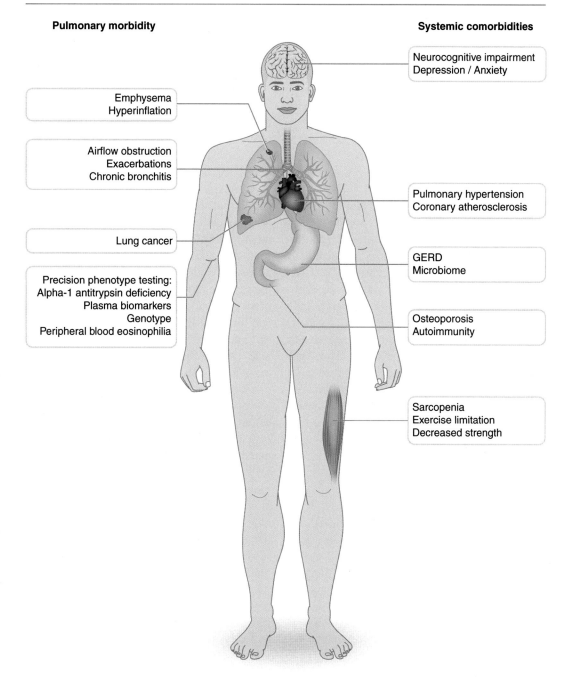

Neurocognitive impairment
Depression / Anxiety

Emphysema
Hyperinflation

Airflow obstruction
Exacerbations
Chronic bronchitis

Pulmonary hypertension
Coronary atherosclerosis

Lung cancer

GERD
Microbiome

Precision phenotype testing:
Alpha-1 antitrypsin deficiency
Plasma biomarkers
Genotype
Peripheral blood eosinophilia

Osteoporosis
Autoimmunity

Sarcopenia
Exercise limitation
Decreased strength

Fig. 15.1 Chronic obstructive pulmonary disease is not only associated with lung phenotypes, including emphysema and chronic bronchitis, but is also associated with numerous non-pulmonary sequelae

muscle weakness that are independently associated with increased mortality in COPD [48, 49]. Decreased fat free mass index (FFMI), as a measure of lean body composition, is also closely associated with lung function impairment and is an independent predictor of mortality in COPD [50, 51]. Pectoralis muscle cross sectional area, captured during CT chest imaging, is emerging as a promising metric of lean body mass that correlates with lung function in those with and without airflow obstruction [52, 53] and has been shown to independently associate with mortality risk in a study derived from two large COPD cohorts [54]. Pulmonary rehabilitation is a particularly important intervention in those with sarcopenia as it improves both muscle function and exercise endurance [55, 56]. Pharmacological therapy to complement traditional rehabilitation approaches is an unmet need in in COPD despite substantial progress in the development of new therapies that augment muscle mass and strength [57].

It is increasingly recognized that the shared pathogenic mechanisms driving comorbid illness in COPD, such as inflammation, oxidative stress, and immune dysfunction, can be therapeutically targeted to deliver benefits that cross over organ-specific boundaries and may classify individual phenotypes to benefit from future therapies [58]. In this era of big data, unsupervised computer learning raises the opportunity to uncover new associations and disease pathways relevant to comorbidities in COPD, thereby improving our understanding of the complex systems biology, and compelling new insights for therapeutic intervention in this disease [59].

Research Approaches to COPD Phenotype Assessment

The development of novel imaging modalities; high-performance platforms for protein, gene, and metabolite assessment; and integrative computational approaches to disease classification have led to the characterization of numerous complex COPD phenotypes over the past decade. Although most widely used in the research domain, technologies such as quantitative CT assessment of emphysema and fissure integrity to inform patients of their emphysema severity or to target subgroups of patients appropriate for bronchoscopic lung volume reduction are examples of how these novel approaches to phenotype assessment are already being used clinically to deliver precision-based therapy in COPD. Further validation against clinical outcomes in different patient populations, particularly in the realm of biomarker discovery, as well as efforts to increase

accessibility of these methods in clinical practice are crucial to the incorporation of these approaches into a precision-based strategy of COPD care delivery.

Radiographic Phenotyping

Two decades ago, Muller and colleagues introduced the density mask method as a way to objectively quantify emphysema using CT imaging of the chest [60]. With this technique, lung tissue voxels within a specified density range are highlighted and the severity of emphysema defined by the quantification of areas of abnormally low attenuation. In this early study, the extent of emphysema defined by the density mask correlated well with pathologic grade and was thought to eliminate both the intra-observer and inter-observer variabilities that impact subjective measurements. Later studies have demonstrated strong correlations between quantitative emphysema, microscopic and macroscopic morphometry [61, 62], and measures of lung function [63, 64]. A change in an alternative quantitative emphysema metric, the 15th percentile lung density (PD15) derived from the CT voxel histogram distribution of the whole lung transformed from Hounsfield units to density (g/L) and adjusted for lung volume, has demonstrated sensitivity to measure longitudinal effects of augmentation therapy in severe AATD [65]. In parallel with the development of methods to quantify radiographic emphysema, numerous image analysis techniques have been developed to measure airway dimensions on CT imaging [66–69]. Both quantitative emphysema and airway measurements have been associated with quality of life and disease outcomes in COPD [70] and are routinely used in research studies. The development of automated software has facilitated the transition of quantitative emphysema analysis from the research realm to clinical practice where it is now used routinely to evaluate emphysema distribution for lung volume reduction and to provide feedback on emphysema severity to smokers undergoing CT lung cancer screening.

Image phenotyping in COPD has continued to evolve to determine not only the severity, but also the lobar distribution of emphysema, fissure integrity, and the degree of small airway involvement, all of which hold prognostic and therapeutic implications. Increased quantitative lower lobe emphysema has been associated with worse lung function whereas increased quantitative upper lobe emphysema has been shown to correlate with greater dyspnea, gas trapping, and 5-year emphysema progression [71]. Emphysema distribution is likewise associated with a differential response to both surgical and bronchoscopic lung volume reduction [72, 73]. In clinical trials, lung fissure integrity on chest CT imaging is associated with response to endobronchial valve lung volume reduction with patients having intact fissures, a surrogate for the absence of collateral airflow, demonstrating a more favorable response to therapy [72, 73]. The determination of fissure integrity is now being used clinically to deliver precision-based bronchoscopic lung volume reduction to a select group of patients with heterogeneous emphysema and intact fissures. Meanwhile, advances in airway analyses have led to greater insight into the contribution of small airway disease in COPD [74]. Parametric response mapping, an imaging technique that pairs registered inspiratory and expiratory CT images to define areas of functional small airways disease and emphysema based on changes in registered voxel Hounsfield unit attenuation with the respiratory cycle [75], has been used to demonstrate associations between functional small airway disease and lung function decline and is a promising radiographic biomarker for COPD progression [76].

Biomarker Discovery

A biomarker is broadly defined as a "measurement that is associated with, and believed to be pathophysiologically related to, a relevant clinical outcome" [77]. Although COPD-related biomarkers may be measured in blood, sputum, or bronchoalveolar lavage fluid, the greatest efforts have focused on the identification of blood biomarkers, given their accessibility. Such markers

have been proposed to define disease pathogenesis, determine prognosis and risk of disease progression, and to further classify individuals with COPD in terms of phenotypic heterogeneity, exacerbation risk, and anticipated response to therapy. Numerous studies report associations of blood biomarkers with COPD outcomes although many of these investigations are limited by only cross-sectional measurements or lack of consistency across cohorts [78], limiting translation to clinical practice. With the exception of fibrinogen, which has been qualified by the Food and Drug Administration as a prognostic biomarker to identify COPD patients at high risk for exacerbations and/or all-cause mortality in clinical trials [77], few blood biomarkers have emerged as single, consistent predictors of COPD outcomes. Interleukin-6 has been shown to improve mortality prediction when combined with clinical predictors [79], and both surfactant protein D (SPD) and soluble receptor for advanced glycation end-products (sRAGE) have generated interest as potential biomarkers for emphysema severity and progression [80, 81]. Some studies have suggested that panels of biomarkers may have greater predictive ability than any one biomarker in isolation [79, 82]. Despite a growing body of COPD biomarker research and the availability of increasingly sophisticated genetic and proteomic technologies, clinical uptake has been minimal.

One biomarker that has gained considerable attention for its promise in guiding clinical management of COPD is blood eosinophil count, which the most recent Global Initiative for Chronic Obstructive Lung Disease guidelines recommend considering when making decisions on the initiation or withdrawal of inhaled corticosteroids [12]. Multiple studies have shown that responsiveness to ICS in terms of acute exacerbation reduction associates with blood eosinophil count [83–89] with levels <100 per cubic milliliter associated with no benefit from ICS and ≥300 per cubic milliliter predictive of the greatest response [84]. Likewise, withdrawal of inhaled corticosteroids in COPD patients with infrequent exacerbations appears to be safest in those with eosinophil counts ≤300 per cubic milliliter [87, 89].

As would be anticipated, biologic therapies targeting key eosinophil cytokines, such as the interleukin-5 monoclonal antibody mepolizumab, have been associated with reduced annual rates of moderate or severe exacerbations in COPD patients with elevated eosinophil counts [90]. The need for further studies establishing efficacy, defining the optimal eosinophil threshold, and further characterizing the responsive patient phenotype has prevented FDA approval of mepolizumab therapy in eosinophilic COPD.

Computational Approaches to Disease Classification

The establishment of several large, longitudinal COPD cohorts in recent years has provided a wealth of physiologic, radiographic, and biologic data coupled with information regarding longitudinal outcomes, disease trajectory, and mortality.

Integrative computational approaches, in some instances, offer an advantage over standard statistical techniques when analyzing data from these cohorts in that they can assimilate large quantities of multimodal data and provide insight into the relationships between multiple, often dependent, variables [91] (Fig. 15.2). Distinct clusters based on clinical variables and inflammatory biomarker levels in smokers have been associated with important COPD outcomes, including hospitalizations and all-cause mortality [92]. Unsupervised clustering of blood microarray expression data has led to the identification of unique, clinically relevant molecular subtypes of COPD that were consistent across both the ECLIPSE and COPDGene study cohorts [93]. In an analysis by Sedgewick and colleagues, multiple sources of clinical, radiographic, and biologic data were combined to create mixed graphical models to provide insight into factors associated with lung function decline [33] (Fig. 15.2).

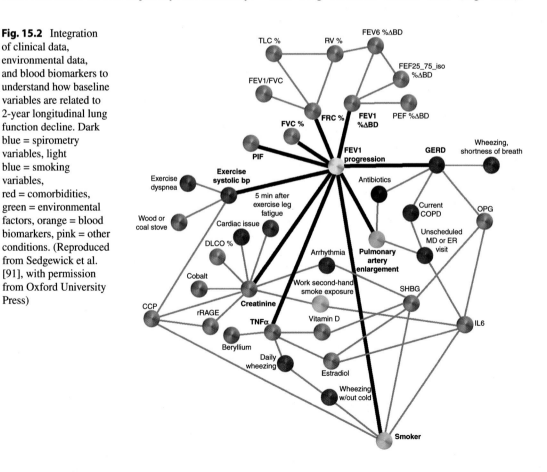

Fig. 15.2 Integration of clinical data, environmental data, and blood biomarkers to understand how baseline variables are related to 2-year longitudinal lung function decline. Dark blue = spirometry variables, light blue = smoking variables, red = comorbidities, green = environmental factors, orange = blood biomarkers, pink = other conditions. (Reproduced from Sedgewick et al. [91], with permission from Oxford University Press)

Further understanding of the pathogenesis of acute exacerbations of COPD and the associated risk factors has been garnered from cluster analyses of sputum and serum biomarkers as well as clinical variables [94, 95]. As computational approaches to rapidly accumulating epidemiologic data evolve, we anticipate further refinement of COPD classification with the development of precision-based management strategies that match distinct phenotypes to individualized therapy.

Selection for Lung Volume Reduction: A Case of Precision Medicine in Clinical Practice #1

A 50-year old female with severe radiographic emphysema and airflow obstruction is evaluated in a pulmonary clinic for persistent dyspnea and severe activity impairment. She is optimized on an inhaler regimen of long-acting beta agonist, long-acting muscarinic antagonist, and inhaled corticosteroids. She is currently attending pulmonary rehabilitation. Despite these therapies, she experiences dyspnea while performing her daily activities and asks if there are any further options. She is not interested in pursuing lung transplantation or other surgical alternatives.

The patient's pulmonary function tests reveal severe airflow obstruction with an FEV1 of 0.65 L (25% predicted). She has severe hyperinflation with a residual volume of 294% predicted and a residual volume to total lung capacity ratio of 0.75. Her diffusion capacity for carbon monoxide is reduced at 30% predicted. A review of her CT scan reveals severe confluent emphysema of the bilateral upper lung lobes with only moderate emphysema in the lower lobes. On visual inspection, the interlobar fissure of her left lung appears complete to the hilum while her right minor fissure is only 70% complete, and R major fissure 85% complete. Further evaluation for bronchoscopic lung volume reduction using endobronchial valve placement is offered.

Lung volume reduction surgery is a viable treatment option demonstrated to improve symptoms and exercise tolerance in individuals with severe emphysema and survival in the subset of individuals with upper lobe dominant emphysema and low exercise capacity [38]. While an acceptable treatment option for some, others, such as this patient, do not wish to undergo surgical management of their lung disease. Bronchoscopic lung volume reduction with the placement of endobronchial valves, to completely occlude the targeted lobe, results in targeted lobe volume reduction and expansion and better ventilation of the ipsilateral nontargeted lobe and is available to a select group of COPD patients with severe lung hyperinflation and heterogeneous emphysema. The initial endobronchial valve trials demonstrated a statistically, but not clinically, significant improvement in FEV1 and 6-minute walk distance [13]. However, subgroup analyses revealed that individuals with intact interlobar fissures, thought to be a surrogate for the absence of inter-lobar collateral airflow, had both a statically and clinically meaningful response to intervention. A subsequent multicenter, randomized controlled trial in this subset of patients showed similar improvement in FEV1, walk distance, and symptoms scores following valve placement [14], leading to recent FDA approval for clinical use.

The severity of airflow obstruction (FEV1 <45% predicted) and hyperinflation (RV >175% predicted), distribution of emphysema (heterogeneous upper lobe dominant), and presence of intact interlobar fissures in this patient suggests that she would be appropriate for bronchoscopic lung volume reduction. Should the patient have had incomplete fissures, indicating inter-lobar collateral channels, surgical lung volume reduction would have been the only option. This case is only one example of how clinical precision-based treatment of COPD already exists in clinical practice.

Alpha-1 Antitrypsin Deficiency: A Case of Precision Medicine in Clinical Practice #2

A 38-year old man was referred to a pulmonologist for evaluation of COPD. He has a 2-year history of progressive shortness of breath and frequent chest infections requiring multiple courses of antibiotics. He is a former smoker of one pack per day who quit 6 months ago. Post-bronchodilator spirometry reveals an obstructive FEV1/FVC ratio with an FEV1 of 43% predicted. On further questioning, he had a history of neonatal jaundice which was uncomplicated. His family history was notable as his mother died of emphysema at 62 years of age and his maternal uncle uses oxygen for emphysema. A chest X-ray demonstrated marked hyperinflation with evidence of basal predominant emphysema. Blood testing revealed a plasma alpha-1 antitrypsin level of 22 mg/dL (normal 100–220 mg/dL), and isoelectric focusing electrophoresis demonstrated a migration pattern consistent with the PiZZ phenotype (normal PiMM), thereby confirming the diagnosis of severe alpha-1 antitrypsin deficiency.

Identification of individuals affected by alpha-1 antitrypsin deficiency remains a major challenge as only a small proportion are detected in clinical practice [96]. Population-based screening is not cost effective though targeted detection strategies for high-risk individuals may be feasible [97, 98]. Due to the identification of a major causative genetic factor to account for the patient's presentation in this case, he received genetic counselling with regard to the autosomal dominant inheritance pattern of the pathogenic Z-allele, and his children and siblings were offered screening for the disease. Informing affected family members who harbor even a single disease allele is an opportunity to detect or prevent the later development of respiratory illness [99]. The patient was offered vaccination, commenced on maintenance dual LAMA/LABA bronchodilator therapy, and referred for pulmonary rehabilitation. Concurrently, he began administration of weekly intravenous human plasma-derived alpha-1 antitrypsin protein, that is, augmentation therapy, a precision therapy that restores plasma levels above a protective threshold and has been shown to slow emphysema progression in randomized controlled trials [65, 100].

Future Directions

The approach to characterizing COPD has evolved over the years from broadly classifying patients based on the presence of emphysema or chronic bronchitis to the identification of multiple, clinically relevant phenotypes. We now know that emphysema distribution and fissure integrity hold clinical implications for selection for surgical or bronchoscopic lung volume reduction [73, 101]. The use of eosinophil counts to direct inhaled corticosteroid therapy has been introduced in the most recent GOLD guidelines for COPD management [12]. Fibrinogen has been qualified as a predictive biomarker for exacerbation risk in COPD clinical trials [77]. However, while we have certainly made progress with COPD phenotyping, this area of research is in many ways still in its infancy as it pertains to clinical translation to precision-based medicine.

Future efforts should focus on further refinement and validation of phenotypes leveraging ongoing data collection from multiple longitudinal epidemiologic cohorts and increasingly sophisticated analysis techniques. In order to translate research findings into clinical practice, initiatives to identify clinically relevant thresholds, such as the eosinophil count most responsive to anti-IL5 therapy [90], should be undertaken. A greater understanding of specific disease phenotypes, for example, the frequent exacerbator or high comorbidity burden phenotypes, is needed to guide future preventative or comorbidity screening strategies, respectively. The translation of research-based radiographic phenotyping strategies to clinical practice will provide the opportunity to extract important, clinically relevant information regarding chronic lung disease as well as other comorbidities from chest CT imaging obtained in smokers undergoing lung cancer screening. Interventional trials are already underway and may continue to extend bronchoscopic approaches to include endobronchial amelioration of mucus production in chronic bronchitis. Only through these efforts and others can we truly achieve a precision-based approach to COPD management.

Key Point Summary

- The application of clinical precision medicine to accurately diagnose phenotypes of COPD is essential for the investigation, development, and delivery of beneficial therapies to populations at risk.
- Identification of frequent exacerbator and emphysema/hyperinflation phenotypes is of particular importance given the availability of precision treatments to ameliorate disease burden in these individuals.
- The application of an integrative approach to combine current physiological, radiographical, and clinical biomarkers with research initiatives that harness advances in basic science, genetics, and computational biology may delineate clinical phenotypes of COPD in the future.

References

1. Abboud RT, Vimalanathan S. Pathogenesis of COPD. Part I. The role of protease-antiprotease imbalance in emphysema [State of the Art Series. Chronic obstructive pulmonary disease in high- and low-income countries. Edited by G. Marks and M. Chan-Yeung. Number 3 in the series]. International Union Against Tuberculosis and Lung Disease; 2008.
2. Jha P, Ramasundarahettige C, Landsman V, Rostron B, Thun M, Anderson RN, et al. 21st-century hazards of smoking and benefits of cessation in the United States. N Engl J Med. 2013;368(4):341–50.
3. Harris HW, Meneely GR, Renzetti AD, Steele JD Jr, Wyatt JP. Chronic bronchitis, asthma, and pulmonary emphysema. Arch Environ Health. Routledge. 1962;5(4):375–82.
4. Petty TL. The history of COPD. Int J Chron Obstruct Pulmon Dis. 2006;1(1):3–14.
5. Calverley PMA, Rennard SI. What have we learned from large drug treatment trials in COPD? Lancet. 2007;370(9589):774–85.
6. Vestbo J, Hurd SS, Agustí AG, Jones PW, Vogelmeier C, Anzueto A, et al. Global strategy for the diagnosis, management, and prevention of chronic obstructive pulmonary disease: GOLD executive summary. Am J Respir Crit Care Med. 2013;187(4):347–65.
7. Laurell CB, Eriksson S. The electrophoretic α; 1-globulin pattern of serum in α; 1-antitrypsin deficiency. Scand J Clin Lab Invest. 1963;15(2):132–40.
8. Rennard SI. The promise of observational studies (ECLIPSE, SPIROMICS, and COPDGene) in achieving the goal of personalized treatment of chronic obstructive pulmonary disease. Semin Respir Crit Care Med. 2015;36(4):478–90.
9. Svanes C, Sunyer J, Plana E, Dharmage S, Heinrich J, Jarvis D, et al. Early life origins of chronic obstructive pulmonary disease. Thorax. BMJ Publishing Group Ltd. 2010;65(1):14–20.
10. De Soyza A, Calverley PMA. Large trials, new knowledge: the changing face of COPD management. Eur Respir J. 2015;45(6):1692–703.
11. Calverley PMA, Rabe KF, Goehring U-M, Kristiansen S, Fabbri LM, Martinez FJ, et al. Roflumilast in symptomatic chronic obstructive pulmonary disease: two randomised clinical trials. Lancet. 2009;374(9691):685–94.
12. Global strategy for the diagnosis, management and prevention of COPD, global initiative for chronic obstructive lung disease (GOLD). 2018. https://goldcoped.org/. Accessed 17 Nov 2018.
13. Kew KM, Seniukovich A. Inhaled steroids and risk of pneumonia for chronic obstructive pulmonary disease. Cochrane Database Syst Rev (Online). 2014;(3):CD010115.
14. Continuous or nocturnal oxygen therapy in hypoxemic chronic obstructive lung disease: a clinical trial. Nocturnal Oxygen Therapy Trial Group. Ann Intern Med. 1980;93(3):391–8.
15. Long term domiciliary oxygen therapy in chronic hypoxic cor pulmonale complicating chronic bronchitis and emphysema. Report of the Medical Research Council Working Party. Lancet. 1981;1(8222):681–6.
16. Long-Term Oxygen Treatment Trial Research Group, Albert RK, Au DH, Blackford AL, Casaburi R, Cooper JA, et al. A randomized trial of long-term oxygen for COPD with moderate desaturation. N Engl J Med. 2016;375(17):1617–27.
17. Rochester CL, Vogiatzis I, Holland AE, Lareau SC, Marciniuk DD, Puhan MA, et al. An official American Thoracic Society/European Respiratory Society policy statement: enhancing implementation, use, and delivery of pulmonary rehabilitation. Am J Respir Crit Care Med. 2015;192:1373–86.
18. Lacasse Y, Goldstein R, Lasserson TJ, Martin S. Pulmonary rehabilitation for chronic obstructive pulmonary disease. Cochrane Database Syst Rev (Online). 2006;(4):CD003793.
19. Puhan MA, Gimeno-Santos E, Cates CJ, Troosters T. Pulmonary rehabilitation following exacerbations of chronic obstructive pulmonary disease. Cochrane Database Syst Rev (Online). 2016;(12):CD005305.
20. Tan WC, Bourbeau J, Hernandez P, Chapman KR, Cowie R, FitzGerald JM, et al. Exacerbation-like respiratory symptoms in individuals without chronic obstructive pulmonary disease: results from

a population-based study. Thorax. BMJ Publishing Group Ltd. 2014;69(8):709–17.

21. Wan ES, Castaldi PJ, Cho MH, Hokanson JE, Regan EA, Make BJ, et al. Epidemiology, genetics, and subtyping of preserved ratio impaired spirometry (PRISm) in COPDGene. Respir Res. 2014;15:89.

22. Woodruff PG, Barr RG, Bleecker E, Christenson SA, Couper D, Curtis JL, et al. Clinical significance of symptoms in smokers with preserved pulmonary function. N Engl J Med. Massachusetts Medical Society. 2016;374(19):1811–21.

23. Tashkin DP, Altose MD, Bleecker ER, Connett JE, Kanner RE, Lee WW, et al. The lung health study: airway responsiveness to inhaled methacholine in smokers with mild to moderate airflow limitation. The Lung Health Study Research Group. Am Rev Respir Dis. 1992;145(2 Pt 1):301–10.

24. van den Berge M, Vonk JM, Gosman M, Lapperre TS, Snoeck-Stroband JB, Sterk PJ, et al. Clinical and inflammatory determinants of bronchial hyperresponsiveness in COPD. Eur Respir J. 2012;40(5):1098–105.

25. Tashkin DP, Altose MD, Connett JE, Kanner RE, Lee WW, Wise RA. Methacholine reactivity predicts changes in lung function over time in smokers with early chronic obstructive pulmonary disease. The Lung Health Study Research Group. Am J Respir Crit Care Med. 1996;153(6 Pt 1):1802–11.

26. Vestbo J, Hansen EF. Airway hyperresponsiveness and COPD mortality. Thorax. 2001;56(Suppl 2):ii11–4.

27. Postma DS, Rabe KF. The asthma-COPD overlap syndrome. N Engl J Med. 2015;373(13):1241–9.

28. Barrecheguren M, Esquinas C, Miravitlles M. The asthma-chronic obstructive pulmonary disease overlap syndrome (ACOS): opportunities and challenges. Curr Opin Pulm Med. 2015;21(1):74–9.

29. Hurst JR, Vestbo J, Anzueto A, Locantore N, Müllerova H, Tal-Singer R, et al. Susceptibility to exacerbation in chronic obstructive pulmonary disease. N Engl J Med. 2010;363(12):1128–38.

30. Pasquale MK, Sun SX, Song F, Hartnett HJ, Stemkowski SA. Impact of exacerbations on health care cost and resource utilization in chronic obstructive pulmonary disease patients with chronic bronchitis from a predominantly Medicare population. COPD. 2012;7:757–64.

31. Wedzicha JA, Miravitlles M, Hurst JR, Calverley PMA, Albert RK, Anzueto A, et al. Management of COPD exacerbations: a European Respiratory Society/American Thoracic Society guideline. Eur Respir J. 2017;49(3):1600791.

32. Niewoehner DE, Rice K, Cote C, Paulson D, Cooper JAD, Korducki L, et al. Prevention of exacerbations of chronic obstructive pulmonary disease with tiotropium, a once-daily inhaled anticholinergic bronchodilator: a randomized trial. Ann Intern Med. 2005;143(5):317–26.

33. Kardos P, Wencker M, Glaab T, Vogelmeier C. Impact of salmeterol/fluticasone propionate versus salmeterol on exacerbations in severe chronic obstructive pulmonary disease. Am J Respir Crit Care Med. 2007;175(2):144–9.

34. Wedzicha JA, Calverley PMA, Seemungal TA, Hagan G, Ansari Z, Stockley RA, et al. The prevention of chronic obstructive pulmonary disease exacerbations by salmeterol/fluticasone propionate or tiotropium bromide. Am J Respir Crit Care Med. 2008;177(1):19–26.

35. Fabbri LM, Calverley PMA, Izquierdo-Alonso JL, Bundschuh DS, Brose M, Martinez FJ, et al. Roflumilast in moderate-to-severe chronic obstructive pulmonary disease treated with longacting bronchodilators: two randomised clinical trials. Lancet. 2009;374(9691):695–703.

36. Leuppi JD, Schuetz P, Bingisser R, Bodmer M, Briel M, Drescher T, et al. Short-term vs conventional glucocorticoid therapy in acute exacerbations of chronic obstructive pulmonary disease: the REDUCE randomized clinical trial. JAMA. American Medical Association. 2013;309(21):2223–31.

37. Han MK, Quibrera PM, Carretta EE, Barr RG, Bleecker ER, Bowler RP, et al. Frequency of exacerbations in patients with chronic obstructive pulmonary disease: an analysis of the SPIROMICS cohort. Lancet Respir Med. 2017;5(8):619–26.

38. Sin DD, Anthonisen NR, Soriano JB, Agusti AG. Mortality in COPD: role of comorbidities. Eur Respir J. 2006;28(6):1245–57.

39. Chatila WM, Thomashow BM, Minai OA, Criner GJ, Make BJ. Comorbidities in chronic obstructive pulmonary disease. Proc Am Thorac Soc. 2008;5(4):549–55.

40. MacNee W. Pathophysiology of cor pulmonale in chronic obstructive pulmonary disease. Part one. Am J Respir Crit Care Med. 1994;150(3):833–52.

41. Hill K, Geist R, Goldstein RS, Lacasse Y. Anxiety and depression in end-stage COPD. Eur Respir J. 2008;31(3):667–77.

42. Barnes PJ, Celli BR. Systemic manifestations and comorbidities of COPD. Eur Respir J. 2009;33(5):1165–85.

43. Schols AMWJ. Pulmonary cachexia. Int J Cardiol. 2002;85(1):101–10.

44. Bernard S, LeBlanc P, Whittom F, Carrier G, Jobin J, Belleau R, et al. Peripheral muscle weakness in patients with chronic obstructive pulmonary disease. Am J Respir Crit Care Med. 1998;158(2):629–34.

45. Allaire J, Maltais F, Doyon JF, Noël M, LeBlanc P, Carrier G, et al. Peripheral muscle endurance and the oxidative profile of the quadriceps in patients with COPD. Thorax. 2004;59(8):673–8.

46. Gosselink R, Troosters T, Decramer M. Peripheral muscle weakness contributes to exercise limitation in COPD. Am J Respir Crit Care Med. 1996;153(3):976–80.

47. Gosker HR, Zeegers MP, Wouters EFM, Schols AMWJ. Muscle fibre type shifting in the vastus lateralis of patients with COPD is associated with disease severity: a systematic review and meta-analysis. Thorax. 2007;62(11):944–9.

48. Marquis K, Debigaré R, Lacasse Y, LeBlanc P, Jobin J, Carrier G, et al. Midthigh muscle cross-sectional area is a better predictor of mortality than body mass index in patients with chronic obstructive pulmonary disease. Am J Respir Crit Care Med. 2002;166(6):809–13.

49. Patel MS, Natanek SA, Stratakos G, Pascual S, Martínez-Llorens J, Disano L, et al. Vastus lateralis fiber shift is an independent predictor of mortality in chronic obstructive pulmonary disease. Am J Respir Crit Care Med. 2014;190(3):350–2.

50. Agusti A, Calverley PMA, Celli B, Coxson HO, Edwards LD, Lomas DA, et al. Characterisation of COPD heterogeneity in the ECLIPSE cohort. Respir Res. 2010;11:122.

51. Schols AMWJ, Broekhuizen R, Weling-Scheepers CA, Wouters EF. Body composition and mortality in chronic obstructive pulmonary disease. Am J Clin Nutr. 2005;82(1):53–9.

52. Diaz AA, Zhou L, Young TP, McDonald M-L, Harmouche R, Ross JC, et al. Chest CT measures of muscle and adipose tissue in COPD: gender-based differences in content and in relationships with blood biomarkers. Acad Radiol. 2014;21(10):1255–61.

53. McDonald M-LN, Diaz AA, Ross JC, San José Estépar R, Zhou L, Regan EA, et al. Quantitative computed tomography measures of pectoralis muscle area and disease severity in chronic obstructive pulmonary disease. A cross-sectional study. Ann Am Thorac Soc. 2014;11(3):326–34.

54. McDonald M-LN, Diaz AA, Rutten E, Lutz SM, Harmouche R, San José Estépar R, et al. Chest computed tomography-derived low fat-free mass index and mortality in COPD. Eur Respir J. 2017;50(6):1701134.

55. Vogiatzis I, Simoes DCM, Stratakos G, Kourepini E, Terzis G, Manta P, et al. Effect of pulmonary rehabilitation on muscle remodelling in cachectic patients with COPD. Eur Respir J. 2010;36(2):301–10.

56. Jones SE, Maddocks M, Kon SSC, Canavan JL, Nolan CM, Clark AL, et al. Sarcopenia in COPD: prevalence, clinical correlates and response to pulmonary rehabilitation. Thorax. 2015;70(3):213–8.

57. Cohen S, Nathan JA, Goldberg AL. Muscle wasting in disease: molecular mechanisms and promising therapies. Nat Rev Drug Discov. 2015;14(1):58–74.

58. Martinez FJ, Donohue JF, Rennard SI. The future of chronic obstructive pulmonary disease treatment--difficulties of and barriers to drug development. Lancet. 2011;378(9795):1027–37.

59. Agusti A, Sobradillo P, Celli B. Addressing the complexity of chronic obstructive pulmonary disease: from phenotypes and biomarkers to scale-free networks, systems biology, and P4 medicine. Am J Respir Crit Care Med. 2011;183(9):1129–37.

60. Müller NL, Staples CA, Miller RR, Abboud RT. "Density mask." An objective method to quantitate emphysema using computed tomography. Chest. 1988;94(4):782–7.

61. Gevenois PA, de Maertelaer V, De Vuyst P, Zanen J, Yernault JC. Comparison of computed density and macroscopic morphometry in pulmonary emphysema. Am J Respir Crit Care Med. 1995;152(2):653–7.

62. Gevenois PA, De Vuyst P, de Maertelaer V, Zanen J, Jacobovitz D, Cosio MG, et al. Comparison of computed density and microscopic morphometry in pulmonary emphysema. Am J Respir Crit Care Med. 1996;154(1):187–92.

63. Kinsella M, Müller NL, Abboud RT, Morrison NJ, DyBuncio A. Quantitation of emphysema by computed tomography using a "density mask" program and correlation with pulmonary function tests. Chest. 1990;97(2):315–21.

64. Nakano Y, Sakai H, Muro S, Hirai T, Oku Y, Nishimura K, et al. Comparison of low attenuation areas on computed tomographic scans between inner and outer segments of the lung in patients with chronic obstructive pulmonary disease: incidence and contribution to lung function. Thorax. 1999;54(5):384–9.

65. Chapman KR, Burdon JGW, Piitulainen E, Sandhaus RA, Seersholm N, Stocks JM, et al. Intravenous augmentation treatment and lung density in severe α1 antitrypsin deficiency (RAPID): a randomised, double-blind, placebo-controlled trial. Lancet. 2015;386(9991):360–8.

66. McNamara AE, Müller NL, Okazawa M, Arntorp J, Wiggs BR, Paré PD. Airway narrowing in excised canine lungs measured by high-resolution computed tomography. J Appl Physiol. 1992;73(1):307–16.

67. Amirav I, Kramer SS, Grunstein MM, Hoffman EA. Assessment of methacholine-induced airway constriction by ultrafast high-resolution computed tomography. J Appl Physiol. 1993;75(5):2239–50.

68. Okazawa M, Müller N, McNamara AE, Child S, Verburgt L, Paré PD. Human airway narrowing measured using high resolution computed tomography. Am J Respir Crit Care Med. 1996;154(5):1557–62.

69. McNitt-Gray MF, Goldin JG, Johnson TD, Tashkin DP, Aberle DR. Development and testing of image-processing methods for the quantitative assessment of airway hyperresponsiveness from high-resolution CT images. J Comput Assist Tomogr. 1997;21(6):939–47.

70. Martinez CH, Chen Y-H, Westgate PM, Liu LX, Murray S, Curtis JL, et al. Relationship between quantitative CT metrics and health status and BODE in chronic obstructive pulmonary disease. Thorax. 2012;67(5):399–406.

71. Boueiz A, Chang Y, Cho MH, Washko GR, San José Estépar R, Bowler RP, et al. Lobar emphysema distribution is associated with 5-year radiological disease progression. Chest. 2018;153(1):65–76.

72. Sciurba FC, Ernst A, Herth FJF, Strange C, Criner GJ, Marquette CH, et al. A randomized study of endobronchial valves for advanced emphysema. N Engl J Med. 2010;363(13):1233–44.

73. Criner GJ, Sue R, Wright S, Dransfield M, Rivas-Perez H, Wiese T, et al. A multicenter randomized controlled trial of Zephyr endobronchial valve treatment in heterogeneous emphysema (LIBERATE). Am J Respir Crit Care Med. 2018 ed. 2018;198(9):1151–64.

74. Hogg JC, McDonough JE, Suzuki M. Small airway obstruction in COPD: new insights based on micro-CT imaging and MRI imaging. Chest. 2013;143(5):1436–43.

75. Galbán CJ, Han MK, Boes JL, Chughtai KA, Meyer CR, Johnson TD, et al. Computed tomography-based biomarker provides unique signature for diagnosis of COPD phenotypes and disease progression. Nat Med. 2012;18(11):1711–5.

76. Bhatt SP, Soler X, Wang X, Murray S, Anzueto AR, Beaty TH, et al. Association between functional small airway disease and FEV1 decline in chronic obstructive pulmonary disease. Am J Respir Crit Care Med. 2016;194(2):178–84.

77. Mannino DM, Tal-Singer R, Lomas DA, Vestbo J, Graham Barr R, Tetzlaff K, et al. Plasma fibrinogen as a biomarker for mortality and hospitalized exacerbations in people with COPD. Chronic Obstr Pulm Dis. 2015;2(1):23–34.

78. Keene JD, Jacobson S, Kechris K, Kinney GL, Foreman MG, Doerschuk CM, et al. Biomarkers predictive of exacerbations in the SPIROMICS and COPDGene cohorts. Am J Respir Crit Care Med. 3rd ed. American Thoracic Society. 2017;195(4):473–81.

79. Celli BR, Locantore N, Yates J, Tal-Singer R, Miller BE, Bakke P, et al. Inflammatory biomarkers improve clinical prediction of mortality in chronic obstructive pulmonary disease. Am J Respir Crit Care Med. 2012;185(10):1065–72.

80. Cheng DT, Kim DK, Cockayne DA, Belousov A, Bitter H, Cho MH, et al. Systemic soluble receptor for advanced glycation endproducts is a biomarker of emphysema and associated with AGER genetic variants in patients with chronic obstructive pulmonary disease. Am J Respir Crit Care Med. 2013;188(8):948–57.

81. Coxson HO, Dirksen A, Edwards LD, Yates JC, Agusti A, Bakke P, et al. The presence and progression of emphysema in COPD as determined by CT scanning and biomarker expression: a prospective analysis from the ECLIPSE study. Lancet Respir Med. 2013;1(2):129–36.

82. Zemans RL, Jacobson S, Keene J, Kechris K, Miller BE, Tal-Singer R, et al. Multiple biomarkers predict disease severity, progression and mortality in COPD. Respir Res. 2017;18(1):117.

83. Lipson DA, Barnhart F, Brealey N, Brooks J, Criner GJ, Day NC, et al. Once-daily single-inhaler triple versus dual therapy in patients with COPD. N Engl J Med. 2018;378(18):1671–80.

84. Bafadhel M, Peterson S, De Blas MA, Calverley PM, Rennard SI, Richter K, et al. Predictors of exacerbation risk and response to budesonide in patients with chronic obstructive pulmonary disease: a post-hoc analysis of three randomised trials. Lancet Respir Med. 2018;6(2):117–26.

85. Siddiqui SH, Guasconi A, Vestbo J, Jones P, Agusti A, Paggiaro P, et al. Blood eosinophils: a biomarker of response to extrafine beclomethasone/formoterol in chronic obstructive pulmonary disease. Am J Respir Crit Care Med. 2015;192(4):523–5.

86. Papi A, Vestbo J, Fabbri L, Corradi M, Prunier H, Cohuet G, et al. Extrafine inhaled triple therapy versus dual bronchodilator therapy in chronic obstructive pulmonary disease (TRIBUTE): a double-blind, parallel group, randomised controlled trial. Lancet. 2018;391(10125):1076–84.

87. Watz H, Tetzlaff K, Wouters EFM, Kirsten A, Magnussen H, Rodriguez-Roisin R, et al. Blood eosinophil count and exacerbations in severe chronic obstructive pulmonary disease after withdrawal of inhaled corticosteroids: a post-hoc analysis of the WISDOM trial. Lancet Respir Med. 2016;4(5):390–8.

88. Calverley PMA, Tetzlaff K, Vogelmeier C, Fabbri LM, Magnussen H, Wouters EFM, et al. Eosinophilia, frequent exacerbations, and steroid response in chronic obstructive pulmonary disease. Am J Respir Crit Care Med. 2017;196(9):1219–21.

89. Chapman KR, Hurst JR, Frent S-M, Larbig M, Fogel R, Guerin T, et al. Long-term triple therapy de-escalation to indacaterol/glycopyrronium in patients with chronic obstructive pulmonary disease (SUNSET): a randomized, double-blind, triple-dummy clinical trial. Am J Respir Crit Care Med. 2018;198(3):329–39.

90. Pavord ID, Chanez P, Criner GJ, Kerstjens HAM, Korn S, Lugogo N, et al. Mepolizumab for eosinophilic chronic obstructive pulmonary disease. N Engl J Med. 2017;377(17):1613–29.

91. Sedgewick AJ, Buschur K, Shi I, Ramsey JD, Raghu VK, Manatakis DV, et al. Mixed graphical models for integrative causal analysis with application to chronic lung disease diagnosis and prognosis. Wren J, editor. Bioinformatics. 2018;183:1129.

92. Rennard SI, Locantore N, Delafont B, Tal-Singer R, Silverman EK, Vestbo J, et al. Identification of five chronic obstructive pulmonary disease subgroups with different prognoses in the ECLIPSE cohort using cluster analysis. Ann Am Thorac Soc. 2015;12(3):303–12.

93. Chang Y, Glass K, Liu Y-Y, Silverman EK, Crapo JD, Tal-Singer R, et al. COPD subtypes identified by network-based clustering of blood gene expression. Genomics. 2016;107(2–3):51–8.

94. Bafadhel M, McKenna S, Terry S, Mistry V, Reid C, Haldar P, et al. Acute exacerbations of chronic obstructive pulmonary disease: identification of biologic clusters and their biomarkers. Am J Respir Crit Care Med. 2011;184(6):662–71.

95. Le Rouzic O, Roche N, Cortot AB, Tillie-Leblond I, Masure F, Perez T, et al. Defining the "frequent exacerbator" phenotype in COPD: a hypothesis-free approach. Chest. 2018;153(5):1106–15.

96. Aboussouan LS, Stoller JK. Detection of alpha-1 antitrypsin deficiency: a review. Respir Med. 2009;103(3):335–41.

97. Gildea TR, Shermock KM, Singer ME, Stoller JK. Cost-effectiveness analysis of augmentation therapy for severe alpha1-antitrypsin deficiency. Am J Respir Crit Care Med. 2003;167(10):1387–92.

98. Bals R, Koczulla R, Kotke V, Andress J, Blackert K, Vogelmeier C. Identification of individuals with alpha-1-antitrypsin deficiency by a targeted screening program. Respir Med. 2007;101(8):1708–14.

99. Molloy K, Hersh CP, Morris VB, Carroll TP, O'Connor CA, Lasky-Su JA, et al. Clarification of the risk of chronic obstructive pulmonary disease in α1-antitrypsin deficiency PiMZ heterozygotes. Am J Respir Crit Care Med. 2014; 189(4):419–27.

100. McElvaney NG, Burdon J, Holmes M, Glanville A, Wark PAB, Thompson PJ, et al. Long-term efficacy and safety of α1 proteinase inhibitor treatment for emphysema caused by severe α1 antitrypsin deficiency: an open-label extension trial (RAPID-OLE). Lancet Respir Med. 2017;5(1):51–60.

101. Fishman A, Martinez F, Naunheim K, Piantadosi S, Wise R, Ries A, et al. A randomized trial comparing lung-volume-reduction surgery with medical therapy for severe emphysema. N Engl J Med. 2003;348(21):2059–73.

Precision Medicine in Pulmonary Hypertension

Inderjit Singh, William M. Oldham, and Farbod Nick Rahaghi

Introduction

Pulmonary hypertension (PH) is defined by an elevated mean pulmonary arterial pressure of greater than or equal to 25 mmHg at rest as measured by pulmonary arterial catheterization. Importantly, this hemodynamic criterion incorporates a heterogeneous group of diseases characterized by distinct etiologies, pathophysiologies, and management strategies. Currently, patients diagnosed with PH are subclassified into one of five World Health Organization (WHO) groups on the basis of hemodynamic measurements and medical comorbidities (Table 16.1). Regardless of the underlying etiology, elevated pulmonary artery pressures confer an increased risk of morbidity and mortality [1].

WHO Group 1 pulmonary arterial hypertension (PAH) is defined clinically by an elevated pulmonary vascular resistance and pathologically as a primary pulmonary vasculopathy resulting from a number of complex pathophysiologic processes (Table 16.1). Despite recent therapeutic advances, the prognosis of PAH remains poor [2] which likely reflects, in part, delayed detection of the disease [3] and, in part, the heterogeneity of the underlying pathophysiology. Indeed, the current clinical classification scheme places all PAH patients together into the same treatment algorithm whether the cause is heritable, toxin-induced, or associated with connective tissue disease (Table 16.1). While the notion of precision medicine in pulmonary vascular disease dates to the recognition of the value of pulmonary vasodilator testing in selection of patients for calcium channel blocker therapy, the future diagnosis and management of patients with pulmonary vascular disease will rely on a more sophisticated diagnostic and treatment paradigms based on each patient's disease phenotype. This chapter reviews the evolving approaches to subphenotype patients with PH based on clinical, imaging, and molecular signatures that will form the basis of personalized clinical classification schemes and management strategies.

Resting Hemodynamic Phenotyping

All patients suspected of having PH should be referred for pulmonary arterial catheterization for diagnosis. Pulmonary arterial catheterization allows direct measurements of pulmonary artery

I. Singh (✉)
Division of Pulmonary, Critical Care and Sleep Medicine, Division of Applied Hemodynamics, Yale New Haven Hospital, New Haven, CT, USA
e-mail: Inderjit.singh@yale.edu

W. M. Oldham · F. N. Rahaghi
Division of Pulmonary and Critical Care Medicine, Brigham and Women's Hospital, Boston, MA, USA
e-mail: woldham@bwh.harvard.edu; frahaghi@bwh.harvard.edu

© Springer Nature Switzerland AG 2020
J. L. Gomez et al. (eds.), *Precision in Pulmonary, Critical Care, and Sleep Medicine*, Respiratory Medicine, https://doi.org/10.1007/978-3-030-31507-8_16

Table 16.1 Comprehensive clinical classification of pulmonary hypertension

1. Pulmonary arterial hypertension

1.1 Idiopathic

1.2 Heritable

    1.2.1 BMPR2 mutation

    1.2.2 Other mutations

1.3 Drug and toxins induced

1.4 Associated with:

    1.4.1 Connective tissue disease

    1.4.2 Human immunodeficiency virus (HIV) infection

    1.4.3 Portal hypertension

    1.4.4 Congenital heart disease

    1.4.5 Schistosomiasis

1′. Pulmonary veno-occlusive disease and/or pulmonary capillary hemangiomatosis

1′.1 Idiopathic

1′.2 Heritable

    1′.2.1 EIF2AK4 mutation

    1′.2.2 Other mutations

1′.3 Drugs, toxins, and radiation induced

1′.4 Associated with:

    1′.4.1 Connective tissue disease

    1′.4.2 Human immunodeficiency virus (HIV) infection

1″. Persistent pulmonary hypertension of the newborn

2. Pulmonary hypertension due to left heart disease

2.1 Left ventricular systolic dysfunction

2.2 Left ventricular diastolic dysfunction

2.3 Valvular disease

2.4 Congenital/acquired left heart inflow/outflow tract obstruction and congenital cardiomyopathies

2.4 Congenital/acquired pulmonary vein stenosis

3. Pulmonary hypertension due to lung disease and/or hypoxia

3.1 Chronic obstructive pulmonary disease

3.2 Interstitial lung disease

3.3 Other pulmonary diseases with mixed restrictive and obstructive pattern

3.4 Sleep disordered breathing

3.5 Alveolar hypoventilation disorder

3.6 Chronic exposure to high altitude

3.7 Developmental lung disease

4. Chronic thromboembolic pulmonary hypertension and other pulmonary artery obstructions

4.1 Chronic thromboembolic pulmonary hypertension

4.2 Other pulmonary artery obstructions

    4.2.1 Angiosarcoma

    4.2.2 Other intra-vascular tumors

    4.2.3 Arteritis

    4.2.4 Congenital pulmonary artery stenoses

    4.2.5 Parasites (hydatidosis)

5. Pulmonary hypertension with unclear and/or multifactorial mechanisms

5.1 Hematological disorders: chronic hemolytic anemia, myeloproliferative disorders, splenectomy

5.2 Systemic disorders: sarcoidosis, pulmonary histiocytosis, lymphangioleiomyomatosis, neurofibromatosis

5.3 Metabolic disorders: glycogen storage disorders, Gaucher disease, thyroid disorders

5.4 Others: pulmonary tumor thrombotic microangiopathy, fibrosing mediastinitis, chronic renal failure (with/without dialysis), segmental pulmonary hypertension

BMPR2 bone morphogenetic protein receptor, type 2, *EIFK2A4* eukaryotic translation initiation factor 2 alpha kinase 4, *HIV* human immunodeficiency virus

pressures from which the mean pulmonary artery pressure (mPAP), left atrial filling pressures by balloon occlusion of distal pulmonary arteries (pulmonary artery wedge pressure [PAWP]), and cardiac output (CO) by thermodilution or the Fick equation are determined. From these parameters, the pulmonary vascular resistance (PVR) may be calculated according to the ohmic Starling resistor model [4]:

$$PVR = \frac{\text{Mean pulmonary artery pressure} - \text{PA wedge pressure}(PAWP)}{\text{Cardiac output}(CO)} \qquad (a)$$

Pulmonary arterial hypertension (PAH) is defined by both an increased mPAP and an increased PVR >3 Wood units. Increased PVR is a consequence of proliferative remodeling of the small pulmonary arterial resistance vessels [5]. This remodeling process involves all three layers of the vessel wall (intima, media, and adventitia) and is the consequence of cellular hypertrophy, hyperplasia, inflammation, abnormal cellular metabolism, defects in cellular differentiation and apoptosis, excessive migration, and accumulation of extracellular matrix components [6]. This pro-proliferative and anti-apoptotic phenotype reduces vessel distensibility and causes luminal narrowing, impairing the ability of pulmonary vasculature to accommodate increases in pulmonary blood flow.

Once the diagnosis of PAH is made during pulmonary arterial catheterization study, all patients undergo vasoreactivity testing. This involves the acute administration of a short-acting pulmonary arterial vasodilator such as inhaled nitric oxide or intravenous adenosine followed by repeat measurement of the hemodynamic response. Patients are considered vasoreactive if, following acute vasodilator testing, there is a reduction in mPAP by 10 mmHg to a value less than 40 mmHg with an increase or no change in cardiac output [7]. The main purpose of vasoreactivity testing is to identify a phenotype of PAH patients who are candidates for calcium channel blocker therapy. The use of calcium channel blockers in PAH is associated with a significant survival benefit compared to patients who are not vasoreactive [8].

The diagnosis of PH due to left heart disease (WHO Group 2) is defined by both an increased mPAP greater than or equal to 25 mmHg and a PAWP greater than or equal to 15 mmHg. Hemodynamic phenotyping in PH due to left heart disease is challenging because of the uncertainty surrounding the best measure to differentiate between isolated retrograde transmission of elevated PAWP, known as passive or isolated post-capillary PH (IpC-PH), and the concomitant development of pre-capillary pulmonary vascular disease, known as combined pre- and post-capillary PH (CpC-PH) [9–11].

Why is the distinction between Ipc-PH and Cpc-PH important? One of the major determinants of the poor outcome observed in patients with PH due to left heart disease is the presence of RV dysfunction [12]. Patients with CpC-PH are more likely to have a significantly higher RV afterload that is comparable to patients with idiopathic PAH [13] and have worse RV function compared to their IpC-PH counterparts [14]. Therefore, the ability to distinctly phenotype and ascertain the relative contributions of PAWP (or pulsatile RV afterload) and PVR (or resistive RV afterload) is an intriguing prospect that would allow for dedicated interventions directed at either the left heart or the remodeled pre-capillary pulmonary vasculature. However, the use of PAH-specific therapies in PH due to left heart disease thus far has yielded mixed results [15–18].

There have been a number of hemodynamic parameters implemented to help distinguish between IpC-PH and CpC-PH. These include the trans-pulmonary gradient (i.e., TPG = mean pulmonary artery pressure – PAWP) and the diastolic pressure gradient (i.e., DPG = diastolic pulmonary artery pressure – PAWP). In the setting of IpC-PH, the elevated PAWP can spuriously increase the TPG without any coexistent pulmonary vascular remodeling or vasoconstriction [19]. The DPG, therefore, may be more preferable as it is less sensitive to changes in PA compliance, stroke volume, and PAWP [19]. However, studies utilizing DPG for a diagnosis of CpC-PH have yielded mixed prognostic results. These discrepancies can be explained by inaccuracies in the measurement of diastolic pulmonary arterial pressure owing to motion artifacts, the influence of large v-waves on DPG values, and insufficient or excessive flushing of the fluid-filled catheter system [19, 20]. Previous studies have shown that PVR strongly predicts outcomes in PH due to left heart disease [21, 22]. Accordingly, recent guidelines have reincorporated PVR into the CpC-PH definition. In the latest iteration of the European Society of Cardiology / European Respiratory Society guidelines, CpC-PH was defined as DPG ≥7 mmHg, mPAP ≥25 mmHg, and PVR >3 Wood units (WU) [10].

Exercise Hemodynamic Phenotyping

Exercise intolerance is one of the earliest manifestations of PAH, and reduced exercise capacity has important implications for prognosis and mortality in PAH [23]. Since the essential stress of exercise imposed on the pulmonary circulation is an increase in pulmonary blood flow, provocative testing such as the cardiopulmonary exercise test (CPET) is able to demonstrate early [24–28] and reproducible [29, 30] abnormalities seen in PH. Additionally, factors that contribute to exercise intolerance in PAH are not simply confined to the central cardiopulmonary system and include peripheral factors such as impaired mitochondrial and respiratory muscle function (Fig. 16.1). In fact, pharmacotherapies such as dicholoroacetate [31] and ranolazine [32] that restitute mitochondrial oxidative metabolism have shown promise in the management of PAH.

CPET provides a comprehensive and dynamic assessment, integrating the cardiovascular, pulmonary, muscular, and cellular oxidative metabolism systems during exercise. The two modalities of CPET are noninvasive (niCPET) and invasive CPET (iCPET). The former is equipped with continuous 12-lead electrocardiogram, cuff blood pressure monitoring, breath-by-breath gas exchange assessment, and pulse oximetry while the latter also includes systemic and pulmonary arterial catheters for continuous systemic and pulmonary arterial, and right ventricular (RV) pressure measurements as well as intermittent measurement of PAWP [33]. Combining exercise

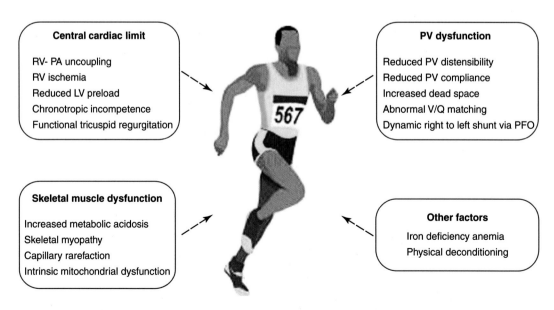

Fig. 16.1 Factors implicated in exercise intolerance in patients with pulmonary arterial hypertension (PAH). RV right ventricle, PA pulmonary artery, PV pulmonary vascular, V/Q ventilation/perfusion, PFO patent foramen ovale

hemodynamics with CPET is gaining prominence, particularly for its ability to potentially identify with early pulmonary vascular disease such as exercise PH.

Exercise PH is increasingly being recognized as an early phase of PH that is a potential target for PAH-specific therapy [34–36] (Table 16.2). Although further studies are needed to refine its diagnosis, exercise PH has been shown to be a major risk factor for the development of PAH in patients with systemic sclerosis [27, 28] and in healthy carriers of the bone morphogenetic receptor-2 (*BMPR2*) mutation [38]. In addition, patients with systemic sclerosis and exercise PH have a similarly reduced transplant-free survival compared to patients with established PAH [26].

Exercise PH is typically diagnosed in patients with exertional dyspnea or exercise intolerance without obvious underlying pulmonary or cardiac etiology. In patients with exercise PH, the data gathered from iCPET demonstrates an inverse relationship between the slope of mPAP-CO with a depressed maximal O_2 uptake, suggesting impaired RV adaptation to increasing afterload with resulting reduced aerobic exercise capacity [39]. Recently, cumulative evidence from invasive as well as noninvasive studies have shown that the slope of linearized mPAP–CO relationship should not exceed 3 mmHg.L^{-1}.min^{-1}. Hence, an mPAP/CO slope of >3 mmHg.L^{-1}.min^{-1} may be used to define exercise PH (Fig. 16.2). Similarly, a PAWP/CO slope of 2 mmHg/L/min can be used to define the potential contribution from left-sided heart disease [40, 41].

CPET can also be used to extract individualized parameters related to pulmonary vascular remodeling. Using CPET, the ability of the pulmonary vasculature to distend and accommodate the ejected RV stroke volume can be quantified by estimating the resistive vessel distensibility coefficient, α [42]. α or pulmonary distensibility is an intrinsic mechanical property of the vasculature and is defined as the percent change in vessel diameter per unit mmHg increase in distending pressure. By including different pressure and flow measurements during exercise, this assessment of pulmonary vascular distensibility accounts for the significant variation in pulmonary pressures and flow encountered during exercise [42]:

Table 16.2 Summary of studies evaluating exercise pulmonary hypertension

Study (Author, year)	Studied population	No. of patients	ePH Definition	Main findings
Oliveira et al., [37]	Borderline PH (mPAP 21–24 mmHg)	35 ePH 224 non-PH	≤50 years old: peak mPAP >30 mmHg and peak PVR >1.34 WU >50 years old: peak mPAP >33 mmHg and peak PVR >2.10 WU	ePH is common in borderline PH (27%) and its presence substantially affects aerobic exercise capacity
Tolle et al., 2008 [24]	Unexplained dyspnea who have ePH	78 ePH 15 PAH 16 non-PH	mPAP >30 mmHg	ePH has reduced peak exercise aerobic capacity compared to controls
Condliffe et al., [28]	SSc	42 ePH 259 PAH	mPAP >30 mmHg with mPAP/CO >3 mmHg/min/L^{-1} and PAWP <20 mmHg	14% of ePH patients died within 3 years of diagnosis with a 3-year survival rate of 86%. 19% of ePH patients progressed to over PAH
Stamm et al., 2016 [26]	SSc	17 PAH 28 ePH 27 non-PH	mPAP >30 mmHg with mPAP/CO >3 mmHg/min/L^{-1} and PAWP <20 mmHg	ePH associated with reduced survival and abnormal exercise hemodynamics rather than resting hemodynamics predicts transplant-free survival

PH pulmonary hypertension, *mPAP* mean pulmonary arterial pressure, *PVR* pulmonary vascular resistance, *ePH* exercise pulmonary hypertension, *PAH* pulmonary arterial hypertension, *SSc* systemic sclerosis

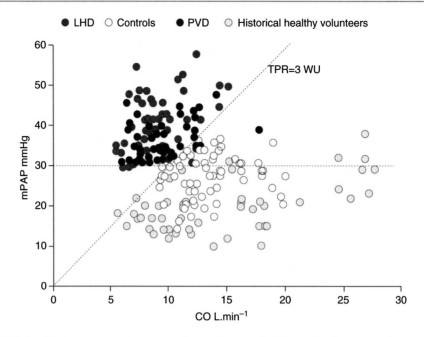

Fig. 16.2 Relationship between exercise mean pulmonary artery pressure (mPAP) and cardiac output (CO). Individual data points represent mPAP and CO reached at maximal exercise stratified by subjects with pulmonary vascular disease (PVD), left heart disease (LHD), control subjects and historical healthy volunteers. It can be seen that the total pulmonary resistance (TPR) line with a slope of 3 Wood units (WU) differentiated the diseased (PVD and LHD) and non-diseased groups (controls and historical volunteers). (Reproduced with permission of the © ERS 2019: Herve et al. [103], Published 31 August 2015)

$$mPAP = \frac{\left[\left(1 + \alpha PAWP\right)^5 + 5\alpha . PVR.CO\right]^{\frac{1}{5}} - 1}{\alpha}$$

Invasive studies and noninvasive echocardiography have shown that the normal value of α is between 1% and 2% per mmHg [39]. Reduced vessel distensibility has been demonstrated in patients with early PH (i.e., those with normal resting pulmonary hemodynamics who later evolve into resting PAH or have lung biopsy consistent with pulmonary vascular disease) [43] and in healthy carriers of the *BMPR2* mutation [44].

Another use of CPET is to quantify the degree of RV dysfunction which is closely linked to survival in patients with PH [45]. Exercise hemodynamics allows for dynamic assessment of RV contractile function (termed Ees, end-systolic elastance) to its afterload (termed Ea, arterial elastance). The matching of RV contractility (Ees) and RV afterload (Ea) describes RV–PA coupling, and a normal RV Ees to Ea ratio (Ees/Ea) of between 1.5 and 2.0

allows for optimal RV functioning at minimal energy cost while a value of <0.8 is associated with RV failure [46]. RV-PA coupling can be determined using single-beat pressure waveform analysis or multi-beat pressure volume loop analysis (Figs. 16.3 and 16.4).

The initial response of the RV to an increased afterload is to increase its contractility (Ees) to match the increasing afterload (Ea). When the RV no longer is able to augment its contractility in the face of increasing afterload, RV–PA uncoupling ensues. The RV then relies on volumetric adaptation (i.e., Frank Starling's mechanism) to sustain its flow output in response to increasing metabolic demand leading to RV dilatation and associated poor prognosis [47, 48].

Exercise hemodynamics may play an important role in identifying early pulmonary vascular disease in subjects who are at risk of overt PAH due to established risk factors such as systemic sclerosis or *BMPR2* mutation. It can be used to examine the relative contribution of pulmonary

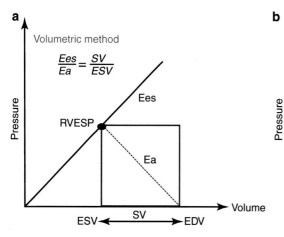

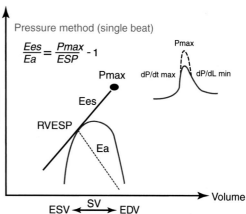

Fig. 16.3 Single-beat methods to estimate right ventricle–pulmonary artery (RV-PA) coupling. In the (**a**) volumetric method and (**b**) pressure method, pulmonary arterial elastance (Ea) is calculated from the ratio of RV end-systolic pressure (RVESP) to stroke volume (SV). The mean PA pressure can be used as surrogates for the RV-ESP. End-systolic elastance (Ees) in the volume method is estimated by the ratio of RV-ESP to end-systolic volume. The Ees/Ea is, therefore, simplified as SV/ESV. In the pressure method, Pmax was estimated by nonlinear extrapolation of early and late isovolumic portions of an RV pressure curve from the point of maximum (dp/dt max) and minimum (dp/dt min) pressure derivation. End-systolic elastance is then determined by a tangent from Pmax to the RV-ESP point. Ees/Ea in the pressure method is then determined by the ratio of (Pmax-RVESP) divided by SV or (Pmax/ESP – 1)

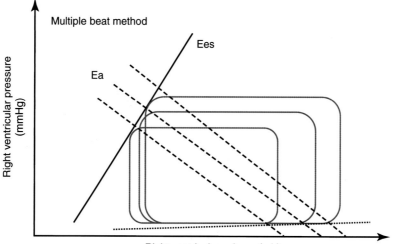

Fig. 16.4 Multi-beat method to estimate right ventricle–pulmonary artery (RV-PA) coupling. End-systolic elastance (Ees) is determined by a tangent fitted on the end-systolic portions of a series of pressure–volume loops produced by alteration in venous return or preload. Pulmonary arterial elastance (Ea) is calculated from the ratio of the RV-end systolic pressure to stroke volume. RV-PA coupling is then determined from the ratio of Ees to Ea (Ees/Ea)

vascular remodeling and left-sided heart disease to exercise impairment. Additionally, it allows to identify maladaptive RV phenotype response during exercise in patients with established PAH and exercise PH. This may prove useful in harnessing therapies aimed at improving RV contractility and potentially serve as endpoints for clinical prevention trials.

Phenotyping by Cardiopulmonary Imaging

Imaging can be used to quantify structural and functional changes to the pulmonary circulation allowing for detection, classification, and monitoring of PH. Thus, significant efforts have focused on utilizing imaging in defining individualized parameters of PH that have clinical utility.

Although the initial insult in PAH implicates the pulmonary vasculature, the functional state, exercise capacity, and survival of patients with PAH is closely linked to RV function [45]. While right heart catheterization provides important information about the hemodynamic impact of PH and the ability of the heart to provide cardiac output in that context, RV imaging using echocardiogram and cMRI provide significant information about the structure and function of the heart. Echocardiography remains the most important tool for screening patients for PH and monitoring RV function in no small part because of its relative availability, owing mainly to low cost of deployment [49]. Echocardiography can be used to estimate RV systolic pressures and evaluate RV systolic function [50]. It additionally provides information about other structural cardiac issues such as valvular dysfunction and left-sided heart failure, all of which have a very important impact on RV function. Beyond these well-established methods, current development is focusing on 3D reconstruction of RV geometry and estimation of the strain on the RV [51, 52], which can be combined together to aid with prognostication [53].

Cardiac magnetic resonance imaging (cMRI) provides a versatile set of tools with which many structural and functional parameters of the RV and its interactions with the proximal pulmonary artery can be measured [54]. As a noninvasive modality, cMRI is an attractive tool for monitoring patients with PAH. Standard cMRI imaging provides accurate information about changes in RV mass and volumes, RV function, as well as RV/LV interactions [49, 51, 54]. cMRI measures of ventricular volume and mass have been shown to be reproducible and superior to standard echocardiography [55]. Furthermore, specific techniques applied in the context of cMRI can provide information about cardiac mechanics and cardiac tissue remodeling. For example, the presence of late gadolinium enhancement can be used to assess degree of RV fibrosis [56] while phase-contrast imaging can be used to study cardiac output and assess PA stiffness and pulsatility [56–58]. Additionally, fluid dynamics models can utilize imaging data to study the impact of the remodeling of the proximal pulmonary circulation on vorticity of flow [59].

Computed tomography (CT) imaging has long been used as a screening tool for PH. Dilation of the pulmonary artery has been appreciated as a sign of pulmonary vascular disease [60]. Additionally, measurements of the size and dimensions of the chambers of the heart from CT imaging have potential utility in screening for PH [61] and distinguishing subtypes of PH [62–64]. Remodeling and loss of distal vascular volume have been quantified as markers of disease using CT imaging in multiple etiologies of PH [65–68]. Furthermore, changes in intraparenchymal blood vessel volumes have been noted with interventions [69]. Given the ubiquity of CT imaging in most patients with shortness of breath, as well as smokers, derived predictive models for PH are a promising tool for screening and evaluating patients prior to invasive measures [70].

Perfusion, which conceptually represents the flow of blood through the lung microvasculature, has also been the subject of great interest in PH given that the extent and spatial heterogeneity may provide insight into disease stage and phenotype. Nuclear imaging has been used to assess perfusion patterns in PH [71–73]. For example, utilizing 3′-deoxy-3′-[^{18}F]-fluorothymidine positron emission tomography (^{18}FLT-PET) imaging technique allows for the identification of a hyperproliferative PH phenotype. Unlike 2-deoxy-2-[^{18}F]-fluoro-D-glucose (^{18}F-FDG), which reports both inflammation and cellular proliferation, ^{18}FLT serves primarily as a marker of cell proliferation and can be used as a direct measure of pulmonary endothelial cell growth and, therefore, can be used to assess disease activity directly. In fact, treatment with anti-proliferative agents such as dichloroacetate and the tyrosine kinase inhibitor imatinib has been shown to attenuate [18]FLT uptake on PET imaging [74].

While MRI often lacks the spatial resolution of CT scan in the lung parenchyma, functional data and the ability to distinguish between materials permit spatial quantification of perfusion. These properties have been used to study perfusion in chronic thromboembolic pulmonary hypertension (CTEPH) [75] as well as in chronic obstructive pulmonary disease (COPD) [76]. Dual-energy computed tomography (DECT) utilizes multiple X-ray sources to help quantify molecular density without significant exposure to additional radiation. The spatial density of iodine tracer can then be derived from DECT, giving a high-resolution spatial map related to perfusion. This has been deployed largely in the study of CTEPH [77, 78] and can be used to study impact of intervention [71]. Recent studies have also evaluated its use in the detection of parenchymal perfusion in PAH [79].

In summary, imaging methods have been well established for individualized diagnosis, subtyping, and prognostication in pulmonary hypertension. Improved resolutions, image processing, and quantification algorithms along with development of new methods of marking the site of disease continue to expand the initial role of each imaging into better understanding of the entirety of the pulmonary circulation.

Molecular Phenotyping

Genetics

A "familial tendency" for the development of PAH was first suggested in 1954 [80] and, subsequently, mutations in the gene encoding *BMPR2*, a member of the transforming growth factor β (TGF-β) family of receptors, were linked to several families with heritable PAH in 2000 [81, 82]. Approximately 70% of patients with familial PAH carry mutations in *BMPR2*, which confer only a 20% lifetime risk for the development of the disease (14% for males and 42% for females). Remarkably, up to 25% of patients with non-heritable PAH also carry somatic mutations in

BMPR2 [83]. Since the identification of *BMPR2* mutations, approximately 20 other genes have been implicated in the development of PAH, including several additional members of the BMP/TGF receptor signaling family (*BMPR2*, *ACVRL1*, *CAV1*, *ENG*, *SMAD9*) [84]. More recently, autosomal recessive inheritance of *EIF2AK4* mutations encoding for eukaryotic translation initiation factor 2 alpha kinase 4 predisposes to pulmonary veno-occlusive disease (PVOD) / pulmonary capillary hemangiomatosis (PCH) [85].

PAH patients with *BMPR2* mutations develop the disease approximately 7–10 years earlier than noncarriers, have more severe hemodynamic compromise at time of diagnosis, and are less likely to respond to calcium channel blocker therapy [86]. Furthermore, in patients with idiopathic, anorexigen-associated, and heritable PAH, the presence of *BMPR2* mutation is associated with increased risk of death or lung transplantation [87]. In contrast to *BMPR2* mutation carriers, patients with *ALK1* mutations tend to be younger and have less severe hemodynamic changes at time of diagnosis. However, *ALK1* mutations are associated with poorer survival compared to noncarriers despite receiving similar treatment [88].

In the future, genetic testing in PAH may play an important role in guiding a phenotypic management strategy. In patients with heritable and idiopathic PAH, genetic testing allows for early detection of a progressive disease phenotype. This would allow for early implementation of specific pharmacotherapies, which has been shown to improve clinical outcomes and prevent deterioration in patients with PAH [89–91]. For example, low-dose tacrolimus, a potent *BMPR2* activator has been shown to reverse experimental PAH [92] and improve clinical and functional outcomes in a small cohort of PAH patients with advanced disease [93]. In a Phase 2a safety and tolerability trial, tacrolimus was shown to be well tolerated. Although the trial was under-powered for outcomes assessment, some patients demonstrated marked improvement in functional capacity as measured by 6-minute walk distance. Importantly, those patients with improved functional capacity tended to have larger increases in leukocyte *BMPR2* expression in response to tacrolimus [94]. This suggests that tacrolimus therapy may be tailored to patient subsets based on the recruitment of *BMPR2* signaling.

Genetic testing also allows to distinguish PVOD/PCH from PAH in patients with pre-capillary pulmonary vascular disease, a distinction that is challenging given the similarities in clinical and hemodynamic presentation between these two diseases. Patients with PVOD/PCH have a poor prognosis compared to those patients with PAH, respond poorly to PAH-specific therapies, and lung transplantation is the only curative treatment. Early diagnosis by genetic testing allows timely referral for patients with PVOD/PCH [95] for lung transplant evaluation.

Omics

The advent of omics-based technologies has provided a means to measure tens of thousands of parameters that can be utilized to provide a molecular signature of disease. While most omics studies in PAH have focused on identifying novel features of disease pathobiology or characterizing patients at-risk for developing the disease [96], investigators have recently begun to apply these technologies to address important clinical questions related to outcomes. For example, whole-exome sequencing of PAH patients with and without vasodilator response identified enrichment of vascular smooth muscle cell contraction pathways in vasodilator-responsive patients [97]. Similarly, a single-nucleotide polymorphism (SNP) in the G protein γ subunit 2 gene, *GNG2*, was associated with functional improvement among patients treated with an endothelin receptor antagonist [98]. A recent trial of dichloroacetate in PAH demonstrated that a lack of clinical response to the drug was associated with functional variants of *SIRT3* and *UCP2* [31]. In addition to providing meaningful pathobiological insights, these three studies demonstrate the value of genomic approaches to subclassifying PAH patients based on responsiveness to specific therapies. While genetic testing is unlikely to supplant clinical vasodilator testing, once prospectively validated, it may be very helpful to tailor current medical therapy or guide enrollment in clinical trials of novel agents.

In addition to genomics, proteomic and metabolomic approaches have been employed to identify circulating biomarkers to aid in the diagnosis and prognosis of patients with PAH. Using an aptamer-based assay of 1129 plasma proteins, Rhodes and colleagues identified a panel of nine circulating proteins that identifies PAH patients with a high risk of mortality, independent of existing clinical assessments [99]. Similarly, iTRAQ proteomics identified decreases in plasma carbamoyl-phosphate synthetase I and complement factor H-related protein associated with PAH in patients with congenital heart disease [100]. Plasma metabolomics has also identified circulating small molecules that distinguish PAH patients from healthy subjects and prognosticate outcomes [101]. At the present moment, these findings may have more impact by directing further investigation of novel disease mechanisms rather than guiding clinical management of PAH patients; however, as the therapeutic armamentarium increases in size, these approaches will become invaluable for customizing treatment.

Future Directions

As with many areas of medicine, the foundations are currently being poured for the implementation of sophisticated clinical, imaging, and molecular phenotyping of patients with PAH. Two limitations of the studies described above, however, are the relatively small sample sizes studied and the incorporation of relatively limited clinical data. Moreover, how these disparate datasets can be meaningfully synthesized is a critical issue for leveraging their full potential. These areas may be addressed by the ongoing Redefining Pulmonary Hypertension through Pulmonary Vascular Disease Phenomics (PVDomics) sponsored by the National Heart, Lung, and Blood Institute of the National Institutes of Health [102]. This clinical trial seeks to enroll 1500 incident cases of PH who undergo a battery of diagnostic testing, including pulmonary artery catheterization, polysomnography, pulmonary function tests, exercise testing, echocardiography, cMRI, lung imaging, ventilation/perfusion scanning, and plasma omic profiling (genome, transcriptome, proteome, and metabolome), the results of which are linked to clinical parameters such as medical history, exam, vital signs, and quality-of-life survey results. The goal of this program is to use all of these parameters to define new subclassifications of PH patients, leveraging the tools of systems biology and network medicine to facilitate earlier diagnosis, more targeted at-risk screening, and personalized approaches for intervention. Certainly, the field has come a long way since its first foray into personalized medicine with pulmonary vasodilator testing with many exciting new discoveries on the horizon.

References

1. Maron BA, Hess E, Maddox TM, Opotowsky AR, Tedford RJ, Lahm T, et al. Association of borderline pulmonary hypertension with mortality and hospitalization in a large patient cohort: insights from the veterans affairs clinical assessment, reporting, and tracking program. Circulation. 2016;133(13):1240–8.
2. Benza RL, Miller DP, Barst RJ, Badesch DB, Frost AE, McGoon MD. An evaluation of long-term survival from time of diagnosis in pulmonary arterial hypertension from the REVEAL Registry. Chest. 2012;142(2):448–56.
3. Badesch DB, Raskob GE, Elliott CG, Krichman AM, Farber HW, Frost AE, et al. Pulmonary arterial hypertension: baseline characteristics from the REVEAL Registry. Chest. 2010;137(2):376–87.
4. Singh I, Ma KC, Berlin DA. Pathophysiology of pulmonary hypertension in chronic parenchymal lung disease. Am J Med. 2016;129(4):366–71.
5. Bloodworth NC, West JD, Merryman WD. Microvessel mechanobiology in pulmonary arterial hypertension: cause and effect. Hypertension. 2015;65(3):483–9.
6. Guignabert C, Tu L, Le Hiress M, Ricard N, Sattler C, Seferian A, et al. Pathogenesis of pulmonary arterial hypertension: lessons from cancer. Eur Respir Rev. 2013;22(130):543–51.
7. McLaughlin VV, Archer SL, Badesch DB, Barst RJ, Farber HW, Lindner JR, et al. ACCF/AHA 2009 expert consensus document on pulmonary hypertension a report of the American College of Cardiology Foundation Task Force on expert consensus documents and the American Heart Association developed in collaboration with the American College of Chest Physicians; American Thoracic Society, Inc.; and the Pulmonary Hypertension Association. J Am Coll Cardiol. 2009;53(17):1573–619.
8. Rich S, Kaufmann E, Levy PS. The effect of high doses of calcium-channel blockers on survival in primary pulmonary hypertension. N Engl J Med. 1992;327(2):76–81.
9. Vachiery JL, Adir Y, Barbera JA, Champion H, Coghlan JG, Cottin V, et al. Pulmonary hypertension due to left heart diseases. J Am Coll Cardiol. 2013;62(25 Suppl):D100–8.
10. Galie N, Humbert M, Vachiery JL, Gibbs S, Lang I, Torbicki A, et al. 2015 ESC/ERS guidelines for the diagnosis and treatment of pulmonary hypertension. Kardiol Pol. 2015;73(12):1127–206.
11. Rosenkranz S, Gibbs JS, Wachter R, De Marco T, Vonk-Noordegraaf A, Vachiery JL. Left ventricular heart failure and pulmonary hypertension. Eur Heart J. 2016;37(12):942–54.
12. Gorter TM, Hoendermis ES, van Veldhuisen DJ, Voors AA, Lam CS, Geelhoed B, et al. Right ventricular dysfunction in heart failure with preserved ejection fraction: a systematic review and meta-analysis. Eur J Heart Fail. 2016;18(12):1472–87.
13. Gerges C, Gerges M, Fesler P, Pistritto AM, Konowitz NP, Jakowitsch J, et al. In-depth haemodynamic phenotyping of pulmonary hypertension due to left heart disease. Eur Respir J. 2018;51(5):1800067.
14. Gerges M, Gerges C, Pistritto AM, Lang MB, Trip P, Jakowitsch J, et al. Pulmonary hypertension in heart failure. Epidemiology, right ventricular function, and survival. Am J Respir Crit Care Med. 2015;192(10):1234–46.
15. Guazzi M, Vicenzi M, Arena R, Guazzi MD. Pulmonary hypertension in heart failure with preserved ejection fraction: a target of phosphodiesterase-5 inhibition in a 1-year study. Circulation. 2011;124(2):164–74.
16. Lewis GD, Lachmann J, Camuso J, Lepore JJ, Shin J, Martinovic ME, et al. Sildenafil improves exercise hemodynamics and oxygen uptake in patients with systolic heart failure. Circulation. 2007;115(1):59–66.
17. Hussain I, Mohammed SF, Forfia PR, Lewis GD, Borlaug BA, Gallup DS, et al. Impaired right ventricular-pulmonary arterial coupling and effect of sildenafil in heart failure with preserved ejection fraction: an ancillary analysis from the phosphodiesterase-5 inhibition to improve clinical status and exercise capacity in diastolic heart failure (RELAX) trial. Circ Heart Fail. 2016;9(4):e002729.
18. Vachiery JL, Delcroix M, Al-Hiti H, Efficace M, Hutyra M, Lack G, et al. Macitentan in pulmonary hypertension due to left ventricular dysfunction. Eur Respir J. 2018;51(2):1701886.
19. Naeije R, Vachiery JL, Yerly P, Vanderpool R. The transpulmonary pressure gradient for the diagnosis of pulmonary vascular disease. Eur Respir J. 2013;41(1):217–23.
20. Tampakakis E, Tedford RJ. Balancing the positives and negatives of the diastolic pulmonary gradient. Eur J Heart Fail. 2017;19(1):98–100.

21. Khush KK, Tasissa G, Butler J, McGlothlin D, De Marco T, Investigators E. Effect of pulmonary hypertension on clinical outcomes in advanced heart failure: analysis of the evaluation study of congestive heart failure and pulmonary artery catheterization effectiveness (ESCAPE) database. Am Heart J. 2009;157(6):1026–34.

22. Aronson D, Eitan A, Dragu R, Burger AJ. Relationship between reactive pulmonary hypertension and mortality in patients with acute decompensated heart failure. Circ Heart Fail. 2011;4(5):644–50.

23. Weatherald J, Farina S, Bruno N, Laveneziana P. Cardiopulmonary exercise testing in pulmonary hypertension. Ann Am Thorac Soc. 2017;14(Supplement_1):S84–92.

24. Tolle JJ, Waxman AB, Van Horn TL, Pappagianopoulos PP, Systrom DM. Exercise-induced pulmonary arterial hypertension. Circulation. 2008;118(21):2183–9.

25. Steen V, Chou M, Shanmugam V, Mathias M, Kuru T, Morrissey R. Exercise-induced pulmonary arterial hypertension in patients with systemic sclerosis. Chest. 2008;134(1):146–51.

26. Stamm A, Saxer S, Lichtblau M, Hasler ED, Jordan S, Huber LC, et al. Exercise pulmonary haemodynamics predict outcome in patients with systemic sclerosis. Eur Respir J. 2016;48(6):1658–67.

27. Saggar R, Khanna D, Furst DE, Shapiro S, Maranian P, Belperio JA, et al. Exercise-induced pulmonary hypertension associated with systemic sclerosis: four distinct entities. Arthritis Rheum. 2010;62(12):3741–50.

28. Condliffe R, Kiely DG, Peacock AJ, Corris PA, Gibbs JS, Vrapi F, et al. Connective tissue disease-associated pulmonary arterial hypertension in the modern treatment era. Am J Respir Crit Care Med. 2009;179(2):151–7.

29. Barron A, Dhutia N, Mayet J, Hughes AD, Francis DP, Wensel R. Test-retest repeatability of cardiopulmonary exercise test variables in patients with cardiac or respiratory disease. Eur J Prev Cardiol. 2014;21(4):445–53.

30. Hansen JE, Sun XG, Yasunobu Y, Garafano RP, Gates G, Barst RJ, et al. Reproducibility of cardiopulmonary exercise measurements in patients with pulmonary arterial hypertension. Chest. 2004;126(3):816–24.

31. Michelakis ED, Gurtu V, Webster L, Barnes G, Watson G, Howard L, et al. Inhibition of pyruvate dehydrogenase kinase improves pulmonary arterial hypertension in genetically susceptible patients. Sci Transl Med. 2017;9(413):eaao4583.

32. Gomberg-Maitland M, Schilz R, Mediratta A, Addetia K, Coslet S, Thomeas V, et al. Phase I safety study of ranolazine in pulmonary arterial hypertension. Pulm Circ. 2015;5(4):691–700.

33. Maron BA, Cockrill BA, Waxman AB, Systrom DM. The invasive cardiopulmonary exercise test. Circulation. 2013;127(10):1157–64.

34. Segrera SA, Lawler L, Opotowsky AR, Systrom D, Waxman AB. Open label study of ambrisentan in patients with exercise pulmonary hypertension. Pulm Circ. 2017;7(2):531–8.

35. Saggar R, Khanna D, Shapiro S, Furst DE, Maranian P, Clements P, et al. Brief report: effect of ambrisentan treatment on exercise-induced pulmonary hypertension in systemic sclerosis: a prospective single-center, open-label pilot study. Arthritis Rheum. 2012;64(12):4072–7.

36. Wallace WD, Nouraie M, Chan SY, Risbano MG. Treatment of exercise pulmonary hypertension improves pulmonary vascular distensibility. Pulm Circ. 2018;8(3):2045894018787381.

37. Oliveira RKF, Faria-Urbina M, Maron BA, Santos M, Waxman AB, Systrom DM. Functional impact of exercise pulmonary hypertension in patients with borderline resting pulmonary arterial pressure. Pulm Circ. 2017;7(3):654–65.

38. Hinderhofer K, Fischer C, Pfarr N, Szamalek-Hoegel J, Lichtblau M, Nagel C, et al. Identification of a new intronic BMPR2-mutation and early diagnosis of heritable pulmonary arterial hypertension in a large family with mean clinical follow-up of 12 years. PLoS One. 2014;9(3):e91374.

39. Naeije R, Saggar R, Badesch D, Rajagopalan S, Gargani L, Rischard F, et al. Exercise-induced pulmonary hypertension: translating pathophysiological concepts into clinical practice. Chest. 2018;154(1):10–5.

40. Esfandiari S, Wright SP, Goodman JM, Sasson Z, Mak S. Pulmonary artery wedge pressure relative to exercise work rate in older men and women. Med Sci Sports Exerc. 2017;49(7):1297–304.

41. Eisman AS, Shah RV, Dhakal BP, Pappagianopoulos PP, Wooster L, Bailey C, et al. Pulmonary capillary wedge pressure patterns during exercise predict exercise capacity and incident heart failure. Circ Heart Fail. 2018;11(5):e004750.

42. Reeves JT, Linehan JH, Stenmark KR. Distensibility of the normal human lung circulation during exercise. Am J Physiol Lung Cell Mol Physiol. 2005;288(3):L419–25.

43. Lau EMT, Chemla D, Godinas L, Zhu K, Sitbon O, Savale L, et al. Loss of vascular distensibility during exercise is an early hemodynamic marker of pulmonary vascular disease. Chest. 2016;149(2):353–61.

44. Pavelescu A, Vanderpool R, Vachiery JL, Grunig E, Naeije R. Echocardiography of pulmonary vascular function in asymptomatic carriers of BMPR2 mutations. Eur Respir J. 2012;40(5):1287–9.

45. Vonk-Noordegraaf A, Haddad F, Chin KM, Forfia PR, Kawut SM, Lumens J, et al. Right heart adaptation to pulmonary arterial hypertension: physiology and pathobiology. J Am Coll Cardiol. 2013;62(25 Suppl):D22–33.

46. Tello K, Dalmer A, Axmann J, Vanderpool R, Ghofrani HA, Naeije R, et al. Reserve of right ventricular-arterial coupling in the setting of chronic overload. Circ Heart Fail. 2019;12(1):e005512.

47. Spruijt OA, de Man FS, Groepenhoff H, Oosterveer F, Westerhof N, Vonk-Noordegraaf A, et al. The effects of exercise on right ventricular contractility and right ventricular-arterial coupling in pulmonary hypertension. Am J Respir Crit Care Med. 2015;191(9):1050–7.

48. Hsu S, Houston BA, Tampakakis E, Bacher AC, Rhodes PS, Mathai SC, et al. Right ventricular functional reserve in pulmonary arterial hypertension. Circulation. 2016;133(24):2413–22.

49. Grunig E, Peacock AJ. Imaging the heart in pulmonary hypertension: an update. Eur Respir Rev. 2015;24(138):653–64.

50. Bossone E, D'Andrea A, D'Alto M, Citro R, Argiento P, Ferrara F, et al. Echocardiography in pulmonary arterial hypertension: from diagnosis to prognosis. J Am Soc Echocardiogr. 2013;26(1):1–14.

51. Rengier F, Melzig C, Derlin T, Marra AM, Vogel-Claussen J. Advanced imaging in pulmonary hypertension: emerging techniques and applications. Int J Cardiovasc Imaging. 2019;35:1407–20.

52. Sachdev A, Villarraga HR, Frantz RP, McGoon MD, Hsiao JF, Maalouf JF, et al. Right ventricular strain for prediction of survival in patients with pulmonary arterial hypertension. Chest. 2011;139(6):1299–309.

53. Vitarelli A, Mangieri E, Terzano C, Gaudio C, Salsano F, Rosato E, et al. Three-dimensional echocardiography and 2D-3D speckle-tracking imaging in chronic pulmonary hypertension: diagnostic accuracy in detecting hemodynamic signs of right ventricular (RV) failure. J Am Heart Assoc. 2015;4(3):e001584.

54. Freed BH, Collins JD, Francois CJ, Barker AJ, Cuttica MJ, Chesler NC, et al. MR and CT imaging for the evaluation of pulmonary hypertension. JACC Cardiovasc Imaging. 2016;9(6):715–32.

55. Peacock AJ, Vonk Noordegraaf A. Cardiac magnetic resonance imaging in pulmonary arterial hypertension. Eur Respir Rev. 2013;22(130):526–34.

56. Dellegrottaglie S, Ostenfeld E, Sanz J, Scatteia A, Perrone-Filardi P, Bossone E. Imaging the right heart-pulmonary circulation unit: The role of MRI and computed tomography. Heart Fail Clin. 2018;14(3):377–91.

57. Ray JC, Burger C, Mergo P, Safford R, Blackshear J, Austin C, et al. Pulmonary arterial stiffness assessed by cardiovascular magnetic resonance imaging is a predictor of mild pulmonary arterial hypertension. Int J Cardiovasc Imaging. 2018;35(10):1881–92.

58. Schafer M, Myers C, Brown RD, Frid MG, Tan W, Hunter K, et al. Pulmonary arterial stiffness: toward a new paradigm in pulmonary arterial hypertension pathophysiology and assessment. Curr Hypertens Rep. 2016;18(1):4.

59. Reiter G, Reiter U, Kovacs G, Olschewski H, Fuchsjager M. Blood flow vortices along the main pulmonary artery measured with MR imaging for diagnosis of pulmonary hypertension. Radiology. 2015;275(1):71–9.

60. Ng CS, Wells AU, Padley SP. A CT sign of chronic pulmonary arterial hypertension: the ratio of main pulmonary artery to aortic diameter. J Thorac Imaging. 1999;14(4):270–8.

61. Rahaghi FN, Vegas-Sanchez-Ferrero G, Minhas JK, Come CE, De La Bruere I, Wells JM, et al. Ventricular geometry from non-contrast non-ECG-gated CT scans: an imaging marker of cardiopulmonary disease in smokers. Acad Radiol. 2017;24(5):594–602.

62. Colin GC, Gerber BL, de Meester de Ravenstein C, Byl D, Dietz A, Kamga M, et al. Pulmonary hypertension due to left heart disease: diagnostic and prognostic value of CT in chronic systolic heart failure. Eur Radiol 2018, 28, 4643.

63. Currie BJ, Johns C, Chin M, Charalampopolous T, Elliot CA, Garg P, et al. CT derived left atrial size identifies left heart disease in suspected pulmonary hypertension: derivation and validation of predictive thresholds. Int J Cardiol. 2018;260:172–7.

64. Aviram G, Rozenbaum Z, Ziv-Baran T, Berliner S, Topilsky Y, Fleischmann D, et al. Identification of pulmonary hypertension caused by left-sided heart disease (World Health Organization Group 2) based on cardiac chamber volumes derived from chest CT imaging. Chest. 2017;152(4):792–9.

65. Rahaghi FN, Ross JC, Agarwal M, Gonzalez G, Come CE, Diaz AA, et al. Pulmonary vascular morphology as an imaging biomarker in chronic thromboembolic pulmonary hypertension. Pulm Circ. 2016;6(1):70–81.

66. Matsuoka S, Washko GR, Yamashiro T, Estepar RS, Diaz A, Silverman EK, et al. Pulmonary hypertension and computed tomography measurement of small pulmonary vessels in severe emphysema. Am J Respir Crit Care Med. 2010;181(3):218–25.

67. Helmberger M, Pienn M, Urschler M, Kullnig P, Stollberger R, Kovacs G, et al. Quantification of tortuosity and fractal dimension of the lung vessels in pulmonary hypertension patients. PLoS One. 2014;9(1):e87515.

68. Moledina S, de Bruyn A, Schievano S, Owens CM, Young C, Haworth SG, et al. Fractal branching quantifies vascular changes and predicts survival in pulmonary hypertension: a proof of principle study. Heart. 2011;97(15):1245–9.

69. Rahaghi FN, Winkler T, Kohli P, Nardelli P, Marti-Fuster B, Ross JC, et al. Quantification of the pulmonary vascular response to inhaled nitric oxide using noncontrast computed tomography imaging. Circ Cardiovasc Imaging. 2019;12(1):e008338.

70. Aviram G, Shmueli H, Adam SZ, Bendet A, Ziv-Baran T, Steinvil A, et al. Pulmonary hypertension: a nomogram based on CT pulmonary angiographic data for prediction in patients without pulmonary embolism. Radiology. 2015;277(1):236–46.

71. Koike H, Sueyoshi E, Sakamoto I, Uetani M, Nakata T, Maemura K. Comparative clinical and predictive value of lung perfusion blood volume CT, lung perfusion SPECT and catheter pulmonary angi-

ography images in patients with chronic thromboembolic pulmonary hypertension before and after balloon pulmonary angioplasty. Eur Radiol. 2018;28(12):5091–9.

72. Marsboom G, Wietholt C, Haney CR, Toth PT, Ryan JJ, Morrow E, et al. Lung (1)(8)F-fluorodeoxyglucose positron emission tomography for diagnosis and monitoring of pulmonary arterial hypertension. Am J Respir Crit Care Med. 2012;185(6):670–9.

73. Zhao L, Ashek A, Wang L, Fang W, Dabral S, Dubois O, et al. Heterogeneity in lung (18) FDG uptake in pulmonary arterial hypertension: potential of dynamic (18)FDG positron emission tomography with kinetic analysis as a bridging biomarker for pulmonary vascular remodeling targeted treatments. Circulation. 2013;128(11):1214–24.

74. Ashek A, Spruijt OA, Harms HJ, Lammertsma AA, Cupitt J, Dubois O, et al. 3′-deoxy-3′-[18F]fluorothymidine positron emission tomography depicts heterogeneous proliferation pathology in idiopathic pulmonary arterial hypertension patient lung. Circ Cardiovasc Imaging. 2018;11(8):e007402.

75. Schoenfeld C, Cebotari S, Hinrichs J, Renne J, Kaireit T, Olsson KM, et al. MR imaging-derived regional pulmonary parenchymal perfusion and cardiac function for monitoring patients with chronic thromboembolic pulmonary hypertension before and after pulmonary endarterectomy. Radiology. 2016;279(3):925–34.

76. Hueper K, Parikh MA, Prince MR, Schoenfeld C, Liu C, Bluemke DA, et al. Quantitative and semi-quantitative measures of regional pulmonary microvascular perfusion by magnetic resonance imaging and their relationships to global lung perfusion and lung diffusing capacity: the multiethnic study of atherosclerosis chronic obstructive pulmonary disease study. Investig Radiol. 2013;48(4):223–30.

77. Nallasamy N, Bullen J, Karim W, Heresi GA, Renapurkar RD. Evaluation of vascular parameters in patients with pulmonary thromboembolic disease using dual-energy computed tomography. J Thorac Imaging. 2019;4(6):367–72.

78. Renapurkar RD, Bolen MA, Shrikanthan S, Bullen J, Karim W, Primak A, et al. Comparative assessment of qualitative and quantitative perfusion with dual-energy CT and planar and SPECT-CT V/Q scanning in patients with chronic thromboembolic pulmonary hypertension. Cardiovasc Diagn Ther. 2018;8(4):414–22.

79. Ameli-Renani S, Ramsay L, Bacon JL, Rahman F, Nair A, Smith V, et al. Dual-energy computed tomography in the assessment of vascular and parenchymal enhancement in suspected pulmonary hypertension. J Thorac Imaging. 2014;29(2):98–106.

80. Dresdale DT, Michtom RJ, Schultz M. Recent studies in primary pulmonary hypertension, including pharmacodynamic observations on pulmonary vascular resistance. Bull N Y Acad Med. 1954;30(3):195–207.

81. Deng Z, Morse JH, Slager SL, Cuervo N, Moore KJ, Venetos G, et al. Familial primary pulmonary hypertension (gene PPH1) is caused by mutations in the bone morphogenetic protein receptor-II gene. Am J Hum Genet. 2000;67(3):737–44.

82. International PPHC, Lane KB, Machado RD, Pauciulo MW, Thomson JR, Phillips JA 3rd, et al. Heterozygous germline mutations in BMPR2, encoding a TGF-beta receptor, cause familial primary pulmonary hypertension. Nat Genet. 2000; 26(1):81–4.

83. Thomson JR, Machado RD, Pauciulo MW, Morgan NV, Humbert M, Elliott GC, et al. Sporadic primary pulmonary hypertension is associated with germline mutations of the gene encoding BMPR-II, a receptor member of the TGF-beta family. J Med Genet. 2000;37(10):741–5.

84. Garcia-Rivas G, Jerjes-Sanchez C, Rodriguez D, Garcia-Pelaez J, Trevino V. A systematic review of genetic mutations in pulmonary arterial hypertension. BMC Med Genet. 2017;18(1):82.

85. Aldred MA, Comhair SA, Varella-Garcia M, Asosingh K, Xu W, Noon GP, et al. Somatic chromosome abnormalities in the lungs of patients with pulmonary arterial hypertension. Am J Respir Crit Care Med. 2010;182(9):1153–60.

86. Rosenzweig EB, Morse JH, Knowles JA, Chada KK, Khan AM, Roberts KE, et al. Clinical implications of determining BMPR2 mutation status in a large cohort of children and adults with pulmonary arterial hypertension. J Heart Lung Transplant. 2008;27(6):668–74.

87. Evans JD, Girerd B, Montani D, Wang XJ, Galie N, Austin ED, et al. BMPR2 mutations and survival in pulmonary arterial hypertension: an individual participant data meta-analysis. Lancet Respir Med. 2016;4(2):129–37.

88. Girerd B, Montani D, Coulet F, Sztrymf B, Yaici A, Jais X, et al. Clinical outcomes of pulmonary arterial hypertension in patients carrying an ACVRL1 (ALK1) mutation. Am J Respir Crit Care Med. 2010;181(8):851–61.

89. Galie N, Barbera JA, Frost AE, Ghofrani HA, Hoeper MM, McLaughlin VV, et al. Initial use of ambrisentan plus tadalafil in pulmonary arterial hypertension. N Engl J Med. 2015;373(9):834–44.

90. Humbert M, Sitbon O, Chaouat A, Bertocchi M, Habib G, Gressin V, et al. Survival in patients with idiopathic, familial, and anorexigen-associated pulmonary arterial hypertension in the modern management era. Circulation. 2010;122(2):156–63.

91. Galie N, Rubin L, Hoeper M, Jansa P, Al-Hiti H, Meyer G, et al. Treatment of patients with mildly symptomatic pulmonary arterial hypertension with bosentan (EARLY study): a double-blind, randomised controlled trial. Lancet. 2008;371(9630):2093–100.

92. Spiekerkoetter E, Tian X, Cai J, Hopper RK, Sudheendra D, Li CG, et al. FK506 activates BMPR2, rescues endothelial dysfunction, and

reverses pulmonary hypertension. J Clin Invest. 2013;123(8):3600–13.

93. Spiekerkoetter E, Sung YK, Sudheendra D, Bill M, Aldred MA, van de Veerdonk MC, et al. Low-dose FK506 (tacrolimus) in end-stage pulmonary arterial hypertension. Am J Respir Crit Care Med. 2015;192(2):254–7.

94. Spiekerkoetter E, Sung YK, Sudheendra D, Scott V, Del Rosario P, Bill M, et al. Randomised placebo-controlled safety and tolerability trial of FK506 (tacrolimus) for pulmonary arterial hypertension. Eur Respir J. 2017;50(3):1602449.

95. Montani D, Jais X, Price LC, Achouh L, Degano B, Mercier O, et al. Cautious epoprostenol therapy is a safe bridge to lung transplantation in pulmonary veno-occlusive disease. Eur Respir J. 2009;34(6):1348–56.

96. Rhodes CJ, Batai K, Bleda M, Haimel M, Southgate L, Germain M, et al. Genetic determinants of risk in pulmonary arterial hypertension: international genome-wide association studies and meta-analysis. Lancet Respir Med. 2019;7:227–38.

97. Hemnes AR, Zhao M, West J, Newman JH, Rich S, Archer SL, et al. Critical genomic networks and vasoreactive variants in idiopathic pulmonary arterial hypertension. Am J Respir Crit Care Med. 2016;194(4):464–75.

98. Benza RL, Gomberg-Maitland M, Demarco T, Frost AE, Torbicki A, Langleben D, et al. Endothelin-1 pathway polymorphisms and outcomes in pulmonary arterial hypertension. Am J Respir Crit Care Med. 2015;192(11):1345–54.

99. Rhodes CJ, Wharton J, Ghataorhe P, Watson G, Girerd B, Howard LS, et al. Plasma proteome analysis in patients with pulmonary arterial hypertension: an observational cohort study. Lancet Respir Med. 2017;5(9):717–26.

100. Zhang X, Hou HT, Wang J, Liu XC, Yang Q, He GW. Plasma proteomic study in pulmonary arterial hypertension associated with congenital heart diseases. Sci Rep. 2016;6:36541.

101. Rhodes CJ, Ghataorhe P, Wharton J, Rue-Albrecht KC, Hadinnapola C, Watson G, et al. Plasma metabolomics implicate modified transfer RNAs and altered bioenergetics in the outcome of pulmonary arterial hypertension. Circulation. 2017;135:460–75.

102. Hemnes AR, Beck GJ, Newman JH, Abidov A, Aldred MA, Barnard J, et al. PVDOMICS: a multi-center study to improve understanding of pulmonary vascular disease through phenomics. Circ Res. 2017;121(10):1136–9.

103. Herve P, Lau EM, Sitbon O, Savale L, Montani D, Godinas L, Lador F, Jaïs X, Parent F, Günther S, Humbert M, Simonneau G, Chemla D. Criteria for diagnosis of exercise pulmonary hypertension. Eur Respir J. 2015;46(3):728–37. https://doi.org/10.1183/09031936.00021915.

Identifying Subtypes of Obstructive Sleep Apnea

Allan I. Pack

Obstructive sleep apnea (OSA) is an extremely common disorder [1]. The main risk factor is obesity and, as a result of increases in obesity rates, the prevalence of OSA is increasing [1]. It is a world-wide problem [2]. In Asian populations, craniofacial restriction plays a larger role than in Caucasian populations [3] and increases their vulnerability to increases in weight. With the increasing rates of obesity in China [4, 5], there could be an epidemic of OSA there. There has been a rapid growth of the fast food industry in China [6]. The infrastructure for sleep medicine in China is very underdeveloped and the country is not well positioned to deal with this epidemic.

Obstructive sleep apnea has multiple adverse consequences. Apneas (cessation of breathing) and hypopneas (breathing decrements) are followed by an arousal (sudden change in sleep state) and/or result in oxygen desaturation and resaturation. Thus, sleep apnea results in sleep fragmentation, loss of deep stages of sleep, and/or cyclical intermittent hypoxia [7]. Hence, it is a systemic disorder [7] since all tissues are subject to cyclical intermittent hypoxia although the dynamic changes in oxygen varies between tissues depending on their blood flow [8].

As a result of inadequate sleep, both in terms of amount of deep sleep and sleep continuity, OSA results in excessive sleepiness [9], impaired quality of life [10], and increased risk of car crashes [11]. The systemic effects result in OSA being an independent risk factor for cardiovascular disease (for reviews, see [12, 13]), including myocardial infarction [14, 15], stroke [16, 17], and atrial fibrillation [18] in both cross-sectional and longitudinal follow-up studies. OSA also leads to insulin resistance [19–22], and untreated patients with OSA and pre-diabetes have higher rates of conversion to diabetes compared to those on effective CPAP therapy [23]. Subjects with OSA have an increased incidence of cancer [24], more aggressive melanoma [25], and an increased mortality in subjects with cancer [26]. Thus, obstructive sleep apnea is a major public health problem not only in the United States but worldwide.

While there are many downstream consequences, not all subjects with OSA develop them. Thus, OSA is a heterogeneous disorder. Recent efforts have sought to identify subtypes using unsupervised clustering approaches. The goal is to identify subgroups in which individuals are highly similar within a cluster but as different as possible between clusters. I now describe the different strategies that have been employed and what we have learned.

A. I. Pack (✉)
Division of Sleep Medicine/Department of Medicine, University of Pennsylvania Perelman School of Medicine, Translational Research Laboratories, Philadelphia, PA, USA
e-mail: pack@pennmedicine.upenn.edu

© Springer Nature Switzerland AG 2020
J. L. Gomez et al. (eds.), *Precision in Pulmonary, Critical Care, and Sleep Medicine*, Respiratory Medicine, https://doi.org/10.1007/978-3-030-31507-8_17

Studies Employing Cluster Analysis Using Data from Multiple Dimensions

Some approaches to investigating the heterogeneity of OSA have used cluster analyses based on data from different dimensions. Not surprisingly, the results of the cluster analysis depend on the input variables employed. A study from Greece utilized as input variables the severity of obstructive sleep apnea as assessed by the apnea-hypopnea index (AHI), BMI as a measure of obesity as well as substantial information about associated comorbidities [27]. They utilized the Charlson Cormorbidity Index (CCI) [28]. They found, using a two-step clustering strategy, that the optimal solution was six clusters [27]. Not surprisingly, the clusters had different degrees of severity of OSA, degrees of obesity, and different amounts of comorbidity.

A similar approach was employed by investigators from Italy [29] who again included variables extracted from the sleep study, BMI, and comorbidities. The sample size was small ($n = 198$). They identified what they called three "communities." Community one (the largest one) consisted of younger patients with severe OSA and high prevalence of comorbidities such as hypertension (64%). Community two included patients with moderate-to-severe OSA and lower risk of nocturnal hypoxia. Community three included older patients who were overweight or with mild obesity with severe OSA but a lower risk of nocturnal hypoxemia and less sleepy.

While the sample size in these studies from single sleep centers was relatively small, the sample size from a French study was large [30].

This study was based on the French National Registry of Sleep Apnea. They used as input variables data from the sleep study, age, BMI, OSA symptoms, Pichot fatigue and depression scales, subjective sleep duration, blood pressure, waist circumference, and comorbidities (cardiovascular, metabolic, and respiratory). OSA symptoms included snoring, self-declared sleepiness, morning fatigue, nocturia, headaches, and near-miss accidents. Unfortunately, symptoms did not include symptoms of insomnia, e.g., difficulty staying asleep. This study used a hierarchical clustering approach and found six clusters (see Table 17.1). It is evident that when age and BMI are included as input variables they play a major role in determining the outcome of cluster analyses.

While these approaches are of interest, they have not led to definitions of subtypes that have provided major new insights about heterogeneity. The results of cluster analysis are largely determined by the choice of input variables. Including age, gender, BMI, and measure of sleep apnea severity will determine the outcomes of the clustering approach.

Using More Focused Approaches: Examining for Physiological Subtypes

An alternative strategy, and one that has proved more fruitful, is to do cluster analysis based on input variables from one specific domain. This leads to a more specific question that can be addressed by this approach. Zinchuk et al. [31] asked a specific question—are there specific

Table 17.1 Some characteristics of the six clusters that were identified

	All subjects	Cluster 1 N = 1823	Cluster 2 N = 4200	Cluster 3 N = 3363	Cluster 4 N = 2715	Cluster 5 N = 3511	Cluster 6 N = 2642
Age (years)	59	48	63	66	49	56	60
Gender, male (%)	73.8	78.3	74.7	69.8	81.4	69.3	72.3
BMI (kg/mg^2)	31	29	31	33	28	31	33
AHI (events/h)	35	31.6	34	40	31	34	39
Epworth Sleepiness Score	10	12	8	9	10	11	11

The six clusters were: (1) the young symptomatic, (2) the old obese, (3) the multi-disease old obese, (4) the young snorers, (5) the drowsy obese, and (6) the multi-disease obese symptomatic physiological subtypes; if so, do they associate differently with cardiovascular events?

They used data from the DREAM Study—Determining Risk of Vascular Events by Apnea Monitoring. This was a collaborative study with three Veterans Affairs Medical Centers that enrolled 2041 subjects [32]. They underwent overnight sleep studies between 2000 and 2004 and were followed through 2012. They divided subjects with respect to their CPAP use into regular and non-regular users.

The investigators used a two-step variable reduction analysis. The input variables were all metrics typically derived from an overnight sleep study. First, principal component-based clustering was used to identify groups of variables highly correlated within their own cluster and uncorrelated with others. Second, features extracted from the overnight sleep study were selected to retain >75% of total variance within each domain using the least number of features that were judged to be "clinically interpretable." They used K-mean analysis to generate clusters.

Seven clusters were found (see Table 17.2) [31]. Two (A and B) would be considered to have mild OSA (AHI <15 events/hour), one of which (B) had a large number of periodic limb movements (PLMS). Two clusters (C and D) would be considered to have moderate OSA while three (E, F and G) had severe OSA (i.e., AHI >30 events/hour).

There were differences between these subtypes in the probability of no CV events based on a composite of acute coronary syndrome, transient ischemic attack, stroke, or death (see Fig. 17.1). No differences were found using the more accepted subtypes, i.e., mild OSA (AHI ≥5 and <15 events/hour), moderate OSA (AHI ≥15 and <30 events/hour), and severe OSA (AHI ≥30 events/hour).

When they examined the impact of CPAP use by comparing events (again using a composite score) in regular CPAP users to non-regular, they found that CPAP use only reduced event rates in two of the seven subtypes, i.e., mild OSA with PLMS (labeled PLMS) and in the group with severe OSA with hypopnea and hypoxia (see Fig. 17.2).

This result is somewhat surprising. There are data that periodic limb movements are themselves associated with cardiovascular disease [33, 34]. This could explain the significantly increased risk of cardiovascular events but not the effect of CPAP therapy.

This study was based on traditional metrics derived from overnight sleep studies. New approaches to analysis of sleep study data have emerged. These include the following: (a) intensity of arousal [35, 36]; (b) heart rate response to arousal [37], this trait is heritable [38]; event duration [39, 40], which has also been shown to be heritable [41]; (c) desaturation area, which is

Table 17.2 Description of labels for the polysomnographic clusters based on distinguishing features

Cluster(n)	Cluster label	Median AHI[a] (events/hour)	Conventional OSA severity[a]
A (533)	Mild	4	None/mild
B (119)	PLMS	10	
C (186)	NREM and poor sleep	19	Moderate
D (168)	REM and hypoxia	19	
E (75)	Hypopnoea and hypoxia	44	Severe
F (42)	Arousal and poor sleep	68	
G (124)	Combined severe	84	

Reproduced from Zinchuk AV et al. [31], with permission from BMJ Publishing Group, Ltd

AHI apnoea–hypopnoea index, *NREM* non-rapid eye movement, *OSA* obstructive sleep apnoea, *PLMS* periodic limb movements of sleep, *REM* rapid eye movement

[a]OSA severity definitions none/mild (AHI <15), moderate (15 ≤ AHI < 30) and severe (AHI ≥30). AHI was not used in generating patient clusters. Median AHIs and severity categories based on median AHI for each cluster are shown for descriptive purposes only (mean AHIs were 7.5, 13.6, 24.0, 25.0, 47.6, 72.6 and 82.4 for clusters A, B, C, D, E, F and G, respectively)

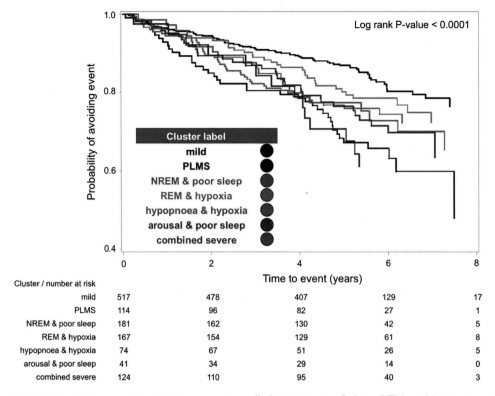

Cluster / number at risk					
mild	517	478	407	129	17
PLMS	114	96	82	27	1
NREM & poor sleep	181	162	130	42	5
REM & hypoxia	167	154	129	61	8
hypopnoea & hypoxia	74	67	51	26	5
arousal & poor sleep	41	34	29	14	0
combined severe	124	110	95	40	3

Fig. 17.1 Kaplan-Meier survival probability curves for risk of acute coronary syndrome, transient ischemic attack, stroke, or death for seven polysomnographic clusters. NREM, non-rapid eye movement; PLMS, periodic limb movements of sleep; REM, rapid eye movement. (Reproduced from Zinchuk et al. [31], with permission from BMJ Publishing Group, Ltd)

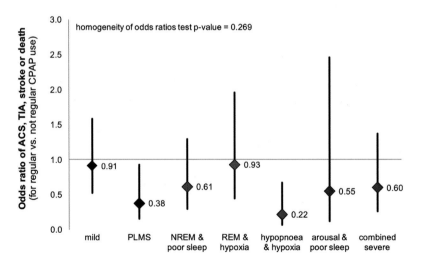

Fig. 17.2 Risk (odds ratio, OR) of acute coronary syndrome (ACS), TIA, stroke, or death for those with regular versus not regular CPAP use for each cluster. ACS, acute coronary syndrome; CPAP, continuous positive airway pressure; NREM, non-rapid eye movement; PLMS, periodic limb movements of sleep; REM, rapid eye movement; TIA, transient ischemic attack. p value is for Breslow-Day homogeneity of ORs test. OR and 95% CI reported for those with regular CPAP use versus not regular CPAP use. In only two groups did CPAP reduce CV event rates (PLMS and hypopnoea & hypoxia). Cluster label same as in Fig. 17.1. (Reproduced from Zinchuk et al. [31], with permission from BMJ Publishing Group, Ltd)

a new measure of the total hypoxic burden resulting from sleep-disordered breathing [42]. This measure is associated with cardiovascular mortality [42]; (d) odds ratio product, a continuous measure of sleep depth [43]; (e) cardiopulmonary coupling, another measure of sleep depth [44]; abnormalities of this measure are heritable in subjects with sleep apnea [45]; and (f) odds ratio product 9, this is the depth of sleep 9 seconds after an arousal. It reflects sleep drive and the ability to return to sleep following an arousal [46].

Moving forward, there is the opportunity to determine if these new metrics provide additional information that is of clinical value. Moreover, there is the opportunity to identify the gene variants that underlie the heritability of several of these new metrics.

Clinical Subtypes Based on Symptoms

Another more focused approach to elucidating heterogeneity is to assess symptoms that patients with OSA have. This approach was initiated in Iceland based on the Icelandic Sleep Apnea Cohort [47]. In the small country of Iceland, home sleep studies for diagnosis of OSA are carried out at several locations around the island. However, all patients requiring CPAP therapy are referred to the University Hospital in Reykjavik for initiation of therapy. This is a wonderful opportunity for clinical research. These patients are enrolled in the Icelandic Sleep Apnea Cohort (ISAC), and all patients assessed are invited to be involved in research and to complete questionnaires about their symptoms.

Using questionnaire data as input variables and based on unsupervised cluster analysis, three distinct subtypes emerged [48]. They are: (a) insomnia (32.7% of total) – a group where the main symptom is difficulty initiating or maintaining sleep; (b) relatively asymptomatic group (24.7% of total); (c) an excessively sleepy group (42.6% of total). This group has quite marked excessive sleepiness with an Epworth Sleepiness Score of 15.7 ± 0.6 (mean ± SE).

These three groups of patients with different symptoms do not differ in terms of age, gender, BMI, or severity of OSA. All three groups have on average severe OSA. Their apnea-hypopnea indices are 43.8 ± 20.4, 43.1 ± 18.9, and 46.7 ± 21.7 events/hour (mean ± SD), respectively.

While of interest, it is conceivable that these subtypes might be unique to Iceland and reflect clinical referral patterns [49]. Thus, efforts have been made to replicate these findings. In the Korean Genomic Cohort, a population-based cohort, the same subtypes are found [50]. However, the prevalence of the asymptomatic group is higher than in the cohort of clinical patients. This is not surprising. In population-based studies, the prevalence of sleep-disordered breathing is high but the symptom burden relatively low [51].

The findings have also been replicated using data from the Sleep Apnea Global Interdisciplinary Consortium (SAGIC). This is an effort by clinical sleep centers in many countries to develop new approaches to diagnosis and management of OSA (for description, see [2]). While the three major subtypes found in the Iceland study are replicated, the optimal cluster solution had five subtypes [52]. The new subtypes were a group with excessive sleepiness but a relative absence of symptoms of upper airway obstruction and a group whose symptoms are dominated by indications of upper airway obstruction [52]. They had high rates of snoring, witnessed apneas, and waking up suddenly unable to breathe [52].

Not surprisingly, individuals with these different clinical subtypes benefit differently from CPAP therapy. All three primary groups show significant improvements in Epworth Sleepiness scores, but the magnitude of change is much larger in the excessively sleepy group. The least symptomatic improvement is in the relatively asymptomatic group with the largest symptomatic change being in the excessively sleepy group. There is improvement in insomnia symptoms with CPAP in the "insomnia" group, but even with successful CPAP therapy there is still a high prevalence of individuals with insomnia symptoms [53]. This likely means that the insomnia in such individuals is not related directly to their obstructive sleep apnea.

It is also of interest to determine whether the outcomes of OSA differ between the clinical subtypes, in particular, cardiovascular disease. To address this, studies were done using data from the Sleep Heart Health Study (SHHS) [54, 55]. Subjects in this community-based study were recruited from 1995 to 1998 and the mean period of follow-up was 11.8 years. Subjects had full sleep studies, with EEG recording, conducted at home as part of their initial evaluation. Data on 5804 subjects were available through the National Sleep Research Resource [56, 57].

Although the questionnaires used in the SHHS are not identical to those used in the other studies described above, there was sufficient information on symptoms to allow unsupervised clustering to be performed. The same three subtypes were identified, i.e., insomnia, relatively asymptomatic, and excessively sleepy. As with the SAGIC study, the optimal solution for clusters was higher than 3; in this case 4. The additional cluster was subjects with moderate sleepiness [58].

The incidence of cardiovascular events was significantly different between the four groups [58]. To evaluate the different risk for CV disease, analyses were done comparing the incidence of different types of CV diseases in subjects with at least moderate OSA (i.e., apnea-hypopnea index >15 events/hour) in the four clinical subtypes compared to that in controls without OSA, i.e., AHI <5 events/hour. Analyses were done unadjusted and after adjusting for age, gender, BMI, and other cardiovascular risk factors (see Fig. 17.3). There was an increased risk for coronary artery disease, heart failure, and all cardiovascular events in the excessively sleepy group (see Fig. 17.3) [58]. There was no increased risk in the other groups (see Fig. 17.3) [58].

This is not the first study to argue that the presence of excessive sleepiness in patients with OSA increases the risk for CV events. Studies of patients who had sleep studies following a myocardial infarction found that subjects with at least moderate OSA, who were excessively sleepy as defined as an Epworth Sleepiness Score of >11, had higher re-infarction rates and significantly more major cardiovascular events than those with

the same degree of OSA who were not excessively sleepy [59]. Few patients in this study identified with OSA were treated for the condition.

This finding that cardiovascular risk for OSA occurs in excessively sleepy subjects has important clinical and research implications [60]. It first raises the important question as to whether the relatively asymptomatic group of patients with OSA, who are very common in population-based studies [51], do need to be treated. Also, these results lead to a plausible hypothesis as to why the large multi-site randomized trial (SAVE) assessing effect of CPAP on CV events was negative [61]. In the SAVE study, excessively sleepy patients, defined by an Epworth Sleepiness Score >15, were excluded. Their exclusion was related to concerns about not treating such patients who are expected to be at increased risk of car crashes [11]. But excluding these subjects likely removed the very group who were at most risk for CV events.

This indicates that new strategies need to be adopted to allow excessively sleepy patients to be included in such clinical trials. One such strategy is to compare outcomes in full users of CPAP with those who did not use CPAP. But this approach raises concerns that non-users may be different in other ways that affect the outcomes. This can be addressed by propensity score matching to ensure equal distribution of key covariates in each group (full users, non-users) [62]. This necessitates trimming to balance groups, i.e., removal of specific patients to allow covariate matches to occur [62]. This approach has been used in a study of the effect of CPAP on levels of lipids [63].

While these observations are important, we also do not know the basis for these differences. They are not explained by severity of disease, as assessed by the apnea-hypopnea index, and degree of obesity. It could be that the physiological response to sleep-disordered breathing could be different between patients in different groups. For example, could excessively sleepy subjects have more fragmented and less deep sleep? Could differences be genetic, epigenetic, and/or are there other molecular differences between groups? A small pilot metabolomics study found low levels of choline in patients with OSA who

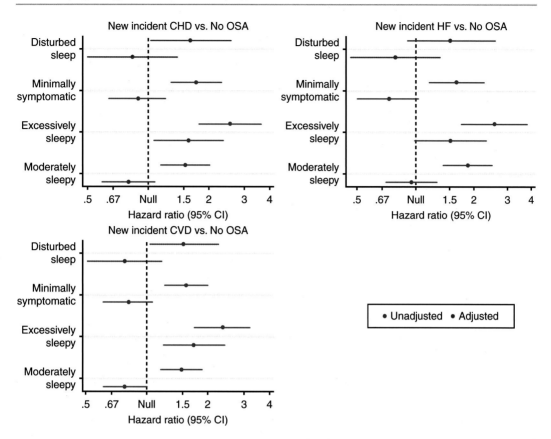

Fig. 17.3 The figure shows the hazard ratio (95% CI) compared to controls without OSA for each of the four symptomatic groups in the Sleep Heart Health Study. The data shown are for incident coronary heart disease (CHD; top left panel), heart failure (HF; top right panel), and incident all cardiovascular disease (CVD; bottom left panel). After adjustment, the increased risk for each of the three cardiovascular outcomes occurs only in the excessively sleep group. *Covariates in adjusted analyses*: age, sex, body mass index, type 2 diabetes, hypertension, HDL, total cholesterol, triglycerides, alcohol use, and smoking status

were excessively sleepy compared to patients with OSA who were not sleepy [64].

It seems likely that it is not the excessive sleepiness itself that contributes to CV risk but rather processes that underlie CV risk in patients with OSA also result in excessive sleepiness.

This is likely to be a fruitful area for research and will require discovery strategies across multiple domains.

Conclusions

There is no doubt that OSA is a heterogeneous disorder. New approaches are beginning to elucidate the nature of the heterogeneity. Efforts based on obtaining data in large numbers of subjects together with unsupervised clustering approaches have proven to be fruitful. However, the value of these approaches depends on the input variables. Studies that have involved input variables from multiple sources, including age, gender, BMI and severity of OSA as assessed by the apnea-hypopnea index, have not been particularly fruitful. Rather, more focused studies whether based on physiological differences [31] or symptomatic differences [48] have been much more helpful. Moving forward, we can anticipate much more work in this area leading to development of a personalized approach to the very common disorder—obstructive sleep apnea [65].

Acknowledgments Original research described in this review was supported by NIH Program Project Grant P01 HL094307. The concepts described in this review arose in helpful discussions with my colleagues: Thorarinn Gislason, Brendan Keenan, Jinyoung Kim, Diane Lim, Greg Maislin, Diego Mazzotti, Bhajan Singh, Magdy Younes, and other participants in the Sleep Apnea Global Interdisciplinary Consortium.

References

1. Peppard PE, Young T, Barnet JH, Palta M, Hagen EW, Hla KM. Increased prevalence of sleep-disordered breathing in adults. Am J Epidemiol. 2013;177(9):1006–14.
2. Sutherland K, Keenan BT, Bittencourt L, Chen NH, Gislason T, Leinwand S, et al. A global comparison of anatomic risk factors and their relationship to obstructive sleep apnea severity in clinical samples. J Clin Sleep Med. 2019;15(4):629–39.
3. Lee RW, Vasudavan S, Hui DS, Prvan T, Petocz P, Darendeliler MA, et al. Differences in craniofacial structures and obesity in Caucasian and Chinese patients with obstructive sleep apnea. Sleep. 2010;33(8):1075–80.
4. Wang Y, Mi J, Shan XY, Wang QJ, Ge KY. Is China facing an obesity epidemic and the consequences? The trends in obesity and chronic disease in China. Int J Obes. 2007;31(1):177–88.
5. Ji CY, Chen TJ, Working Group on Obesity in China (WGOC). Empirical changes in the prevalence of overweight and obesity among Chinese students from 1985 to 2010 and corresponding preventive strategies. Biomed Environ Sci. 2013;26(1):1–12.
6. Wang Y, Wang L, Xue H, Qu W. A review of the growth of the fast food industry in China and its potential impact on obesity. Int J Environ Res Public Health. 2016;13(11):1112.
7. Lim DC, Pack AI. Obstructive sleep apnea: update and future. Annu Rev Med. 2017;68:99–112.
8. Reinke C, Bevans-Fonti S, Drager LF, Shin MK, Polotsky VY. Effects of different acute hypoxic regimens on tissue oxygen profiles and metabolic outcomes. J Appl Physiol (1985). 2011;111(3):881–90.
9. Jenkinson C, Davies RJ, Mullins R, Stradling JR. Comparison of therapeutic and subtherapeutic nasal continuous positive airway pressure for obstructive sleep apnoea: a randomised prospective parallel trial. Lancet. 1999;353(9170):2100–5.
10. Ye L, Liang ZA, Weaver TE. Predictors of health-related quality of life in patients with obstructive sleep apnoea. J Adv Nurs. 2008;63(1):54–63.
11. Sassani A, Findley LJ, Kryger M, Goldlust E, George C, Davidson TM. Reducing motor-vehicle collisions, costs, and fatalities by treating obstructive sleep apnea syndrome. Sleep. 2004;27(3):453–8.
12. Pack AI, Gislason T. Obstructive sleep apnea and cardiovascular disease: a perspective and future directions. Prog Cardiovasc Dis. 2009;51(5):434–51.
13. Javaheri S, Barbe F, Campos-Rodriguez F, Dempsey JA, Khayat R, Javaheri S, et al. Sleep apnea: types, mechanisms, and clinical cardiovascular consequences. J Am Coll Cardiol. 2017;69(7):841–58.
14. Marin JM, Carrizo SJ, Vicente E, Agusti AG. Long-term cardiovascular outcomes in men with obstructive sleep apnoea-hypopnoea with or without treatment with continuous positive airway pressure: an observational study. Lancet. 2005;365(9464):1046–53.
15. Aronson D, Nakhleh M, Zeidan-Shwiri T, Mutlak M, Lavie P, Lavie L. Clinical implications of sleep disordered breathing in acute myocardial infarction. PLoS One. 2014;9(2):e88878.
16. Li M, Hou WS, Zhang XW, Tang ZY. Obstructive sleep apnea and risk of stroke: a meta-analysis of prospective studies. Int J Cardiol. 2014;172(2):466–9.
17. Yaggi HK, Concato J, Kernan WN, Lichtman JH, Brass LM, Mohsenin V. Obstructive sleep apnea as a risk factor for stroke and death. N Engl J Med. 2005;353(19):2034–41.
18. Mehra R, Benjamin EJ, Shahar E, Gottlieb DJ, Nawabit R, Kirchner HL, et al. Association of nocturnal arrhythmias with sleep-disordered breathing: the Sleep Heart Health Study. Am J Respir Crit Care Med. 2006;173(8):910–6.
19. Harsch IA, Schahin SP, Radespiel-Troger M, Weintz O, Jahreiss H, Fuchs FS, et al. Continuous positive airway pressure treatment rapidly improves insulin sensitivity in patients with obstructive sleep apnea syndrome. Am J Respir Crit Care Med. 2004;169(2):156–62.
20. Schahin SP, Nechanitzky T, Dittel C, Fuchs FS, Hahn EG, Konturek PC, et al. Long-term improvement of insulin sensitivity during CPAP therapy in the obstructive sleep apnoea syndrome. Med Sci Monit. 2008;14(3):CR117–21.
21. Punjabi NM, Sorkin JD, Katzel LI, Goldberg AP, Schwartz AR, Smith PL. Sleep-disordered breathing and insulin resistance in middle-aged and overweight men. Am J Respir Crit Care Med. 2002;165(5):677–82.
22. Ip MS, Lam B, Ng MM, Lam WK, Tsang KW, Lam KS. Obstructive sleep apnea is independently associated with insulin resistance. Am J Respir Crit Care Med. 2002;165(5):670–6.
23. Botros N, Concato J, Mohsenin V, Selim B, Doctor K, Yaggi HK. Obstructive sleep apnea as a risk factor for type 2 diabetes. Am J Med. 2009;122(12):1122–7.
24. Campos-Rodriguez F, Martinez-Garcia MA, Martinez M, Duran-Cantolla J, Pena Mde L, Masdeu MJ, et al. Association between obstructive sleep apnea and cancer incidence in a large multicenter Spanish cohort. Am J Respir Crit Care Med. 2013;187(1):99–105.
25. Martinez-Garcia MA, Campos-Rodriguez F, Nagore E, Martorell A, Rodriguez-Peralto JL,

Riveiro-Falkenbach E, et al. Sleep-disordered breathing is independently associated with increased aggressiveness of cutaneous melanoma: a multicenter observational study in 443 patients. Chest. 2018;154(6):1348–58.

26. Nieto FJ, Peppard PE, Young T, Finn L, Hla KM, Farre R. Sleep-disordered breathing and cancer mortality: results from the Wisconsin sleep cohort study. Am J Respir Crit Care Med. 2012;186(2):190–4.

27. Vavougios GD, George DG, Pastaka C, Zarogiannis SG, Gourgoulianis KI. Phenotypes of comorbidity in OSAS patients: combining categorical principal component analysis with cluster analysis. J Sleep Res. 2016;25(1):31–8.

28. Brusselaers N, Lagergren J. The Charlson Comorbidity Index in registry-based research. Methods Inf Med. 2017;56(5):401–6.

29. Lacedonia D, Carpagnano GE, Sabato R, Storto MM, Palmiotti GA, Capozzi V, et al. Characterization of obstructive sleep apnea-hypopnea syndrome (OSA) population by means of cluster analysis. J Sleep Res. 2016;25(6):724–30.

30. Bailly S, Destors M, Grillet Y, Richard P, Stach B, Vivodtzev I, et al. Obstructive sleep apnea: a cluster analysis at time of diagnosis. PLoS One. 2016;11(6):e0157318.

31. Zinchuk AV, Jeon S, Koo BB, Yan X, Bravata DM, Qin L, et al. Polysomnographic phenotypes and their cardiovascular implications in obstructive sleep apnoea. Thorax. 2018;73(5):472–80.

32. Koo BB, Won C, Selim BJ, Qin L, Jeon S, Redeker NS, et al. The Determining Risk of Vascular Events by Apnea Monitoring (DREAM) study: design, rationale, and methods. Sleep Breath. 2016;20(2):893–900.

33. Xie J, Chahal CAA, Covassin N, Schulte PJ, Singh P, Srivali N, et al. Periodic limb movements of sleep are associated with an increased prevalence of atrial fibrillation in patients with mild sleep-disordered breathing. Int J Cardiol. 2017;241:200–4.

34. Winkelman JW, Blackwell T, Stone K, Ancoli-Israel S, Redline S. Associations of incident cardiovascular events with restless legs syndrome and periodic leg movements of sleep in older men, for the outcomes of sleep disorders in older men study (MrOS sleep study). Sleep. 2017;40(4). https://doi.org/10.1093/sleep/zsx023.

35. Amatoury J, Azarbarzin A, Younes M, Jordan AS, Wellman A, Eckert DJ. Arousal intensity is a distinct pathophysiological trait in obstructive sleep apnea. Sleep. 2016;39(12):2091–100.

36. Azarbarzin A, Ostrowski M, Younes M, Keenan BT, Pack AI, Staley B, et al. Arousal responses during overnight polysomnography and their reproducibility in healthy young adults. Sleep. 2015;38(8):1313–21.

37. Azarbarzin A, Ostrowski M, Hanly P, Younes M. Relationship between arousal intensity and heart rate response to arousal. Sleep. 2014;37(4):645–53.

38. Gao X, Azarbarzin A, Keenan BT, Ostrowski M, Pack FM, Staley B, et al. Heritability of heart rate response to arousals in twins. Sleep. 2017;40(6):zsx055.

39. Koch H, Schneider LD, Finn LA, Leary EB, Peppard PE, Hagen E, et al. Breathing disturbances without hypoxia are associated with objective sleepiness in sleep apnea. Sleep. 2017;40(11):zsx152.

40. Leppanen T, Toyras J, Mervaala E, Penzel T, Kulkas A. Severity of individual obstruction events increases with age in patients with obstructive sleep apnea. Sleep Med. 2017;37:32–7.

41. Liang J, Cade BE, Wang H, Chen H, Gleason KJ, Larkin EK, et al. Comparison of heritability estimation and linkage analysis for multiple traits using principal component analyses. Genet Epidemiol. 2016;40(3):222–32.

42. Azarbarzin A, Sands SA, Stone KL, Taranto-Montemurro L, Messineo L, Terrill PI, et al. The hypoxic burden of sleep apnoea predicts cardiovascular disease-related mortality: the Osteoporotic Fractures in Men Study and the Sleep Heart Health Study. Eur Heart J. 2019;40(14):1149–57.

43. Younes M, Ostrowski M, Soiferman M, Younes H, Raneri J, Hanly P. Odds ratio product of sleep EEG as a continuous measure of sleep state. Sleep. 2015;38(4):641–54.

44. Thomas RJ, Mietus JE, Peng CK, Guo D, Gozal D, Montgomery-Downs H, et al. Relationship between delta power and the electrocardiogram-derived cardiopulmonary spectrogram: possible implications for assessing the effectiveness of sleep. Sleep Med. 2014;15(1):125–31.

45. Ibrahim LH, Jacono FJ, Patel SR, Thomas RJ, Larkin EK, Mietus JE, et al. Heritability of abnormalities in cardiopulmonary coupling in sleep apnea: use of an electrocardiogram-based technique. Sleep. 2010;33(5):643–6.

46. Younes M, Hanly PJ. Immediate postarousal sleep dynamics: an important determinant of sleep stability in obstructive sleep apnea. J Appl Physiol (1985). 2016;120(7):801–8.

47. Arnardottir ES, Maislin G, Schwab RJ, Staley B, Benediktsdottir B, Olafsson I, et al. The interaction of obstructive sleep apnea and obesity on the inflammatory markers C-reactive protein and interleukin-6: the Icelandic Sleep Apnea Cohort. Sleep. 2012;35(7):921–32.

48. Ye L, Pien GW, Ratcliffe SJ, Bjornsdottir E, Arnardottir ES, Pack AI, et al. The different clinical faces of obstructive sleep apnoea: a cluster analysis. Eur Respir J. 2014;44(6):1600–7.

49. Ryan CM, Kendzerska T, Wilton K, Lyons OD. The different clinical faces of obstructive sleep apnea (OSA), OSA in older adults as a distinctly different physiological phenotype, and the impact of OSA on cardiovascular events after coronary artery bypass surgery. Am J Respir Crit Care Med. 2015;192(9):1127–9.

50. Kim J, Keenan BT, Lim DC, Lee SK, Pack AI, Shin C. Symptom-based subgroups of Koreans with obstructive sleep apnea. J Clin Sleep Med. 2018;14(3):437–43.

51. Arnardottir ES, Bjornsdottir E, Olafsdottir KA, Benediktsdottir B, Gislason T. Obstructive sleep apnoea in the general population: highly prevalent but minimal symptoms. Eur Respir J. 2016;47(1):194–202.

52. Keenan BT, Kim J, Singh B, Bittencourt L, Chen NH, Cistulli PA, et al. Recognizable clinical subtypes of obstructive sleep apnea across international sleep centers: a cluster analysis. Sleep. 2018;41(3):zsx214.

53. Pien GW, Ye L, Keenan BT, Maislin G, Bjornsdottir E, Arnardottir ES, et al. Changing faces of obstructive sleep apnea: treatment effects by cluster designation in the Icelandic Sleep Apnea Cohort. Sleep. 2018;41(3):zsx201.

54. Gottlieb DJ, Yenokyan G, Newman AB, O'Connor GT, Punjabi NM, Quan SF, et al. Prospective study of obstructive sleep apnea and incident coronary heart disease and heart failure: the sleep heart health study. Circulation. 2010;122(4):352–60.

55. Redline S, Yenokyan G, Gottlieb DJ, Shahar E, O'Connor GT, Resnick HE, et al. Obstructive sleep apnea-hypopnea and incident stroke: the sleep heart health study. Am J Respir Crit Care Med. 2010;182(2):269–77.

56. Dean DA 2nd, Goldberger AL, Mueller R, Kim M, Rueschman M, Mobley D, et al. Scaling up scientific discovery in sleep medicine: the National Sleep Research Resource. Sleep. 2016;39(5):1151–64.

57. Zhang GQ, Cui L, Mueller R, Tao S, Kim M, Rueschman M, et al. The National Sleep Research Resource: towards a sleep data commons. J Am Med Inform Assoc. 2018;25(10):1351–8.

58. Mazzotti DR, Keenan BT, Lim DC, Gottlieb DJ, Kim J, Pack AI. Symptom subtypes of obstructive sleep apnea predict incidence of cardiovascular outcomes. Am J Respir Crit Care Med. 2019;200:493–506.

59. Xie J, Sert Kuniyoshi FH, Covassin N, Singh P, Gami AS, Chahal CAA, et al. Excessive daytime sleepiness independently predicts increased cardiovascular risk after myocardial infarction. J Am Heart Assoc. 2018;7(2):e007221.

60. Zinchuk A, Yaggi HK. Sleep apnea heterogeneity, phenotypes, and cardiovascular risk: implications for trial design and precision sleep medicine. Am J Respir Crit Care Med. 2019;200:412.

61. McEvoy RD, Antic NA, Heeley E, Luo Y, Ou Q, Zhang X, et al. CPAP for prevention of cardiovascular events in obstructive sleep apnea. N Engl J Med. 2016;375(10):919–31.

62. Maislin G, Rubin DB. Design of non-randomized medical device trials based on sub-classification using propensity score quintiles. Proc Joint Stat Meet. 2010:2182–96.

63. Keenan BT, Maislin G, Sunwoo BY, Arnardottir ES, Jackson N, Olafsson I, et al. Obstructive sleep apnoea treatment and fasting lipids: a comparative effectiveness study. Eur Respir J. 2014;44(2):405–14.

64. Pak VM, Dai F, Keenan BT, Gooneratne NS, Pack AI. Lower plasma choline levels are associated with sleepiness symptoms. Sleep Med. 2018;44:89–96.

65. Edwards BA, Redline S, Sands SA, Owens RL. More than the sum of the respiratory events: personalized medicine approaches for obstructive sleep apnea. Am J Respir Crit Care Med. 2019;200:691.

Precision Medicine in Critical Illness: Sepsis and Acute Respiratory Distress Syndrome

18

Angela J. Rogers and Nuala J. Meyer

Key Point Summary
- Disease heterogeneity in ARDS and sepsis has challenged the conduct of omics studies involving these syndromes, yet precision medicine approaches are sorely needed to improve outcomes.
- Genomics studies of ARDS and sepsis are challenged by small sample sizes and the difficulty in identifying appropriate controls.
- Gene expression studies have identified biologically distinct expression signatures that retroactively identify differential response to routine treatments applied in the ICU. In sepsis, a signature of dysregulated adaptive immune signaling has evidence to stratify patients according to a differential response to systemic steroid therapy. In ARDS,

patients with a hyperinflammatory pattern identified in plasma using targeted proteomics responded more favorably to randomized interventions including high positive end-expiratory pressure, volume conservative fluid therapy, and simvastatin therapy.
- Fewer ARDS and sepsis metabolomics and unbiased proteomics studies exist, but as these approaches become more standardized, additional biomarkers may be identified.

A. J. Rogers
Department of Medicine, Stanford University, Palo Alto, CA, USA
e-mail: ajrogers@stanford.edu

N. J. Meyer (✉)
Pulmonary, Allergy, and Critical Care Division, University of Pennsylvania Perelman School of Medicine, Hospital of the University of Pennsylvania, Philadelphia, PA, USA
e-mail: nuala.meyer@pennmedicine.upenn.edu

Introduction

Sepsis and the acute respiratory distress syndrome (ARDS) are two syndromes causing a sobering proportion of deaths in the intensive care unit (ICU). By one estimate, sepsis was responsible for between one third and one half of inpatient deaths [1], whereas ARDS has been observed to complicate almost one quarter of critical care admissions requiring mechanical ventilation, with a mortality rate exceeding 35% [2]. Despite significant advances in our understanding of the pathologic mechanisms contributing to each of these syndromes, neither sepsis nor ARDS can boast specific pharmacologic therapy with a consistently proven effect. Numerous trials in sepsis

© Springer Nature Switzerland AG 2020
J. L. Gomez et al. (eds.), *Precision in Pulmonary, Critical Care, and Sleep Medicine*, Respiratory Medicine, https://doi.org/10.1007/978-3-030-31507-8_18

[3–5] and ARDS [6–8] have failed to establish drug therapy for these deadly syndromes. One major factor that may contribute to this treatment gap is the profound heterogeneity encompassed by patients meeting criteria for each syndrome. A valid concern is that our syndromic definitions [9–11], although useful in identifying patients who share clinical factors and who may benefit from standardized care [12–15], may have almost no utility in predicting a patient's biologic subclassification nor in predicting mortality, expected complications, or response to therapy. Precision medicine options for these syndromes, whereby the correct drug could be targeted to the patients most likely to be helped and least likely to be harmed, are sorely needed.

For complex traits such as asthma or cystic fibrosis, the knowledge of a patient's biologic endotype provides clues about a patient's prognosis, pathophysiology, and expected response to therapy [16–20], yet such a breakthrough has yet to arrive for sepsis or ARDS. In this chapter, we review the contributions of genomic medicine to identifying potential biologic subgroups in sepsis and ARDS, a necessary first step for precision medicine. In addition, we consider specific challenges to pursuing omics approaches in each of these traits, as well as potential opportunities we envision in the near future.

Targeted Proteomics: Laying the Foundation for Precision Medicine of Sepsis and ARDS

Increasingly, we have objective evidence that response to therapy is nonuniform and potentially predictable by factors beyond clinical features. In ARDS, this has been consistently demonstrated among clinical trial populations using an analytic method known as latent class analysis (LCA) to uncover potentially unobserved subpopulations while remaining agnostic to outcomes. In analyses considering clinical variables including vital signs, ventilator data, and laboratory values in addition to exploratory plasma biomarkers representing inflammation, vascular dysfunction, or alveolar injury, a latent

class model consistently identified two classes of ARDS trial subjects that differed in their plasma expression of inflammatory biomarkers epitomized by interleukin (IL-) 8 or IL-6, and by their degree of systemic illness, characterized by low blood pressure and low serum bicarbonate [21–24].

Not only were subjects in the "hyperinflammatory" subphenotype group more likely to die, but the LCA group assignment (hyperinflammatory versus non-hyperinflammatory) exhibited significant statistical interaction with randomized treatment effects (Table 18.1) [21, 22, 24]. Thus, when the randomized interventions of higher positive end-expiratory pressure (PEEP), conservative fluid strategy, or simvastatin therapy were analyzed in groups stratified by LCA assignment, each therapy seemed to have a mortality benefit only observed in the hyperinflammatory group, with no signal for improvement in the non-hyperinflamed group [21, 22, 24]. In each trial, there was no evidence for heterogeneity in treatment effect by baseline severity of illness, as defined by the Acute Physiology and Chronic Health Evaluation (APACHE) score, nor by the severity of ARDS, as defined by the ratio of arterial partial pressure of oxygen to fraction of inspired oxygen ($PaO_2:FiO_2$).

Reproducible biologically defined ARDS subgroups based on plasma protein expression patterns were also reported in a population of sepsis-associated ARDS subjects from a prospective sepsis cohort applying a Ward clustering algorithm [25]. Showing remarkable similarity to the LCA-derived subgroups, the clustering algorithm detected two classes of ARDS, one "reactive" defined by high plasma concentrations of markers of inflammation, coagulation, and endothelial activation compared to the "noninflamed" group, and a significantly higher mortality was observed for the reactive subgroup. Although the overlap in plasma protein signatures between the Calfee "hyperinflamed" and Bos "reactive" subgroups is striking [21–23, 25], both studies sampled fairly similar candidate biomarkers that have previously performed well in human and animal studies of sepsis-associated ARDS [26, 27], so the overlap is less surprising than if the authors

Table 18.1 Apparent heterogeneous response to therapy that may be predictable by biologic testing

Population	Potential classifier	Intervention	Study findings
Pediatric sepsis	Gene expression subtype A vs B	Corticosteroids	Subtype A with higher mortality when treated with steroids Subtype B plus a high predicted mortality displayed a mortality benefit from steroids [117, 118]
Adult sepsis	Plasma IL1RA level	Recombinant IL1RA	High plasma IL1RA subjects with a mortality benefit when randomized to rhIL1RA; low plasma IL1RA no benefit [35]
Adult septic shock	Gene expression subtype SRS1 vs SRS2	Corticosteroids	SRS2 subjects with increased mortality with steroids; SRS1 no effect of steroids [124]
Adult ARDS	Latent class assignment (clinical and plasma protein expression)	High PEEP (positive end-expiratory pressure)	Hyperinflammatory subjects with a mortality benefit when randomized to high PEEP; no benefit in non-hyperinflammatory patients [21]
Adult ARDS	Latent class assignment (clinical and plasma protein expression)	Conservative IV fluid therapy	Hyperinflammatory patients with a mortality benefit when randomized to conservative (dry) fluid strategy; non-hyperinflammatory without benefit [22]
Adult ARDS	Latent class assignment (clinical and plasma protein expression)	Simvastatin therapy	Hyperinflammatory patients with a mortality benefit when randomized to simvastatin; non-hyperinflammatory subjects with no benefit from simvastatin [23]

As evidence for the potential of precision medicine to better target therapy to patients, each study listed describes an apparent statistical interaction between an intervention and study outcome (mortality). Because these were all retrospective studies and many were subgroup analyses, a prospective validation study is needed before altering clinical care
SRS sepsis response signature, *PEEP* positive end-expiratory pressure, *IV* intravenous

had used unbiased discovery or untargeted proteomics approaches.

Similarly, in sepsis, it is conceivable that heterogeneity of treatment effect may underlie some of the negative overall findings for such drugs as recombinant human interleukin-1 receptor antagonist (rhIL1RA) [28–30], antitumor necrosis factor [31, 32], or activated protein C [4, 33, 34]. In a subgroup reanalysis of a randomized trial of rhIL1RA for sepsis [29], the mortality benefit of rhIL1RA differed significantly between subjects with high baseline endogenous plasma interleukin-1 receptor antagonist (IL1RA), who seemed to benefit from the drug, and those without elevated plasma IL1RA in whom there was no effect [35]. A separate subgroup reanalysis of the same rhIL1RA trial demonstrated a very strong signal for benefit among subjects with clinically defined macrophage activation syndrome [36]. Although subgroup analyses must be viewed with caution due to underpowering and the risk of unstable effect estimates [37–39], these reports nonethe-

less highlight the potential for precision application of sepsis therapy if replicated in prospectively defined studies.

What Can Be Learned from Genetic Approaches in Complex, Non-Mendelian Traits?

Neither sepsis nor ARDS is considered a classic monogenic or "Mendelian" trait, whereby the expression of the trait is easily predictable by parsing the inheritance of one genetic locus through several generations. However, multiple lines of evidence support a major interplay between genetic variation and patterned responses to injury and infection. Primary, or inherited, immunodeficiency diseases (PIDD) include over 330 specific disorders caused by at least 320 monogenetic changes [40, 41] and span broad subgroups that include defects in just one aspect of the immune system (e.g., antibody, innate,

T-cell, natural killer cell, neutrophil) to combined immunodeficiencies, autoimmune diseases, or autoinflammatory disorders. Some syndromes present as an inherited susceptibility to one particular type of infection, such as mycobacteria, fungi, or certain bacteria, and thus, elucidation of the respective genetic underpinnings has helped to pinpoint critical host responses to specific pathogens [42–46]. Further, the identification of monogenic conditions causing auto-inflammatory conditions that mimic the clinical features of sepsis while remaining culture-negative [47–49] highlight the primacy of host response in driving shock and organ failure.

Further, there is ample evidence that historic infectious threats likely shaped genetic architecture through natural selection [50, 51]. The single missense variant in the beta-globin gene responsible for sickle cell anemia (rs334) persists at a frequency of 5–10% in genotyped African populations [52, 53], a frequency much higher than expected for such a deleterious mutation. However, because individuals who carry only one copy of rs334 seem to be protected from malarial infection [51, 54], this variant is common in populations where malaria has been, or continues to be, a threat. Similar examples may explain the striking variation in genes encoding cytokines [55], or genes that control activation of the complement syndrome, some of which have also been strongly implicated in inflammatory traits like age-related macular degeneration [56–58].

Accepting that our genes influence response to infection or injury, and that such historic threats have in turn shaped genetic architecture, it remains true that most patients with sepsis do not harbor a single genetic variant that explains their risk for sepsis or sepsis death. Nonetheless, there exists strong evidence that sepsis death exhibits significant heritability. In a classic study merging genealogic records and population health information, biologic parents and their children displayed a much stronger concordance for premature death from infection than did adopted parents and their children, suggesting that genes play a stronger role in response to infection than does environment [59]. The relative risk (RR) of dying prematurely from infection when one parent had also

died from infection was almost 6 (95% CI 2.47–13.7), a larger risk than was observed for cancer or even vascular disease [59]. Just as unraveling the monogenic PIDD have suggested precision treatment options that sometimes obviate the need for bone marrow transplantation [47], it may be that better recognition of dysregulated genes contributing to sepsis outcomes suggests novel treatment paradigms for this deadly disease.

Similar data do not exist to support the inherited susceptibility to ARDS, in part because ARDS was only described with the advent of modern ICU care [60], but one might consider the syndrome of acute hypoxia and bilateral lung opacities following a potential insult – ARDS [10] – to be a patterned response to injury or infection. Although to our knowledge no pedigrees exist of ARDS, genetic investigations have suggested novel pathophysiologic processes. Recognizing that we are unlikely to explain a large proportion of the variance in the risk for sepsis or ARDS by one or even a small handful of genes, the dissection of trait-associated pathways may still suggest individuals predisposed to these syndromes via specific mechanisms and, thus, suggest groups who are likely to respond to specific interventions.

Knowledge- and Discovery-Based Genomics Studies

In general terms, there are two major approaches to identify inherited variation that may influence a trait (Fig. 18.1). Knowledge-based approaches, sometimes referred to as candidate gene studies, select specific genes or pathways already hypothesized to contribute to a disease and test for a higher frequency of genetic variants in disease-positive subjects compared to subjects without the disease. Advantages of the candidate approach include the straightforward design, typically as either a case-control or cohort study, low cost, and the fact that next steps after a positive finding are relatively clear. However, precisely because candidate gene studies are predicated on existing knowledge of sepsis or ARDS pathophysiology, these studies have a high risk of failure. For com-

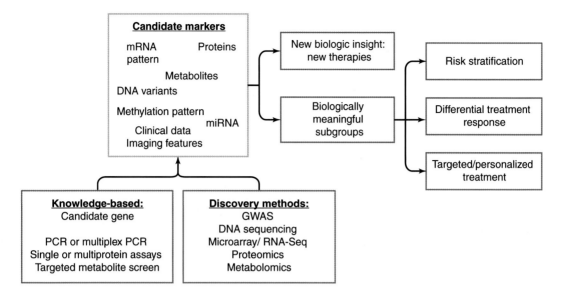

Fig. 18.1 Both knowledge-based and discovery-based methods can identify new candidate markers that span all aspects of biology and clinical features. Novel analytic techniques can then combine clinical, genetic, transcriptomic, metabolomic, and proteomic data to achieve the goals of precision medicine: identifying new therapies via refined mechanistic insight and unpacking clinical heterogeneity into biologically meaningful subgroups. PCR polymerase chain reaction, GWAS genome-wide association study, RNA-Seq RNA sequencing, mRNA messenger RNA

plex traits like sepsis or ARDS, the expected effect size of any given genetic variant is modest, with an odds ratio less than 1.4, and consequently most studies are statistically underpowered to detect an effect even if one exists. Further, even if the selected candidate gene does play a central role in ARDS pathophysiology, researchers still need to genotype the causal part of the gene responsible for the trait or, leveraging linkage disequilibrium [61], a variant in linkage with the causal variant. We are only beginning to understand the complexities of genetic regulation beyond the traditional paradigm of *cis* regulation, whereby local DNA sequence dictates local messenger RNA (mRNA) sequence, which in turn explains protein sequence. With the application of next-generation sequencing techniques to better understand DNA-protein binding, noncoding RNA regulatory elements, epigenetic changes that may silence or activate gene expression, and the impact of three-dimensional chromatin organization [62–66], it is now apparent that early genotyping strategies may have been too simplistic. Thus, the failure to detect associations does not exonerate a gene from playing a significant role. Finally, the candidate gene approach now seems highly inefficient in the era of next generation sequencing approaches.

Genome-wide association studies (GWAS) assay single nucleotide polymorphisms (SNPs) at over 500,000 loci across the genome using nanofabricated arrays of oligonucleotide probes specific for individual SNPs. Then, using knowledge of linkage disequilibrium between SNPs based on large-scale genotyping of multiple populations [52, 67, 68], investigators can impute genotypes at loci that were not genotyped, allowing dense characterization of genetic variation for less than 100 US dollars per sample. However, though the array-based GWAS does characterize DNA variation "across the genome" and is considered a discovery approach, it is not truly bias-free, as the arrays are built using oligonucleotide probes for known SNPs and imputation steps rely upon preexisting knowledge of LD relationships between SNPs. The technology that yields data closest to truly bias-free genome sequences is next-generation sequencing (NGS), in which massively parallel sequencing of fragmented input DNA occurs. NGS is the preferred method to discover new variants or private variants that occur in only one family, or only one individual, as well as to study rare variants [69].

Factors beyond the inherited genomic DNA sequence influence the expression of genes. Profiling of messenger RNA (mRNA) or, more broadly, entire transcriptomes (i.e., transcriptomics) has enabled major advances in the understanding of cancer and complex traits like asthma [16, 70, 71]. Gene expression studies also can be thought of as following either knowledge-based or discovery-based paths. To understand the mRNA abundance or expression pattern of a specific transcript, one could use traditional polymerase chain reaction (PCR) methods using an oligonucleotide probe or probes complementary to the sequence(s) of interest. When roughly 20–30 thousand probes are arrayed onto a single nanofabricated platform to assess global gene expression, we term this a whole genome microarray, which is a discovery method, albeit based on probes and, thus, not bias-free. For broader unbiased characterization of transcriptomes, investigators can use RNA-sequencing (RNA-Seq), a NGS approach that sequences a complementary DNA (cDNA) library prepared from input RNA. Gene expression studies have unique challenges compared to genomics in that the former are cell type and context specific and highly dynamic. Beyond mRNA, multiple noncoding RNA species have been identified and demonstrated to influence transcription, translation, message stability, splicing, enhancing/silencing, epigenetic regulation, and even molecular scaffolding [72]. Bias-free sequencing has elucidated the breadth of the noncoding RNA landscape, and the study of noncoding RNA in critical illness remains in its infancy. Epigenetic changes, which describe inherited but modifiable DNA-protein interactions, such as histone modifications or DNA methylation patterns, also modify gene expression and can be assessed in targeted, high-throughput, or bias-free applications.

Unique Challenges to Achieving Precision Medicine in Critical Care

Although the promise of omics techniques to contribute to precision medicine options is undeniable, specific challenges complicate the application of these methods to sepsis and ARDS. Both syndromes are complex genetic traits, requiring both an extreme environmental insult like infection or exposure to a ventilator and host susceptibility. This gene-by-environment interaction can be complex to study and poses unique barriers to identifying omics signals even when present.

First, the genomic signature of sepsis or ARDS will never occur in isolation. Sepsis by definition is a systemic disease, and multiple organ dysfunction is often central to its diagnosis. Dissecting out the signature of sepsis from that of secondary kidney, lung, brain, or liver injury requires unique analytic tools as well as potentially arbitrary decisions classifying changes as sepsis related or not. With genomic material from the infecting microbe potentially circulating in blood, sequencing techniques might amplify bacterial, viral, parasitic, or fungal genomes rather than the patient's cells. ARDS is also frequently complicated by coincident non-lung organ failure and frequently occurs on the background of sepsis, such that identifying the specific ARDS signature may be difficult. Further, liver and kidney dysfunction can alter the clearance of proteins and metabolites. When metabolic or proteomic changes seem to distinguish ARDS cases from non-cases, these could represent an important feature of the causal pathway in sepsis or may simply reflect end-organ dysfunction with impaired clearance.

Second is the problem of identifying a suitable control population and appropriately designing the study. In many diseases, large convenience cohorts of healthy adults can be used as controls, and large-scale genomic resources such as the UK Biobank can be very powerful to detect a genetic signal [73]. For ICU diseases, however, the use of healthy controls may be problematic, precisely because of the gene-by-environment interaction that requires a severe environmental insult to manifest sepsis or ARDS. A person's genome may contain multiple risk variants for ARDS, but if she never develops sepsis, exposure to a ventilator, or another ARDS precipitant, she may never exhibit lung flooding. The presence of such a subject in the control group would attenuate any signal for ARDS risk, even if multiple ARDS cases carry the same variant. Similar issues arise when designing a sepsis study. In a case-control design, should controls be a group of patients who never had pneumonia or, instead, a group infected with pneumonia and thus at risk to develop sepsis, but who remained relatively well? For this reason, many critical care investigators choose a cohort design, which alleviates the concern for selection bias, but comes at increased cost and lower efficiency. Design issues may complicate the analytic phase as well. A frequent criticism of a potential new prognostic marker for sepsis or ARDS is that it merely reflects severity of illness, and investigators are asked to confirm that associations remain independent of illness severity characterized by simplified acute physiology or APACHE scores [74–76]. While appropriate adjusting for potential confounders has face validity for any analysis, there is a counterargument that the very processes driving acute physiologic derangement and captured by such scores may be in the causal path influencing sepsis or ARDS risk and outcome. Observing that an association persists across multiple levels of illness severity or predicted mortality can sometimes mitigate this concern [77].

Third, timing of biospecimen sampling is both critically important and yet challenging to enact. For both sepsis and ARDS, genomic, proteomic, and metabolomic signatures change substantially within hours to days, and the timeframe to collect samples is highly compressed. Whereas genomic DNA samples should be stable over time and could be collected after the acute event, RNA, protein, or metabolite profiling often requires specific collection strategies and is only relevant if collected during the illness itself. At the same time, critically ill patients are frequently unable to consent for themselves, suffer from anemia [78], and have multiple competing clinical needs that may limit the ability to conduct observational research in the early hours of ICU admission. Furthermore, it is challenging to define "time zero" for sepsis; is it when the patient presents to the emergency room, the first low blood pressure, or the first fever? The importance of

time-course analysis in sepsis was highlighted by gene expression work by Sweeney et al. [79], in which a clear sepsis gene expression signature emerged in early sepsis, but was later swamped by recovery signals. For ARDS, does the clock start when exogenous oxygen exceeds 4 liters per minute, when the chest radiograph is first abnormal, or when the patient is intubated and meeting all consensus criteria [10, 80]? For each omics study, these issues should be carefully considered and protocolized to ensure the highest possible scientific rigor.

Finally, there is the issue of which tissue warrants profiling. Peripheral blood – easily obtained by a blood draw and either left whole or segmented into constituent blood cells – is convenient, widely available, and relevant, as a potential snapshot of circulating host response. Buffy coat gene expression signatures reproducibly separate sepsis cases from controls [81, 82], and circulating inflammatory cells may be the critical actor in sepsis pathology. However, peripheral blood has numerous limitations. Genes that are expressed exclusively by endothelium, epithelium, stromal tissue, or tissue specific to the infected organ will not be captured by whole blood or leukocyte gene expression profiling. Though there may be strong interest to evaluate vascular mRNA, a vessel biopsy will remain highly unlikely and circulating endothelial cells are difficult to collect and may be fundamentally distinct compared to intact vasculature [83]. For ARDS, there is general consensus that lung tissue would provide the maximal utility for gene, protein, and metabolite expression. However, patients with ARDS are rarely subjected to lung biopsy due to their tenuous stability and the risk of the procedure [84]. Easily obtained peripheral blood is not a consistent surrogate for omics states in the lung. In ARDS, peripheral blood gene expression may be swamped by sepsis severity rather than lung injury per se [85]. Even when limiting analysis to only the mononuclear cell fraction and carefully timing blood draws to coincide with bronchoalveolar lavage (BAL), the signature of alveolar macrophages in ARDS is markedly distinct from synchronous peripheral blood monocytes [86]. Despite these formidable challenges, there are numerous examples of incremental and occasionally transformational progress toward precision medicine that speak to tremendous potential of omics approaches in sepsis and ARDS (Table 18.1).

Sepsis Genetics: Hints at Heterogeneous Treatment Effects

Although the promise of genetics to contribute to precision medicine options for sepsis remains strong, progress to date has been relatively modest. Candidate gene association studies have yielded a number of variants that reliably associate with increased susceptibility to specific infections and occasionally with a higher frequency of hypotension or death [87–89]. As candidate gene studies extend from our preexisting paradigm of sepsis, most of the interrogated genes have been those influencing host response, immune regulation, or vascular regulation. Genome-wide studies of sepsis outcome – a highly heritable trait [59] – have also been published and suggest novel pathways that merit consideration.

In one of the first published GWAS for sepsis survival, investigators from the Genetics of Sepsis and Septic Shock in Europe (GenOSept) consortium used a discovery population of approximately 1000 subjects with community-acquired pneumonia and replicated findings in an additional 1000 individuals from clinical trials or an ongoing pneumonia cohort. The GenOSept authors reported a fairly convincing LD peak on chromosome 5 in the *FER* gene encoding Fps/Fes-related tyrosine kinase that associated with lower risk of death (meta-analysis odds ratio 0.56, 95% confidence interval 0.41–0.66) with a *p*-value robust to multiple comparison testing ($p = 5.6 \times 10^{-8}$) [90]. Interestingly, the association with death was attenuated by expanding the population to include septic subjects with abdominal infections, suggesting that the protective association may be relevant only to pulmonary sepsis. The *FER* gene encodes a non-receptor protein tyrosine kinase implicated in actin cytoskeleton regulation as well as chemotaxis and leukocyte migration – areas already of interest in

sepsis pathophysiology [91–93] – thus, it is an attractive sepsis candidate gene. Mortality was 25% for homozygous carriers of the dominant allele compared to 10% in homozygous recessive carriers [90], suggesting that genotype might act as a prognostic enrichment tool to help select a high-risk population [11]. However, as is often the case with genomic findings, replication of this variant has been inconsistent, and it was not associated with mortality in a smaller population of septic subjects enrolled in clinical trials in Germany [94]. A second GWAS found that a rare missense variant in gene *VSP13A* was associated with very high risk for mortality, and this *VSP13A* SNP was associated with higher sequential organ failure assessment score in a separate pneumonia study, providing possible replication. *VSP13A* encodes for vacuolar protein sorting 13 homolog A and has been implicated in autophagy, another pathway relevant to sepsis [95].

Examples of genetic studies contributing to precision therapy in sepsis are indirect, but a few do exist. Meyer et al. identified a synonymous coding SNP in the gene *IL1RN* encoding interleukin-1 receptor antagonist (IL1RA) that associated with reduced ARDS risk in both trauma and sepsis populations, as well as with reduced sepsis mortality in the VASST septic shock trial [96–98]. The SNP seemed to be functional, associating with increased plasma IL1RA among patients at risk for ARDS, lower plasma interleukin-1 beta (IL1β) during septic shock, and as a site of allelic imbalance with more efficient *IL1RN* gene expression following endotoxin challenge. As these data suggested that more efficient plasma IL1RA generation might be protective in sepsis, Meyer and colleagues used plasma from a completed clinical trial of recombinant human IL1RA (rhIL1RA) for sepsis to phenotype sepsis patients for pre-randomization plasma IL1RA and IL1β expression. They detected a differential effect of rhIL1RA on mortality based on plasma IL1RA expression, such that rhIL1RA seemed to reduce mortality among "IL1RA-high" subjects [adjusted risk difference (ARD) −12%, 95% CI −23% to −1%], $p = 0.044$, but not among "IL1RA-low" subjects (ARD +7%, 95% CI −4% to +17%), resulting in a statistically significant

Table 18.2 Genetic associations with sepsis or ARDS with potential impact on therapeutic response

Gene (Official gene ID)	Population	Outcome associated with gene variant	Potential therapy with pharmacogenetic response
Interleukin-1 receptor antagonist (*IL1RN*)	Adult sepsis trial populations Adult trauma cohort	Reduced sepsis death; reduced ARDS risk [97, 98]	Recombinant human interleukin-1 receptor antagonist (rhIL1RA)
Leucyl/cystinyl aminopeptidase or vasopressinase (*LNPEP*)	Adults with septic shock	Higher sepsis mortality [132]	Vasopressin
Protein C (*PROC*)	Adults with sepsis	Higher sepsis mortality, higher organ failure score [133, 134]	Drotrecogin alpha (activated protein C)
Pre-elafin (*PI3*)	Adult at risk for ARDS	ARDS [135, 136]	Human neutrophil elastase inhibitors
Angiotensin-converting enzyme (*ACE*)	Adults with ARDS compared to at-risk or healthy controls	ARDS risk ARDS mortality [137, 138]	ACE inhibitors, angiotensin receptor blockers, or ACE2 analogs
Surfactant protein B (*SFPTB*)	Adults with ARDS compared to at-risk or healthy controls; children with pneumonia	ARDS risk [139], mechanical ventilation risk [140]	Exogenous surfactant
Angiopoietin-2 (*ANGPT2*)	Adult trauma at-risk ARDS Adult sepsis	ARDS; plasma Angiopoietin-2 level [103, 114]	Anti-angiopoietin-2 agent; TIE2 agonist

In each case, a genetic association has been reported in at least one population, and drugs exist to target the gene's pathway

interaction term [35]. As a subgroup analysis, the observation of lower mortality was insufficient evidence to change practice [77, 99] yet it demonstrates that individualized sepsis treatment based on plasma biomarker expression is possible. Given numerous potential genetic associations with sepsis in pathways associated with drug targets (Table 18.2), testing for heterogeneous treatment effect by genotype or plasma protein expression as a routine addition to interventional trials is an approach that, if adequately powered, could be promising to identify precision targets.

ARDS Genetics and the Search for Causal Intermediates

Numerous candidate gene studies have been undertaken in ARDS populations to elucidate key factors associated with either risk of ARDS or ARDS mortality [100, 101]. Among the best replicated loci, genes contributing to inflammatory response (*IL6, IL10, IL1RN, PI3, MBL2, NFKB1, TLR1*), vascular regulation (*ACE, VEGFA, MYLK, ANGPT2, SERPINE1*), oxidant stress (*NFE2L2, HMOX1*), and lung epithelial function (*SFTPB*) are overrepresented. Discovery approaches have also been published [102] and have contributed new candidate genes such as *PPFIA1*, which encodes for liprin alpha 1, a gene expressed in lung and numerous tissues that plays a role in regulating focal adhesions and cell-matrix interactions. As previously mentioned, medium-throughput candidate gene DNA array studies identified risk variants in ARDS that may have potential therapeutic implications, as for *IL1RN*, the gene encoding IL1RA, or *ANGPT2*, the angiopoietin-2 gene that contributes to vascular permeability [98, 103].

Given results of GWAS over the past decade, it is usually unreasonable to expect that common variants will be associated with complex diseases with effect sizes large enough to be statistically significant in studies involving fewer than 2000 cases. In complex traits where numerous relatively frequent SNPs are hypothesized to alter risk with modest effect sizes (odds ratio 1.1–1.5) [104], a well-powered study should include many thousands of cases and non-cases, and no such ARDS population yet exists. Nonetheless, an approach by which genetics may help advance a precision medicine platform is by integrating genetic association results with those of other omics studies to prioritize candidate biomarkers. For example, plasma markers could be prioritized based on genetic results to identify those with the most direct relationships with ARDS risk or mortality. To borrow from a cardiology example, genetics provided strong inferential evidence that plasma concentration of low-density lipoprotein cholesterol (LDL) was the major risk factor for coronary artery disease (CAD) risk and mortality. Plasma LDL is strongly genetically regulated and variants that influence plasma LDL strongly associate with CAD in a consonant fashion; genetic variants that lower LDL associate with reduced lifetime CAD risk and those that elevate LDL associate with high CAD and mortality [105–107]. Thus, drugs targeting LDL are a mainstay of CAD prevention and treatment, and we term LDL a "causal" marker for CAD. Causal markers are lacking for ARDS, but if a causal marker were identified, it could speed drug development via the design of high-throughput screens to identify compounds that alter the marker.

A few examples of leveraging genetics to infer causal ARDS intermediates are worth highlighting. Recognizing that platelets contribute to both microvascular and immune system activation during ARDS and that the lung is a major site of platelet biogenesis [108–110], Wei and colleagues focused on genes shown to strongly associate with platelet counts in healthy subjects and verified that variants in the gene *LRRC16A* also associate with platelet count in a critically ill population. Further, the same platelet-associated variant is also associated with ARDS risk, and a small but significant portion of the ARDS risk was mediated through platelet count, implicating thrombocytopenia as a causal intermediate for ARDS risk [111]. The same group then identified an independent locus in the *LRRC16A* gene associated with both a falling platelet trajectory in the

ICU and ARDS mortality [112] and statistically demonstrated that declining platelet count mediated the association between *LRRC16A* and death. These examples of genetic mediation analysis are one demonstration of using genetic data to adapt causal inference methodology for the identification of causal disease intermediates. By mathematically disassembling an association between an explanatory variable (gene variant) and outcome (ARDS) into direct (gene-ARDS) and indirect (gene-platelet and platelet-ARDS) effects, one can infer the relative proportion of effect for the candidate mediator. The concept of using drugs to target platelet abundance or platelet trajectory to modify ARDS risk or mortality may seem unfamiliar, yet there was strong rationale for the LIPS-A study that tested whether aspirin reduced ARDS risk and found that it reduced ARDS risk though with a smaller effect size than anticipated [113]. Future work in this area may be fruitful.

A complementary approach termed Mendelian randomization (MR) leverages the association between genetic variants and intermediates such as plasma biomarkers to infer a biomarker's causality. Each individual's genetic variants are independently assigned by random assortment of parental alleles, according to the law of independent assortment, and alleles are distributed independently of any potential confounder. MR leverages this independence and applies the instrumental variable method to reduce a potential predictor variable to the portion that is least confounded, least susceptible to measurement error, and least vulnerable to reverse causation. Reilly and colleagues used MR to infer a potential causal role for plasma angiopoietin-2 (ANG2) and ARDS risk following sepsis; ANG2 was selected as a marker based on a genetic association between the angiopoietin-2 gene (*ANGPT2*) and ARDS they had previously identified [114]. Further, via mediation analysis, they found that plasma ANG2 mediated a substantial proportion (>34%) of the association between *ANGPT2* variants and ARDS risk [114], whereas no direct effect between *ANGPT2* and ARDS was observed. Together, these data highlight the potential for drugs that block ANG2 signaling to improve ARDS outcomes and the promise of applying a similar study design to prioritize interventions in future trials.

Sepsis Gene Expression Studies: Ready for Clinical Launch?

Gene expression studies are close to yielding findings that can be clinically translated into prognostic and predictive biomarkers in sepsis. Much of the early work demonstrating the power of whole blood, or peripheral leukocyte, gene expression signatures to discriminate biologically meaningful sepsis subgroups originated with Hector Wong's work in pediatric populations. Using unsupervised hierarchical clustering, his group consistently identified three patterns of gene expression among pediatric patients with septic shock [82, 115, 116]: "subclass A" patients, characterized by repression of adaptive immunity genes and glucocorticoid receptor signaling, who exhibited higher severity of illness, fewer ICU-free days, and higher mortality.

Given that glucocorticoids are frequently administered to patients with septic shock, the same group then asked whether the effect of glucocorticoids on sepsis mortality was associated with baseline gene expression patterns. They reported a potential interaction ($p = 0.089$) with steroids increasing mortality in subclass A patients with an odds ratio of 4.1 (95% CI: 1.4–12.0), but not in subclass B patients [117]. Further, by using a plasma biomarker risk stratification tool as a prognostic marker that reliably identified high risk for mortality [11], along with the glucocorticoid-response gene expression subclassification signature, Wong and colleagues established preliminary proof that the gene expression signature could be used to identify subjects who respond favorably to glucocorticoids among those with high predicted mortality [118].

This work set the stage for a precision clinical trial of corticosteroids leveraging the PERSEVERE pediatric biomarker risk model [119], which is based on plasma expression of five biomarkers (C-C chemokine ligand 3, interleukin 8, heat shock protein 70 kDa 1B, gran-

zyme B, and matrix metallopeptidase 8), to identify high-risk subjects. Subsequently, a 100-gene mRNA classifier was used to identify sepsis subclass and limit enrollment to subclass B patients. By focusing on high-risk individuals, the prognostic approach seeks to improve trial efficiency, whereas the predictive approach, in theory, will limit the potential for the intervention to harm patients predicted to do worse with corticosteroid treatment. The Stress Hydrocortisone in Pediatric Septic Shock (SHIPSS) is a phase III randomized double-blind placebo-controlled trial to test whether steroids are beneficial in refractory septic shock; the trial will use plasma and gene expression classifiers to determine whether the above approach is ready for clinical use.

Similar efforts have been undertaken in adult sepsis, with the results of several large, highly cited adult sepsis trials highlighted in Table 18.3. In every case, authors were able to identify a subset of patients at increased risk of death, though the precise method of detecting classes and the number of clusters varied. The UK Genomic Advances in Sepsis (GAiNS) group performed whole blood gene expression profiling by microarray on a discovery cohort of 265 subjects with severe pneumonia, with replication in a second pneumonia population of 106 [120]. Using unsupervised hierarchical cluster analysis of the most variable 10% of transcript probes, they identified two dominant clusters which they termed "sepsis response signatures 1 and 2" (SRS1, SRS2). The SRS1 subtype had a 27% mortality at 28 days, while SRS2 had 17% mortality. Although SRS1 subjects were more likely to require vasoactive medications and had higher Sequential Organ Failure Assessment (SOFA) scores at baseline, there was no statistically significant difference in baseline APACHE II score, need for mechanical ventilation, or use of renal replacement therapy. Combinations of clinical covariates performed poorly at predicting SRS membership with misclassification rates of 20–40%. Thus, SRS grouping seemed to add prognostic value beyond typical clinical scoring systems [120]. Investigators were able to reduce their classifier to seven transcripts that predicted SRS classification in both discovery and validation cohorts. In pathway analysis annotating the genes

Table 18.3 Sepsis gene expression cohort studies

Author, population	Population	Sepsis source	N Dis[a]	N Rep[b]	RNA source	Statistical approach	Subphenotype identified	Gene set, highlighted genes
Scicluna, *MARS* [121]	Adults with sepsis	CAP	306	216/265	Whole blood RNA, first 24 hours	Unsupervised clustering	4 MARS clusters	140 gene classifier *BPGM, TAP2*
Davenport *UK GAiNS* [120]	Adults with sepsis	CAP	265	106	Peripheral blood leukocyte RNA, first 5 days	Unsupervised hierarchical clustering	2 clusters, SRS1 and SRS2	7-gene classifier *DYRK2, TDRD9, CCNB1IP1, ZAP70, ARL14EP, MDC1,*
Burnham, *UK GAiNS* [141]	Adults with sepsis	CAP	73	53	Peripheral blood leukocyte RNA, first 5 days	Unsupervised hierarchical clustering	2 clusters, SRS1 high mortality	*ADGRE3*
Burnham, *UK GAiNS* [141]	Adults with sepsis	Fecal peritonitis	64	53	Peripheral blood leukocyte RNA, first 5 days	Unsupervised hierarchical clustering	2 clusters SRS1 and SRS2; very similar to CAP profile	
Wong [116]	Children <age 11 in ICU	Diverse bacterial and virus	98	82	Whole blood RNA, 24 hours	Clustering via computer-based image analysis of gene expression mosaics	3 clusters; type "A" with increased mortality	Dysregulated adaptive immunity, repressed GC receptor signaling
Sweeney; *meta-analysis* [123]	14 datasets, diverse ages, <48 h	Bacterial (diverse)	700	600 (9 datasets)	Whole blood or leukocyte RNA	COMMUNAL multiple clustering	3 clusters: adaptive, coagulopathic, inflammopathic	500-gene classifier inflammopathic-IL-1 receptor, PRP activity, complement activity; Adaptive: adaptive immunity, interferon signaling; Coagulopathic: platelet degranulation, coagulation cascade, GAG binding

Study populations are named by their published acronyms

CAP community-acquired pneumonia, *IL-1* interleukin 1, *PRP* pattern recognition receptor, *GAG* glycosaminoglycan

[a]Discovery population

[b]Replication population

that were most differentially expressed between SRS1 and SRS2 groups, the high-mortality SRS1 group did not exhibit increased expression of cytokine or inflammatory genes, but, rather, exhibited dysregulation of genes related to T-cell activation, cell death, apoptosis, necrosis, cytotoxicity, and phagocyte movement, in addition to upregulation of genes that characterize endotoxin tolerance [121, 122], suggesting a defective adaptive immune signature characterized SRS1 subjects.

In consonant fashion, a group from the Netherlands created the observational Molecular Diagnosis and Risk Stratification of Sepsis (MARS) cohort and applied slightly different clustering methodology to identify four clusters of sepsis subjects [121]. A 140-gene classifier reliably identified cluster membership when applied to two additional adult sepsis populations, and it identified three of four clusters in a pediatric sepsis population. Although the particular genes that best discriminated the high-risk cohort varied by study, this may be due to high correlation among many dysregulated genes, rather than a failure to replicate. Indeed, a meta-analysis by Sweeney et al. [123] that included mortality data from 14 diverse datasets of bacterial infection, including both adult and child cohorts, identified three clusters (a high-mortality "inflammopathic" cluster, a low-mortality "adaptive" cluster, and an additional "coagulopathic" cluster characterized by abnormal coagulation profiles) that could be distinguished with an 11-gene signature. They assessed overlap of their signature-based clusters with the high-mortality clusters identified in the MARS and Wong et al. pediatric cohorts, and they found substantial overlap in patients identified by each cohort's high-mortality/high-inflammation endotype.

Thus, while the specific genes selected for gene expression signatures vary, across numerous populations, a high-mortality subset of septic patients with dysregulated adaptive immunity can be identified, and "high-risk" gene expression status enhances mortality prediction over the APACHE score [121]. As mentioned above, the PERSEVERE trial is using these methods for targeted enrollment into a personalized trial of corticosteroid therapy for high-risk patients,

demonstrating the potential such signatures have for personalized medicine trials. Adults with sepsis may also exhibit heterogeneous response to glucocorticoids, and one study has suggested that response may be predicted by whole blood gene expression patterns. Using a parsimonious classifier based on the expression of seven transcripts that distinguished the high-mortality, adaptive immune dysregulated SRS1 group [120], Antcliffe et al. retrospectively assigned SRS classification to subjects with septic shock in the VANISH trial [124, 125]. Although there was no mortality benefit observed for corticosteroids in the overall trial, a statistical interaction was detected between steroid allocation and SRS grouping, such that SRS2 subjects exhibited a higher risk of death from sepsis when randomized to steroids [124]. As SRS2 is classically the low-mortality group of sepsis characterized by higher levels of adaptive immune signaling, it may be that corticosteroids disrupt an otherwise favorable host response to infection in some patients.

Gene Expression Studies in ARDS

Four groups have published whole blood gene expression studies in ARDS to date (including a pediatric cohort of acute respiratory failure), and an additional two publicly available datasets from the GLUE grant of trauma also include ARDS phenotyping. Each cohort is individually small (13–67 cases) and heterogeneous in terms of timing of sampling. In each case, a unique set of ARDS-associated genes has been identified, and the ability to rigorously replicate the genes identified in other cohorts has been modest [126]. Sweeney et al. performed a meta-analysis study of all six publicly available datasets to attempt to find a common gene expression signature across the disparate cohorts, but in contrast to the clear signal found with these methods in septic cohorts [79, 127], no expression signature could robustly distinguish ARDS cases from controls [85]. Limiting the ARDS cohorts to more homogenous groups (e.g., only adults with sepsis, excluding those with trauma) did not enhance the classifier signal. Interestingly, the top ARDS-associated genes in the meta-analysis are related to sepsis according to Gene Ontology classifiers, suggesting a potential overwhelming signal from sepsis and severity of illness may have obscured any lung-specific ARDS signals.

Metabolomics Studies in Sepsis and ARDS

Metabolomics is the study of all small molecules in an organism or tissue, including peptides, lipids, nucleic acids, and carbohydrates. Metabolite levels can change rapidly in response to cellular perturbations, such as the switch to anaerobic metabolism in exercise or sepsis that leads to lactate production. Thus, metabolites are particularly promising targets for personalized medicine because they reflect dynamic changes in the host. In contrast to well-established profiling methods for gene expression or SNP assessment, metabolomic profiling methods are rapidly evolving. The number of detected and quantified human metabolites included in the human metabolome database (HMDB) has increased from 8000 in 2010 to 18,000 in 2019, and the presumed number of actual metabolites is likely >100,000 [128]. This growth in the number of identifiable metabolites, and the parallel growth of metabolomic analytic and statistical methods, makes it difficult to compare studies across years and cohorts.

Metabolic changes in sepsis are widely recognized, as lactate, the end product of anaerobic metabolism, is the most widely used sepsis biomarker. Lactate measurement is a Centers for Medicare & Medicaid Services quality measure for patients with sepsis. Elevated lactate (>4 mmol/L) defines septic shock in the most recent sepsis guidelines, and serial lactate measurement and clearance can be used to assess adequacy of resuscitation [9, 129]. In addition to lactate, numerous metabolites are measured in basic chemistry (e.g., serum bilirubin, creatinine) that are followed as part of standard ICU care and comprise critical elements of our ICU scoring systems [74, 76].

Broad profiling of the plasma metabolome in sepsis has shown promise for biomarker identification. Langley et al. performed nontargeted profiling of plasma in 63 sepsis survivors and 31 non-survivors and identified widespread metabolic abnormalities between the two groups, involving pathways such as fatty acid transport, β-oxidation, gluconeogenesis, and the citric acid cycle. This group identified a biomarker panel of five metabolites, along with age and hematocrit, that outperformed lactate and APACHE score in mortality prediction in several studies [130]. Interestingly, when Rogers et al. examined the same populations with different metabolomics analytic strategies, a separate predictive biomarker panel was identified, likely a result of the high correlation among many metabolites [131] and emphasizing the lack of consistency among different metabolomics analysis strategies.

ARDS metabolomics studies are summarized in Table 18.4. These studies vary widely in terms of fluid studied (plasma, free edema, exhaled breath condensate, bronchoalveolar lavage), control population, and metabolic profiling techniques. All are fairly small, involving fewer than 50 ARDS patients in any individual study. Although an ideal control population might have respiratory failure and a condition that mimics the hypoxia of ARDS, such as hydrostatic pulmonary edema or pneumonia, in practice, most studies used convenience or noncritically ill controls. Not surprisingly, the ARDS-associated metabolites in such disparate populations are far from conclusive in terms of either pathway or individual metabolite. Further, given the extent of heterogeneity in sample type and control population, these data are not amenable to meta-analysis. Larger ARDS metabolomics studies are needed, with a focus on careful phenotyping and consistent sample preparation methods.

Table 18.4 Published metabolomic studies in ARDS

Author, year	Sample type	N Cases/ control	Control population	N Metabolites profiled	Major findings	Ref
ARDS vs control						
Schubert, 1998	Exhaled breath	19/18	Surgical ICU patients	9	Decreased isoprene	[142]
Stringer, 2011	Plasma	13/8	Healthy	40	4 metabolites: total glutathione, adenosine, phosphatidylserine, sphingomyelin	[143]
Rai, 2013	Mini-BAL	21/9	Ventilated ICU	>100	11 metabolites including arginine, glycine, aspartic acid, glutamate, muscle breakdown	[144]
Evans, 2014	BAL	18/8	Healthy	>500 untargeted	37 metabolites; amino acid metabolism, glycolysis/ gluconeogenesis, fatty acid synthesis, phospholipids, purine metabolism	[145]
Bos, 2014	Exhaled breath	23/30 19/29	Ventilated ICU (some with CHF or pneumonia)	>500	Octane, acetaldehyde, 3-methylheptane; improved ability to discriminate ARDS	[146]
Singh, 2014	Serum	26/19	Ventilated ICU	>100	Many differ, focus on lipids	[147]
Rogers, 2017	Undilute edema fluid	16/13	Hydrostatic edema	>700	2 subsets of ARDS, higher mortality	[148]
Izquierdo-Garcia, 2018	Serum	12/18 13/13	H1N1 without ARDS	>100	7 metabolites: 90% discrimination of ARDS; correlates w SOFA	[149]
Within ARDS variability						
Viswan, 2017	Mini-BAL	36 ARDS 23 severe vs 12 non-severe		29 metabolites	6 metabolites ➔ ~80% classification	[150]
Maille, 2018	Plasma	30 ARDS 22 survivors vs 8 fatality		359 lipids	90 lipids, >90% increased	[151]

For each study the biofluid profiled (sample type), the number of ARDS cases and controls (*N* cases/controls), characteristics of the control population, the number (*N*) of metabolites profiled, and major findings are shown
Ref reference, *Mini-BAL* bronchoalveolar lavage using small volume of saline, *BAL* bronchoalveolar lavage, *H1N1* a strain of influenza known to be virulent and an ARDS precipitant

Conclusion

Despite unique challenges in sepsis and ARDS, the past 10 years have shown substantial advances in the prospect of precision medicine for these deadly diseases. Large-scale gene expression and targeted proteomics plasma studies are identifying biologically distinct patterns of expression that at least retroactively identify a differential response to routine treatments applied in the ICU. Once metabolomics and proteomics approaches become more standardized, investigators may identify additional biomarkers for use in clinical trials that serve either as enrollment criteria to enrich for high-risk subgroups or for potential predictive enrichment to select a population for whom an intervention is more likely to have a positive effect. Prospective randomized trials based on biologic classification will be a reality in the near future, and the era of critical illness precision medicine might thus begin.

References

1. Liu V, Escobar GJ, Greene JD, et al. Hospital deaths in patients with sepsis from 2 independent cohorts. JAMA. 2014;312(1):90–2.
2. Bellani G, Laffey JG, Pham T, et al. Epidemiology, patterns of care, and mortality for patients with acute respiratory distress syndrome in intensive care units in 50 countries. JAMA. 2016;315(8):788–800.

3. Zeni F, Freeman B, Natanson C. Anti-inflammatory therapies to treat sepsis and septic shock: a reassessment. Crit Care Med. 1997;25(7):1095–100. PubMed PMID: 9233726. Epub 1997/07/01. eng.

4. Ranieri VM, Thompson BT, Barie PS, Dhainaut J-F, Douglas IS, Finfer S, et al. Drotrecogin alfa (activated) in adults with septic shock. N Engl J Med. 2012;366(22):2055–64. PubMed PMID: 22616830.

5. Opal SM, Laterre PF, Francois B, LaRosa SP, Angus DC, Mira JP, et al. Effect of eritoran, an antagonist of MD2-TLR4, on mortality in patients with severe sepsis: the ACCESS randomized trial. JAMA. 2013;309(11):1154–62. PubMed PMID: 23512062.

6. Rice TW, Wheeler AP, Thompson BT, de Boisblanc BP, Steingrub J, Rock P. Enteral omega-3 fatty acid, gamma-linolenic acid, and antioxidant supplementation in acute lung injury. JAMA. 2011;306(14):1574–81. PubMed PMID: 21976613. Epub 2011/10/07. eng.

7. Smith FG, Perkins GD, Gates S, Young D, McAuley DF, Tunnicliffe W, et al. Effect of intravenous β-2 agonist treatment on clinical outcomes in acute respiratory distress syndrome (BALTI-2): a multicentre, randomised controlled trial. Lancet. 2012;379(9812):229–35.

8. National Heart, Lung, and Blood Institute ARDS Clinical Trials Network, Truwit JD, Bernard GR, Steingrub J, Matthay MA, et al. Rosuvastatin for sepsis-associated acute respiratory distress syndrome. N Engl J Med. 2014;370(23):2191–200. PubMed PMID: 24835849. Pubmed Central PMCID: 4241052.

9. Singer M, Deutschman CS, Seymour C, et al. The third international consensus definitions for sepsis and septic shock (sepsis-3). JAMA. 2016;315(8):801–10.

10. Force ADT, Ranieri VM, Rubenfeld GD, Thompson BT, Ferguson ND, Caldwell E, et al. Acute respiratory distress syndrome: the Berlin definition. JAMA. 2012;307(23):2526–33. PubMed PMID: 22797452.

11. Prescott HC, Calfee CS, Thompson BT, Angus DC, Liu VX. Toward smarter lumping and smarter splitting: rethinking strategies for sepsis and acute respiratory distress syndrome clinical trial design. Am J Respir Crit Care Med. 2016;194(2):147–55.

12. The Acute Respiratory Distress Syndrome Network. Ventilation with lower tidal volumes as compared with traditional tidal volumes for acute lung injury and the acute respiratory distress syndrome. The Acute Respiratory Distress Syndrome Network. N Engl J Med. 2000;342(18):1301–8. PubMed PMID: 10793162.

13. Ouellette DR, Patel S, Girard TD, Morris PE, Schmidt GA, Truwit JD, et al. Liberation from mechanical ventilation in critically ill adults: an official American College of Chest Physicians/American Thoracic Society clinical practice guideline: inspiratory pressure augmentation during spontaneous breathing trials, protocols minimizing sedation, and noninvasive ventilation immediately after extubation. Chest. 2017;151(1):166–80.

14. Girard TD, Alhazzani W, Kress JP, Ouellette DR, Schmidt GA, Truwit JD, et al. An official American Thoracic Society/American College of Chest Physicians clinical practice guideline: liberation from mechanical ventilation in critically ill adults. Rehabilitation protocols, ventilator liberation protocols, and cuff leak tests. Am J Respir Crit Care Med. 2017;195(1):120–33. PubMed PMID: 27762595.

15. Girard TD, Kress JP, Fuchs BD, Thomason JWW, Schweickert WD, Pun BT, et al. Efficacy and safety of a paired sedation and ventilator weaning protocol for mechanically ventilated patients in intensive care (Awakening and Breathing Controlled trial): a randomised controlled trial. Lancet. 2008;371(9607):126–34.

16. Woodruff PG, Boushey HA, Dolganov GM, Barker CS, Yang YH, Donnelly S, et al. Genome-wide profiling identifies epithelial cell genes associated with asthma and with treatment response to corticosteroids. Proc Natl Acad Sci. 2007;104(40):15858–63.

17. Ortega HG, Liu MC, Pavord ID, Brusselle GG, FitzGerald JM, Chetta A, et al. Mepolizumab treatment in patients with severe eosinophilic asthma. N Engl J Med. 2014;371(13):1198–207. PubMed PMID: 25199059.

18. Wenzel S, Ford L, Pearlman D, Spector S, Sher L, Skobieranda F, et al. Dupilumab in persistent asthma with elevated eosinophil levels. N Engl J Med. 2013;368(26):2455–66. PubMed PMID: 23688323.

19. Wainwright CE, Elborn JS, Ramsey BW, Marigowda G, Huang X, Cipolli M, et al. Lumacaftor–ivacaftor in patients with cystic fibrosis homozygous for Phe508del CFTR. N Engl J Med. 2015;373(3):220–31. PubMed PMID: 25981758.

20. Ramsey BW, Davies J, McElvaney NG, Tullis E, Bell SC, Dřevínek P, et al. A CFTR Potentiator in patients with cystic fibrosis and the G551D mutation. N Engl J Med. 2011;365(18):1663–72. PubMed PMID: 22047557.

21. Calfee CS, Delucchi K, Parsons PE, Thompson BT, Ware LB, Matthay MA. Subphenotypes in acute respiratory distress syndrome: latent class analysis of data from two randomised controlled trials. Lancet Respir Med. 2014;2(8):611–20. Pubmed Central PMCID: PMC4154544.

22. Famous KR, Delucchi K, Ware LB, Kangelaris KN, Liu KD, Thompson BT, et al. Acute respiratory distress syndrome subphenotypes respond differently to randomized fluid management strategy. Am J Respir Crit Care Med. 2017;195(3):331–8. PubMed PMID: 27513822.

23. Calfee CS, Delucchi KL, Sinha P, Matthay MA, Hackett J, Shankar-Hari M, et al. Acute respiratory distress syndrome subphenotypes and differential response to simvastatin: secondary analysis of a randomised controlled trial. Lancet Respir Med.

2018;6(9):691–8. PubMed PMID: 30078618. Pubmed Central PMCID: 6201750.

24. Sinha P, Delucchi KL, Thompson BT, McAuley DF, Matthay MA, Calfee CS, et al. Latent class analysis of ARDS subphenotypes: a secondary analysis of the statins for acutely injured lungs from sepsis (SAILS) study. Intensive Care Med. 2018;44(11):1859–69. PubMed PMID: 30291376.

25. Bos LD, Schouten LR, van Vught LA, Wiewel MA, Ong DSY, Cremer O, et al. Identification and validation of distinct biological phenotypes in patients with acute respiratory distress syndrome by cluster analysis. Thorax. 2017;72(10):876–83.

26. Ware LB, Matthay MA, Parsons PE, Thompson BT, Januzzi JL, Eisner MD. Pathogenetic and prognostic significance of altered coagulation and fibrinolysis in acute lung injury/acute respiratory distress syndrome*. Crit Care Med. 2007;35:1821–8. PubMed PMID: 17581482. Epub 2007/06/22. Eng.

27. Parsons PE, Eisner MD, Thompson BT, Matthay MA, Ancukiewicz M, Bernard GR, et al. Lower tidal volume ventilation and plasma cytokine markers of inflammation in patients with acute lung injury. Crit Care Med. 2005;33(1):1–6; discussion 230–2. PubMed PMID: 15644641. Epub 2005/01/13. eng.

28. Opal SM, Fisher CJ, Dhainaut JF, Vincent JL, Brase R, Lowry SF, et al. Confirmatory interleukin-1 receptor antagonist trial in severe sepsis: a phase III, randomized, double-blind, placebo-controlled, multicenter trial. Crit Care Med. 1997;25(7):1115–24.

29. Fisher CJ Jr, Dhainaut JF, Opal SM, Pribble JP, Balk RA, Slotman GJ, et al. Recombinant human interleukin 1 receptor antagonist in the treatment of patients with sepsis syndrome. Results from a randomized, double-blind, placebo-controlled trial. Phase III rhIL-1ra Sepsis Syndrome Study Group. JAMA. 1994;271(23):1836–43. PubMed PMID: 8196140. Epub 1994/06/15. eng.

30. Fisher CJ Jr, Slotman GJ, Opal SM, Pribble JP, Bone RC, Emmanuel G, et al. Initial evaluation of human recombinant interleukin-1 receptor antagonist in the treatment of sepsis syndrome: a randomized, open-label, placebo-controlled multicenter trial. Crit Care Med. 1994;22(1):12–21. PubMed PMID: 8124953. Epub 1994/01/01. eng.

31. Panacek EA, Marshall JC, Albertson TE, Johnson DH, Johnson S, MacArthur RD, et al. Efficacy and safety of the monoclonal anti-tumor necrosis factor antibody F(ab')2 fragment afelimomab in patients with severe sepsis and elevated interleukin-6 levels. Crit Care Med. 2004;32(11):2173–82. PubMed PMID: 15640628. Epub 2005/01/11. eng.

32. Reinhart K, Menges T, Gardlund B, Harm Zwaveling J, Smithes M, Vincent JL, et al. Randomized, placebo-controlled trial of the anti-tumor necrosis factor antibody fragment afelimomab in hyperinflammatory response during severe sepsis: the RAMSES Study. Crit Care Med. 2001;29(4):765–9. PubMed PMID: 11373466.

33. Bernard GR, Vincent J-L, Laterre P-F, LaRosa SP, Dhainaut J-F, Lopez-Rodriguez A, et al. Efficacy and safety of recombinant human activated protein C for severe sepsis. N Engl J Med. 2001;344(10):699–709. PubMed PMID: 11236773.

34. Man M, Close SL, Shaw AD, Bernard GR, Douglas IS, Kaner RJ, et al. Beyond single-marker analyses: mining whole genome scans for insights into treatment responses in severe sepsis. Pharmacogenomics J. 2012;13(3):218–26.

35. Meyer NJ, Reilly JP, Anderson BJ, Palakshappa JA, Jones TK, Dunn TG, et al. Mortality benefit of recombinant human interleukin-1 receptor antagonist for sepsis varies by initial interleukin-1 receptor antagonist plasma concentration. Crit Care Med. 2018;46:21–8. PubMed PMID: 28991823. Pubmed Central PMCID: PMC5734955. Epub 2017/10/11. eng.

36. Shakoory B, Carcillo JA, Chatham WW, Amdur RL, Zhao H, Dinarello CA, et al. Interleukin-1 Receptor blockade is associated with reduced mortality in sepsis patients with features of macrophage activation syndrome: reanalysis of a prior phase III trial*. Crit Care Med. 2016;44(2):275–81. PubMed PMID: 00003246-201602000-00005.

37. Wang R, Lagakos SW, Ware JH, Hunter DJ, Drazen JM. Statistics in medicine--reporting of subgroup analyses in clinical trials. N Engl J Med. 2007;357:2189.

38. Hernandez AV, Boersma E, Murray GD, Habbema JD, Steyerberg EW. Subgroup analyses in therapeutic cardiovascular clinical trials: are most of them misleading? Am Heart J. 2006;151:257.

39. Rothwell PM. Treating individuals 2. Subgroup analysis in randomised controlled trials: importance, indications, and interpretation. Lancet. 2005;365:176–86.

40. Picard C, Bobby Gaspar H, Al-Herz W, Bousfiha A, Casanova J-L, Chatila T, et al. International Union of Immunological Societies: 2017 primary immunodeficiency diseases committee report on inborn errors of immunity. J Clin Immunol. 2018;38(1):96–128.

41. Stray-Pedersen A, Sorte HS, Samarakoon P, Gambin T, Chinn IK, Coban Akdemir ZH, et al. Primary immunodeficiency diseases: genomic approaches delineate heterogeneous Mendelian disorders. J Allergy Clin Immunol. 2017;139(1):232–45.

42. Wang Z, Sun Y, Fu X, Yu G, Wang C, Bao F, et al. A large-scale genome-wide association and meta-analysis identified four novel susceptibility loci for leprosy. Nature Commun. 2016;7:13760.

43. Rowe PC, McLean RH, Wood RA, Leggiadro RJ, Winkelstein JA. Association of homozygous C4B deficiency with bacterial meningitis. J Infect Dis. 1989;160(3):448–51. PubMed PMID: 2788199.

44. Bustamante J, Boisson-Dupuis S, Abel L, Casanova J-L. Mendelian susceptibility to mycobacterial disease: genetic, immunological, and clinical features of inborn errors of IFN-γ immunity. Semin Immunol. 2014;26(6):454–70.

45. Ling Y, Cypowyj S, Aytekin C, Galicchio M, Camcioglu Y, Nepesov S, et al. Inherited IL-17RC deficiency in patients with chronic mucocutaneous candidiasis. J Exp Med. 2015;212(5):619–31.

46. von Bernuth H, Picard C, Jin Z, Pankla R, Xiao H, Ku CL, et al. Pyogenic bacterial infections in humans with MyD88 deficiency. Science. 2008;321(5889):691–6. PubMed PMID: 18669862. Pubmed Central PMCID: 2688396. Epub 2008/08/02. eng.

47. Kuemmerle-Deschner JB, Tyrrell PN, Koetter I, Wittkowski H, Bialkowski A, Tzaribachev N. Efficacy and safety of anakinra therapy in pediatric and adult patients with the autoinflammatory Muckle-Wells syndrome. Arthritis Rheum. 2011;63:840.

48. Reddy S, Jia S, Geoffrey R, Lorier R, Suchi M, Broeckel U, et al. An autoinflammatory disease due to homozygous deletion of the IL1RN locus. N Engl J Med. 2009;360(23):2438–44.

49. Aksentijevich I, Masters SL, Ferguson PJ, Dancey P, Frenkel J, van Royen-Kerkhoff A, et al. An autoinflammatory disease with deficiency of the interleukin-1 receptor antagonist. N Engl J Med. 2009;360(23):2426–37.

50. Akey JM, Eberle MA, Rieder MJ, Carlson CS, Shriver MD, Nickerson DA, et al. Population history and natural selection shape patterns of genetic variation in 132 genes. PLoS Biol. 2004;2(10):e286. PubMed PMID: 15361935. Pubmed Central PMCID: 515367. Epub 2004/09/14. eng.

51. Elguero E, Délicat-Loembet LM, Rougeron V, Arnathau C, Roche B, Becquart P, et al. Malaria continues to select for sickle cell trait in Central Africa. Proc Natl Acad Sci. 2015;112(22):7051–4.

52. Consortium TGP. An integrated map of genetic variation from 1,092 human genomes. Nature. 2012;491(7422):56–65.

53. Lek M, Karczewski KJ, Minikel EV, Samocha KE, Banks E, Fennell T, et al. Analysis of protein-coding genetic variation in 60,706 humans. Nature. 2016;536:285.

54. Piel FB, Patil AP, Howes RE, Nyangiri OA, Gething PW, Williams TN, et al. Global distribution of the sickle cell gene and geographical confirmation of the malaria hypothesis. Nat Commun. 2010;1:104.

55. Van Dyke AL, Cote ML, Wenzlaff AS, Land S, Schwartz AG. Cytokine SNPs: comparison of allele frequencies by race and implications for future studies. Cytokine. 2009;46(2):236–44.

56. de Vries RR, Meera Khan P, Bernini LF, van Loghem E, van Rood JJ. Genetic control of survival in epidemics. J Immunogenet. 1979;6(4):271–87. PubMed PMID: 521665. Epub 1979/08/01. eng.

57. Maller J, George S, Purcell S, Fagerness J, Altshuler D, Daly MJ, et al. Common variation in three genes, including a noncoding variant in CFH, strongly influences risk of age-related macular degeneration. Nat Genet. 2006;38(9):1055–9. PubMed PMID: 16936732. Epub 2006/08/29. eng.

58. Klein R, Zeiss C, Chew E, Tsai J, Sackler R, Haynes C, et al. Complement factor H polymorphism in age-related macular degeneration. Science. 2005;308(5720):385–9 . PubMed PMID. https://doi.org/10.1126/science.1109557.

59. Sorensen TI, Nielsen GG, Andersen PK, Teasdale TW. Genetic and environmental influences on premature death in adult adoptees. N Engl J Med. 1988;318(12):727–32. PubMed PMID: 3347221. Epub 1988/03/24. eng.

60. Ashbaugh DG, Bigelow DB, Petty TL, Levine BE. Acute respiratory distress in adults. Lancet. 1967;2(7511):319–23. PubMed PMID: 4143721.

61. Frazer KA, Murray SS, Schork NJ, Topol EJ. Human genetic variation and its contribution to complex traits. Nat Rev Genet. 2009;10(4):241–51. PubMed PMID: 19293820. Epub 2009/03/19. eng.

62. ENCODE_Project_Consortium. An integrated encyclopedia of DNA elements in the human genome. Nature. 2012;489(7414):57–74.

63. ENCODE_Project_Consortium. A user's guide to the encyclopedia of DNA elements (ENCODE). PLoS Biol. 2011;9(4):e1001046.

64. Berdasco M, Esteller M. Clinical epigenetics: seizing opportunities for translation. Nat Rev Genet. 2019;20(2):109–27.

65. Rowley MJ, Corces VG. Organizational principles of 3D genome architecture. Nat Rev Genet. 2018;19(12):789–800.

66. Uszczynska-Ratajczak B, Lagarde J, Frankish A, Guigó R, Johnson R. Towards a complete map of the human long non-coding RNA transcriptome. Nat Rev Genet. 2018;19(9):535–48.

67. Genomes Project Consortium, Abecasis GR, Altshuler D, Auton A, Brooks LD, Durbin RM, et al. A map of human genome variation from population-scale sequencing. Nature. 2010;467(7319):1061–73. PubMed PMID: 20981092. Pubmed Central PMCID: 3042601.

68. The International HapMap Consortium. Integrating common and rare genetic variation in diverse human populations. Nature. 2010;467(7311):52–8.

69. Goodwin S, McPherson JD, McCombie WR. Coming of age: ten years of next-generation sequencing technologies. Nat Rev Genet. 2016;17:333.

70. Golub TR, Slonim DK, Tamayo P, Huard C, Gaasenbeek M, Mesirov JP, et al. Molecular classification of cancer: class discovery and class prediction by gene expression monitoring. Science. 1999;286(5439):531–7. PubMed PMID: 10521349.

71. Mosse YP, Laudenslager M, Longo L, Cole KA, Wood A, Attiyeh EF, et al. Identification of ALK as a major familial neuroblastoma predisposition gene. Nature. 2008;455(7215):930–5.

72. Strobel EJ, Yu AM, Lucks JB. High-throughput determination of RNA structures. Nat Rev Genet. 2018;19(10):615–34.

73. Bycroft C, Freeman C, Petkova D, Band G, Elliott LT, Sharp K, et al. The UK Biobank resource

with deep phenotyping and genomic data. Nature. 2018;562(7726):203–9.

74. Knaus WA, Wagner DP, Draper EA, Zimmerman JE, Bergner M, Bastos PG, et al. The APACHE III prognostic system. Risk prediction of hospital mortality for critically ill hospitalized adults. Chest. 1991;100(6):1619–36. PubMed PMID: 1959406. Epub 1991/12/01. eng.

75. Knaus WA, Draper EA, Wagner DP, Zimmerman JE. APACHE II: a severity of disease classification system. Crit Care Med. 1985;13:818.

76. Le Gall J-R, Lemeshow S, Saulnier F. A new simplified acute physiology score (SAPS II) based on a European/North American Multicenter Study. JAMA. 1993;270(24):2957–63.

77. Kent DM, Rothwell PM, Ioannidis JP, Altman DG, Hayward RA. Assessing and reporting heterogeneity in treatment effects in clinical trials: a proposal. Trials. 2010;11(1):1–11.

78. Hébert PC, Wells G, Blajchman MA, Marshall J, Martin C, Pagliarello G, et al. A multicenter, randomized, controlled clinical trial of transfusion requirements in critical care. N Engl J Med. 1999;340(6):409–17. PubMed PMID: 9971864.

79. Sweeney TE, Shidham A, Wong HR, Khatri P. A comprehensive time-course-based multicohort analysis of sepsis and sterile inflammation reveals a robust diagnostic gene set. Sci Transl Med. 2015;7(287):287ra71. PubMed PMID: 25972003. Pubmed Central PMCID: 4734362.

80. Levitt JE, Bedi H, Calfee CS, Gould MK, Matthay MA. Identification of early acute lung injury at initial evaluation in an acute care setting prior to the onset of respiratory failure. Chest. 2009;135(4):936–43. PubMed PMID: 19188549. Pubmed Central PMCID: 2758305. Epub 2009/02/04. eng.

81. Cazalis M-A, Lepape A, Venet F, Frager F, Mougin B, Vallin H, et al. Early and dynamic changes in gene expression in septic shock patients: a genome-wide approach. Intensive Care Med Exp. 2014;2(1):20. PubMed PMID: 26215705.

82. Wong HR, Cvijanovich N, Allen GL, Lin R, Anas N, Meyer K, et al. Genomic expression profiling across the pediatric systemic inflammatory response syndrome, sepsis, and septic shock spectrum. Crit Care Med. 2009;37(5):1558–66. PubMed PMID: 19325468. Pubmed Central PMCID: 2747356.

83. Dolan JM, Meng H, Sim FJ, Kolega J. Differential gene expression by endothelial cells under positive and negative streamwise gradients of high wall shear stress. Am J Physiol Cell Physiol. 2013;305(8):C854–66. PubMed PMID: 23885059. Epub 07/24.

84. Palakshappa JA, Meyer NJ. Which patients with ARDS benefit from lung biopsy? Chest. 2015;148(4):1073–82. PubMed PMID: 25950989. Epub 2015/05/08. eng.

85. Sweeney TE, Thomas NJ, Howrylak JA, Wong HR, Rogers AJ, Khatri P. Multicohort analysis of whole-blood gene expression data does not form a robust diagnostic for acute respiratory distress syndrome. Crit Care Med. 2018;46(2):244–51. PubMed PMID: 29337789. Pubmed Central PMCID: PMC5774019. Epub 2018/01/18.

86. Morrell ED, Radella F 2nd, Manicone AM, Mikacenic C, Stapleton RD, Gharib SA, et al. Peripheral and alveolar cell transcriptional programs are distinct in acute respiratory distress syndrome. Am J Respir Crit Care Med. 2018;197(4):528–32. PubMed PMID: 28708019. Pubmed Central PMCID: PMC5821902. Epub 2017/07/15.

87. Sutherland AM, Walley KR. Bench-to-bedside review: association of genetic variation with sepsis. Crit Care. 2009;13(2):210.

88. Villar J, Maca-Meyer N, Pérez-Méndez L, Flores C. Bench-to-bedside review: understanding genetic predisposition to sepsis. Critical Care Lond Engl. 2004;8(3):180–9. PubMed PMID: 15153236. Epub 04/29.

89. Lu H, Wen D, Wang X, Gan L, Du J, Sun J, et al. Host genetic variants in sepsis risk: a field synopsis and meta-analysis. Crit Care. 2019;23(1):26.

90. Rautanen A, Mills TC, Gordon AC, Hutton P, Steffens M, Nuamah R, et al. Genome-wide association study of survival from sepsis due to pneumonia: an observational cohort study. Lancet Respir Med. 2015;3(1):53–60.

91. Jacobson JR, Dudek SM, Birukov KG, Ye SQ, Grigoryev DN, Girgis RE, et al. Cytoskeletal activation and altered gene expression in endothelial barrier regulation by simvastatin. Am J Respir Cell Mol Biol. 2004;30(5):662–70. PubMed PMID: 14630613.

92. Petrache I, Verin AD, Crow MT, Birukova A, Liu F, Garcia JG. Differential effect of MLC kinase in TNF-alpha-induced endothelial cell apoptosis and barrier dysfunction. Am J Physiol Lung Cell Mol Physiol. 2001;280(6):L1168–78. PubMed PMID: 11350795.

93. Garcia JG, Davis HW, Patterson CE. Regulation of endothelial cell gap formation and barrier dysfunction: role of myosin light chain phosphorylation. J Cell Physiol. 1995;163(3):510–22. PubMed PMID: 7775594.

94. Schöneweck F, Kuhnt E, Scholz M, Brunkhorst FM, Scherag A. Common genomic variation in the FER gene: useful to stratify patients with sepsis due to pneumonia? Intensive Care Med. 2015;41(7):1379–81.

95. Lee S, Lee SJ, Coronata AA, Fredenburgh LE, Chung SW, Perrella MA, Nakahira K, Ryter SW, Choi AM. Carbon monoxide confers protection in sepsis by enhancing beclin 1-dependent autophagy and phagocytosis. Antioxid Redox Signal. 2014;20(3):432–42. PubMed PMID: 23971531.

96. Russell JA, Walley KR, Singer J, Gordon AC, Hebert PC, Cooper DJ, et al. Vasopressin versus norepinephrine infusion in patients with septic shock. N Engl J Med. 2008;358(9):877–87. PubMed PMID: 18305265. Epub 2008/02/29. eng.

97. Meyer NJ, Ferguson JF, Feng R, Wang F, Patel PN, Li M, et al. A functional synonymous coding variant in the IL1RN gene is associated with survival in septic shock. Am J Respir Crit Care Med. 2014;190(6):656–64. PubMed PMID: 25089931. Pubmed Central PMCID: PMC4214110. Epub 2014/08/05. eng.

98. Meyer NJ, Feng R, Li M, Zhao Y, Sheu CC, Tejera P, et al. IL1RN coding variant is associated with lower risk of acute respiratory distress syndrome and increased plasma IL-1 receptor antagonist. Am J Respir Crit Care Med. 2013;187(9):950–9. PubMed PMID: 23449693. Epub 2013/03/02. Eng.

99. Freidlin B, Korn EL. Biomarker enrichment strategies: matching trial design to biomarker credentials. Nat Rev Clin Oncol. 2014;11(2):81–90.

100. Reilly JP, Christie JD, Meyer NJ. Fifty years of research in ARDS. Genomic contributions and opportunities. Am J Respir Crit Care Med. 2017;196(9):1113–21. PubMed PMID: 28481621. Pubmed Central PMCID: PMC5694838. Epub 2017/05/10. eng.

101. Acosta-Herrera M, Pino-Yanes M, Perez-Mendez L, Villar J, Flores C. Assessing the quality of studies supporting genetic susceptibility and outcomes of ARDS. Front Genet. 2014;5:20. PubMed PMID: 24567738. Pubmed Central PMCID: 3915143.

102. Christie JD, Wurfel MM, Feng R, O'Keefe GE, Bradfield J, Ware LB, et al. Genome wide association identifies PPFIA1 as a candidate gene for acute lung injury risk following major trauma. PLoS One. 2012;7(1):e28268.

103. Meyer NJ, Li M, Feng R, Bradfield J, Gallop R, Bellamy S, et al. ANGPT2 genetic variant is associated with trauma-associated acute lung injury and altered plasma angiopoietin-2 isoform ratio. Am J Respir Crit Care Med. 2011;183:1344–53. PubMed PMID: 21257790. Epub 2011/01/25. eng.

104. Manolio TA, Collins FS, Cox NJ, Goldstein DB, Hindorff LA, Hunter DJ, et al. Finding the missing heritability of complex diseases. Nature. 2009;461(7265):747–53. PubMed PMID: 19812666. Pubmed Central PMCID: 2831613. Epub 2009/10/09. eng.

105. Cohen JC, Boerwinkle E, Mosley TH, Hobbs HH. Sequence variations in PCSK9, low LDL, and protection against coronary heart disease. N Engl J Med. 2006;354(12):1264–72. PubMed PMID: 16554528.

106. Cohen J, Pertsemlidis A, Kotowski IK, Graham R, Garcia CK, Hobbs HH. Low LDL cholesterol in individuals of African descent resulting from frequent nonsense mutations in PCSK9. Nat Genet. 2005;37(2):161–5.

107. Linsel-Nitschke P, Götz A, Erdmann J, Braenne I, Braund P, Hengstenberg C, et al. Lifelong reduction of LDL-cholesterol related to a common variant in the LDL-receptor gene decreases the risk of coronary artery disease—a Mendelian Randomisation study. PLoS One. 2008;3(8):e2986.

108. Wu J, Sheng L, Wang S, Li Q, Zhang M, Xu S, et al. Analysis of clinical risk factors associated with the prognosis of severe multiple-trauma patients with acute lung injury. J Emerg Med. 2012;43(3):407–12.

109. Wang T, Liu Z, Wang Z, Duan M, Li G, Wang S, et al. Thrombocytopenia is associated with acute respiratory distress syndrome mortality: an international study. PLoS One. 2014;9(4):e94124.

110. Lefrançais E, Ortiz-Muñoz G, Caudrillier A, Mallavia B, Liu F, Sayah DM, et al. The lung is a site of platelet biogenesis and a reservoir for haematopoietic progenitors. Nature. 2017;544:105.

111. Wei Y, Wang Z, Su L, Chen F, Tejera P, Bajwa EK, et al. Platelet count mediates the contribution of a genetic variant in LRRC 16A to ARDS risk. Chest. 2015;147(3):607–17.

112. Wei Y, Tejera P, Wang Z, Zhang R, Chen F, Su L, et al. A missense genetic variant in LRRC16A/CARMIL1 improves acute respiratory distress syndrome survival by attenuating platelet count decline. Am J Respir Crit Care Med. 2017;195(10):1353–61. PubMed PMID: 27768389. Pubmed Central PMCID: 5443896.

113. Kor DJ, Carter RE, Park PK, et al. Effect of aspirin on development of ards in at-risk patients presenting to the emergency department: the lips-a randomized clinical trial. JAMA. 2016;315(22):2406–14.

114. Reilly JP, Wang F, Jones TK, Palakshappa JA, Anderson BJ, Shashaty MGS, et al. Plasma angiopoietin-2 as a potential causal marker in sepsis-associated ARDS development: evidence from Mendelian randomization and mediation analysis. Intensive Care Med. 2018;44(11):1849–58.

115. Wong HR, Cvijanovich N, Lin R, Allen GL, Thomas NJ, Willson DF, et al. Identification of pediatric septic shock subclasses based on genome-wide expression profiling. BMC Med. 2009;7:34. PubMed PMID: 19624809. Pubmed Central PMCID: 2720987. Epub 2009/07/25. eng.

116. Wong HR, Cvijanovich NZ, Allen GL, Thomas NJ, Freishtat RJ, Anas N, et al. Validation of a gene expression-based subclassification strategy for pediatric septic shock. Crit Care Med. 2011;39(11):2511–7. PubMed PMID: 21705885. Pubmed Central PMCID: 3196776. Epub 2011/06/28. eng.

117. Wong HR, Cvijanovich NZ, Anas N, Allen GL, Thomas NJ, Bigham MT, et al. Developing a clinically feasible personalized medicine approach to pediatric septic shock. Am J Respir Crit Care Med. 2015;191(3):309–15. PubMed PMID: 25489881.

118. Wong HR, Atkinson SJ, Cvijanovich NZ, Anas N, Allen GL, Thomas NJ, et al. Combining prognostic and predictive enrichment strategies to identify children with septic shock responsive to corticosteroids. Crit Care Med. 2016;44(10):e1000–3. PubMed PMID: 27270179. Pubmed Central PMCID: 5026540.

119. Wong H, Salisbury S, Xiao Q, Cvijanovich N, Hall M, Allen G, et al. The pediatric sepsis biomarker risk

model. Crit Care. 2012;16(5):R174. PubMed PMID. https://doi.org/10.1186/cc11652.

120. Davenport EE, Burnham KL, Radhakrishnan J, Humburg P, Hutton P, Mills TC. Genomic landscape of the individual host response and outcomes in sepsis: a prospective cohort study. Lancet Respir Med. 2016;4:259.

121. Scicluna BP, van Vught LA, Zwinderman AH, Wiewel MA, Davenport EE, Burnham KL, et al. Classification of patients with sepsis according to blood genomic endotype: a prospective cohort study. Lancet Respir Med. 2017;5(10):816–26. PubMed PMID: 28864056. Epub 2017/09/03.

122. Pena OM, Pistolic J, Raj D, Fjell CD, Hancock REW. Endotoxin tolerance represents a distinctive state of alternative polarization (M2) in human mononuclear cells. J Immunol. 2011;186(12):7243–54.

123. Sweeney TE, Azad TD, Donato M, Haynes WA, Perumal TM, Henao R, et al. Unsupervised analysis of transcriptomics in bacterial sepsis across multiple datasets reveals three robust clusters. Crit Care Med. 2018;46(6):915–25. PubMed PMID: 29537985. Pubmed Central PMCID: PMC5953807. Epub 2018/03/15.

124. Antcliffe DB, Burnham KL, Al-Beidh F, Santhakumaran S, Brett SJ, Hinds CJ, et al. transcriptomic signatures in sepsis and a differential response to steroids: from the VANISH Randomized Trial. Am J Respir Crit Care Med. 2019;199:980–6. PubMed PMID: 30365341.

125. Gordon AC, Mason AJ, Thirunavukkarasu N, Perkins GD, Cecconi M, Cepkova M, et al. Effect of early vasopressin vs norepinephrine on kidney failure in patients with septic shock: the VANISH randomized clinical trial early vasopressin vs norepinephrine on kidney failure in septic shock patients early vasopressin vs norepinephrine on kidney failure in septic shock patients. JAMA. 2016;316(5):509–18.

126. Kangelaris KN, Prakash A, Liu KD, Aouizerat B, Woodruff PG, Erle DJ, et al. Increased expression of neutrophil-related genes in patients with early sepsis-induced ARDS. Am J Physiol Lung Cell Mol Physiol. 2015;308(11):L1102–13. PubMed PMID: 25795726. Pubmed Central PMCID: 4451399.

127. Sweeney TE, Wong HR, Khatri P. Robust classification of bacterial and viral infections via integrated host gene expression diagnostics. Sci Transl Med. 2016;8(346):346ra91. PubMed PMID: 27384347.

128. Wishart DS, Feunang YD, Marcu A, Guo AC, Liang K, Vazquez-Fresno R, et al. HMDB 4.0: the human metabolome database for 2018. Nucleic Acids Res. 2018;46(D1):D608–17. PubMed PMID: 29140435. Pubmed Central PMCID: PMC5753273. Epub 2017/11/16.

129. Nguyen HB, Rivers EP, Knoblich BP, Jacobsen G, Muzzin A, Ressler JA, et al. Early lactate clearance is associated with improved outcome in severe sepsis and septic shock. Crit Care Med. 2004;32(8):1637–42. PubMed PMID: 15286537.

130. Langley RJ, Tsalik EL, van Velkinburgh JC, Glickman SW, Rice BJ, Wang C, et al. An integrated clinico-metabolomic model improves prediction of death in sepsis. Sci Transl Med. 2013;5(195):195ra95. PubMed PMID: 23884467.

131. Rogers AJ, McGeachie M, Baron RM, Gazourian L, Haspel JA, Nakahira K, et al. Metabolomic derangements are associated with mortality in critically ill adult patients. PLoS One. 2014;9(1):e87538. PubMed PMID: 24498130. eng.

132. Nakada T-A, Russell JA, Wellman H, Boyd JH, Nakada E, Thain KR, et al. Leucyl/cystinyl aminopeptidase gene variants in septic shock. Chest J. 2011;139(5):1042–9.

133. Chen QX, Wu SJ, Wang HH, Lv C, Cheng BL, Xie GH, et al. Protein C -1641A/-1654C haplotype is associated with organ dysfunction and the fatal outcome of severe sepsis in Chinese Han population. Hum Genet. 2008;123(3):281–7.

134. Walley KR, Russell JA. Protein C -1641 AA is associated with decreased survival and more organ dysfunction in severe sepsis. Crit Care Med. 2007;35(1):12–7. PubMed PMID: 17080006. Epub 2006/11/03. eng.

135. Tejera P, Wang Z, Zhai R, Su L, Sheu C-C, Taylor DM, et al. Genetic polymorphisms of peptidase inhibitor 3 (elafin) are associated with acute respiratory distress syndrome. Am J Respir Cell Mol Biol. 2009;41(6):696–704.

136. Wang Z, Beach D, Su L, Zhai R, Christiani DC. A genome-wide expression analysis in blood identifies pre-elafin as a biomarker in ARDS. Am J Respir Cell Mol Biol. 2008;38(6):724–32. PubMed PMID: 18203972. Pubmed Central PMCID: 2396250. Epub 2008/01/22. eng.

137. Marshall RP, Webb S, Bellingan GJ, Montgomery HE, Chaudhari B, McAnulty RJ, et al. Angiotensin converting enzyme insertion/deletion polymorphism is associated with susceptibility and outcome in acute respiratory distress syndrome. Am J Respir Crit Care Med. 2002;166(5):646–50. PubMed PMID: 12204859.

138. Marshall RP, Webb S, Hill MR, Humphries SE, Laurent GJ. Genetic polymorphisms associated with susceptibility and outcome in ARDS. Chest. 2002;121(3 Suppl):68S–9S. PubMed PMID: 11893690.

139. Lin Z, Pearson C, Chinchilli V, Pietschmann SM, Luo J, Pison U, et al. Polymorphisms of human SP-A, SP-B, and SP-D genes: association of SP-B Thr131Ile with ARDS. Clin Genet. 2000;58(3):181–91. PubMed PMID: 11076040.

140. Dahmer MK, O'Cain P, Patwari PP, Simpson P, Li SH, Halligan N, et al. The influence of genetic variation in surfactant protein B on severe lung injury in African American children. Crit Care Med. 2011;39(5):1138–44. PubMed PMID: 21283003. Epub 2011/02/02. eng.

141. Burnham KL, Davenport EE, Radhakrishnan J, Humburg P, Gordon AC, Hutton P, et al. Shared and

distinct aspects of the sepsis transcriptomic response to fecal peritonitis and pneumonia. Am J Respir Crit Care Med. 2017;196(3):328–39. PubMed PMID: 28036233. Pubmed Central PMCID: PMC5549866. Epub 2016/12/31.

142. Schubert JK, Muller WP, Benzing A, Geiger K. Application of a new method for analysis of exhaled gas in critically ill patients. Intensive Care Med. 1998;24(5):415–21. PubMed PMID: 9660254.

143. Stringer KA, Serkova NJ, Karnovsky A, Guire K, Paine R 3rd, Standiford TJ. Metabolic consequences of sepsis-induced acute lung injury revealed by plasma (1)H-nuclear magnetic resonance quantitative metabolomics and computational analysis. Am J Physiol Lung Cell Mol Physiol. 2011;300(1):L4–L11. PubMed PMID: 20889676. Pubmed Central PMCID: 3023293.

144. Rai RK, Azim A, Sinha N, Sahoo JN, Singh C, Ahmed A, et al. Metabolic profiling in human lung injuries by high-resolution nuclear magnetic resonance spectroscopy of bronchoalveolar lavage fluid (BALF). Metabolomics. 2013;9(3):667–76.

145. Evans CR, Karnovsky A, Kovach MA, Standiford TJ, Burant CF, Stringer KA. Untargeted LC–MS metabolomics of bronchoalveolar lavage fluid differentiates acute respiratory distress syndrome from health. J Proteome Res. 2014;13(2):640–9.

146. Bos LD, Weda H, Wang Y, Knobel HH, Nijsen TM, Vink TJ, et al. Exhaled breath metabolomics as a noninvasive diagnostic tool for acute respiratory distress syndrome. Eur Respir J. 2014;44(1):188–97. PubMed PMID: 24743964. Epub 2014/04/20.

147. Singh C, Rai RK, Azim A, Sinha N, Ahmed A, Singh K, et al. Metabolic profiling of human lung injury by H-1 high-resolution nuclear magnetic resonance spectroscopy of blood serum. Metabolomics. 2015;11(1):166–74. PubMed PMID: WOS:000348343300016. English.

148. Rogers AJ, Contrepois K, Wu M, Zheng M, Peltz G, Ware LB, et al. Profiling of ARDS pulmonary edema fluid identifies a metabolically distinct subset. Am J Physiol Lung Cell Mol Physiol. 2017;312(5):L703–L9. PubMed PMID: 28258106. Pubmed Central PMCID: PMC5451591. Epub 2017/03/05.

149. Izquierdo-Garcia JL, Nin N, Jimenez-Clemente J, Horcajada JP, Arenas-Miras MDM, Gea J, et al. Metabolomic profile of ARDS by nuclear magnetic resonance spectroscopy in patients with H1N1 influenza virus pneumonia. Shock. 2018;50(5):504–10. PubMed PMID: 29293175. Epub 2018/01/03.

150. Viswan A, Singh C, Rai RK, Azim A, Sinha N, Baronia AK. Metabolomics based predictive biomarker model of ARDS: a systemic measure of clinical hypoxemia. PLoS One. 2017;12(11):e0187545. PubMed PMID: 29095932. Pubmed Central PMCID: PMC5667881. Epub 2017/11/03.

151. Maile MD, Standiford TJ, Engoren MC, Stringer KA, Jewell ES, Rajendiran TM, et al. Associations of the plasma lipidome with mortality in the acute respiratory distress syndrome: a longitudinal cohort study. Respir Res. 2018;19(1):60. PubMed PMID: 29636049. Pubmed Central PMCID: PMC5894233. Epub 2018/04/11.

Mobile Applications and Wearables for Chronic Respiratory Disease Monitoring

19

Ann Chen Wu, Sze Man Tse, and Fabio Balli

Key Point Summary
- mHealth increases access to health knowledge and allows monitoring at any time and at any location, which can help enable precision medicine.
- Most of the relatively few mobile apps and wearables that are dedicated to respiratory health focus on providing medical information, messaging services, diaries, lung function self-assessment, and educational games.
- Challenges to the widespread adoption of mHealth include limited access to technology by all patients, decreased adoption over time, and data privacy concerns.

A. C. Wu (✉)
PRecisiOn Medicine Translational Research (PROMoTeR) Center, Department of Population Medicine, Harvard Medical School, Boston, MA, USA
e-mail: ann.wu@childrens.harvard.edu

S. M. Tse
Department of Pediatrics, Sainte-Justine University Hospital Center, Montreal, QC, Canada

University of Montreal, Montreal, QC, Canada
e-mail: sze.man.tse@umontreal.ca

F. Balli
Breathing Games, Geneva, Switzerland

Concordia University, Montreal, QC, Canada
e-mail: info@fabioballi.net

Introduction

The omnipresence of connected mobile devices has great potential to transform the relationship between patient and healthcare provider. *mHealth* is "the use of mobile devices [...] for medical and public health practice" [1], and one of its components is "the cost-effective and secure use of information communication technologies in support of health and health-related fields, including healthcare services, health surveillance, health literature, and health education, knowledge and research" [2]. mHealth not only provides access to health knowledge anytime and anywhere; it can also collect unprecedented amounts and types of data about patients' daily lives. At every step in the treatment process, mHealth increases patients' autonomy in self-assessing their health and acting to preserve their well-being. These technologies can facilitate the ability of healthcare providers to track their patients' progress and modify treatments appropriately, thereby reducing the need for office visits and decreasing the burden on the healthcare system. Three key reasons for patients to adopt mHealth are more effective provider access, reduced costs of care, and improved health self-management. For physicians, key reasons to recommend mHealth are enhanced health outcomes, facilitated access for the care of patients, and decreased time required for administrative tasks [6]. According to the

© Springer Nature Switzerland AG 2020
J. L. Gomez et al. (eds.), *Precision in Pulmonary, Critical Care, and Sleep Medicine*,
Respiratory Medicine, https://doi.org/10.1007/978-3-030-31507-8_19

World Health Organization, mHealth is a central element to achieve universal health coverage [1].

Today, over 325,000 mobile applications, or apps, provide health and well-being services [3]. The majority of these apps are limited to sending information. Fitness, lifestyle, coping with stress, or nutrition is the focus of 65%, while 23% focus on treatment. Social media is a feature in 65% of the apps and only 2% currently connect to a healthcare system. While most apps are free to download, one third of them require purchasing a device, and one tenth require payment [4].

More than half of currently available apps have been downloaded less than 5000 times, while 3% have been downloaded over a million times, reaching a total of 3.7 billion yearly downloads. Only 2% of the apps recommended by healthcare providers focus on respiratory health, and this group of respiratory apps has the lowest fill-and-sustain rate among all apps [4]. Apps recommended by clinicians have a retention increase of 10–30%, and one in three physicians has recommended a mHealth app to their patients [4]. However, the larger system continues to fall short, only 2% of hospitals promote the use of apps [5], and apps developed by healthcare providers often fail to satisfy the functionalities patients seek: access to medical records, appointment management, and prescription renewals [5]. Less than 1% of people living with asthma use an asthma app [3]. Wearables are devices worn on the body to track bodily functions. They have become a part of daily life, with 232 million objects sold in 2015 [4]. Most wearables are worn on a wrist (55%) or chest (23%) [4] and focus on improving overall well-being by tracking exercise, weight loss, and sleep and coping with stress [7], among other functions. In the USA, the main users of wearables are 18–34-year-olds [8].

mHealth from the Patient's Perspective

The majority of mHealth apps dedicated to treatment are designed to optimize self-management of chronic diseases by providing greater patient autonomy [9], reducing healthcare utilization [10], and improving clinical outcomes [9–11]. Improved self-management occurs by increasing a patient's awareness of symptoms, self-measuring objective parameters such as pulmonary function, maintaining a symptom diary, and proving guidance for symptom management. Wearables can monitor body functions, measure physiological changes, and capture environmental data [12]. Smartwatches and sensors worn daily could facilitate the embedding of biofeedback into diaries of a patient's daily routine. Disease self-management with mHealth apps requires the active participation and engagement of the patient. It is therefore not surprising that the majority of studies evaluating mHealth apps do so from the patients' perspective. Figure 19.1 summarizes the major aspects of mHealth that are necessary for the development of successful tools. Next, we focus on some of these factors, including apps' usability and perceived benefits and concerns, with a focus on research pertaining to chronic respiratory disease apps.

Usability and Engagement

Usability refers to how well an app functions and serves its intended purposes in a target population [13]. It includes user satisfaction and app operability, flexibility, ease of learning, and visual interface attractiveness [14]. Usability can be assessed through expert inspection of the app, user observation, surveys, and experimental evaluation to gather user feedback [15, 16]. Although international standards and frameworks for software quality evaluation exist, namely, those from the International Organization for Standardization (ISO) (ISO/IEC 25010 [17] and ISO 9241 [18]), few apps are empirically evaluated for their usability [19]. Successful apps are first and foremost characterized by their ability to engage the user, a key element underlying user satisfaction. Without user engagement, user boredom and loss of interest quickly ensue. Apps that can sustain positive behavior are more likely to have sustained use [20]. Attrition rates in respiratory disease app use can be as high as 28% [21]. User

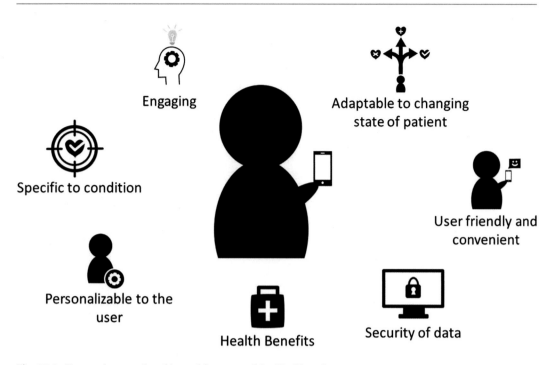

Fig. 19.1 Factors that must be addressed for successful mHealth tools

engagement can be optimized by integrating game design elements (gamification), including using points or leveling systems, creating leaderboards, using rewards such as badges or trophies, implementing challenges, and integrating social features so users can interact with each other [22, 23]. A review of 38 asthma apps (up to April 2016) demonstrated considerable differences between apps, and most apps used little gamification [24]. While 74% of the tested apps allowed users to see and "compete" against their own records, a reward system was only implemented in 8% of them. When the apps' quality was evaluated by the standardized Mobile Application Rating Scale, a measure of health app quality using five subscales (engagement, functionality, aesthetics, information, and subjective quality) [25], asthma apps performed poorest in user engagement. Researchers suggested that reward systems, which have recognized effectiveness in psychology theories and can be implemented easily, should be integrated in future apps.

User engagement matters because integration of mHealth into a patient's self-management routine requires long-term use of the technology, particularly for chronic lung disease care which requires long-term management [26]. mHealth apps need to be flexible and adaptable to a user's changing needs. Thus, the design of apps for chronic diseases should consider how the patient interacts with their condition over time (e.g., frequency and length of treatments, changes in the condition) [23]. Some research has demonstrated that most participants using health apps reduced or stopped using their app when they became familiar with the self-management techniques or did not learn anything further from the app [20]. Moreover, while long-term engagement is essential in determining an app's value in chronic disease management, few studies have evaluated user engagement over time. Among those that did, the testing period was usually not long term and under 6 months [21, 27–29].

Wearables may offer improved opportunities for mHealth. Smartwatches have limited sensing and computing capability, but their location on the body and extensive patient contact have potential to transform health function monitoring into an automatism, increasing retention in the long run. Ways to improve the interactivity and user experience of such devices have not been studied [30]. Wearables, such as clothing, seem currently only adapted to specific contexts in lung health such as chronic obstructive pulmonary disease (COPD) monitoring [31–33]. Lighter and less constraining tattoo-like sensor films have some promise in extending the power of mHealth apps [34]. Such easy-to-carry devices could indeed increase patient adoption and use [35]. Medication trackers such as inhaler-based monitoring devices could also help patients log their treatment intakes. Combined with physiological data, such trackers could help personalize treatment to each patient [36, 37]. Despite their promise, clinical research remains very limited regarding wearables. Most apps that have been clinically tested report few technological or operability issues [38]. Adults using health apps report an appreciation for automation of in-app functions such as automatic data entry via a sensor or a wearable device [20].

Perceived Benefits

A few mHealth studies documented users' perceived benefits, an important consideration for app users. Specifically, users reported greater self-awareness of their condition, improved self-confidence in chronic disease monitoring, easier integration of self-management techniques, and increased feelings of being "in control" [39]. Patients also reported decreased anxiety due to knowing that their health symptoms were being monitored [39]. A pilot study of an app encouraging home-based pre-lung transplant rehabilitation to treat frailty found summarily positive feedback from users [40]. Participants felt in control of their physical status and felt that they could take some action to improve their health rather than just waiting for their next appointment. Benefits were also perceived for apps that provided alert systems reminding users to take medications [41, 42] or informing users when health indicators reached a critical range and prompted them to call their health professional [42]. Specifically, in designing an app to promote medication adherence in adolescent solid organ

recipients, field-test users requested the function of alerts and felt that the app was helpful in tracking their medication intake [41]. Other apps transmitted patients' data to their health professionals, a feature that was valued by users because it avoided repeated healthcare visits [20]. The limited number of available studies has reported perceived benefits of mHealth tools although clinical studies are needed to determine actual health benefits to the user.

Parents' Point of View

Parents see benefits in using mHealth to manage their children's chronic respiratory disease. A survey-based study demonstrated that a majority of parents believed the use of an app would help them better monitor and manage their child's asthma. Specifically, parents ranked an app's ability to generate reports for the doctor, input symptoms into a diary, and complete a self-check quiz as the most useful features [43]. Parents also appreciated reminder messages to their teenagers to take their medication or to get refills, benefits reiterated by the teenagers as well [44], as parents felt less need to continuously remind their teenagers to take their medications [41], potentially decreasing parent-adolescent conflict. Given the increasing societal concern of screen time in children [45], the adoption of mHealth by parents is an important aspect in apps aimed at children. Future studies should consider parental input in creating mHealth apps aimed at children, in addition to ensuring user involvement.

Patients' Concerns

While patients usually have a positive view of mHealth, some concerns remain that may affect acceptability of apps and wearables. Data security is a primary concern, particularly with regard to transmission of sensitive information that may be accessed by health insurers [20]. Additionally, when using a short message service (SMS) system for asthma self-management, some patients raised concerns about the lack of feedback and unnecessary medicalization [39]. Further, while some apps offered distance support [29], most apps did not offer specific training on their use, which led to user engagement issues in some studies where technical barriers inhibited use of the apps [46, 47]. In addition to technical difficulties, literacy barriers, language, and connectivity issues are potential barriers to mHealth.

Summary

mHealth is a patient-centered means to promote self-management of chronic conditions, and its efficacy is highly user dependent. Thus, understanding mHealth from the patient's perspective is essential. In fact, studies suggest an iterative design process with multiple user experience testing sessions in the development of mHealth apps optimizes user engagement of the final product [38, 48]. Several studies documented a generally high usability, acceptability, and user satisfaction of mHealth tools, with most users perceiving benefits. However, few studies have assessed long-term user engagement and health benefits. Furthermore, the theoretical framework behind positive behavioral change resulting from using mHealth is poorly understood. Integrating the user early in the design process will maximize user engagement and address their concerns, which could in turn lead to the development of better apps and wearables that better meet patients' needs.

mHealth from the Healthcare Provider's Perspective

mHealth Apps

Although few studies have focused on chronic respiratory disease monitoring, general studies have reported benefits and barriers to mHealth apps from the viewpoint of providers. A systematic review of 33 studies examining factors influencing healthcare professional adoption of mHealth apps found that their adoption was more often seen as a benefit than a barrier [49]. Notable factors that led to increased adoption included perceived utility of app over current practice and ease of technology use in the working environment [49]. Benefits to providers include the potential saving of time, better patient engagement, and enhanced care. Saving of time is the result of healthcare providers being able to access patient-reported symptoms in electronic health records and reviewing them before in-person visits [50]. A study of a mobile portal application for hospitalized patients reported that providers felt the portal improved patient engagement in care and identification of errors [51]. Research on a sensor-based mobile intervention for asthma identified mHealth technology as enhancing the patient-centered medical home [52]. Further, in a qualitative study asking providers about their views of a sensor-based mobile intervention for asthma patients, providers were enthusiastic for the mobile health technology if it could provide adherence to prescribed inhaler therapy and data on inhaler technique [52]. Providers hoped data gathered would be available prior to scheduled clinic visits and that the app would provide inter-visit alerts for excessive use of rescue therapy, while pulmonologists were interested in inter-visit lung function data [52].

mySinusitusCoach

mySinusitusCoach (Fig. 19.2) is a mobile app that helps patients with chronic rhinosinusitis log their symptoms and treatments, get recommendations, and learn about the disease. The longitudinal data collected can improve physician follow-up, such as early identification of the need for surgery. Initiated by the *European Forum for Research and Education in Allergy and Airway diseases*, the app was conceived by medical care professionals with input from patients, primary care physicians, and pharmacists. The app is currently available in three countries, and research on its health outcomes is ongoing [53].

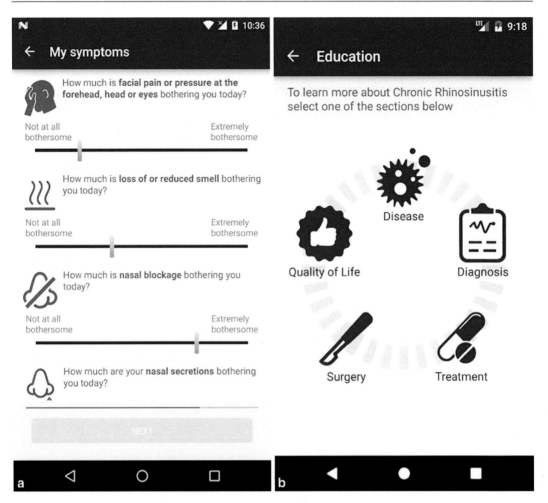

Fig. 19.2 (a) Screenshot of a questionnaire to assess one's symptoms in the mySinusitusCoach app. (b) Screenshot of themes available on the mySinusitusCoach app. (Images from https://play.google.com/store/apps/ details?id=nl.euforea.sinusitishealth&hl=en. Used with permission of EUFOREA-European Forum for Research and Education in Allergy and Airway Diseases)

Beyond standalone apps, mHealth interventions that involve remote monitoring can supplement traditional care usefully. Researchers in the United Kingdom conducted semi-structured interviews with providers to learn about their views of a telehealth care program for patients with chronic conditions, including chronic heart disease, COPD, and diabetes [54]. This telehealth monitoring system included the installation of equipment, such as pulse oximeter and weighing scales, in the patient's home; patients recorded their biometric readings which were transmitted to healthcare professionals and monitored remotely by nurses or community matrons. When parametrics were outside of normal ranges, providers contacted the patients and/or referred them to other healthcare professionals, such as physicians. The majority of providers felt that this telehealth monitoring system empowered patients and was a good supplement for traditional patient care [54].

mHealth offers many favorable facets to providers, yet obstacles remain, primarily regarding the disruption of workflow: organizations were not designed or created to accommodate mHealth, so adapting to new workflow demands can bring challenges [55]. Of primary concern is the increase in workload involved with mHealth implementation [54, 56, 57]. Undefined and changed roles occur when an mHealth app leads to different providers being responsible for a workflow task or no responsibilities are assigned [58], and providers may have to invest a significant amount of time with patients to teach them how to use apps and interpret the data reported [59]. Additionally, workflow is disrupted as providers are unable to complete the work process in a linear and smooth manner [57]. Lack of alignment with existing clinical processes poses a barrier when mHealth apps do not integrate with, or support, workflow systems that are in place [54]. Another concern for department-specific mHealth protocols is provider turnover: every time providers change departments, whether via rotations between departments or because they are short-term hires, they may need to learn new mHealth implementation strategies [55].

Provider concerns beyond workflow issues have also been identified. First, face-to-face communication may be undermined as direct personal contact between patient and provider may decrease with adoption of mHealth [60]. Moreover, concerns exist regarding safeguarding protected health information, data accuracy in the case, for example, in which sensor-based mobile interventions are used by families who share inhalers, and lack of access to smartphones [51]. In the study of a mobile portal application for hospitalized patients, providers worried that additional features might result in a volume and complexity of information that could be overwhelming for patients, as well as a high percentage of false-positive tests resulting from a potentially high volume of tests performed, which could lead to unnecessary concerns, particularly due to patients' limited ability to interpret results in the context of their acute illness [52].

Wearables

Few studies to date have evaluated wearables for chronic respiratory disease management, and none have found evidence supporting sustained use of wearables or effects on health outcomes. Most of the existing studies have focused on

development and feasibility of monitoring activity for pulmonary rehabilitation [61], detecting wheeze [62], and monitoring pulmonary edema in adult respiratory distress syndrome [63]. One study sought to improve the care of individuals with COPD and reduce hospitalizations by using smartwatches to detect early exacerbations in time for intervention [64]. Specifically, the smartwatch collected sensor data, including heart rate, accelerometer, and gyroscope recordings. Researchers concluded that individuals wanted to actively engage with the smartwatch and receive feedback about their activity, heart rate, and how to better manage their COPD, but further work is necessary to improve the patient experience [64].

mHealth from the Healthcare System's Perspective

Three salient issues to address from the healthcare system's perspective are cost-effectiveness, privacy, and widespread diffusion of mHealth. Cost-effectiveness analyses help policy makers decide how to allocate limited resources, and insurers often use cost-effectiveness analyses to decide whether to cover health interventions [65, 66]. Risks to privacy with mHealth are an important consideration by the healthcare system as mHealth technologies collect detailed personal data; communication of these risks for the purposes of informed consent is critical [67]. As mHealth is essential to achieve universal health coverage [1], its widespread diffusion is critical yet challenged by factors such as geographic and financial accessibility [68].

Cost-Effectiveness

Cost-effectiveness is a method of economic evaluation that can be helpful in health technology assessment and is often expressed in terms of the ratio of the cost associated with health gain divided by gain in health from a measure [69]. The gain in health from a measure is often calculated as quality-adjusted life year (QALY) so that multiple interventions can be compared [65, 66]. Cost-effectiveness analysis produces the incremental cost-effectiveness ratio in units of dollars per QALY [65, 66]. Cost is an important component that will determine the success or failure of mHealth. On a broad level, many expect that mHealth will bring cost reductions, but because most studies report on the implementation process rather than measuring costs and financial benefits after implementation of mHealth, most studies have not yet addressed actual costs [59]. Healthcare system representatives believe that costs are the most important component contributing to the success or failure of mHealth apps: a review paper concluded that institutional adoption of mHealth apps can be considered when organizations break even or profit, but is more difficult to consider with a financial loss [59]. Thus, national policy investments and health insurer reimbursement to providers for mHealth adoption and usage will play a critical role in their adoption [59].

While no studies specifically studied cost-effectiveness of mHealth and chronic respiratory diseases, we can learn from the general mHealth literature. In addition to costs related to development and implementation of mHealth, there are the costs related to equipment, staffing, and communication [70]. One study that assessed the cost-effectiveness of outpatient pulmonary subspecialty consultations in rural populations found that telemedicine was more cost-effective compared to routine care when patients travel from a remote site to a hub site to receive care; the main driver of cost-effectiveness was the ability to cost share, as providers shared telemedicine infrastructure while patients suffered fewer costs from lost productivity [71].

Studies of mHealth effectiveness are needed to help inform its cost-effectiveness. One review of mobile apps for asthma found that only two randomized controlled trials compared patient self-management asthma interventions delivered via smartphone apps to those delivered via traditional methods [73]. Based on these two studies, the authors concluded that there was not enough

evidence to advise providers to use asthma self-management programs via smartphone and table computer apps [73]. In order for effectiveness studies to be conducted, participation is important. One study that attempted to examine a remote clinical monitoring tool following palliative radiotherapy for lung cancer found that only one of 17 providers contacted agreed to participate in the study, so the benefits of the technology could not be assessed [74]. The lack of providers accepting participation in this study suggests that there are still uncertainties about adoption of mHealth.

Privacy

The health information that can be collected via mHealth has great potential value, but there are special privacy risks that need to be addressed. These include the potential for discrimination from insurers, such as the nonpurposeful collection of data of family members [75]. In medical settings, the Common Rule and the Health Insurance Portability and Accountability Act (HIPAA) require high standards for the protection of patient and research participant data [76]. However, mHealth technologies used for medical care often come from the commercial sector; thus, ensuring those mHealth technologies meet the high standards of privacy protection is important and challenging [77, 78]. Commercially developed technologies usually have long informed consent forms, sometimes stipulating the release or selling of personal identifiable data. Furthermore, commercial data collection, transmission, storage, access, and use are underregulated and not standardized [76], while healthcare systems need to use strategies to protect privacy of patients.

Widespread Diffusion of mHealth

mHealth is essential to achieve universal health coverage by 2030, a United Nations Global

Goal [69]. mHealth can widen the number of individuals who can access health services, increase the amount of services available, and reduce the cost of access to such services [79]. In 2016, 109 countries reported having at least one mHealth program. The most common services offered were free calls to emergency and medical services, as well as appointment reminders—an effective means to reduce no-shows in consultations. Only 25 countries, however, reported evaluations on the safety, quality, and reliability of mHealth programs. Access to mHealth was also difficult to assess. Indicators of access should thus be implemented in every mHealth project, with special consideration to priority audiences such as vulnerable and marginalized populations [1].

In addition to addressing disease management, mHealth should encompass health promotion and primary prevention. In the European Union alone, respiratory mHealth apps could help 4 million Europeans quit smoking, and 1 million Europeans reduce the risk of developing COPD [80]. In Europe, mHealth could reduce the cost of medical care by 99 billion euros when all diseases are considered. Such potential remains theoretical until a large audience adopts and uses mHealth over the long term.

To ensure that mHealth provides high quality of care and meets local needs, individuals and communities must be involved in the conception, production, and evaluation of such technologies [69]. Unfortunately, most projects use standard copyright licenses, which forbid individuals and communities to take ownership of the innovation. Alternative licenses such as the GNU Affero General Public License [81] or the CERN Open Hardware License [82] could encourage populations to engage in mHealth projects by ensuring usability is high, as well as improving source code of apps or design of wearables. Projects released under fair use licenses or in the public domain could foster an approach where the individual (before and beyond their disease) is at the core and where medical experts or researchers become partners. Free and open source projects also increase reproducibility of work, allow people from different countries to join their knowledge and experience to reach a common goal (crowdsourcing), and enable design of tools that are appropriate even in low resource settings. Combined with new ways of doing research [83], free mHealth apps and open source mHealth wearables could accelerate the pace of innovation [84], stimulate individuals to contribute to the respiratory health of their communities, democratize

Respi Heroes

Respi Heroes is a mobile game that aims to make respiratory health accessible and fun through learning by playing (Fig. 19.3). The player can explore different environments (mountain, city field of pampas, etc.), interact with characters who provide cultural and health knowledge (the air, the lung system, nutrition, food, physical activity, etc.), and play different mini-games according to their health condition (memorizing asthma triggers, matching the inhaler with the correct situation, self-assessing one's lung capacity, reducing one's stress, etc.).

The game and game controller that transform the breath into data (game input and self-assessment of lung function) are developed in a participatory action research approach. Research is ongoing in Canada, France, Switzerland, and Italy on user experience, health outcomes, and the co-creation process. The game and reproducible controller are expected to be publicly available mid-2019, covering asthma, cystic fibrosis, and respiratory health promotion. Unlike most mHealth projects, the source code of the game and design of the controller are documented and released under fair use licenses to allow interested communities to enhance and adapt the work done. This open science approach allows the reduction of cost of access by mutualizing resources across countries. The initiative is led by the *Breathing Games* commons, a participant of the *Global Alliance Against Respiratory Diseases* [72].

respiratory health knowledge, and reduce the burden on the healthcare system.

- Images: Reuse permitted. Credit to www. breathinggames.net
- Legend 1: Screenshot of a region to explore in the game Respi Heroes
- Legend 2: Screenshot of a mini-game to self-assess one's lung capacity in Respi Heroes
- Legend 3: 3D-printed enclosure with a pressure sensor that is part of the reproducible game controller used with the games

Conclusion

Widespread adoption of mHealth will occur over time. mHealth can help individuals adopt healthy lifestyles, deepen their knowledge about health, and get support to self-assess and manage diseases. mHealth can help medical care providers improve follow-up care of their patients and increase their efficiency by allowing for earlier diagnosis and remote consultations. At the level of healthcare systems, mHealth can help achieve universal health coverage (Fig. 19.4).

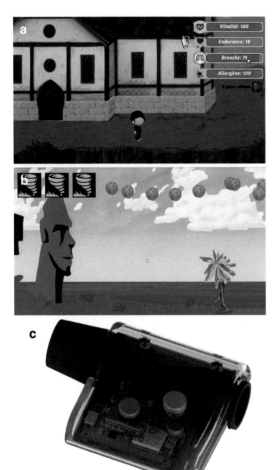

Fig. 19.3 Screenshots from the Respi Heroes game. (**a**) Game scene in which the player learns how to avoid and manage asthma crisis in the game. (**b**) Game scene in which the player self-assesses their lung capacity (peak flow). (**c**) Game controller that can be used to play the games and self-assess one's lung capacity. (Images reproduced with permission from Fabio Balli, Lead Coordinator, Breathing Games, as content under Creative Commons BY-SA 4.0 International license)

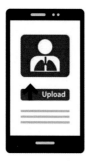

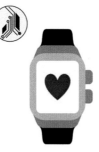

» 325,000 health / wellbeing apps
» 2% on respiratory health

» 232 million objects sold in 2015
» no inventory on respi. health

» medical information
» interactive, rewarding contents
» messaging service
» symptoms / treatment diary
» lung function assessment

» monitoring of physiological
   or / and environmental data
» hands-on biofeedback

For the user
» improved access to medical information and provider
» increased autonomy for the prevention and management of diseases
» ability to contribute to one's health technologies and knowledge

For the medical care provider
» closer follow up, ability to better track changes and adapt treatment
» increased efficiency via early screening, alerts, remote consultations
» support to increase adherence

For the medical care system
» increased coverage and access to care for the population
» reduced costs
» key to universal health coverage

Icons adapted from Freepik, Alfredo Hernandez from flaticon.com

Fig. 19.4 Mobile apps and wearables in short: amount, uses, benefits

References

1. World Health Organization. Global diffusion of eHealth: making universal health coverage achievable. Report of the third global survey on eHealth. Global Observatory for eHealth; 2016.
2. World Health Assembly resolution 58.28. 2005. Available from: http://www.who.int/healthacademy/media/WHA58-28-en.pdf.
3. Research 2 Guidance. mHealth app economics 2017/2018: current status and future trends in mobile health 2017, 1–27 pp. Available from: https://research-2guidance.com/wp-content/uploads/2017/11/R2G-mHealth-Developer-Economics-2017-Status-And-Trends.pdf.
4. IMS Institute for Healthcare Informatics. Patient adoption of mHealth: use, evidence and remaining barriers to mainstream acceptance 2015, 1–63 pp. Available from: https://www.iqvia.com/-/media/iqvia/pdfs/institute-reports/patient-adoption-of-mhealth.pdf?la=en&hash=B3ACFA8ADDB143F29EAC0C33D533BC5D7AABD689.
5. Accenture. Losing patience: why healthcare providers need to up their mobile game. 2015, 1–4 pp. Available from: https://www.accenture.com/t20151112T042615__w__/us-en/_acnmedia/Accenture/Conversion-Assets/DotCom/Documents/Global/PDF/Dualpub_24/Accenture-Losing-Patience.pdf#zoom=50.
6. PwC. Emerging mHealth: paths for growth 2014, 1–44 pp. Available from: https://www.pwc.com/gx/en/healthcare/mhealth/assets/pwc-emerging-mhealth-full.pdf.
7. Zweig M, Shen J, Jug L. Healthcare consumers in a digital transition. 2018. https://rockhealth.com/reports/healthcare-consumers-in-a-digital-transition/ (accessed October 25, 2019).
8. Adams A, Shankar M, Tecco H. 50 things we now know about digital health consumers. 2016. https://rockhealth.com/reports/digital-health-consumer-adoption-2016/ (accessed October 25, 2019).
9. Coulter A, Entwistle VA, Eccles A, Ryan S, Shepperd S, Perera R. Personalised care planning for adults with chronic or long-term health conditions. Cochrane Database Syst Rev. 2015;(3):Cd010523.
10. Lorig KR, Ritter P, Stewart AL, Sobel DS, Brown BW Jr, Bandura A, et al. Chronic disease self-management program: 2-year health status and health care utilization outcomes. Med Care. 2001;39(11):1217–23.
11. Chodosh J, Morton SC, Mojica W, Maglione M, Suttorp MJ, Hilton L, et al. Meta-analysis: chronic disease self-management programs for older adults. Ann Intern Med. 2005;143(6):427–38.
12. Aliverti A. Wearable technology: role in respiratory health and disease. Breathe (Sheff). 2017;13(2):e27–36.
13. Jake-Schoffman DE, Silfee VJ, Waring ME, Boudreaux ED, Sadasivam RS, Mullen SP, et al. Methods for evaluating the content, usability, and efficacy of commercial mobile health apps. JMIR Mhealth Uhealth. 2017;5(12):e190.
14. Nassar V. Common criteria for usability review. Work. 2012;41(Suppl 1):1053–7.
15. Jaspers MW. A comparison of usability methods for testing interactive health technologies: methodological aspects and empirical evidence. Int J Med Inform. 2009;78(5):340–53.
16. Moumane K, Idri A, Abran A. Usability evaluation of mobile applications using ISO 9241 and ISO 25062 standards. Springerplus. 2016;5:548.
17. International Organization for Standardization, The International Electrotechnical Commission. Systems and software engineering — Systems and software Quality Requirements and Evaluation (SQuaRE) — System and software quality models. 2011. p. 1–34.
18. International Organization for Standardization. Ergonomics of human-system interaction -- part 11: usability: definitions and concepts. 2018. p. 1–29.
19. Zapata BC, Fernandez-Aleman JL, Idri A, Toval A. Empirical studies on usability of mHealth apps: a systematic literature review. J Med Syst. 2015;39(2):1.
20. Anderson K, Burford O, Emmerton L. Mobile health apps to facilitate self-care: a qualitative study of user experiences. PLoS One. 2016;11(5):e0156164.
21. Liu WT, Huang CD, Wang CH, Lee KY, Lin SM, Kuo HP. A mobile telephone-based interactive self-care system improves asthma control. Eur Respir J. 2011;37(2):310–7.
22. Morford ZH, Witts BN, Killingsworth KJ, Alavosius MP. Gamification: the intersection between behavior analysis and game design technologies. Behav Anal. 2014;37(1):25–40.
23. Giunti G. 3MD for chronic conditions, a model for motivational mHealth design: embedded case study. JMIR Serious Games. 2018;6(3):e11631.
24. Tinschert P, Jakob R, Barata F, Kramer JN, Kowatsch T. The potential of mobile apps for improving asthma self-management: a review of publicly available and well-adopted asthma apps. JMIR Mhealth Uhealth. 2017;5(8):e113.
25. Stoyanov SR, Hides L, Kavanagh DJ, Zelenko O, Tjondronegoro D, Mani M. Mobile app rating scale: a new tool for assessing the quality of health mobile apps. JMIR Mhealth Uhealth. 2015;3(1):e27.
26. Xu W, Huang MC, Liu JJ, Ren F, Shen X, Liu X, et al. mCOPD: mobile phone based lung function diagnosis and exercise system for COPD. In: ACM international conference proceeding series, 2013.
27. Global Initiative for Asthma. 2018 GINA report, Global strategy for asthma management and prevention. 2018.
28. Stukus DR, Farooqui N, Strothman K, Ryan K, Zhao S, Stevens JH, et al. Real-world evaluation of a mobile health application in children with asthma. Ann Allergy Asthma Immunol. 2018;120(4):395–400 e1.
29. Liu WT, Wang CH, Lin HC, Lin SM, Lee KY, Lo YL, et al. Efficacy of a cell phone-based exercise programme for COPD. Eur Respir J. 2008;32(3):651–9.

30. Ryan D, Price D, Musgrave SD, Malhotra S, Lee AJ, Ayansina D, et al. Clinical and cost effectiveness of mobile phone supported self monitoring of asthma: multicentre randomised controlled trial. BMJ. 2012;344:e1756.

31. Rawassizadeh R, Price BA, Petre M. Wearables: has the age of smartwatches finally arrived? Commun ACM. 2015;58(1):45–7.

32. Chetelat O, Wacker J, Rapin M, Porchet J-A, Meier C, Fahli A, et al. New biosensors and wearables for cardiorespiratory telemonitoring. In: The proceedings of the IEEE-EMBS international conference on biomedical and health informatics (BHI). Las Vegas: IEEE; 2016. p. 481–84.

33. Nabhani S, Siva R, Kayyali R, Yagambrun C, Robinson P, Spruit M, et al. M23 the use of wearables for COPD patients: a qualitative study. Thorax. 2015;70(Suppl 3):A236–A7.

34. Grochala D, Kajor M, Kantoch E, editors. A wearable multi-sensor solution for daily activities monitoring with an expanded respiratory part. 2018 Baltic URSI symposium (URSI), 15–17 May 2018.

35. Dunn J, Runge R, Snyder M. Wearables and the medical revolution. Per Med. 2018;15(5):429–48.

36. Crema C, Depari A, Flammini A, Sisinni E, Vezzoli A, Bellagente P. Virtual respiratory rate sensors: an example of a smartphone-based integrated and multiparametric mHealth gateway. IEEE Trans Instrum Meas. 2017;66(9):2456–63.

37. Patel M, Pilcher J, Travers J, Perrin K, Shaw D, Black P, et al. Use of metered-dose inhaler electronic monitoring in a real-world asthma randomized controlled trial. J Allergy Clin Immunol Pract. 2013;1(1):83–91.

38. Kikidis D, Konstantinos V, Tzovaras D, Usmani OS. The digital asthma patient: the history and future of inhaler based health monitoring devices. J Aerosol Med Pulm Drug Deliv. 2016;29(3):219–32.

39. Whitehead L, Seaton P. The effectiveness of self-management mobile phone and tablet apps in long-term condition management: a systematic review. J Med Internet Res. 2016;18(5):e97.

40. Anhoj J, Moldrup C. Feasibility of collecting diary data from asthma patients through mobile phones and SMS (short message service): response rate analysis and focus group evaluation from a pilot study. J Med Internet Res. 2004;6(4):e42.

41. Singer JP, Soong A, Bruun A, Bracha A, Chin G, Hays SR, et al. A mobile health technology enabled home-based intervention to treat frailty in adult lung transplant candidates: a pilot study. Clin Transpl. 2018;32(6):e13274.

42. Shellmer DA, Dew MA, Mazariegos G, DeVito Dabbs A. Development and field testing of Teen Pocket PATH((R)), a mobile health application to improve medication adherence in adolescent solid organ recipients. Pediatr Transplant. 2016;20(1):130–40.

43. DeVito Dabbs A, Dew MA, Myers B, Begey A, Hawkins R, Ren D, et al. Evaluation of a hand-held, computer-based intervention to promote early self-care behaviors after lung transplant. Clin Transpl. 2009;23(4):537–45.

44. Geryk LL, Roberts CA, Sage AJ, Coyne-Beasley T, Sleath BL, Carpenter DM. Parent and clinician preferences for an asthma app to promote adolescent self-management: a formative study. JMIR Res Protoc. 2016;5(4):e229.

45. Panzera AD, Schneider TK, Martinasek MP, Lindenberger JH, Couluris M, Bryant CA, et al. Adolescent asthma self-management: patient and parent-caregiver perspectives on using social media to improve care. J Sch Health. 2013;83(12):921–30.

46. Domingues-Montanari S. Clinical and psychological effects of excessive screen time on children. J Paediatr Child Health. 2017;53(4):333–8.

47. Faridi Z, Liberti L, Shuval K, Northrup V, Ali A, Katz DL. Evaluating the impact of mobile telephone technology on type 2 diabetic patients' self-management: the NICHE pilot study. J Eval Clin Pract. 2008;14(3):465–9.

48. Waki K, Fujita H, Uchimura Y, Omae K, Aramaki E, Kato S, et al. DialBetics: a novel smartphone-based self-management support system for type 2 diabetes patients. J Diabetes Sci Technol. 2014;8(2):209–15.

49. Osborn CY, Mulvaney SA. Development and feasibility of a text messaging and interactive voice response intervention for low-income, diverse adults with type 2 diabetes mellitus. J Diabetes Sci Technol. 2013;7(3):612–22.

50. Gagnon MP, Ngangue P, Payne-Gagnon J, Desmartis M. m-Health adoption by healthcare professionals: a systematic review. J Am Med Inform Assoc. 2016;23(1):212–20.

51. Rudin RS, Fanta CH, Predmore Z, Kron K, Edelen MO, Landman AB, et al. Core components for a clinically integrated mHealth app for asthma symptom monitoring. Appl Clin Inform. 2017;8(4):1031–43.

52. O'Leary KJ, Sharma RK, Killarney A, O'Hara LS, Lohman ME, Culver E, et al. Patients' and healthcare providers' perceptions of a mobile portal application for hospitalized patients. BMC Med Inform Decis Mak. 2016;16(1):123.

53. Hollenbach JP, Cushing A, Melvin E, McGowan B, Cloutier MM, Manice M. Understanding clinicians' attitudes toward a mobile health strategy to childhood asthma management: a qualitative study. J Asthma. 2017;54(7):754–60.

54. Seys SF, Bousquet J, Bachert C, Fokkens WJ, Agache I, Bernal-Sprekelsen M, et al. mySinusitisCoach: patient empowerment in chronic rhinosinusitis using mobile technology. Rhinology. 2018;56(3):209–15.

55. MacNeill V, Sanders C, Fitzpatrick R, Hendy J, Barlow J, Knapp M, et al. Experiences of front-line health professionals in the delivery of telehealth: a qualitative study. Br J Gen Pract. 2014;64(624):e401–7.

56. Appelbaum S, Wohl L. Transformation or change: some prescriptions for health care organizations. Manag Serv Qual Int J. 2000;10:279–98.

57. Solling IK, Caroe P, Mathiesen KS. Development and implementation of IT require focus on user participation, acceptance and workflow. Stud Health Technol Inform. 2014;201:219–26.

58. Steele Gray C, Gill A, Khan AI, Hans PK, Kuluski K, Cott C. The electronic patient reported outcome tool: testing usability and feasibility of a mobile app and portal to support care for patients with complex chronic disease and disability in primary care settings. JMIR Mhealth Uhealth. 2016;4(2):e58.

59. Lamothe L, Fortin JP, Labbe F, Gagnon MP, Messikh D. Impacts of telehomecare on patients, providers, and organizations. Telemed J E Health. 2006;12(3):363–9.

60. Granja C, Janssen W, Johansen MA. Factors determining the success and failure of eHealth interventions: systematic review of the literature. J Med Internet Res. 2018;20(5):e10235.

61. Das A, Faxvaag A, Svanaes D. The impact of an eHealth portal on health care professionals' interaction with patients: qualitative study. J Med Internet Res. 2015;17(11):e267.

62. Chiauzzi E, Rodarte C, DasMahapatra P. Patient-centered activity monitoring in the self-management of chronic health conditions. BMC Med. 2015;13:77.

63. Acharya J, Basu A, Ser W. Feature extraction techniques for low-power ambulatory wheeze detection wearables. In: Conference proceedings: Annual international conference of the IEEE Engineering in Medicine and Biology Society. IEEE Engineering in Medicine and Biology Society annual conference. 2017, p. 4574–7.

64. Michard F. Lung water assessment: from gravimetry to wearables. J Clin Monit Comput. 2019;33:1–4.

65. Wu R, Liaqat D, de Lara E, Son T, Rudzicz F, Alshaer H, et al. Feasibility of using a smartwatch to intensively monitor patients with chronic obstructive pulmonary disease: prospective cohort study. JMIR Mhealth Uhealth. 2018;6(6):e10046.

66. Gold MR, Siegel J, Russell L, Weinstein M. Cost-effectiveness in health and medicine. New York: Oxford University Press; 1996.

67. Granata AV, Hillman AL. Competing practice guidelines: using cost-effectiveness analysis to make optimal decisions. Ann Intern Med. 1998;128(1):56–63.

68. Schairer CE, Rubanovich CK, Bloss CS. How could commercial terms of use and privacy policies undermine informed consent in the age of mobile health? AMA J Ethics. 2018;20(9):E864–72.

69. World Health Organization. Delivering quality health services: a global imperative for universal health coverage. Paris: OECD Publishing; 2018.

70. Bleichrodt H, Quiggin J. Life-cycle preferences over consumption and health: when is cost-effectiveness analysis equivalent to cost-benefit analysis? J Health Econ. 1999;18(6):681–708.

71. de la Torre-Diez I, Lopez-Coronado M, Vaca C, Aguado JS, de Castro C. Cost-utility and cost-effectiveness studies of telemedicine, electronic, and mobile health systems in the literature: a systematic review. Telemed J E Health. 2015;21(2):81–5.

72. Agha Z, Schapira RM, Maker AH. Cost effectiveness of telemedicine for the delivery of outpatient pulmonary care to a rural population. Telemed J E Health. 2002;8(3):281–91.

73. Balli F, Gervais Y, Frangos M, Gaudy T, Valderrama A, Bransi M, et al. Next-gen advocacy for respiratory health: fun, empowering, participatory, freely adaptable. 12th general meeting of the global alliance against respiratory diseases – World Health Organization; 2018 August 31; Helsinki, Finland.

74. Marcano Belisario JS, Huckvale K, Greenfield G, Car J, Gunn LH. Smartphone and tablet self management apps for asthma. Cochrane Database Syst Rev. 2013;(11):Cd010013.

75. Cox A, Illsley M, Knibb W, Lucas C, O'Driscoll M, Potter C, et al. The acceptability of e-technology to monitor and assess patient symptoms following palliative radiotherapy for lung cancer. Palliat Med. 2011;25(7):675–81.

76. Nebeker C, Lagare T, Takemoto M, Lewars B, Crist K, Bloss CS, et al. Engaging research participants to inform the ethical conduct of mobile imaging, pervasive sensing, and location tracking research. Transl Behav Med. 2016;6(4):577–86.

77. Menikoff J. Federal Register Volume 82, Issue 12 (January 19, 2017). Government Publishing Office, Office GP; 2017 Jan 19. Contract No.: 2017-01058.

78. Bloss CS, Wineinger NE, Peters M, Boeldt DL, Ariniello L, Kim JY, et al. A prospective randomized trial examining health care utilization in individuals using multiple smartphone-enabled biosensors. PeerJ. 2016;4:e1554.

79. World Health Organization – Europe. From innovation to implementation: Ehealth in the WHO European Region. 2016. www.euro.who.int/__data/assets/pdf_file/0012/302331/From-Innovation-to-Implementation-eHealth-Report-EU.pdf.

80. PWC. Socio-economic impact of mHealth an assessment report for the European Union. 2013. www.gsma.com/iot/wp-content/uploads/2013/06/Socio-economic_impact-of-mHealth_EU_14062013V2.pdf.

81. GUN Operating System. GNU Affero General Public License. 2016. https://www.gnu.org/licenses/agpl-3.0.en.html.

82. Open Hardware Repository. CERN Open Hardware Licence – Introduction. 2017. https://www.ohwr.org/projects/cernohl/wiki.

83. Swan M. Crowdsourced health research studies: an important emerging complement to clinical trials in the public health research ecosystem. J Med Internet Res. 2012;14(2):e46. https://doi.org/10.2196/jmir.1988.

84. Niezen G, Eslambolchilar P, Thimbleby H. Open-source hardware for medical devices. BMJ Innov. 2016;2:78. https://doi.org/10.1136/bmjinnov-2015-000080.

Personal Environmental Monitoring

20

20

Sherrie Xie and Blanca E. Himes

Key Point Summary

- Several air pollutants, including particulate matter, ozone (O_3), nitrogen dioxide (NO_2), carbon monoxide (CO), sulfur dioxide (SO_2), and volatile organic compounds (VOCs), have deleterious effects on respiratory health.
- Low-cost pollution sensors are becoming widely available, and their ability to capture increasingly finer-scaled geographic differences in pollution is improving our ability to capture personalized measures of pollution.
- Low-cost pollution sensors are currently suitable for research studies that seek to understand relationships between exposures and disease outcomes, but future applications may include their integration into health self-monitoring tools.

Introduction

Air pollution is a major health hazard with a global reach. Population-based studies that relate air pollution measurements to various outcomes have been conducted for decades, contributing to the incontrovertible evidence that pollutants negatively affect health. Recent and continued development of small, portable and low-cost sensors has resulted in a shift towards capturing pollution measures at finer geographic scales to better link pollutant exposures with individual health outcomes. In this chapter, we discuss air pollution, its effects on respiratory health, and instruments available to measure components of air pollution and assess individual-level exposures, with an emphasis on low-cost sensors that can be deployed at scales not previously possible. We offer guidelines for successful sensor deployment, including practical tips for sensor selection and calibration. We end by discussing how low-cost sensors can support respiratory research and precision medicine efforts.

Air Pollution and Respiratory Health

Air pollution is a dynamic and complex mixture of particulate matter (PM) and gaseous chemicals produced by human activity and natural

S. Xie · B. E. Himes (✉)
Department of Biostatistics, Epidemiology and Informatics, University of Pennsylvania, Philadelphia, PA, USA
e-mail: xiex@vet.upenn.edu; bhimes@pennmedicine.upenn.edu

© Springer Nature Switzerland AG 2020
J. L. Gomez et al. (eds.), *Precision in Pulmonary, Critical Care, and Sleep Medicine*, Respiratory Medicine, https://doi.org/10.1007/978-3-030-31507-8_20

processes. PM pollution is composed of airborne particles that are typically classified by size: PM_{10} refers to particles with diameter < 10 μm; $PM_{2.5}$ or *fine particles* have diameter < 2.5 μm; and $PM_{0.1}$ or *ultrafine particles* (UFP) have diameter < 0.1 μm. The adverse effect of PM pollution is inversely proportional to particle size: while *coarse particles* (with diameter > 2.5 μm and < 10 μm) are retained in the nasal passages and upper airways, fine and ultrafine particles can penetrate deep into lung alveoli and may enter the bloodstream, causing increased local and systemic inflammation [1–3]. Gas-phase pollutants include ozone (O_3), nitrogen dioxide (NO_2), carbon monoxide (CO), sulfur dioxide (SO_2) and volatile organic compounds (VOCs). Ozone and NO_2 can induce airway inflammation and hyper-responsiveness [4–7], and all pollutants can increase oxidative stress and damage respiratory tract tissues [8, 9].

The deleterious effects of ambient (i.e., outdoor) air pollution on respiratory health are well documented. Long-term exposures to $PM_{2.5}$ and ozone, even at moderate levels, have been shown to increase all-cause mortality [10, 11] and risk of acute respiratory distress syndrome (ARDS) [12]. Short-term exposures to $PM_{2.5}$, ozone, NO_2, SO_2, and CO increase the risk of exacerbations among patients with asthma [13–15], COPD [16, 17], and cystic fibrosis [18] and can lead to other acute respiratory events [12, 19–21] and even death [16, 22]. Among children, early-life exposure to ambient $PM_{2.5}$ has been associated with reduced lung function [23], increased emergency room visits [24], increased asthma medication use [25], higher asthma prevalence [26, 27], and higher rates of severe acute asthma [28]. Exposure to NO_2 and SO_2 has been associated with increased risk of developing asthma [29–32]. Some constituents of fine particulate matter are more hazardous than others, and sensors specific to these constituents may be preferable than those measuring bulk $PM_{2.5}$. For example, black carbon, which is sourced primarily from combustion engines in urban environments, has been more strongly associated with health outcomes (e.g., pediatric asthma admissions) than $PM_{2.5}$ in

some studies, making it a potentially more useful indicator for the evaluation of health risks due to combustion-related air pollution exposure [33].

Although fewer studies have investigated the effects of indoor than outdoor air pollution due to the challenges involved in monitoring indoor environments at scale, indoor air quality may have a greater impact on health, as people spend approximately 85–90% of their time indoors [34]. Some studies have indeed found that personal exposure to air pollutants is more strongly correlated with indoor than ambient concentrations of PM and gaseous components [35, 36]. Several pollutants originate indoors: cooking, cigarettes, candles, and other combustible products release PM; gas and kerosene appliances release NO_2; and cleaning agents, aerosol sprays, pesticides, paints, and other household products are a source of VOCs [37]. Pollutants from ambient air are another major source of indoor air pollution, as they can enter buildings through the processes of infiltration and ventilation [38]. Indoor PM and NO_2 levels are associated with asthma morbidity among children living in urban environments [39], and high VOC levels in the home have been associated with increased prevalence of asthma and rhinitis [40, 41]. Among the elderly, presence of environmental tobacco smoke and PM have been associated with increased incidence of acute respiratory symptoms and decreased lung function [42].

Regulatory Monitors

In the United States, levels of major air pollutants are monitored by the Environmental Protection Agency (EPA) to reduce their impact on human health in accordance with the Clean Air Act, which established the National Ambient Air Quality Standards (NAAQS) for six criteria pollutants, including PM, ozone, NO_2, SO_2, and CO [43]. NAAQS compliance is assessed via a network of regulatory monitors that meet Federal Reference Method (FRM) or Federal Equivalent Method (FEM) standards [44, 45]. Similar monitoring networks exist in Canada via the National

Air Pollution Surveillance Network [46], and Europe via the European Monitoring and Evaluation Programme [47] and the Automatic Urban and Rural Network (UK only) [48]. Reference monitors are highly accurate and have good temporal resolution, making them well suited for monitoring compliance to air quality legislation. However, their high cost, bulky size, and sophisticated operating and maintenance requirements limit their deployment to a discrete number of fixed locations, resulting in relatively sparse spatial coverage.

Beyond their use in regulatory monitoring, measurements taken by reference monitors support research on the health impact of air pollution, as they can be used to derive population-level and individual-level (i.e., *personal*) exposure estimates. In deriving exposure estimates, pollution measures are typically averaged over a time period that is appropriate for a study (e.g., 1 month), with a typical lower limit of 1–24 hours that is determined by the agency taking the measures, in accordance with the type of pollutant and the time frame during which it is known to impact health. In addition, personal exposures can only be estimated *indirectly* from reference measurements because monitoring sites seldom coincide with locations where exposures take place (e.g., home, work, school). Time-averaged exposure to pollutants has been estimated for individuals based on their location of residence in several ways, including using measurements taken at a reference monitor closest to their home [49], averaging measurements for all monitors within a pre-defined area of residence (e.g., county or zip code) [50], and using spatial interpolation to combine measurements from monitors within a fixed radius (e.g., 50 km) to the home. The latter can be accomplished via inverse-distance-square weighting [12], a straightforward technique that weights measurements taken at sites close to a point of origin more than those of distal sites, or more sophisticated approaches such as kriging [51] and land-use regression modeling [52, 53], techniques that require specialized knowledge and appropriate input data that may not be available for all geographical locations [54]. It is worth noting that even advanced modeling techniques may be unable to capture accurate fine-scale spatial and temporal variations.

While pollution measures taken by regulatory monitors are helpful for deriving coarse exposure estimates, they do not account for the spatial and temporal heterogeneity of personal exposures. Even short exposures to polluted microenvironments, such as bursts experienced during commutes, can account for a large proportion of an individual's exposures and impact health outcomes. Personal exposure studies utilizing sensors found that exposure to black carbon and PM were highest during commute times [53, 55–58] and inside vehicles [59]. In addition, a study comparing children's PM exposure in home, school, and commute microenvironments determined that exposure experienced while commuting was most strongly associated with urinary leukotriene E4 and albuterol use [60]. Because sensors can be used to capture fine-scale exposures missed by traditional regulatory networks, they offer new possibilities for respiratory health research and personal exposure monitoring.

Applications of Low-Cost Air Pollution Sensors

Concern for pollution's effect on health and broad demand for accessible environmental monitoring have led researchers and manufacturers to develop a number of low-cost, portable pollution sensors in recent years. Commercially available sensors include optical-based particle sensors that measure PM, and electrochemical or metal oxide sensors that measure gas-phase pollutants. Uses for low-cost sensors can be grouped loosely into the following categories: (1) supplementing traditional air monitoring networks to increase the spatiotemporal resolution of measurements, (2) evaluating indoor air quality, and (3) measuring both indoor and outdoor personal exposures directly with a portable sensor. In the following sub-sections, we discuss these applications and highlight work done in each area.

Supplementing Traditional Air Monitoring Networks

Pollution measurements taken with low-cost sensors are less accurate and reliable than reference monitors, and there is currently no legislation in place to permit their use for regulatory monitoring [61]. Nevertheless, low-cost sensors are increasingly deployed by researchers and community groups to supplement traditional monitoring, thereby increasing the overall spatiotemporal resolution of measurements. A straightforward application of low-cost sensors is to measure pollution levels at a location of interest, such as near a suspected source. For example, some community groups have utilized sensors for citizen-led "fence-line monitoring" of emissions near refineries or other industrial sites [62, 63].

Several studies have demonstrated the feasibility and validity of using sensors to capture air pollution information across an area by deploying them in a multi-sensor, fixed-location network [64–72]. Such networks enable the capture of local pollution concentrations in areas with poor coverage by existing regulatory networks [67, 69], can identify local source emissions not captured by traditional monitors [70], and can monitor air quality in underdeveloped regions that lack a monitoring infrastructure [66, 71]. In addition, sensor measurements taken at purposefully selected locations can be used to derive more accurate personal exposure estimates than those possible with regulatory monitors alone [72].

In addition to deploying sensors at fixed locations, researchers have attached sensors to moving vehicles traveling on pre-defined routes to increase the spatial coverage of measurements. While mobile sensing presents additional analytical challenges beyond those of fixed-location sensing [73], it has been used successfully by researchers to map pollution distributions at very fine spatial resolutions (i.e., less than a city block) [74–76]. To prevent self-contamination by vehicle exhaust, mobile sensing campaigns have attached sensors to bicycles [75, 77–79] or zero-emission (e.g., electric) automobiles [73, 75, 80, 81] or railcars [82]. Air pollution sensors have also been attached to public transportation vehicles to cut down on personnel and equipment costs, allowing for sustainable mobile monitoring campaigns to be conducted continuously over longer periods [82–84].

Evaluating Indoor Air Quality

Because regulatory monitoring networks capture only ambient pollution levels, they provide limited insight into indoor air quality. Low-cost sensors provide an accessible tool for researchers and citizens to monitor pollution levels within home, school, and work environments. Some indoor pollution sensors, such as the Speck and Awair Glow, are specifically targeted to consumers for home use and feature intuitive dashboards that display easily interpretable measurements. Sensors have also aided research on air quality within schools: motivated by the greater susceptibility of children versus adults to air pollution [85] and the large amount of time children spend in schools, recent studies have installed air sensors in classrooms to determine diurnal and seasonal patterns of pollution exposure experienced by schoolchildren [86–89], with some reports finding significant associations between exposures and poor cognitive development [88, 89]. Researchers have also deployed sensors to study factors contributing to poor air quality in private residences [36, 90] and public spaces, such as subway stations [91, 92], office buildings [93], and restaurants [94]. Finally, sensors have been installed to detect specific indoor source emissions such as secondhand tobacco smoke [34, 95] and gas leaks [96, 97] to aid with behavioral interventions and pipeline monitoring, respectively.

Measuring Personal Exposures Directly

Personal exposure to air pollutants has traditionally been assessed indirectly using ambient air pollution measures, which can lead to significant error [98, 99]. Improvements in the miniaturization and portability of sensors have made it increasingly feasible to use sensors for personal exposure studies. In broad terms, such studies can be classified as scripted or unscripted. In *scripted* or simulated study designs, participants are instructed to perform predetermined activities in set locations, while participants of *unscripted* studies are asked to go about their usual activities. Scripted studies have the advantage of circumventing issues related to environmental monitors impacting a person's usual behaviors and activities [100], while unscripted studies are able to comprehensively assess everyday personal exposures.

Several scripted studies have assessed exposure to pollution during commute activities, allowing capture of highly variable pollution levels during short time periods (e.g., as people move between high-traffic and low-traffic areas). In these scripted studies, study participants were instructed to carry sensor equipment while traveling on a set route to either assess pollution exposures associated with a single mode of transportation (e.g., bicycle [101], automobile [59], or auto-rickshaw [102]) or compare exposures between different transportation modes [103, 104]. Among the latter studies, de Nazelle et al. found $PM_{2.5}$ exposures to be highest for participants traveling by car compared to participants traveling by foot, bicycle, or bus [103], while Apparicio et al. found that cyclists experienced the highest inhaled dose of NO_2 after factoring in their high ventilation rates [104]. Other scripted personal exposure studies have instructed participants to perform physical activities in polluted environments to study the acute effects of air pollution exposure on physiological responses to exercise [105–107].

In contrast to scripted studies, which aim to capture exposures associated with a targeted activity and environment, unscripted studies aim to capture all exposures experienced by an individual in their daily life. As such, unscripted studies are typically longer in duration, although the cumbersome nature of carrying personal monitors have precluded any continuous monitoring period from being longer than 1 week. Early studies were conducted with few (<20) participants over short (18–24 hour) monitoring windows and established the feasibility of using low-cost sensors to

directly measure individual-level pollutant exposures [108–110]. Recent studies have been conducted with over 100 subjects for up to 1 week of continuous monitoring [111–113]. To capture seasonal variation in pollutant exposures, these studies have repeated monitoring of the same subject at different times of year, either across different seasons (e.g., summer versus winter) [111, 113] or across different trimesters in the case of pregnant women [112].

To provide context for personal exposure measurements, air pollution sensors are often deployed concurrently with GPS-enabled devices to link exposures with geographic locations [53, 55–57, 72]. Participants (or their parents, in the case of young children) may also keep a time-activity diary in which they record activities performed during the sampling period [55–58, 72]. Pollution measures paired to GPS and/or time-activity data can provide fine-grained information on the locations (e.g., home, work, commute) and activities (e.g., cooking, burning candles, driving) associated with high exposure levels, which can be helpful in determining appropriate risk mitigation measures [114]. Geographic location data can also be linked to external sources of geospatial data on green spaces, traffic-related noise, and other local environmental conditions to provide a more complete picture of personal environmental exposures [112, 115, 116].

Other monitoring devices that have been deployed alongside air pollution sensors include UV dosimeters, noise dosimeters, personal activity monitors, physiological monitors that track heart and breathing rates, or some combination of the above [53, 56, 108, 113, 117]. Concurrently capturing multiple exposures and physiological parameters holds promise for more precise and efficient evaluations of exposure-health relationships [108, 112].

Considerations for Sensor Selection and Use

In the following section, we present general guidelines for appropriately selecting and deploying low-cost sensors for use in pollution monitoring

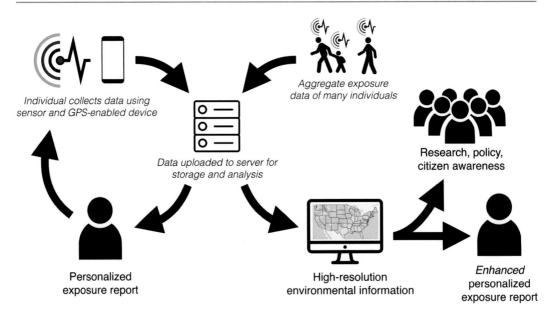

Fig. 20.1 Major aspects of air pollution sensor use for monitoring and improving the health of individuals and communities

and provide an overview of major aspects related to their use (Fig. 20.1). Sensor selection should be guided by the study question, with consideration for the pollutant(s) of interest, expected field conditions (pollutant concentration and temperature/humidity ranges), duration of data collection, type of measurements (mobile versus stationary, site/route-specific versus personal exposure), and data quality requirements. After sensors have been acquired, they must be properly calibrated to ensure measurement validity. More detailed information on these topics can be found in the EPA's Air Sensor Guidebook [118].

Sensor Selection

In addition to differences in specific pollutants measured, sensors vary by their response and sensitivity to given pollutants, detection range, calibration requirements, size, and other specifications that make them more or less suited for a given use. Thus, care should be taken in selecting an appropriate sensor for a desired application and setting. A sensor's *detection range* refers to the range of pollutant levels to which it will respond. Some sensors are sensitive to low- or mid-range concentrations but saturate at high concentrations, while others may be able to resolve high concentrations but not detect low concentrations. Determining the pollutant levels that one expects to encounter at a deployment site(s) should thus precede sensor selection. *Response time* refers to how quickly a sensor responds to local changes in pollutant concentrations; what response times are acceptable will depend on a sensor's intended use. While it may be acceptable for sensors used in stationary monitoring of background pollution concentrations to respond relatively slowly to changes, sensors deployed for dynamic uses, such as mobile sensing or the detection of transient sources, should have more rapid response times (e.g., <1 minute). Other important sensor characteristics include *precision,* the extent to which a sensor reproduces a pollution measurement under identical conditions, and *bias* or systematic measurement error. Sensor accuracy is typically evaluated by comparing sensor measurements to those taken by a reference (e.g., FEM or FRM) monitor, with R^2 reported as the summary correlation measure.

Sensor evaluation programs are valuable resources that offer a good starting point in the sensor selection process. The Air Quality Sensor

Performance Evaluation Center (AQ-SPEC, www.aqmd.gov/aq-spec) operated by the South Coast Air Quality Management District (SCAQMD) evaluates low-cost, commercially available sensors by deploying them outdoors in the SCAQMD monitoring station in southern California. Sensors that perform reasonably well in AQ-SPEC field tests are further tested in controlled laboratory conditions. The EPA Office of Research and Development also conducts field and laboratory evaluations of low-cost air quality sensors and releases these evaluations as part of the EPA Air Sensors Toolbox (www.epa.gov/air-sensor-toolbox). In Europe, the Joint Research Center of the European Commission's science and knowledge service conducts research on sensor performance, including investigations of calibration techniques and long-term sensor performance and drift, which they communicate mostly via publications [119–121]. A separate multi-sensor evaluation program is performed by the European Network on New Sensing Technologies for Air Pollution Control and Environmental Sustainability (EuNetAir), a research collaboration between multiple academic, government, and corporate agencies as part of an urban air quality campaign [122, 123]. Some academic researchers have also evaluated select sensors in various laboratory and field conditions [124–127].

Care should be taken in reviewing sensor performance evaluations. Correlations between sensor and reference measurements should be interpreted in light of the field or laboratory conditions in which instruments were deployed. In addition to the specifications discussed above, sensor performance may be influenced by temperature and relative humidity. In general, evaluations conducted in conditions similar to those of the deployment site will provide the most reliable information about sensor performance. For example, AQ-SPEC field evaluations are performed in the warm and relatively dry climate of southern California with low-to-moderate pollution levels and may not reflect sensor performance in humid or highly polluted environments. It is also important to take into account intended use while considering sensor performance. For example, requirements for measurement accuracy will be lower for sensors intended for educational use, where it may suffice to capture qualitative differences in pollutant concentrations, compared to research use, where even moderate measurement uncertainty may be unacceptable. Other criteria guiding sensor selection include sensor portability, particularly in the case of mobile monitoring and personal exposure studies, and sensor usability, particularly for studies requiring participants to use and maintain sensors without assistance from study personnel.

Specifications for select currently available full sensor platforms are provided in Table 20.1. These platforms, which are referred to by AQ-SPEC as "turnkey" products, are readily deployable sensors that include at least one sensing component that responds to the concentration of a particular pollutant, plus some or all of the following: microprocessor, data-logger, memory card, battery, external packaging, and display. Commercially available sensor platforms use algorithms to filter and transform the electrical signal received by the sensing component to an easily interpretable measurement that can be displayed and stored. While individual sensing components can be purchased for less cost than a full platform, they require considerable technical expertise to set up and calibrate for use in pollution sensing [66, 68, 128]. We do not discuss passive samplers, which provide time-averaged exposure levels rather than real-time measurements, but we note that they are typically more cost-effective than active sensors, do not require power to operate, and may be small enough to be worn on outer clothing [100]. Because passive samplers can only be used to measure time-integrated exposures, they cannot capture short-term or peak exposures, making them unsuitable for mobile sensing or capturing temporal variation in pollution levels at fixed sites.

Sensor Calibration

Calibration, the process of checking and adjusting sensor measurements against a known standard or reference instrument, is crucial to sensor

Table 20.1 Characteristics of select low-cost air pollution sensors

Sensor model (manufacturer)	Pollutant(s) measured	Estimated cost in 2019 (US$)	Size (mm), weight (g)	Suitable for personal sensing
AirBeam2 (HabitatMap)	$PM_{2.5}$, PM_1, PM_{10}	249	$132 \times 98 \times 13$, 142	Yes
PA-II (PurpleAir)	$PM_{2.5}$, PM_1, PM_{10}	229	$50 \times 38 \times 21$, 357	No
DC1100 Pro (Dylos)	$PM_{(0.5-2.5)}$	290	$125 \times 90 \times 185$, 544	No
microAeth AE51 (AethLabs)	Black carbon	5995	$117 \times 66 \times 38$, 280	Yes
AQY 1 (Aeroqual)	$PM_{2.5}$, NO_2, O_3	4000	$215 \times 170 \times 125$, <1000	No
S-500 (Aeroqual)	NO_2, CO, CO_2, SO_2, or O_3	500	$195 \times 122 \times 54$, 460	Yes

performance and should be completed before each deployment. Because sensor response can change over time (a phenomenon known as *drift*), sensors should be calibrated at regular intervals during and after measurement collection. Ideally, calibration should occur under the same conditions (temperature, humidity, pollution composition and concentrations) as the deployment site(s). Additionally, due to imperfect reproducibility in the sensor manufacturing process, each sensor should be calibrated individually, even if multiple sensors of the same model are to be deployed at once [129].

Calibrations can be performed in controlled laboratory environments by introducing sensors to a known standard. Instruments can be "zeroed" using ultra-filtered air containing no particulates or gaseous pollutants, and many gas-phase sensors can be calibrated using gas standards, typically delivered in a compressed gas cylinder. While particle standards are available (e.g., Urban Particulate Matter and Arizona Road Dust), they are less reliable than gas standards as PM composition varies by setting, making it infeasible to create particle suspensions that are universally representative of urban exposures. Differences in PM composition are particularly pronounced for indoor PM pollution, which require calibration to specific sources (e.g., cigarette smoke, cooking, household dust) to ensure measurement precision [95, 124]. In the case of sensors that are to be deployed outdoors, it is important to complement any laboratory calibration with field calibrations because the controlled

laboratory environment is unlikely to reflect actual deployment conditions [118].

Field calibrations, which are typically performed by collocating sensors with FRM/FEM equipment, result in more accurate concentration estimates than laboratory calibrations [130]. Collocated sensors should be positioned so that their inlet is as close to the inlet of the reference monitor as possible, which may require prior communication and approval from local authorities [128]. After collocated sensors have taken measurements for a few days or more, sensor measurements can be normalized to FRM/FEM measurements using a calibration curve [118]. Calibration equations can be linear [128], high-order [66], or power [34, 131] functions, and may include multivariable adjustment for temperature and relative humidity [66, 102]. Adjustment for relative humidity may be particularly important for particle sensors deployed in humid environments as humidity causes hygroscopic particle enlargement, which can result in inflated PM measurements [132, 133].

Practical Considerations for Sensor Deployment

While it is infeasible to discuss all aspects of sensor study design due, in part, to the wide range of study goals and settings possible, we highlight some salient issues here. Even after appropriate testing and calibration have taken place, long-term sensor deployment is not a passive process but rather, one that requires oversight to ensure continual functioning. Batteries may need charging or changing-out every few hours to days, wireless and/or Bluetooth connectivity may falter, and sensors may take erroneous measures due to movement or weather (e.g., falling, intakes blocked) or simply stop working. Because sensor activity must be monitored, any individual using sensors as part of a study must be trained to debug problems and/or have an available resource to assist them. The need for continual attention may also represent a barrier to study participants in that user engagement of technologies tends to substantially decrease after short periods of time [134–136]. While all of these issues impose funding and personnel constraints that have typically limited sensor monitoring campaigns and research studies in duration and scope, there are successful models for sustainable and continuous air quality surveillance; one example is the Imperial County Community Air Network, which involves and trains community members to maintain a low-cost air monitoring network [67].

With regard to sensor study design, there is often some trade-off between measurement validity and acceptability to participants carrying sensors. An ideal personal exposure monitor would be worn near a person's breathing zone without interfering with the wearer's usual behaviors and habits, but most current research-grade sensing devices are too big to be worn directly. Thus, subjects of personal exposure studies are typically asked to carry air sensors inside a bag [113], backpack [58, 108–110, 112], or vest [72]. Early unscripted exposure studies instructed participants to wear monitors during all activities except sleeping and bathing, but subsequent studies have only required participants to carry sensors when they are moving outdoors, allowing them to place sensors in the room they spend most of their time while indoors. While decreasing monitoring burden to study participants can improve long-term study feasibility, doing so may result in exposure misclassification from indoor sources (e.g., cooking exposures not captured due to sensors being in another room).

After raw sensor measurements are obtained, they must be stored and appropriately analyzed to be informative. Some sensors provide onboard data storage, while others require connection to a secondary device either via cable or Bluetooth. A third option is for sensor measures to be sent directly to a cloud service provider via the Internet. Individual measurements taken by sensors tend to be small in size, but because it is common to collect many such measures (e.g., every second or minute for days to weeks), sensor datasets can be very large. Thus, adequate plans to handle streaming of data from many sensors are a requirement for an effective study or monitoring effort. As data arrives to a server, it can be analyzed on-the-fly, stored for future analysis, or both. Storage of data for future analysis is often the route taken by research studies, while real-time data analysis may be preferred by individuals or communities seeking live feedback on personal or neighborhood exposures. Approaches to analyze data from sensors include those discussed above (e.g., spatial interpolation), and various other modeling and visualization techniques that take into account the data's longitudinal nature, the characteristics of persons using sensors, and the environment in which sensors were deployed. To fully leverage all of this information, sophisticated analysis plans designed by statisticians and data scientists are needed. Importantly, if data gathered by sensors will be used for personal monitoring or to provide information to communities, design of web or smartphone applications that provide results should include formal usability testing to ensure the tools are acceptable, informative, and engaging to all relevant stakeholders [137].

Advancing Respiratory Health Through Low-Cost Sensing: Applications and Future Directions

By improving the spatiotemporal resolution of air quality measurements and directly capturing personal environmental exposures, low-cost sensors enable more accurate exposure estimates than those derived using traditional regulatory monitors alone. Figure 20.1 describes in broad terms how low-cost sensors can improve respiratory health. First, individuals can use a sensor in isolation to receive information about their personal exposures via an app. Users may choose to receive alerts of high pollution levels they are encountering in real-time or access reports summarizing their exposure to specific pollutants over time and space to determine when and where their symptoms are at highest risk of being triggered. Second, many individuals can contribute their exposure measures to generate community-level reports suitable for (1) research related to the identification of high-risk areas that can subsequently inform residents and policymakers of local hazards and (2) providing informative background data that enhances personalized exposure reports. For example, by integrating self-reported data with pollution data collected at places and times only other community members have observed, an app may suggest that an individual avoid a specific location at a specific time because it is predicted to have conditions that will induce symptoms in that individual.

Results from previous studies with small samples that targeted specific populations support the plausibility of these scenarios. For example, Alexeef et al. used a 30 m resolution air pollution map generated by a mobile air monitoring campaign conducted using sensors attached to Google Street View Cars to detect an increased risk of cardiovascular events among those residing on blocks with above-average pollution levels [138, 139]. The study's authors noted that they were able to detect significant effects using a much smaller sample than those of traditional environmental epidemiology studies: their elderly subpopulation aged 65 years or older, in which they detected the greatest effect, totaled less than 3500 residents [138, 139]. Donaire-Gonzalez et al. characterized the personal exposome of hundreds of pregnant women and children using air sensors, a GPS-enabled smartphone and other monitors to measure exposure to $PM_{2.5}$, black carbon, physical activity, traffic-related noise, UV-B, and green space [112]. Other small-scale studies have demonstrated the feasibility of pairing personal exposure data from air sensors to physiological activity monitors [113, 117] and mobile health platforms that monitor medication use [140]. While air sensors are currently too costly and cumbersome (Table 20.1) to be deployed at the scale required for large, data-driven studies of environmental exposures, further advances in sensor technology will enable a more nuanced understanding of the environmental drivers of human health [141, 142].

Most commercially available air sensors are targeted for general use, making them accessible to anyone interested in purchasing them, including patients and caretakers. While evidence of their clinical utility is currently lacking, studies have demonstrated the feasibility of using particle sensors, along with an intuitive visual display that provides instantaneous feedback on indoor air quality, to promote changes in smoking behavior [34, 95]. Particle sensors could be used in a similar way by patients and/or caretakers to monitor the effectiveness of exposure mitigation (such as reducing household dust) to reduce symptoms of diseases such as asthma. In the future, pollution data streams may be available to healthcare providers to help them identify individual patient disease risk factors and potentially, intervene to reduce pollutant exposure.

Conclusion

Respiratory research studies that relate pollution to health outcomes have traditionally depended on indirectly measured or modeled estimates of individual pollution exposure, but the increasing availability of low-cost sensors has enabled direct measurement of individual exposures. When properly calibrated and maintained, some low-cost sensors can accurately capture spatiotemporal fluctuations in pollution exposures that are commonly missed by traditional monitoring equipment. As a result, sensors have been helpful for uncovering the health impact of pollution on individuals and communities, thereby advancing knowledge that can improve respiratory health. Further advances in sensor miniaturization and performance will soon enable their use in large cohort studies, and potentially, personalized health interventions.

References

1. Franck U, Odeh S, Wiedensohler A, Wehner B, Herbarth O. The effect of particle size on cardiovascular disorders--the smaller the worse. Sci Total Environ. 2011;409(20):4217–21.
2. Brown JS, Zeman KL, Bennett WD. Ultrafine particle deposition and clearance in the healthy and obstructed lung. Am J Respir Crit Care Med. 2002;166(9):1240–7.
3. Ni L, Chuang CC, Zuo L. Fine particulate matter in acute exacerbation of COPD. Front Physiol. 2015;6:294.
4. Poynter ME, Persinger RL, Irvin CG, Butnor KJ, van Hirtum H, Blay W, et al. Nitrogen dioxide enhances allergic airway inflammation and hyperresponsiveness in the mouse. Am J Physiol Lung Cell Mol Physiol. 2006;290(1):L144–52.
5. Frampton MW, Boscia J, Roberts NJ Jr, Azadniv M, Torres A, Cox C, et al. Nitrogen dioxide exposure: effects on airway and blood cells. Am J Physiol Lung Cell Mol Physiol. 2002;282(1):L155–65.
6. Seltzer J, Bigby BG, Stulbarg M, Holtzman MJ, Nadel JA, Ueki IF, et al. O3-induced change in bronchial reactivity to methacholine and airway inflammation in humans. J Appl Physiol (1985). 1986;60(4):1321–6.
7. Aris RM, Christian D, Hearne PQ, Kerr K, Finkbeiner WE, Balmes JR. Ozone-induced airway inflammation in human subjects as determined by airway lavage and biopsy. Am Rev Respir Dis. 1993;148(5):1363–72.
8. Gowers AM, Cullinan P, Ayres JG, Anderson HR, Strachan DP, Holgate ST, et al. Does outdoor air pollution induce new cases of asthma? Biological plausibility and evidence; a review. Respirology. 2012;17(6):887–98.
9. Kelly FJ. Oxidative stress: its role in air pollution and adverse health effects. Occup Environ Med. 2003;60(8):612–6.
10. Di Q, Wang Y, Zanobetti A, Wang Y, Koutrakis P, Choirat C, et al. Air pollution and mortality in the medicare population. N Engl J Med. 2017;376(26):2513–22.
11. Di Q, Dai L, Wang Y, Zanobetti A, Choirat C, Schwartz JD, et al. Association of short-term exposure to air pollution with mortality in older adults. JAMA. 2017;318(24):2446–56.
12. Reilly JP, Zhao Z, Shashaty MG, Koyama T, Christie JD, Lanken PN, et al. Low to moderate air pollutant exposure and acute respiratory distress syndrome after severe trauma. Am J Respir Crit Care Med. 2019;199(1):62–70.
13. Mirabelli MC, Vaidyanathan A, Flanders WD, Qin X, Garbe P. Outdoor PM2.5, ambient air temperature, and asthma symptoms in the past 14 days among adults with active asthma. Environ Health Perspect. 2016;124(12):1882–90.
14. Orellano P, Quaranta N, Reynoso J, Balbi B, Vasquez J. Effect of outdoor air pollution on asthma exacerbations in children and adults: systematic review and multilevel meta-analysis. PLoS One. 2017;12(3):e0174050.
15. Smargiassi A, Kosatsky T, Hicks J, Plante C, Armstrong B, Villeneuve PJ, et al. Risk of asthmatic episodes in children exposed to sulfur dioxide stack emissions from a refinery point source in Montreal, Canada. Environ Health Perspect. 2008;117(4):653–9.
16. Song Q, Christiani DC, Wang X, Ren J. The global contribution of outdoor air pollution to the incidence, prevalence, mortality and hospital admission for chronic obstructive pulmonary disease: a systematic review and meta-analysis. Int J Environ Res Public Health. 2014;11(11):11822–32.
17. Tsai SS, Chang CC, Yang CY. Fine particulate air pollution and hospital admissions for chronic obstructive pulmonary disease: a case-crossover study in Taipei. Int J Environ Res Public Health. 2013;10(11):6015–26.
18. Goss CH, Newsom SA, Schildcrout JS, Sheppard L, Kaufman JD. Effect of ambient air pollution on pulmonary exacerbations and lung function in cystic fibrosis. Am J Respir Crit Care Med. 2004;169(7):816–21.
19. Peel JL, Tolbert PE, Klein M, Metzger KB, Flanders WD, Todd K, et al. Ambient air pollution and respiratory emergency department visits. Epidemiology. 2005;16(2):164–74.
20. Dominici F, Peng RD, Bell ML, Pham L, McDermott A, Zeger SL, et al. Fine particulate air pollution and hospital admission for cardiovascular and respiratory diseases. JAMA. 2006;295(10):1127–34.
21. Bell ML, McDermott A, Zeger SL, Samet JM, Dominici F. Ozone and short-term mortality in 95 US urban communities, 1987–2000. JAMA. 2004;292(19):2372–8.
22. Fann N, Lamson AD, Anenberg SC, Wesson K, Risley D, Hubbell BJ. Estimating the national public health burden associated with exposure to ambient PM2.5 and ozone. Risk Anal. 2012;32(1):81–95.
23. Neophytou AM, White MJ, Oh SS, Thakur N, Galanter JM, Nishimura KK, et al. Air pollution and lung function in minority youth with asthma in the GALA II (genes-environments and admixture in Latino Americans) and SAGE II (study of African Americans, asthma, genes, and environments) studies. Am J Respir Crit Care Med. 2016;193(11):1271–80.
24. Strickland MJ, Darrow LA, Klein M, Flanders WD, Sarnat JA, Waller LA, et al. Short-term associations between ambient air pollutants and pediatric asthma

emergency department visits. Am J Respir Crit Care Med. 2010;182(3):307–16.

25. Williams AM, Phaneuf DJ, Barrett MA, Su JG. Short-term impact of PM2.5 on contemporaneous asthma medication use: behavior and the value of pollution reductions. Proc Natl Acad Sci U S A. 2019;116(12):5246–53.

26. Keet CA, Keller JP, Peng RD. Long-term coarse particulate matter exposure is associated with asthma among children in medicaid. Am J Respir Crit Care Med. 2018;197(6):737–46.

27. Bowatte G, Lodge C, Lowe AJ, Erbas B, Perret J, Abramson MJ, et al. The influence of childhood traffic-related air pollution exposure on asthma, allergy and sensitization: a systematic review and a meta-analysis of birth cohort studies. Allergy. 2015;70(3):245–56.

28. Silverman RA, Ito K. Age-related association of fine particles and ozone with severe acute asthma in New York City. J Allergy Clin Immunol. 2010;125(2):367–73 e5.

29. Nishimura KK, Galanter JM, Roth LA, Oh SS, Thakur N, Nguyen EA, et al. Early-life air pollution and asthma risk in minority children. The GALA II and SAGE II studies. Am J Respir Crit Care Med. 2013;188(3):309–18.

30. Clark NA, Demers PA, Karr CJ, Koehoorn M, Lencar C, Tamburic L, et al. Effect of early life exposure to air pollution on development of childhood asthma. Environ Health Perspect. 2010;118(2):284–90.

31. Achakulwisut P, Brauer M, Hystad P, Anenberg SC. Global, national, and urban burdens of paediatric asthma incidence attributable to ambient NO2 pollution: estimates from global datasets. Lancet Planet Health. 2019;3(4):e166–e78.

32. Andersson E, Knutsson A, Hagberg S, Nilsson T, Karlsson B, Alfredsson L, et al. Incidence of asthma among workers exposed to sulphur dioxide and other irritant gases. Eur Respir J. 2006;27(4):720–5.

33. Janssen NA, Hoek G, Simic-Lawson M, Fischer P, van Bree L, ten Brink H, et al. Black carbon as an additional indicator of the adverse health effects of airborne particles compared with PM10 and PM2.5. Environ Health Perspect. 2011;119(12):1691–9.

34. Klepeis NE, Hughes SC, Edwards RD, Allen T, Johnson M, Chowdhury Z, et al. Promoting smoke-free homes: a novel behavioral intervention using real-time audio-visual feedback on airborne particle levels. PLoS One. 2013;8(8):e73251.

35. Lai HK, Kendall M, Ferrier H, Lindup I, Alm S, Hanninen O, et al. Personal exposures and micro-environment concentrations of PM2.5, VOC, NO2 and CO in Oxford, UK. Atmos Environ. 2004;38(37):6399–410.

36. Stranger M, Potgieter-Vermaak SS, Van Grieken R. Particulate matter and gaseous pollutants in residences in Antwerp, Belgium. Sci Total Environ. 2009;407(3):1182–92.

37. Franklin PJ. Indoor air quality and respiratory health of children. Paediatr Respir Rev. 2007;8(4):281–6.

38. Chen C, Zhao B. Review of relationship between indoor and outdoor particles: I/O ratio, infiltration factor and penetration factor. Atmos Environ. 2011;45:275–88.

39. Breysse PN, Diette GB, Matsui EC, Butz AM, Hansel NN, McCormack MC. Indoor air pollution and asthma in children. Proc Am Thorac Soc. 2010;7(2):102–6.

40. Billionnet C, Gay E, Kirchner S, Leynaert B, Annesi-Maesano I. Quantitative assessments of indoor air pollution and respiratory health in a population-based sample of French dwellings. Environ Res. 2011;111(3):425–34.

41. Hulin M, Simoni M, Viegi G, Annesi-Maesano I. Respiratory health and indoor air pollutants based on quantitative exposure assessments. Eur Respir J. 2012;40(4):1033–45.

42. Simoni M, Jaakkola MS, Carrozzi L, Baldacci S, Di Pede F, Viegi G. Indoor air pollution and respiratory health in the elderly. Eur Respir J Suppl. 2003;40:15s–20s.

43. National Ambient Air Quality Standards (NAAQS) Table: United States Environmental Protection Agency. Available from: https://www.epa.gov/criteria-air-pollutants/naaqs-table.

44. Process of Reviewing the National Ambient Air Quality Standards United States Environmental Protection Agency. Available from: https://www.epa.gov/criteria-air-pollutants/process-reviewing-national-ambient-air-quality-standards.

45. Hall E, Beaver M, Long R, Vanderpool R. EPA's reference and equivalent methods research program: supporting NAAQS implementation through research, development, and analysis. EM Air Waste Manag Assoc. 2012;5:8–12.

46. Governemnt of Canada. National Air Pollution Surveillance (NAPS) Network 2018. Available from: https://open.canada.ca/data/en/dataset/1b36a356-defd-4813-acea-47bc3abd859b.

47. Torseth K, Aas W, Breivik K, Fjaeraa AM, Feibig M, Hjellbrekke A-G, et al. Introduction to the European Monitoring and Evaluation Programme (EMEP) and observed atmospheric composition change during 1972–2009. Atmos Chem Phys. 2012;12(12):5447–81.

48. UK AIR. Automatic Urban and Rural Network (AURN). Available from: https://uk-air.defra.gov.uk/networks/network-info?view=aurn.

49. Miller KA, Siscovick DS, Sheppard L, Shepherd K, Sullivan JH, Anderson GL, et al. Long-term exposure to air pollution and incidence of cardiovascular events in women. N Engl J Med. 2007;356(5):447–58.

50. Pope CA 3rd, Burnett RT, Thun MJ, Calle EE, Krewski D, Ito K, et al. Lung cancer, cardiopulmonary mortality, and long-term exposure to fine particulate air pollution. JAMA. 2002;287(9):1132–41.

51. Jerrett M, Burnett RT, Ma R, Pope CA 3rd, Krewski D, Newbold KB, et al. Spatial analysis

of air pollution and mortality in Los Angeles. Epidemiology. 2005;16(6):727–36.

52. De Prins S, Dons E, Van Poppel M, Int Panis L, Van de Mieroop E, Nelen V, et al. Airway oxidative stress and inflammation markers in exhaled breath from children are linked with exposure to black carbon. Environ Int. 2014;73:440–6.

53. Nieuwenhuijsen MJ, Donaire-Gonzalez D, Rivas I, de Castro M, Cirach M, Hoek G, et al. Variability in and agreement between modeled and personal continuously measured black carbon levels using novel smartphone and sensor technologies. Environ Sci Technol. 2015;49(5):2977–82.

54. Castell N, Dauge FR, Schneider P, Vogt M, Lerner U, Fishbain B, et al. Can commercial low-cost sensor platforms contribute to air quality monitoring and exposure estimates? Environ Int. 2017;99:293–302.

55. Buonanno G, Stabile L, Morawska L, Russi A. Children exposure assessment to ultrafine particles and black carbon: the role of transport and cooking activities. Atmos Environ. 2013;79:53–8.

56. Dons E, Panis LI, Van Poppel M, Theunis J, Willems H, Torfs R, et al. Impact of time-activity patterns on personal exposure to black carbon. Atmos Environ. 2011;45(21):3594–602.

57. Dons E, Panis LI, Van Poppel M, Theunis J, Wets G. Personal exposure to black carbon in transport microenvironments. Atmos Environ. 2012;55:392–8.

58. Paunescu AC, Attoui M, Bouallala S, Sunyer J, Momas I. Personal measurement of exposure to black carbon and ultrafine particles in schoolchildren from PARIS cohort (Paris, France). Indoor Air. 2017;27(4):766–79.

59. Weichenthal S, Van Ryswyk K, Kulka R, Sun L, Wallace L, Joseph L. In-vehicle exposures to particulate air pollution in Canadian metropolitan areas: the urban transportation exposure study. Environ Sci Technol. 2015;49(1):597–605.

60. Rabinovitch N, Adams CD, Strand M, Koehler K, Volckens J. Within-microenvironment exposure to particulate matter and health effects in children with asthma: a pilot study utilizing real-time personal monitoring with GPS interface. Environ Health. 2016;15(1):96.

61. Clements AL, Griswold WG, Rs A, Johnston JE, Herting MM, Thorson J, et al. Low-cost air quality monitoring tools: from research to practice (a workshop summary). Sensors (Basel). 2017;17(11):2478.

62. Ottinger G. Buckets of resistance: standard and the effectiveness of citizen science. Sci Technol Hum Values. 2010;35(2):244–70.

63. Commodore A, Wilson S, Muhammad O, Svendsen E, Pearce J. Community-based participatory research for the study of air pollution: a review of motivations, approaches, and outcomes. Environ Monit Assess. 2017;189(8):378.

64. Penza M, Suriano D, Villani MG. Towards air quality indices in smart cities by calibrated low-cost sensors applied to networks. Proceedings of IEEE Sensors. 2014;2014-December.

65. Borge R, Narros A, Artíñano B, Yagüe C, Gómez-Moreno FJ, de la Paz D, et al. Assessment of microscale spatio-temporal variation of air pollution at an urban hotspot in Madrid (Spain) through an extensive field campaign. Atmos Environ. 2016;140:432–45.

66. Gao M, Cao J, Seto E. A distributed network of low-cost continuous reading sensors to measure spatiotemporal variations of PM2.5 in Xi'an, China. Environ Pollut. 2015;199:56–65.

67. English PB, Olmedo L, Bejarano E, Lugo H, Murillo E, Seto E, et al. The imperial county community air monitoring network: a model for community-based environmental monitoring for public health action. Environ Health Perspect. 2017;125(7):074501.

68. Mead MI, Popoola OAM, Stewart GB, Landshoff P, Calleja M, Hayes M, et al. The use of electrochemical sensors for monitoring urban air quality in low-cost, high-density networks. Atmos Environ. 2013;70:186–203.

69. Sun L, Wong K, Wei P, Ye S, Huang H, Yang F, et al. Development and application of a next generation air sensor network for the Hong Kong marathon 2015 air quality monitoring. Sensors. 2016;16(2):211.

70. Heimann I, Bright VB, McLeod MW, Mead MI, Popoola OAM, Stewart GB, et al. Source attribution of air pollution by spatial scale separation using high spatial density networks of low cost air quality sensors. Atmos Environ. 2015;113:10–9.

71. Hansel NN, Romero KM, Pollard SL, Bose S, Psoter KJ, J. Underhill L, et al. Ambient air pollution and variation in multiple domains of asthma morbidity among Peruvian children. Ann Am Thorac Soc. 2019;16(3):348–55.

72. Sloan CD, Philipp TJ, Bradshaw RK, Chronister S, Barber WB, Johnston JD. Applications of GPS-tracked personal and fixed-location PM(2.5) continuous exposure monitoring. J Air Waste Manag Assoc. 2016;66(1):53–65.

73. Brantley HL, Hagler GSW, Kimbrough ES, Williams RW, Mukerjee S, Neas LM. Mobile air monitoring data-processing strategies and effects on spatial air pollution trends. Atmos Meas Tech. 2014;7:2169–83.

74. Apte JS, Messier KP, Gani S, Brauer M, Kirchstetter TW, Lunden MM, et al. High-resolution air pollution mapping with Google Street View Cars: exploiting big data. Environ Sci Technol. 2017;51(12):6999–7008.

75. Lee JK, Christen A, Ketler R, Nesic Z. A mobile sensor network to map carbon dioxide emissions in urban environments. Atmos Meas Tech. 2017;10:645–65.

76. Hasenfratz D, Saukh O, Walser C, Hueglin C, Fierz M, Arn T, et al. Deriving high-resolution urban air pollution maps using mobile sensor nodes. Pervasive Mob Comput. 2015;16:268–85.

77. Pattinson W, Longley I, Kingham S. Using mobile monitoring to visualize diurnal variation of traffic pollutants across two near-highway neighborhoods. Atmos Environ. 2014;94:782–92.

78. Peters J, Theunis J, Van Poppel M, Berghmans P. Monitoring PM10 and ultrafine particles in urban environments using mobile measurements. Aerosol Air Qual Res. 2013;13(2):509–22.

79. McKercher GR, Vanos JK. Low-cost mobile air pollution monitoring in urban environments: a pilot study in Lubbock, Texas. Environ Technol. 2018;39(12):1505–14.

80. Choi W, Hu S, He M, Kozawa K, Mara S, Winer AM, et al. Neighborhood-scale air quality impacts of emissions from motor vehicles and aircraft. Atmos Environ. 2013;80:310–21.

81. Padro-Martinez LT, Patton AP, Trull JB, Zamore W, Brugge D, Durant JL. Mobile monitoring of particle number concentration and other traffic-related air pollutants in a near-highway neighborhood over the course of a year. Atmos Environ (1994). 2012;61:253–64.

82. Castellini S, Moroni B, Cappelletti D. PMetro: measurement of urban aerosols on a mobile platform. Measurement. 2014;49:99–106.

83. Castell N, Kobernus M, Liu HY, Schneider P, Lahoz W, Berre AJ, et al. Mobile technologies and services for environmental monitoring: the Citi-Sense-MOB approach. Urban Clim. 2015;14:370–82.

84. Hagemann R, Corsmeier U, Kottmeier C, Rinke R, Wieser A, Vogel B. Spatial variability of particle number concentrations and NOx in the Karlsruhe (Germany) area obtained with the mobile laboratory 'AERO-TRAM'. Atmos Environ. 2014;94:341–52.

85. Salvi S. Health effects of ambient air pollution in children. Paediatr Respir Rev. 2007;8(4):275–80.

86. Fuoco FC, Stabile L, Buonanno G, Vargas Trassiera C, Massimo A, Russi A, et al. Indoor air quality in naturally ventilated Italian classrooms. Atmos. 2016;6:1652–75.

87. Rivas I, Viana M, Moreno T, Pandolfi M, Amato F, Reche C, et al. Child exposure to indoor and outdoor air pollutants in schools in Barcelona, Spain. Environ Int. 2014;69:200–12.

88. Sunyer J, Esnaola M, Alvarez-Pedrerol M, Forns J, Rivas I, Lopez-Vicente M, et al. Association between traffic-related air pollution in schools and cognitive development in primary school children: a prospective cohort study. PLoS Med. 2015;12(3):e1001792.

89. Sunyer J, Suades-Gonzalez E, Garcia-Esteban R, Rivas I, Pujol J, Alvarez-Pedrerol M, et al. Traffic-related air pollution and attention in primary school children: short-term association. Epidemiology. 2017;28(2):181–9.

90. Ramachandran G, Adgate JL, Pratt GC, Sexton K. Characterizing indoor and outdoor 15 minute average PM2.5 concentrations in urban neighborhoods. Aerosol Sci Technol. 2003;37(1):33–45.

91. Moreno T, Perez N, Martins V, de Miguel E, Capdevila M, Centelles S, et al. Subway platform air quality: assessing the influences of tunnel ventilation, train piston effect and station design. Atmos Environ. 2014;92:461–8.

92. Chen YY, Sung FC, Chen ML, Mao IF, Lu CY. Indoor air quality in the metro system in North Taiwan. Int J Environ Res Public Health. 2016;13(12):1200.

93. Choi J-H, Loftness V, Aziz A. Post-occupancy evaluation of 20 office buildings as basis for future IEQ standards and guidelines. Energ Buildings. 2012;46:167–75.

94. Lee SC, Li WM, Chan LY. Indoor air quality at restaurants with different styles of cooking in metropolitan Hong Kong. Sci Total Environ. 2001;279(1–3):181–93.

95. Semple S, Ibrahim AE, Apsley A, Steiner M, Turner S. Using a new, low-cost air quality sensor to quantify second-hand smoke (SHS) levels in homes. Tob Control. 2015;24(2):153–8.

96. van Leeuwen C, Hensen A, Meijer HAJ. Leak detection of CO2 pipelines with simple atmospheric CO2 sensors for carbon capture and storage. Int J Greenhouse Gas Control. 2013;19:420–31.

97. Erden F, Sorey EB, Toreyin BU, Cetin AE. VOC gas leak detection using pyro-electric infrared sensors. IEEE International Conference on Acoustics, Speech and Signal Processing. 2010;1682–5.

98. Meng QY, Svendsgaard D, Kotchmar DJ, Pinto JP. Associations between personal exposures and ambient concentrations of nitrogen dioxide: a quantitative research synthesis. Atmos Environ. 2012;57:322–9.

99. Avery CL, Mills KT, Williams R, McGraw KA, Poole C, Smith RL, et al. Estimating error in using ambient PM2.5 concentrations as proxies for personal exposures: a review. Epidemiology. 2010;21(2):215–23.

100. Steinle S, Reis S, Sabel CE. Quantifying human exposure to air pollution-Moving from static monitoring to spatio-temporally resolved personal exposure assessment. Sci Total Environ. 2013;443:184–93.

101. Weichenthal S, Kulka R, Dubeau A, Martin C, Wang D, Dales R. Traffic-related air pollution and acute changes in heart rate variability and respiratory function in urban cyclists. Environ Health Perspect. 2011;119:1373–8.

102. Apte JS, Kirchstetter TW, Reich AH, Deshpande SJ, Kaushik G, Chel A, et al. Concentrations of fine, ultrafine, and black carbon particles in autorickshaws in New Delhi, India. Atmos Environ. 2011;45:4470–80.

103. de Nazelle A, Fruin S, Westerdahl D, Martinez D, Matamala J, Kubesch N, et al. Traffic exposures and inhalations of Barcelona commuters. Epidemiology. 2011;22(1):S77–S8.

104. Apparicio P, Gelb J, Carrier M, Mathieu M, Kingham S. Exposure to noise and air pollution by mode of transportation during rush hours in Montreal. J Transp Geogr. 2018;70:182–92.

105. Cole-Hunter T, Weichenthal S, Kubesch N, Foraster M, Carrasco-Turigas G, Bouso L, et al. Impact of traffic-related air pollution on acute changes in cardiac autonomic modulation during

rest and physical activity: a cross-over study. J Expo Sci Environ Epidemiol. 2016;26(2):133–40.

106. Strak M, Janssen NA, Godri KJ, Gosens I, Mudway IS, Cassee FR, et al. Respiratory health effects of airborne particulate matter: the role of particle size, composition, and oxidative potential- the RAPTES project. Environ Health Perspect. 2012;120(8):1183–9.

107. Pun VC, Ho KF. Blood pressure and pulmonary health effects of ozone and black carbon exposure in young adult runners. Sci Total Environ. 2019;657:1–6.

108. Nieuwenhuijsen MJ, Donaire-Gonzalez D, Foraster M, Martinez D, Cisneros A. Using personal sensors to assess the exposome and acute health effects. Int J Environ Res Public Health. 2014;11(8):7805–19.

109. Delgado-Saborit JM. Use of real-time sensors to characterise human exposures to combustion related pollutants. J Environ Monit. 2012;14:1824.

110. Steinle S, Reis S, Sabel CE, Semple S, Twigg MM, Braban CF, et al. Personal exposure monitoring of PM2.5 in indoor and outdoor microenvironments. Sci Total Environ. 2015;508:383–94.

111. Dons E, Laeremans M, Orjuela JP, Avila-Palencia I, Carrasco-Turigas G, Cole-Hunter T, et al. Wearable sensors for personal monitoring and estimation of inhaled traffic-related air pollution: evaluation of methods. Environ Sci Technol. 2017;51(3):1859–67.

112. Donaire-Gonzalez D, Curto A, Valentin A, Andrusaityte S, Basagana X, Casas M, et al. Personal assessment of the external exposome during pregnancy and childhood in Europe. Environ Res. 2019;174:95–104.

113. Laeremans M, Dons E, Avila-Palencia I, Carrasco-Turigas G, Orjuela JP, Anaya E, et al. Short-term effects of physical activity, air pollution and their interaction on the cardiovascular and respiratory system. Environ Int. 2018;117:82–90.

114. Koehler KA, Peters TM. New methods for personal exposure monitoring for airborne particles. Curr Environ Health Rep. 2015;2(4):399–411.

115. Donaire-Gonzalez D, Valentin A, van Nunen E, Curto A, Rodriguez A, Fernandez-Nieto M, et al. ExpoApp: an integrated system to assess multiple personal environmental exposures. Environ Int. 2019;126:494–503.

116. Xie S, Himes BE. Approaches to link geospatially varying social, economic, and environmental factors with electronic health record data to better understand asthma exacerbations. AMIA Annu Symp Proc. 2018;2018:1561–70.

117. Laeremans M, Dons E, Avila-Palencia I, Carrasco-Turigas G, Orjuela-Mendoza JP, Anaya-Boig E, et al. Black carbon reduces the beneficial effect of physical activity on lung function. Med Sci Sports Exerc. 2018;50(9):1875–81.

118. Williams R, Kilaru VJ, Snyder EG, Kaufman A, Dye T, Rutter A, et al., editors. Air sensor guidebook. EPA/600/R-14/159. Research Triangle Park: U.S. Enviromental Protection Agency; 2014.

119. Spinelle L, Gerboles M, Villani MG, Aleixandre M, Bonavitacola F. Field calibration of a cluster of low-cost available sensors for air quality monitoring. Part A: ozone and nitrogen dioxide. Sensors Actuators B Chem. 2015;215:249–57.

120. Spinelle L, Gerboles M, Villani MG, Aleixandre M, Bonavitacola F. Field calibration of a cluster of low-cost commercially available sensors for air quality monitoring. Part B: NO, CO and CO2. Sensors Actuators B Chem. 2017;238:706–15.

121. Spinelle L, Gerboles M, Aleixandre M. Performance evaluation of amperometric sensors for the monitoring of O3 and NO2 in ambient air at ppb level. Procedia Eng. 2015;120:480–3.

122. Borrego C, Costa A, Ginja J, Amorim M, Coutinho M, Karatzas K, et al. Assessment of air quality microsensors versus reference methods: the EuNetAir joint exercise. Atmos Environ. 2016;147:246–63.

123. Borrego C, Ginja J, Coutinho M, Ribeiro C, Karatzas K, Sioumis T, et al. Assessment of air quality microsensors versus reference methods: the EuNetAir Joint Exercise–Part II. Atmos Environ. 2018;193:127–42.

124. Singer BC, Delp WW. Response of consumer and research grade indoor air quality monitors to residential sources of fine particles. Indoor Air. 2018;28(4):624–39.

125. Zikova N, Hopke PK, Ferro AR. Evaluation of new low-cost particle monitors for PM2.5 concentration measurements. J Aerosol Sci. 2017;105:25–34.

126. Lin C, Gillespie J, Schuder MD, Duberstein W, Beverland IJ, Heal MR. Evaluation and calibration of Aeroqual series 500 portable gas sensors for accurate measurement of ambient ozone and nitrogen dioxide. Atmos Environ. 2015;100:111–6.

127. Duvall RM, Long RW, Beaver MR, Kronmiller KG, Wheeler ML, Szykman JJ. Performance evaluation and community application of low-cost sensors for ozone and nitrogen dioxide. Sensors (Basel). 2016;16(10):1698.

128. Holstius DM, Pillarisetti A, Smith KR, Seto E. Field calibrations of a low-cost aerosol sensor at a regulatory monitoring site in California. Atmos Meas Tech. 2014;7:1121–31.

129. Cross ES, Williams LR, Lewis DK, Magoon GR, Onasch TB, Kaminsky ML, et al. Use of electrochemical sensors for measurement of air pollution: correcting interference response and validating measurements. Atmos Meas Tech. 2017;10:3575–88.

130. Piedrahita R, Xiang Y, Masson N, Ortega J, Collier A, Jiang Y, et al. The next generation of low-cost personal air quality sensors for quantitative exposure monitoring. Atmos Meas Tech. 2014;7(10):3325–36.

131. Dacunto PJ, Klepeis NE, Cheng K-C, Acevedo-Bolton V, Jiang R-T, Repace JL, et al. Determining PM 2.5 calibration curves for a low-cost particle monitor: common indoor residential aerosols. Environ Sci: Processes Impacts. 2015;17(11):1959–66.

132. Wang Y, Li J, Jing H, Zhang Q, Jiang J, Biswas P. Laboratory evaluation and calibration of three

low-cost particle sensors for particulate matter measurement. Aerosol Sci Technol. 2015;49:1063–77.

133. Jayaratne R, Liu X, Thai P, Dunbabin M, Morawska L. The influence of humidity on the performance of a low-cost air particle mass sensor and the effect of atmospheric fog. Atmos Meas Tech. 2018;11:4883–90.

134. Chan YY, Wang P, Rogers L, Tignor N, Zweig M, Hershman SG, et al. The Asthma Mobile Health Study, a large-scale clinical observational study using ResearchKit. Nat Biotechnol. 2017;35(4):354–62.

135. Karapanos E. Sustaining user engagement with behavior-change tools. Interactions. 2015;22(4):48–52.

136. Serrano KJ, Coa KI, Yu M, Wolff-Hughes DL, Atienza AA. Characterizing user engagement with health app data: a data mining approach. Transl Behav Med. 2017;7(2):277–85.

137. Himes BE, Weitzman ER. Innovations in health information technologies for chronic pulmonary diseases. Respir Res. 2016;17:38.

138. Alexeeff SE, Roy A, Shan J, Liu X, Messier K, Apte JS, et al. High-resolution mapping of traf-

fic related air pollution with Google street view cars and incidence of cardiovascular events within neighborhoods in Oakland, CA. Environ Health. 2018;17(1):38.

139. Beans C. News feature: exposing the exposome to elucidate disease. Proc Natl Acad Sci U S A. 2018;115(47):11859–62.

140. Hosseini A, Buonocore CM, Hashemzadeh S, Hojaiji H, Kalantarian H, Sideris C, et al. Feasibility of a secure wireless sensing smartwatch application for the self-management of pediatric asthma. Sensors (Basel). 2017;17(8):1780.

141. Niedzwiecki MM, Walker DI, Vermeulen R, Chadeau-Hyam M, Jones DP, Miller GW. The exposome: molecules to populations. Annu Rev Pharmacol Toxicol. 2019;59:107–27.

142. Agache I, Miller R, Gern JE, Hellings PW, Jutel M, Muraro A, et al. Emerging concepts and challenges in implementing the exposome paradigm in allergic diseases and asthma: a Practall document. Allergy. 2019;74(3):449–63.

Tele-ICU in Precision Medicine: It's Not What You Do, But How You Do It

21

Peter S. Marshall

Key Points

1. Patient-centered benefits attributed to Tele-ICU can only be achieved with proper implementation that includes not only installation of audiovisual equipment but also introduction of standardized protocols, adherence to best practices, and acceptance by bedside staff.
2. The effect of Tele-ICU implementation on health system outcomes, such as cost and inter-hospital transfers, require further analysis.
3. Newer models of Tele-ICU, new acuity scoring systems and novel technologies should be rigorously studied prior to widespread adoption to ensure that they produce intended outcomes.

Introduction

Tele-intensive care unit (Tele-ICU) is the application of telemedicine to critical care and is defined by the American Telemedicine Association as a "Network of audiovisual communication and computer systems which provide the foundation for a collaborative and interprofessional care model focusing on critically ill patients. Tele-ICU service is not designed to replace local services, but meant to augment care through the leveraging of resources and the standardization of processes" [1].

The concept of applying telemedicine to the intensive care unit (ICU) has been discussed for several decades. In 1906 electrocardiographic data was transmitted via telephone lines [2]. As early as 1924 Radio News suggested that a "radio doctor" may provide direct medical care. In 1977 a trial of "television" consultation with university-based intensivists demonstrated the extended availability of specialist expertise and was superior to telephone consultation [3, 4]. In 1997 the first trial of remote monitoring using computer-based data transmission to communicate with bedside staff for 24 hours was successfully completed. In 2000 a 19-hour trial of remote monitoring, computer data relay and computer-based decision support was conducted. This study demonstrated a reduction in ICU mortality, ICU length of stay and ICU complications compared with historical data [5]. The trial conducted by Rosenfeld et al. [5] used computer-based decision support to assist in patient care. Subsequent advances in Tele-ICU have come in the form

P. S. Marshall (✉)
Yale School of Medicine, Section of Pulmonary, Critical Care & Sleep Medicine, New Haven, CT, USA
e-mail: peter.marshall@med.usc.edu

© Springer Nature Switzerland AG 2020
J. L. Gomez et al. (eds.), *Precision in Pulmonary, Critical Care, and Sleep Medicine*, Respiratory Medicine, https://doi.org/10.1007/978-3-030-31507-8_21

321

of improved hardware (video, audio and data streaming equipment) but also in software designed to identify decompensation early in a wide variety of illnesses.

In theory, application of the Tele-ICU can have benefits for ICU patients, health delivery networks, and individual members of the healthcare team. Early studies have demonstrated improved hospital mortality, reduced ICU length of stay (LOS), reduced complication rates, improved compliance with best practices and improved patient safety [6–9]. A recent meta-analysis by Chen et al. [10] concluded these benefits may be achieved only with proper implementation and are achieved at a high upfront cost.

Epidemiology

The rapid growth of Tele-ICU is, in large part, due to the national shortage of intensivists in the setting of rising costs of critical care and an aging population. The shortage of intensivists is projected to reach 35% by the year 2020 [11]. As of 2012, over 4 million patients were admitted to ICUs each year in the United States, and approximately 540,000 deaths occur yearly in the ICU population [12–15]. ICU utilization in those over 64 is 3.5 times that of younger age groups [16]. The combination of an ever-increasing demographic of those older than 65 years old and ICU services consuming 10% of hospital costs ($65–$81 billion per year) has created a need to find ways of optimizing the use critical care providers and resources. In addition, patient safety continues to be a concern in the fast paced, high stakes realm of critical care. Serious medication errors account for 78% of the errors in the ICU. The use of Tele-ICU is one way that hospitals are addressing the short-fall of intensivists and improving patient safety in the ICU. It is apparent that three factors have driven the adoption of Tele-ICU models: (1) a desire to improve outcomes through standardization and reporting, (2) a desire to address workforce shortages and, (3) a desire to improve patient safety [17].

The total number of hospitals adopting Tele-ICU rose from 0.4% to 4.6% between 2003 and 2010 [18]. The total number of beds covered by Tele-ICU programs increased 10 – fold and corresponded to an increase of beds covered from 0.9% to 7.9% of the total. It should be noted that the rate of adoption of Tele-ICU has decreased over time with most growth (101% per year) occurring from 2003 to 2006 and subsequent growth from 2007 to 2010 dropping to 8.1% per year [18, 19]. One of the reasons for the slowed growth is the start-up cost for Tele-ICU. The central monitoring station (or "command center") costs between $2 and 5 million dollars to create, and an additional $250,000 is needed to add additional ICUs to the program [20]. This may be one reason why the hospitals investing in Tele-ICU tend to be large, non-profit teaching hospitals located in large metropolitan areas [18]. Hospitals without Tele-ICU tend to have fewer resources with respect to major technologies and procedures.

Concepts/Models

There are three models of Tele-ICU, (1) Continuous monitoring or high intensity, (2) Individual/consult/reactive model also known as a low intensity, and (3) Scheduled care model in which care occurs with periodic consultation on a pre-determined schedule [1]. Tele-ICUs are connected to client sites via private secure audio-visual tele-communications and communication systems [21]. In the continuous model data streams from each patient at client sites to the central monitoring station. The central monitoring station is staffed by tele-intensivists (trained critical care physicians working in the Tele-ICU) and other critical care providers. These other critical care providers may be nurse practitioners, physician assistants or critical care nurses. Some larger Tele-ICUs have incorporated other allied health professionals such as pharmacists [22]. In the consultative model bedside providers in the ICU alert tele-intensivists to issues and the Tele-ICU becomes involved. There is little or no real-time monitoring or constant data feed. A systemic review by Ramnath et al. compared the consultative model to the continuous model [23]. The authors found that both the consultative and continuous monitoring models showed improved compliance with best clinical practice adherence. There was little data to find concerning the consultative model and outcomes such as mortality and length of stay. Most of the reported outcomes data on Tele-ICU performance refers to the continuous model. More high-quality studies are needed to assess the efficacy and costs of both the consultative model and scheduled care model.

Another way of describing Tele-ICU is centralized and de-centralized [20, 23]. The centralized Tele-ICU is comprised of a single monitoring station staffed by critical care providers. The model delivers service to several different ICUs at one site or multiple sites. In the de-centralized model multiple medical facilities can be accessed remotely from many different sites which may include home, office, or mobile device. There is no defined central monitoring station, but there is a workflow whereby multiple locations have access to patients with critical care providers monitoring patients from multiple locations. More than one virtual provider may be present in the ICU at any given time [1].

Data and Acuity Scoring Systems

The continuous model offers onstant data streaming that may be real-time unvalidated data (raw data) or data that is confirmed (validated data) prior to being available to the tele-intensivist. All data whether delivered in real time from patient monitoring devices or validated by bedside staff may be analyzed by algorithms prior to being received by the Tele-ICU staff. Interfaces with bedside monitoring systems can alert Tele-ICU staff of deterioration in vital signs in real-time and bring attention to drastic changes in a patient's condition. Relying solely on real-time raw information offers little advantage over bedside providers and is similar to telemetry monitoring stations used in the past.

Algorithms provide a means of assessing severity of illness and risk for deterioration so that the sickest patients are brought to the atten-

tion of Tele-ICU staff prior to drastic chnages in a patient's clinical condition. The Acute Physiologic and Chronic Health Evaluation II (APACHE II) and Sequential Organ Failure Assessment (SOFA) score are assessments of severity used in the ICU population [24, 25]. The APACHE II score and SOFA were not originally designed to be used sequentially during an ICU stay. The APACHE II score was originally designed to estimate risk of death at the time of ICU admission and to objectively quantify severity of illness in ICU populations [25]. The APACHE II score has since been used to assess risk of readmission [25] and predict mortality in individual patients [26]. The SOFA score was originally formulated to quantify organ dysfunction in sepsis and later validated as a marker of mortality risk when repeated during the ICU stay [27, 28].

Badawi et al. [29] compared the predictive abilities of the APACHE II and SOFA along with a third score, the discharge readiness score (DRS) when used as continuous markers for illness severity in a broad ICU population (333 ICUs from 208 hospitals). The DRS was designed to estimate the risk of events after ICU discharge. It does not use the "worst" values during a given period. How it would function as a marker of illness severity during an ICU stay was unknown [30]. The study compared the three predictive models' ability to predict mortality when calculated hourly. Receiver operator curves (ROC) for ICU mortality were determined for each model and the area under the curves (AUC) calculated. The APACHE II score had an AUCROC of 0.81, the SOFA had an AUCROC of 0.76, and the DRS had an AUCROC of 0.86. The investigators concluded that the three models had a high discriminatory value for ICU mortality when calculated hourly. It appears that these familiar models used to assess severity of illness can predict mortality in an environment where there is continuous streaming of data from individual patients such as the Tele-ICU.

Venders of Tele-ICU platforms (Philips VISICU© and Metavision © for example) have scoring systems and algorithms that analyze data [6, 7, 9, 31] specifically for the Tele-ICU environment. Often, it is a series of subtle changes that herald deterioration in an ICU patient. The absolute value of a heart rate, blood pressure or respiratory rate may be late signs of deterioration. The rate of change or increased variability in a given physiologic parameter may provide earlier recognition of deterioration than the discovery of absolute values that fall outside of accepted norms. These algorithms allow Tele-ICU staff to provide surveillance over many ICU patients because early signs of deterioration and high acuity are revealed in an automated fashion. Clinicians can be alerted prior to drastic deterioration and intervene. These "early warning" algorithms make it unnecessary to open individual patient records and search for abnormalities.

Some institutions (Criticalware ©, University of Massachusetts) have created their own acuity systems and refined these to meet the needs of their institutions and patients [7]. The Yale Early Warning System (YEWS) was created within the Epic © EMR Tele-ICU platform and integrates physiological data, rate of change, laboratory data, ventilator data and pharmacological data to produce an acuity score that is constantly recalculated with the most recent information. The YEWS can be updated or modified based on new data or developments in critical care.

Outcomes

Outcomes related to Tele-ICU can be divided into patient-centered outcomes and into outcomes that reflect changes in healthcare delivery (system-centered outcomes). Patient-centered outcomes include mortality, length of stay (LOS), ventilator days and complication rates. System-centered outcomes include cost of care and effects on patient movement/transfers [32]. Many local factors impact the effect of Tele-ICU on outcomes, and it can be difficult to predict how Tele-ICU implementation will affect a given environment.

In general, Tele-ICU implementation is expected to result in reduced ICU LOS, reduced ICU mortality and reduced hospital mortality [6, 7, 9, 33]. Two meta-analyses have been completed [8, 34] and show a reduction in ICU mortality. The systematic review by Young et al. also revealed a reduction in ICU LOS but no effect on in-hospital mortality. It is important to note that not all implementations have resulted in improved patient-centered outcomes [34–36]. Variable outcomes may be explained by the method of implementation. The Wilcox and Adhikari [8] meta-analysis categorized outcomes by quality of study and the intensity of Tele-ICU intervention. High-intensity ICU intervention was defined by continuous patient monitoring with or without computer-generated alerts. Low-intensity ICU intervention was defined as the absence of continuous monitoring and the absence of computer-generated alerts. When analyzed as a group the high-intensity Tele-ICU studies revealed favorable outcomes and the low-intensity Tele-ICU studies failed to show benefit. In other words, there is a dose-response relationship between the level of Tele-ICU intervention and beneficial outcomes.

The ability of the Tele-ICU to alter patient care (also referred to as autonomy) also affects the ability of the intervention to alter outcomes. Research has demonstrated that the acceptance of the Tele-ICU by bedside staff was a key factor in the success of the Tele-ICU. A study by Nassar et al. [37] demonstrated variability between ICUs in their acceptance of Tele-ICU implementation. Poor acceptance along with low baseline mortality, resulted in no change in ICU mortality or LOS after Tele-ICU implementation. Thomas et al. [36] noted that no improvement in patient-centered outcomes was detected in their study but that only 31% of physicians yielded full management of their patients to the Tele-ICU. These examples illustrate that to impact patient care, Tele-ICUs need to have decision-making capacity and authority to make significant management changes.

ICUs with adequate staffing may benefit less from Tele-ICU implementation. Some have pointed to the role of nighttime intensivists as similar to that of nighttime Tele-ICU coverage. Studies conducted in ICUs with strong daytime intensivist presence or nighttime resident physician (with telephone access to intensivists) presence have failed to demonstrate benefit of nighttime intensivist presence [38, 39]. Similarly, nighttime Tele-ICU coverage may have little impact on well-staffed ICUs.

The level of acuity of the ICUs being covered will also affect the impact of the Tele-ICU on patient outcomes. One study showed no difference in ICU LOS or mortality with Tele-ICU implementation, but when patients with higher acuity were analyzed, the survival among these patients was improved [36]. This observation reflects the inability of any intervention to have an impact on populations where the outcomes of interest are rare.

The ability of Tele-ICU to improve outcomes is dependent on several factors that include intensity of Tele-ICU implementation, level of Tele-ICU autonomy, acuity of patient population, quality of bedside ICU staffing, and acceptance by ICU bedside staff. When starting a Tele-ICU program all these factors need to be taken into consideration and addressed if successful implementation is to be achieved.

Implementation is a multi-faceted process that includes not only the installation of audiovisual technology and algorithms. Implementation often brings along standardization of protocols and real-time audits [40, 41]. Lilly describes not only the introduction of audiovisual equipment and monitoring algorithms but also outlined the introduction of standardized protocols, clinical bundles and clinical pathways. The holistic implementation of Tele-ICU results in increased compliance with best practice which likely explains some of the improved patient-centered outcomes described with Tele-ICU implementation [6, 7, 42].

Tele-ICUs have demonstrated an ability to improve adherence with best practices [7, 33, 43–45] by standardizing protocols and encouraging adherence. Best practices where the Tele-ICU has improved adherence include prevention of ventilator associated pneumonia (VAP) bundles, venous thromboembolism (VTE) prophylaxis, stress ulcer prophylaxis (SUP), glycemic control, cardiovascular protection, spontaneous breathing trial (SBT) protocols, prevention of catheter related blood stream infections, and sepsis bundles. Other best practices where the Tele-ICU may help improve adherence is prompt removal of indwelling urinary catheters and delirium prevention measures. Mechanisms to improve compliance with best practices must

be incorporated into successful Tele-ICU programs and are part of the holistic implementation noted above.

Sepsis is a disease that dominates the census of most ICUs and may occur in 50–75% of critically ill patients [46, 47]. It is common and potentially lethal, especially if unrecognized and if treatment delays occur [46, 48, 49]. It is now established that having a protocolized approach to recognition of sepsis can promote early diagnosis, thereby decreasing mortality [50, 51]. A few key variables can identify a patient with systemic inflammatory response syndrome (SIRS), and in the presence of a suspected infection, the diagnosis of sepsis is made [51].

Rincon et al. [43] used a Tele-ICU screening tool that conformed to the Surviving Sepsis Campaign [48] criteria for the identification and treatment of sepsis. The screening tool presented data in a useful format that facilitated recognition and analysis. Screens were performed on admission to the ICU and once per shift on any ICU patient suspected of infection. 2–3 RNs were able to perform 194 screens in a 24-hour period and on average identified five new cases of severe sepsis. Thus, screening performed by the Tele-ICU unburdened bedside staff.

Follow-up to ensure that sepsis best practices were adhered to was performed by the Tele-ICU. The study demonstrated an increase in prompt antibiotic administration, fluid bolus, lactate measurement, and central line placement. Improved compliance with sepsis best practices has been shown to improve survival [52–54]. Implementation of Tele-ICU algorithms and screening tools can improve the efficiency of sepsis screening, improve compliance with severe sepsis bundles and improve survival in ICU patients with severe sepsis and septic shock.

Concerning to governments, regulatory agencies and payors is that the implementation of Tele-ICUs (providing service to smaller and less equipped hospitals) will result in patients being transferred to tertiary centers with greater frequency. Alternatively, one could argue that the leveraging of expertise with the assistance of Tele-ICU will encourage patients with high acuity to remain at outlying hospitals. Some have estimated that between 25 and 75% of transfers from rural hospitals could remain at the hospital of admission with appropriate consultation [55]. Panlaqui et al. studied the impact of a low-intensity model of Tele-ICU on inter-hospital transfers as well as patient-centered outcomes [35]. Outcomes were compared before and after Tele-ICU implementation. They found a 12% risk reduction in inter-hospital transfer (RR = 0.88, 95% CI 0.80–0.98, p = 0.03). Interestingly, the proportion of transferred patients who died in the Tele-ICU group was higher than in the non-Tele ICU group (11.6% versus 2.8%, p = 0.03), and suggests that patients selected for transfer in the Tele-ICU group had higher acuity.

In a study of Veteran's Administration ICU patients Fortis et al. [56] concurrently studied transfer rates in hospitals provided Tele-ICU and those without the intervention. In addition, they were able to classify the illness severity of the transfers. The overall transfer rate was reduced (RR 0.79, 95% CI 0.71–0.87; $p < 0.001$) and the reduction was mainly in moderate to high illness severity patients. The 30-day mortality was similar in both Tele-ICU and non-Tele ICU groups. With the Tele-ICU smaller hospitals were able to care for moderate and high severity patients without resulting in excessive mortality.

Pannu et al. [57] studied the Mayo healthcare system ICUs before and after Tele-ICU implementation. The number of inter-hospital transfers to the quaternary referral center increased after implementation (3.03% versus 2.43%, p = 0.04). The authors suggested that the trend was not explained by an increase in severity of illness. The authors raised the possibility that "transfer bias" was present. The study was conducted within an established healthcare system and barriers to transfer are minimal. This results in a low threshold to transfer patients with perceived high acuity. The presence of transfer bias is supported by the fact that there was no measurable increase in severity of illness after the implementation of Tele-ICU. Based on the current literature we cannot conclude that implementation of Tele-ICU reduces (or increases) the rate of inter-hospital transfer. Much like patient-centered outcomes, the impact of Tele-ICU on inter-hospital transfers

will probably be determined by several factors (yet to be identified) related to the functioning of the Tele-ICU, client ICUs and health systems.

Overall, implementation of Tele-ICUs under the appropriate circumstances can reduce ICU mortality and in-hospital mortality. The effects on ICU LOS and hospital LOS are more variable but trend toward the Tele-ICU having a favorable effect. Effective Tele-ICU implementation requires a holistic approach and should include the introduction (and reinforcement) of evidence-based best practices. Tele-ICUs are most likely to succeed if they can actively manage patients, there is "buy-in" from the bedside staff, and there is high-intensity Tele-ICU surveillance. The effect of Tele-ICU implementation on inter-hospital transfers is somewhat controversial and requires greater study. These outcomes have financial implications, and it is the economic impact of the Tele-ICU that will determine its viability as an option for healthcare systems.

Financial Considerations

Direct Reimbursement/Revenue

Reimbursement by payors is minimal for Tele-ICU. In 2013 the Centers for Medicare and Medicaid Services (CMS) assigned category III Current Procedural Terminology (CPT) codes 0188 T and 0189 T [58]. These codes were generally used for data collection purposes only. In the fall of 2018, these codes were updated to G0508 and G0509 (Table 21.1). These codes refer to critical care services and require a minimum investment of 50–60 minutes per patient. The time invested on one patient for a busy tele-intensivist is often impractical and is not consistent with the workflow of most Tele-ICUs. Most of the interventions are of shorter duration and made efficient by acuity scoring and synergy of the EMR with Tele-ICU technical support. Tele-ICU clinicians do not spend as much time on data collection and analysis as their bedside counterparts. While these interventions are of shorter duration than conventional interactions, they are just as important. Telemedicine CPT codes (Table 21.1) for initial consultations and

Table 21.1 Tele-ICU codes recognized by Medicare[a]

CPT code	Descriptor	Duration (mins)	Comments
G0508	Telehealth/initial consult	60	Critical care
G0509	Telehealth/follow-up	50	Critical care
G0406	Telehealth/inpatient/consult follow- up	15	
G0407	Telehealth/inpatient/consult follow- up	25	
G0408	Telehealth/inpatient/consult follow- up	35	
G0425	Telehealth/ED or initial inpatient	30	
G0426	Telehealth/ED or initial inpatient	50	
G0427	Telehealth/ED or initial inpatient	70	
99231	Inpatient follow-up/progress	15	Use 02 modifier for Telehealth
99232	Inpatient follow-up/progress	25	Use 02 modifier for Telehealth
99233	Inpatient follow-up/progress	35	Use 02 modifier for Telehealth
99356	Inpatient follow-up/prolonged service	>70	Use 02 modifier for Telehealth

[a]https://hub.americantelemed.org/home, https://www.excellusbcbs.com/wps/wcm/connect (Medical Policy – Excellus – 12/31/2018) accessed 01/23/2019

for follow-up consultations are now available and do not require the same time commitments as the critical care CPT codes. One may even use the appropriate inpatient follow-up/progress codes and add a telemedicine modifier to bill for Tele-ICU services that do not qualify for critical care by time or acuity. Some insurers are starting to recognize and reimburse these codes, but total collection is a small proportion of services rendered [42, 58].

Some Tele-ICUs have been able to charge client ICUs a per bed fee or per unit fee for coverage [42]. This fee may include capital costs, costs for operation of the Tele-ICU and payment for Tele-ICU staff salaries. Additional charges for consultations or as needed interventions may be added on a case by case basis or billed using an estimate agreed upon prior to initiation of services. Client ICUs and payors may find this form of direct payment attractive if they anticipate the presence of the Tele-ICU will significantly reduce the cost of caring for ICU patients. Stand-alone Tele-ICU companies likely obtain most of their revenue from contracts such as this. Direct reimbursement via a contractual arrangement is imprecise and subject to over or underestimation of the value of services provided. Contracts would likely have to be renegotiated based on the performance of the Tele-ICU, changes in Tele-ICU operating costs, changes in client ICU practice patterns and changes in patient acuity. These contracts, may in part, be based on an estimation of indirect revenue.

Indirect Revenue

While direct billing by Tele-ICU providers is small, cost savings are potentially great if proper implementation of the Tele-ICU is achieved. Investigators have documented the increased direct cost of caring for patients with Tele-ICU [59, 60]. Lilly et al. [61] tried to quantify the cost savings (or cost avoidance) using a concept referred to as the annual direct contribution margin (ADCM) which is defined as the aggregated net case revenue minus the direct costs of care. The direct cost of care includes the expense of operating the Tele-ICU. The study compared three different groups of patients: (1) non-Tele ICU patients, (2) Tele-ICU with full monitoring and intensivist intervention, and (3) full Tele-ICU with additional logistic center support. The logistic center support was comprised of 51 care-standardization and quality improvement projects. Both Tele-ICU groups provided coverage 24/7. The investigators found that the presence of both Tele-ICU models resulted in reduced hospital LOS and increased case volume. This meant that more patients were admitted to and discharged from the ICU in a given period. The reduced LOS and increased case volume resulted in a steep rise in per case revenue with only a small rise in per case cost. Earlier investigators [5, 62] found a similar relationship between increased revenues and reduced ICU LOS.

Lilly et al. observed an aggregate annual cost of $142 million pre-Tele-ICU, $182 million in the full Tele-ICU group and $200 million in the Tele-ICU logistic center group [61]. The ADCM (aggregate annual income minus aggregate annual cost) was $7.9 million in the pre-Tele-ICU group, $37 million in the full Tele-ICU group and $60 million in the Tele-ICU logistic center group. Not only did this study demonstrate that Tele-ICUs can quickly bring a return on investment (start-up costs were recovered after 2¾ months of full Tele-ICU operation) but it also demonstrated the dose-response aspect of Tele-ICU. The largest ADCM was achieved in the Tele-ICU model with the greatest involvement in the operations of the ICU. It is likely that the significant implementation costs and uncertain financial benefits of the Tele-ICU may be limiting wider adoption of an intervention with proven benefits. The results of the study are encouraging for proponents of the Tele-ICU but will have to be repeated by other investigators if more healthcare systems are to adopt a Tele-ICU solution.

Conclusions/Future Challenges

With holistic implementation of Tele-ICU (specifically the centralized, continuous model) to moderate and high acuity ICU patients, the improvements in ICU mortality and in-hospital mortality are clear. The impact on ICU LOS is probably also real. Several areas require more study regarding the impact of Tele-ICU on outcomes. The most robust data exists for the continuous and centralized models for Tele-ICU [23]. Decentralized and consultative models exist and are in use. It is less clear how these models will impact patient-centered outcomes and system-centered outcomes (such as cost and inter-hospital transfers). The assumption that decentralized, consultative models function as well as the centralized-continuous may not be valid.

It is becoming clear that acuity scoring systems such as APACHE II, SOFA and DRS can be used for continuous assessment of illness severity in the Tele-ICU environment. Further assessment of acuity scoring systems and proprietary algorithms are needed to ensure that the scoring systems are performing as intended. Do these constructs all have the impact on patient-centered outcomes as the tools used in the original studies [6, 7, 40]?

Sepsis is an ideal critical illness where application of illness severity systems is possible. Data obtained from the EMR, and laboratory can be used by acuity scoring systems to identify patients with severe sepsis. This data is presented in an automated fashion to Tele-ICU staff thus reducing the need for labor intensive chart review. The Tele-ICU can improve outcomes by screening large numbers, promoting adherence to best practice and providing ongoing surveillance for adverse events [45].

Newer technology such as mobile Tele-ICU units (or avatars and robots) can take two-way audiovisual technology to the bedside at any unit in a hospital. This capability is attractive because it can reduce costs as less up-front capital is used to equip rooms with cameras, speakers and microphones. In areas where there is unpredictability regarding which beds are used for the critically ill (such as EDs), mobile units offer flexibility. Mobile units could also participate in work rounds in or outside of patient rooms. As attractive as this new technology appears, careful analysis during implementation is required to assess its actual impact on critical care.

Improvements in fee for service billing in the Tele-ICU may not significantly increase the proportion of direct revenue generated by the Tele-ICU but will help document effort. Documentation in the medical record [63] can offer an estimate of Tele-ICU effort. However, it is reasonable to suspect that use of CPT codes will formalize documentation and contribute to the relative value unit (RVU) calculations that are used to assess providers. Even if there is no reimbursement by payors, use of CPT codes will provide valuable data to assist in future assessments of Tele-ICU outcomes and usage.

With respect to indirect revenue, more studies which adjust income estimates for the cost savings (related improved outcomes attributable to Tele-ICU) need to be performed [61]. Other investigators will need to obtain similar results to establish the generalizability of the financial outcomes. Decentralized and consultative models should be subjected to the same analysis to establish favorable cost–benefit ratios of these models.

References

1. Davis TM, Barden C, Dean S, Gavish A, Goliash I, Goran S, Graley A, Herr P, Jackson W, Loo E, Marcin JP. American telemedicine association guidelines for tele-ICU operations. Telemed e-Health. 2016;22(12):971–80.
2. Lilly CM, Zubrow MT, Kempner KM. Critical care telemedicine: evolution and state of the art. Crit Care Med. 2014;42(11):2429–36.
3. Grundy BL, Crawford P, Jones PK, Kiley ML, Reisman A, Pao YH, Wilkerson EL, Gravenstein JS. Telemedicine in critical care: an experiment in health care delivery. JACEP. 1977;6(10):439–44.
4. Grundy BL, Jones PK, Lovitt A. Telemedicine in critical care: problems in design, implementation, and assessment. Crit Care Med. 1982;10(7):471–5.
5. Rosenfeld BA, Dorman T, Breslow MJ, Pronovost P, Jenckes M, Zhang N, Anderson G, Rubin H. Intensive care unit telemedicine: alternate paradigm for providing continuous intensivist care. Crit Care Med. 2000;28(12):3925–31.
6. McCambridge M, Jones K, Paxton P, Baker K, Sussman EJ, Etchason J, et al. Association of health information technology and teleintensivist coverage with decreased mortality and ventilator use in critically ill patients. Arch Intern Med. 2010;170(7):648–53.
7. Lilly CM, Cody S, Zhao H, Landry L, Baker SP, McIlwaine J, Chandler MW, et al. For the University of Massachusetts Memorial Critical Care Operations Group. Hospital mortality, length of stay, and preventable complications among critically ill patients before and after tele-ICU reengineering of critical care processes. JAMA. 2011;305(21):2175–83.
8. Wilcox ME, Adhikari NK. The effect of telemedicine in critically ill patients: systematic review and meta-analysis. Crit Care. 2012;16:R127.
9. Sadaka F, Palagiri A, Trottier S, Deibert W, Gudmestad D, Sommer SE, Veremakis C. Telemedicine intervention improves ICU outcomes. Crit Care Res Pract. 2013; https://doi.org/10.1155/2013/456389.
10. Chen J, Sun D, Yang W, Liu M, Zhang S, Peng J, Ren C. Clinical and economic outcomes of telemedicine programs in the intensive care unit: a systematic review and meta-analysis. J Intensive Care Med. 2017;33:383–93.
11. Angus DC, Shorr AF, White A, Dremsizov TT, Schmitz RJ, Kelley MA. Committee on Manpower for Pulmonary Critical Care Societies. Current and projected workforce requirements for care of the critically ill and patients with pulmonary disease: can we meet the requirements of an aging population? JAMA. 2000;284:2762–70.
12. Philip R Lee Institute for Health Policy Studies. ICU outcomes (mortality and length of stay) methods, data collection tool and data [Internet]. University of California, San Francisco. 2012. https://healthpolicy. ucsf.edu/icu-outcomes.
13. Angus DC, Barnato AE, Linde-Zwirble WT, et al. Robert Wood Johnson Foundation ICU End-Of Life Peer Group. Use of intensive care at the end of life in the United States: an epidemiologic study. Crit Care Med. 2004;32(3):63843. https://doi.org/10.1097/01. CCM.0000114816.62331.08.
14. Mayr VD, Dünser MW, Greil V, Jochberger S, Luckner G, Ulmer H, Friesenecker BE, Takala J, Hasibeder WR. Causes of death and determinants of outcome in critically ill patients. Crit Care. 2006;10(6):R154. https://doi.org/10.1186/cc5086.
15. Angus DC, Barnato AE, Linde-Zwirble WT, Wessfield LA, Watson RS, Rickert T, et al. Robert Wood Johnson Foundation ICU End-Of Life Peer Group. Use of intensive care at the end of life in the United States: an epidemiologic study. Crit Care Med. 2004;32(3):63843. https://doi.org/10.1097/01. CCM.0000114816.62331.08.
16. Scurlock C, D'Ambrosio C. Telemedicine in the intensive care unit. Crit Care Clin. 2015;31:187–95.
17. Lilly C, Fuhrman S. ICU telemedicine solutions. Clin Chest Med. 2015;36:L401–7.
18. Kahn JM, Cicero BD, Wallace DJ, Iwashyna TJ. Adoption of intensive care unit telemedicine in the United States. Crit Care Med. 2014;42:362–8.
19. Wenham T, Pittard A. Intensive care unit environment. Contin Educ Anaesth Crit Care Pain. 2009;9(6):178–83. https://doi.org/10.1093/bjaceaccp/mkp036.
20. Coustasse A, Deslich S, Bailey D, Hairston A, Paul D. A business case for tele-intensive care units. Perm J. 2014;18:76–84.
21. Reynolds HN, Bander J, McCarthy M. Different systems and formats for tele-ICU coverage: designing a tele-ICU system to optimize functionality and investment. Crit Care Nurs Q. 2012;35(4):364–77. https://doi.org/10.1097/CNQ.0b013e318266bc26.
22. Forni A, Skehan N, Hartman CA, Yogaratnam D, Njoroge M, Schifferdecker C, Lilly CM. Evaluation of the impact of a tele-ICU pharmacist on the management of sedation in critically III mechanically ventilated patients. Ann Pharmacother. 2010;44:432–8.
23. Ramnath V, Khazeni N. Centralized monitoring and virtual consultant models of tele-ICU care: a systematic review. Telemed e-Health. 2014;20:936–61.
24. Vincent JL, Moreno R, Takala J, Willatts S, De Mendonça A, Bruining H, Reinhart CK, Suter PM, Thijs LG. The SOFA (Sepsis-related Organ Failure Assessment) score to describe organ dysfunction/failure. On behalf of the Working Group on Sepsis-Related Problems of the European Society of Intensive Care Medicine. Intensive Care Med. 1996;22:707–10.

25. Chen YC, Lin MC, Lin YC, Chang HW, Huang CC, Tsai YH. ICU discharge APACHE II scores help to predict post-ICU death. Chang Gung Med J. 2007;30:142–50.

26. Rogers J, Fuller HD. Use of daily Acute Physiology and Chronic Health Evaluation (APACHE) II scores to predict individual patient survival rate. Crit Care Med. 1994;22:1402–5.

27. Ferreira FL, Bota DP, Bross A, Mélot C, Vincent JL. Serial evaluation of the SOFA score to predict outcome in critically ill patients. JAMA. 2001;286:1754–8.

28. Holder L, Elizabeth O, Lyu P, Kempker JA, Nemati S, Razmi F, Martin GS, et al. Serial daily organ failure assessment beyond ICU day 5 does not independently add precision to ICU risk-of-death prediction. Crit Care Med. 2017;45:2014–22.

29. Badawi O, Liu X, Hassan E, Amelung PJ, Swami S. Evaluation of ICU risk models adapted for use as continuous markers of severity of illness throughout the ICU stay. Crit Care Med. 2018;46(3):361–7.

30. Badawi O, Breslow MJ. Readmissions and death after ICU discharge: development and validation of two predictive models. PLoS One. 2012;7:e48758. https://doi.org/10.1371/journal.pone.0048758.

31. Willmitch B, Golembeski S, Kim SS, Nelson LD, Gidel L. Clinical outcomes after telemedicine intensive care unit implementation. Crit Care Med. 2012;40(2):450–4. https://doi.org/10.1097/CCM.0b013e318232d694.

32. Venkataraman R, Ramakrishnan N. Outcomes related to telemedicine in the ICU: what we know and would like to know. Crit Care Clin. 2015;31:225–37.

33. Kalb T, Raikhelkar J, Meyer S, Ntimba F, Thuli J, Gorman MJ, Kopec I, Scurlock C. A multicenter population-based effectiveness study of teleintensive care unit-directed ventilator rounds demonstrating improved adherence to a protective lung strategy, decreased ventilator duration, and decreased. J Crit Care. 2014;29(4):691.e7–14. https://doi.org/10.1016/j.jcrc.2014.02.017.

34. Young LB, Chan PS, Lu X, Nallamothu BK, Sasson C, Cram PM. Impact of telemedicine intensive care unit coverage on patient outcomes: a systematic review and meta-analysis. Arch Intern Med. 2011;171(6):498–506. https://doi.org/10.1001/archinternmed.2011.61.

35. Panlaqui OM, Broadfield E, Champion R, Edington JP, Kennedy S. Outcomes of telemedicine intervention in a regional intensive care unit: a before and after study. Anaesth Intensive Care. 2017;45(5):605–10.

36. Thomas EJ, Lucke JF, Wueste L, Weavind L, Patel B. Association of telemedicine for remote monitoring of intensive care patients with mortality, complications, and length of stay. JAMA. 2009;302(24):2671–8.

37. Nassar BS, Vaughan-Sarrazin MS, Jiang L, Reisinger HS, Bonello R, Cram P. Impact of an intensive care unit telemedicine program on patient outcomes in an integrated health care system. JAMA Intern Med. 2014;174(7):1160–7. https://doi.org/10.1001/jamainternmed.2014.1503.

38. Wallace DJ, Angus DC, Barnato AE, Kramer AA, Kahn JM. Nighttime intensivist staffing and mortality among critically ill patients. N Engl J Med. 2012;366. https://doi.org/10.1056/NEJMsa1201918.

39. Kerlin MP, Small DS, Cooney E, Fuchs BD, Bellini LM, Mikkelsen ME, Schweickert WD, Bakhru RN, Gabler NB, Harhay MO, Hansen-Flaschen J, Halpern SD. A randomized trial of nighttime physician staffing in an intensive care unit. N Engl J Med. 2013;368(23):2201–9. https://doi.org/10.1056/NEJMoa1302854.

40. Lilly CM, Fisher KA, Ries M, Pastores SM, Vender J, Pitts JA, Hanson CW 3rd. A national telemedicine survey: validation and results. Chest. 2012;142:40–7. https://doi.org/10.1378/chest.12-0310.

41. Lilly CM, McLaughlin JM, Zhao H, Baker SP, Cody S, Irwin RS. UMass Memorial Critical Care Operations Group. A multicenter study of ICU telemedicine reengineering of adult critical care. Chest. 2014;145(3):500–7. https://doi.org/10.1378/chest.13-1973.

42. Fortis S, Weinert C, Bushinski R, Koehler AG, Beilman G. A health system-based critical care program with a novel tele-ICU: implementation, cost, and structure details. J Am Coll Surg. 2014;219(4):676–83. https://doi.org/10.1016/j.jamcollsurg.2014.04.015.

43. Rincon TA, Bourke G, Seiver A. Standardizing sepsis screening and management via a tele-ICU program improves patient care. Telemed e-Health. 2011;17(7):560–4. https://doi.org/10.1089/tmj.2010.0225.

44. Olff C, Clark-Wadkins C. Tele-ICU partners enhance evidence based practice – ventilator weaning initiative. AACN Adv Crit Care. 2012;23(3):312–22.

45. Badawi O, Hassan E. Telemedicine and the patient with sepsis. Crit Care Clin. 2015;31:291–304. https://doi.org/10.1016/j.ccc.2014.12.007.

46. Kaukonen KM, Bailey M, Suzuki S, Pilcher D, Bellomo R. Mortality related to severe sepsis and septic shock among critically ill patients in Australia and New Zealand, 2000–2012. JAMA. 2014;311(13):1308–16. https://doi.org/10.1001/jama.2014.2637.

47. Vincent JL, Rello J, Marshall J, Silva E, Anzueto A, Martin CD, Moreno R, Lipman J, Gomersall C, Sakr Y, Reinhart K. EPIC II Group of Investigators. International study of prevalence of outcomes of infection in intensive care units. JAMA. 2009;302(21):2323–9. https://doi.org/10.1001/jama.2009.1754.

48. Dellinger RP, Levy MM, Carlet JM, Bion J, Parker MM, Jaeschke R, et al. Surviving sepsis campaign: international guidelines for management of severe sepsis and septic shock. Crit Care Med. 2008;36:296–327.

49. Jawad I, Luksic I, Rafnsson SB. Assessing available information on the burden of sepsis: global estimates of incidence, prevalence and mortality. J Glob Health. 2012;2:010404. https://doi.org/10.7189/jogh.01.010404.

50. Moore LJ, Jones SL, Kreiner LA, McKinley B, Sucher JF, Todd SR, Turner KL, Valdivia A, Moore FA. Validation of a screening tool for the early identification of sepsis. J Trauma. 2009;66(6):1539–4. https://doi.org/10.1097/TA.0b013e3181a3ac4b.

51. Levy MM, Rhodes A, Phillips GS, Townsend SR, Schorr CA, Beale R, Osborn T, Lemeshow S, Chiche JD, Artigas A, Dellinger RP. Surviving Sepsis Campaign: association between performance metrics and outcomes in a 7.5-year study. Crit Care Med. 2015;43(1):3–12. https://doi.org/10.1097/CCM.0000000000000723.

52. Hooper MH, Weavind L, Wheeler AP, Martin JB, Gowda SS, Semler MW, et al. Randomized trial of automated, electronic monitoring to facilitate early detection of sepsis in the intensive care unit. Crit Care Med. 2012;40(7):2096–10.

53. Barochia AV, Cui X, Vitberg D, Suffredini AF, O'Grady NP, Banks SM, Minneci P, Kern SJ, Danner RL, Natanson C, Eichacker PQ. Bundled care for septic shock: an analysis of clinical trials. Crit Care Med. 2010;38(2):668–78.

54. van Zanten AR, Brinkman S, Arbous MS, Abu-Hanna A, Levy MM, de Keizer NF. Netherlands Patient Safety Agency Sepsis Expert Group. Guideline bundles adherence and mortality in severe sepsis and septic shock. Crit Care Med. 2014;42(8):1890–8.

55. Yeo W, Ahrens SL, Wright T. A new era in the ICU: the case of telemedicine. Crit Care Nurs Q. 2012;35:316–21.

56. Fortis S, Sarrazin MV, Beck BF, Panos RJ, Reisinger HS. ICU telemedicine reduces interhospital ICU transfers in the veterans health administration. Chest. 2018;154(1):69–76. https://doi.org/10.1016/j.chest.2018.04.021.

57. Pannu J, Sanghavi D, Sheley T, Schroeder DR, Kashyap R, Marquez A, et al. Impact of telemedicine monitoring of community ICUs on inter-hospital transfers. Crit Care Med. 2017;45(8):1344–51.

58. Kruklitis R, Tracy JA, McCambridge MM. Clinical and financial considerations for implementing an ICU telemedicine program. Chest. 2014;145(6):1392–6. https://doi.org/10.1378/chest.13-0868.

59. Franzini L, Sail KR, Thomas EJ, Wueste L. Costs and cost-effectiveness of a tele-ICU program in six intensive care units in a large healthcare system. J Crit Care. 2011;26(3):329.e1–6. https://doi.org/10.1016/j.jcrc.2010.12.004.

60. Kumar G, Falk DM, Bonello RS, Kahn JM, Perencevich E, Cram P. The costs of critical care telemedicine programs: a systematic review and analysis. Chest. 2013;143(1):19–29. https://doi.org/10.1378/chest.11-3031.

61. Lilly CM, Motzkus C, Rincon T, Cody SE, Landry K, Irwin RS. UMass Memorial Critical Care Operations Group. ICU telemedicine program financial outcomes. Chest. 2017;151(2):286–97. https://doi.org/10.1016/j.chest.2016.11.029.

62. Breslow MJ, Rosenfeld BA, Doerfler M, Burke G, Yates G, Stone DJ, Tomaszewicz P, Hochman R, Plocher DW. Effect of a multiple-site intensive care unit telemedicine program on clinical and economic outcomes: an alternative paradigm for intensivist staffing. Crit Care Med. 2004;32(1):31–8.

63. O'Shea AMJ, Sarrazin MV, Nassar B, Cram P, Johnson L, Bonello R, Panos RJ, Reisinger HS. Using electronic medical record notes to measure ICU telemedicine utilization. J Am Med Inform Assoc. 2017;24(5):969–74. https://doi.org/10.1093/jamia/ocx029.

Part VI

Precision Therapeutics

Lung Transplantation and Precision Medicine

22

Hanne Beeckmans, Berta Saez, Anke Van Herck,
Annelore Sacreas, Janne Kaes, Tobias Heigl,
Arno Vanstapel, Sofie Ordies, Anna E. Frick,
Stijn E. Verleden, Geert M. Verleden, Robin Vos,
and Bart M. Vanaudenaerde

Abbreviations

AATD	Alpha-1 antitrypsin deficiency
AFOP	Acute fibrinous and organizing pneumonia
ALAD	Acute lung allograft dysfunction
AMR	Antibody-mediated rejection
ARAD	Azithromycin responsive allograft dysfunction
ARDS	Acute respiratory distress syndrome
BAL	Bronchoalveolar lavage
BOS	Bronchiolitis obliterans syndrome
CF	Cystic fibrosis
CLAD	Chronic lung allograft dysfunction
COPD	Chronic obstructive pulmonary disease
CT	Computed tomography
DAD	Diffuse alveolar damage
DSA	Donor-specific antibodies
ECD	Extended-criteria donor
EVLP	Ex-vivo lung perfusion
FEV_1	Forced expiratory volume in 1 second
FiO_2	Fractional inspired oxygen
FVC	Forced vital capacity
HLA	Human leukocyte antigen
HRCT	High resolution computed tomography
ICU	Intensive care unit
IPF	Idiopathic pulmonary fibrosis
ISHLT	International Society of Heart and Lung Transplantation
LB	Lymphocytic bronchiolitis
MMF	Mycophenolate mofetil
NRAD	Neutrophilic reversible allograft dysfunction
OB	Obliterative bronchiolitis
PAH	Pulmonary arterial hypertension
PaO_2	Arterial partial pressure of oxygen
PEEP	Positive end-expiratory pressure
PGD	Primary graft dysfunction
PPFE	Pleuroparenchymal fibroelastosis
QoL	Quality of life
RAS	Restrictive allograft dysfunction

H. Beeckmans · B. Saez · A. Van Herck · A. Sacreas ·
J. Kaes · T. Heigl · A. Vanstapel · S. Ordies · A. E.
Frick · S. E. Verleden · G. M. Verleden · R. Vos
KU Leuven and University Hospitals Leuven,
Department of Chronic Diseases, Metabolism and
Ageing (CHROMETA), Division of Respiratory
Diseases, Lung Transplant Unit, Leuven, Belgium
e-mail: bsaez@vhebron.net;
anke.vanherck@kuleuven.be;
annelore.sacreas@kuleuven.be;
janne.kaes@kuleuven.be; tobias.heigl@kuleuven.be;
arno.vanstapel@kuleuven.be; sofie.ordies@kuleuven.be;
annaelisabeth.frick@uzleuven.be;
stijn.verleden@kuleuven.be;
geert.verleden@kuleuven.be; robin.vos@uzleuven.be

B. M. Vanaudenaerde (✉)
Department of Chronic Diseases, Metabolism and
Ageing (CHROMETA), Lab of Respiratory Diseases,
Lung Transplantation Unit, KU Leuven and UZ
Leuven, Leuven, Belgium
e-mail: bart.vanaudenaerde@kuleuven.be; bart.
vanaudenaerde@med.kuleuven.be

© Springer Nature Switzerland AG 2020
J. L. Gomez et al. (eds.), *Precision in Pulmonary, Critical Care, and Sleep Medicine*,
Respiratory Medicine, https://doi.org/10.1007/978-3-030-31507-8_22

r-CLAD   Restrictive chronic lung allograft
          dysfunction
SCD   Standard-criteria donor

Introduction

The history of lung transplantation starts in the 1940s: researchers tried to perform lung transplantation, initially in laboratory animals followed by human to human. Many of these early attempts were unsuccessful, and even after successful lung transplantation, most lungs were ultimately rejected despite the use of various immunosuppressants available at that time. The first human single lung transplantation was performed in 1963 by James Hardy in Mississippi, using the left lung of a circulatory death donor. The patient survived for 18 days before dying of renal failure. Over the next decade, many more lung transplantations were performed, with limited success: few patients survived over 2 weeks. At that time, the leading causes of death were peri-operative problems. Subsequent improvements in surgical techniques and especially the introduction of immunosuppressive drugs such as cyclosporin and tacrolimus resulted in rapid progress in the 1980s, with the first successful heart-lung

transplantation in 1981 in Stanford by Bruce Reitz and the first single lung transplantation in Toronto in 1983 by Joel Cooper [1]. The second successful lung transplantation from a circulatory death donor was reported by Steen [2]. These advances led to higher success rates and transplant centers all over the world started developing their programs. Today over 100 transplant centers in Europe and North America are active, although the majority of lung transplantations is still performed in a small number of highly specialized centers (see Fig. 22.1). As short-term survival improved substantially, more patients developed long-term complications [3]. These long-term complications compromised the initially increased quality of life (QoL) due to restored normal pulmonary function [4].

Nowadays, lung transplantation is an accepted therapeutic option for many end-stage lung diseases like chronic obstructive pulmonary disease (COPD), Alpha-1 antitrypsin deficiency (AATD), cystic fibrosis (CF), idiopathic pulmonary fibrosis (IPF), pulmonary fibrosis due to other causes (i.e. hypersensitivity pneumonitis, sarcoidosis, scleroderma, rheumatoid arthritis) and pulmonary arterial hypertension (PAH) [5]. There are four main types of lung transplantation; the choice of transplantation type depends on the indication, age, and patient characteris-

Fig. 22.1 Average center volume for lung transplantation (not including heart-lung transplants)

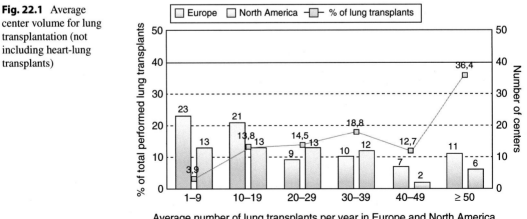

Average number of lung transplants per year in Europe and North America. Based on data from the International Society of Heart and Lung transplantation from January 2009 till June 2017

Table 22.1 Indications and contraindications for lung transplantation [13, 14]

Indications
Clinically and physiologically severe disease for which medical therapy is ineffective or unavailable
>50% risk of death from lung disease without transplantation within 2 years
>80% likelihood of surviving ≥90 days after lung transplantation
>80% predicted 5 years survival if preserved graft function
Absence of nonpulmonary medical comorbidity that would be expected to limit life expectancy substantially in the first 5 years after transplantation
Satisfactory psychosocial profile and support system
Contraindications
Absolute
Malignancy in the last 2 years
Uncontrolled or untreatable pulmonary or extrapulmonary infection
Active Mycobacterium tuberculosis infection
Significant dysfunction of other vital organs (e.g., heart, liver, kidney, and brain)
Significant coronary heart disease not amenable to revascularization
Uncorrectable bleeding diathesis
Significant chest wall/spinal deformity expected to cause severe restriction after transplantation
Active tobacco smoking
Drug or alcohol dependency
BMI ≥35 kg/m²
Unresolved psychosocial problems or noncompliance with medical therapy
Relative
Age > 65 years (if associated by other relative contraindications)
HIV infection
Ongoing hepatitis B or C viral infection
Colonization or infection with highly resistant or highly virulent bacteria, fungi, and certain strains of mycobacteria (e.g., in CF or bronchiectasis)
Extensive prior thoracic surgery with lung resection
Severe or progressive malnutrition
Severe, symptomatic osteoporosis
30 < BMI < 35 kg/m²
Absence of a consistent or reliable social support system

BMI body mass index, *HIV* human immunodeficiency virus, *CF* cystic fibrosis

tics. First, heart-lung transplantation is performed with the assistance of cardiopulmonary bypass, and mainly for pulmonary arterial hypertension. The second type is unilateral lung transplantation, which is increasingly rarer, where the least functional lung is replaced, mainly used for older pulmonary fibrosis or COPD patients. Third and most practiced, double lung transplantation, where both lungs are sequentially replaced by a donor lung, which can sometimes be performed without the use of a cardiopulmonary bypass. Finally, lobar lung transplantation is even more seldom performed than unilateral lung transplantation. For example, when young patients with CF undergo living donor lobar transplant from their parents in the event of lacking a suitable donor (living-related donor transplantation), or when there is a considerable size mismatch between a large donor and a small receptor. In 2016, the International Society of Heart and Lung Transplantation (ISHLT) reported 62 heart-lung transplantations, 3.748 bilateral lung transplantations, and 913 single lung transplantations.

Lung transplantation is not possible without donors. Due to the lack of experience, donor's lungs were initially selected very strictly [6]. However, over the last decade, with increased experience, leading transplant centers started to progressively use more donor lungs that do not fully meet these criteria, to make up for the shortage of lung donors [7, 8]. Also, the donor lung was initially preserved on ice, inducing cold ischemia, and consequently leading to damage of the donor lung. Some centers reported good results using ex-vivo lung perfusion (EVLP), in which the lung is perfused outside of the body [9, 10]. Immediately after lung transplantation, numerous complications can occur, varying from primary graft dysfunction (PGD), infection to acute rejection, among others. The major long-term complication still consists of gradually increasing shortness of breath, due to progressive deterioration of pulmonary function, known as chronic lung allograft dysfunction (CLAD). CLAD is regarded as the main limitation to long-term survival after lung transplantation, namely 57% 5-year survival, which is still limited compared to other solid organ transplantations (i.e., after kidney transplantation a 10-year all-cause graft failure of 51.6% is reported) [11, 12]. The best-studied phenotypes of CLAD are bronchiolitis obliterans syndrome (BOS) and restrictive allograft dysfunction (RAS).

This chapter will discuss the many specialized procedures involved in lung transplantation, starting with the selection of donors and recipients, care for the donor lung, acute complications, and their prevention; and finally the most pressing issue in lung transplantation today: CLAD.

Table 22.2 Standard-criteria lung donor [6]

Age < 55 years
ABO compatibility
Clear serial chest X-ray
Normal gas exchange (PaO$_2$ > 300 mm Hg on FiO$_2$ 1.0, PEEP 5 cm H$_2$O)
≤20-pack-year smoking history
Absence of chest trauma
No previous surgery on side(s) of harvest
No evidence of aspiration or sepsis
Absence of purulent secretions at bronchoscopy
Absence of organisms on sputum gram stain
Appropriate size match with prospective recipient

PaO$_2$ arterial partial pressure of oxygen, *FiO$_2$* fractional inspired oxygen, *PEEP* positive end-expiratory pressure

Surgical Issues

Lung transplantation is considered for patients with end-stage lung diseases who, despite maximal medical or surgical therapy, experience a decline in clinical status. This usually means patients who have a limited life expectancy over the next 2 years and are symptomatic during activities of daily living. Indications and contraindications for lung transplantation have been developed by the ISHLT and are listed in Table 22.1 [13, 14].

Not all organ donors are suitable to be lung donors. Strict criteria of the "standard-criteria lung donor" (SCD) have previously been defined; donors meeting these criteria are considered "ideal" (Table 22.2) [6]. Only 15–25% of all multi-organ donors are suitable for lung transplantation, due to injury from cardio-pulmonary resuscitation, lung contusion, airway aspiration, and pulmonary infection at the time of brain insult, as well as underlying lung disease [15]. This scarcity of suitable donor organs leads to persistent mortality of patients on the waiting list; and thus these criteria have been liberalized to "extended-criteria lung donors" (ECD) in order to increase the number of transplantable donor organs [7, 8]. ECD are lung donors not matching the strict criteria of an SCD, for example, because of pre-existing conditions, a smoking history of more than 20 pack-years or hepatitis, among others. There is no consensus about ECD, and multiple centers report different criteria [16–20]. This increase of transplantable lungs is associated with a negative impact on early outcome: prevalence of severe PGD, length of stay in intensive care unit (ICU) and duration of mechanical ventilation [16, 18]. There is still debate about whether the use of ECD lungs compromises long-term clinical outcomes [17–20]. Figure 22.2 shows the increased use of ECD lungs in lung transplantation [16].

Up till now, donor's lungs were mainly stored on ice; EVLP is an alternative to cold static lung preservation and a new form of isolated lung perfusion in normothermic conditions. It is achieved using a pump-driven perfusion machine that recirculates a preservation solution through the

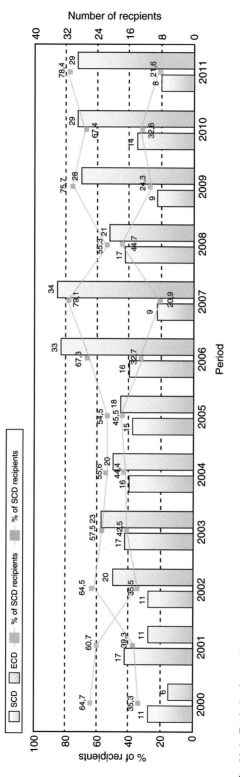

Fig. 22.2 Evolution in numbers and percentage of extended-criteria lung donors [16]. SCD standard-criteria donor, ECD extended-criteria lung donor

vasculature of the lung in addition to protective mechanical ventilation. The main potential benefit is, in the first place, longer storage time (up to 18 hours, compared to cold storage preservation, which can only preserve the lung up to 6 hours) and the resultant optimization of logistics for lung transplantation [9, 10]. Secondly, the possibility of reconditioning the lung and, therefore, the possibility of transplantation of lungs that otherwise would not be used [21–25]. However, in several centers, many of the lungs initially not considered transplantable are already transplanted as an ECD lung without the use of EVLP, with comparable results in large experienced centers [16, 26]. Thus, clinical trials still have to demonstrate if the potential advantages weigh against the costs of the EVLP.

Another new development in lung transplantation is the use of extracorporeal lung support, which can be utilized to bridge deteriorating patients to lung transplantation. This is not a commonly used technique, although there are promising results, with bridging up to 140 days, which could reduce mortality on the waiting list [27–30].

Acute Lung Allograft Dysfunction

Every lung transplantation patient receives lifelong treatment with immunosuppressive drugs in order to avoid rejection of the graft by the immune system. Standard maintenance therapy consists of triple-drug therapy, including a calcineurin inhibitor (cyclosporin or tacrolimus), an antiproliferative agent (azathioprine or mycophenolate mofetil (MMF)) and a corticosteroid (e.g., prednisolone), although protocols may vary from center to center [31].

In the years after transplantation, patients may develop an acute deterioration of pulmonary function status, with a rapid increase in shortness of breath. This is known as acute lung allograft dysfunction (ALAD). Many conditions causing ALAD are known and can be treated, after which the FEV_1 and forced vital capacity (FVC) should usually restore to baseline values. If, however, the pulmonary function decline is not restored to

>90% of baseline and maintains for at least 3 weeks, CLAD may be suspected [32].

First, primary graft dysfunction (PGD) is a common complication that occurs immediately after lung transplantation, resulting in acute failure of the graft. In the past, it was also referred to as ischemia-reperfusion injury, early graft dysfunction, primary graft failure or re-implantation edema. PGD occurs within the first 72 hours after lung transplantation and is characterized by severe hypoxemia, lung edema with diffuse alveolar damage and radiographic evidence of diffuse pulmonary infiltration without other identifiable cause (Fig. 22.3). The radiographic and histological findings resemble acute respiratory distress syndrome (ARDS) [33–37]. Several harmful events may contribute to the development of PGD, such as prolonged mechanical ventilation, prolonged warm ischemia, cold ischemia during storage in cold preservation solution, reperfusion, and peri-operative insults. Several risk factors exist and are summarized up in Table 22.3 [38–40]. This complication leads to prolonged length of mechanical ventilation, prolonged ICU stays, prolonged hospital stay and even increased short-term mortality, but may also have an impact on long-term survival, as it might impact the later development of BOS, a phenotype of CLAD [41–45]. This long-term impact may, however, be modified by accurate treatment. Only supportive

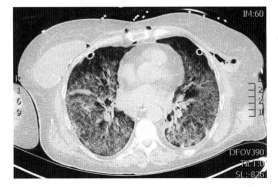

Fig. 22.3 CT at 72 hours posttransplantation of a patient diagnosed with PGD. PGD scores were 1, 3, and 2 at 24, 48, and 72 hours of posttransplantation, respectively, according to the ISHLT grading system of PGD [37]. CT computed tomography, PGD primary graft dysfunction, ISHLT International Society for Heart and Lung Transplantation

Table 22.3 Risk factors for development of primary graft dysfunction [38–40]

Donor-related factors
Donor smoking (especially >20 pack years)
Operative-related factors
Single-lung transplant
Prolonged cold ischemic time
High fractional inspired oxygen upon reperfusion
Poly-transfusion
Intracellular type preservation solutions
Use of cardiopulmonary bypass
Recipient-related factors
BMI ≥ 25
Sarcoidosis
IPF
Primary PAH
Increased pulmonary arterial pressures

BMI body mass index, *IPF* idiopathic pulmonary fibrosis, *PAH* pulmonary arterial hypertension

Table 22.4 Category of infections in function of time [50]

First post-operative month
Infections with microbes present in the donor or recipient
Nosocomial infections
Infections related to technical problems (e.g., catheter infections)
1–6 months after transplantation
Opportunistic infections
Reactivation of latent infections
6 months or more after transplantation
Infections due to community-acquired pathogens

treatment is available for PGD, including lung-protective ventilation, restrictive fluid balance, inhaled nitric oxide (iNO), and finally extracorporeal membrane oxygenation (ECMO) [38, 46–48]. No preventive treatment options have proven to be effective, and retransplantation can be considered, but predicted survival in this setting is poor, and therefore retransplantation for severe PGD is not recommended [49].

Moreover, as a result of the mandatory lifelong immunosuppression and its resultant immune system impairment, lung transplant patients are more vulnerable to infectious agents, both bacterial, viral and fungal [50]. Infection should therefore always be excluded before a diagnosis of acute allograft rejection is made [51]. There are four main clinical scenarios resulting in an infection in a lung transplant patient. First of all, recipients can host infections from a wide range of microorganisms prior to transplantation (especially patients with CF). Second, colonization with nosocomial organisms occurs frequently during hospitalization. Third, lung grafts could transfer infections from donors to recipients. Finally, transplanted patients are, as previously mentioned, more prone to severe community-acquired or nosocomial infections with relatively innocuous infectious [52]. Time affects which type of infection a lung transplant patient can develop (Table 22.4) [50]. However, infections are more difficult to diagnose in lung transplant patients as classic symptoms such as fever, loss of appetite, fatigue, chills, night sweats and pain may be unremarkable or absent, whereas white blood cell count is commonly altered due to immunosuppressive therapy; also, loss of lung function may be observed in lung infection but is also a common trait in acute and chronic rejection. The main technical investigations that should be undertaken to diagnose an infection and differentiate between infection and rejection are a bronchoalveolar lavage (BAL) with culture, transbronchial biopsies and chest computed tomography (CT).

Another frequent complication is acute lung allograft rejection, especially during the first year after lung transplantation, which does not cause mortality per se is frequently treatable with a short pulse of IV steroids. However, mortality should not be neglected as 3.6% of deaths among adult lung transplant recipients within the first 30 days, respectively, and 1.8% up to 1-year posttransplant are attributable to acute rejection. Twenty-nine percent of adult patients experience at least one episode of treated acute rejection between discharge from the hospital and 1-year follow-up after transplant [51, 53]. This complication should not be underestimated as patients who suffer one or more episodes of acute rejection already have a higher risk for later CLAD [51]. Symptoms are nonspecific and may include cough, dyspnea, fever, leukocytosis, and an increased alveolar-

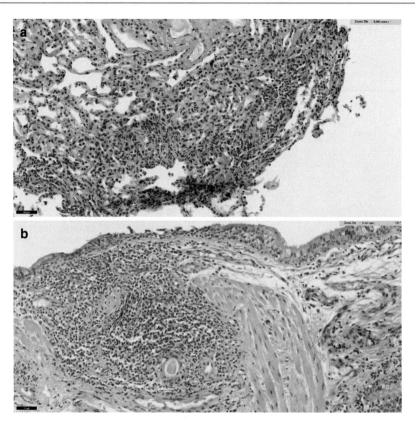

Fig. 22.4 Histopathological findings in patients with acute lung allograft rejection [55]. (**a**) Minimal acute cellular rejection (grade A1, ×40). The hallmark feature of acute cellular rejection is the presence of truly circumferential perivascular cellular infiltrates around blood vessels in the alveolar parenchyma, particularly small veins. These perivascular cuffs consist of mononuclear cells, two to three cells in thickness. Eosinophililic infiltration, endothelialitis or expansion of the cellular infiltrate into the alveolar septa is absent in minimal acute rejection. (**b**) High-grade lymphocytic bronchiolitis (grade B2R). The lamina propria contains a prominent infiltrate of activated lymphocytes; admixed with some plasmacytoid cells, neutrophils, and eosinophils. This mononuclear infiltrate extends into the epithelium, with the presence of prominent intra-epithelial lymphocytes. The overlying epithelium further shows signs of epithelial damage, evidenced by necrosis and apoptosis. (Representative pictures from selected cases from the KULeuven Lung Transplant Unit)

arterial oxygen gradient. High resolution computed tomography (HRCT) of the chest may show ground-glass opacities and septal thickening, which are nonspecific features [54]. Risk factors for acute rejection are genetic predisposition, human leukocyte antigen (HLA) mismatch and the type of immunosuppressive treatment [54]. Transbronchial biopsies remain the gold standard for diagnosis of acute allograft rejection and to discriminate it from aspiration, infection, drug toxicity, or recurrent disease [51]. There are different types of acute lung allograft rejection, first the classic and most frequent form of acute lung allograft rejection:

acute cellular rejection, which is divided into A-grade rejection and B-grade rejection: lymphocytic bronchiolitis (LB). A-grade rejection is characterized by perivascular rejection and is mediated by T lymphocytes that recognize foreign HLAs or other antigens. Transbronchial biopsy displays perivascular and interstitial mononuclear cell infiltrates (Fig. 22.4a), whereas BAL presents elevated lymphocyte and neutrophil counts [54]. LB is considered an acute rejection of the small airways mediated by T-lymphocytes, peribronchial mononuclear cell infiltration and sometimes epithelial damage of the airways can be observed on concurrent transbronchial biopsies (Fig. 22.4b) [55]. Second, antibody-mediated rejection (AMR), which is a rejection of the allograft by the production of antibodies directed to donor HLA molecules [56]. These antibodies may be formed prior to transplantation or de novo. Findings on transbronchial biopsies are mostly non-specific: capillary inflammation and acute lung injury, with or without diffuse alveolar damage (DAD) and endothelialitis, sometimes with evidence of endothelial capillary complement 4d staining. In addition to clinical findings and transbronchial biopsies, diagnosis of AMR can be suspected when donor-specific antibodies (DSA) are found in the blood [51, 57]. Also, there is a form of AMR known as hyperacute rejection, which occurs minutes to hours after transplantation and is mediated by preformed antibodies directed toward donor HLA and ABO molecules [58].

Another cause of ALAD is azithromycin responsive allograft dysfunction (ARAD), which was previously also referred to as neutrophilic reversible allograft dysfunction (NRAD) or azithromycin responsive BOS [32]. It is characterized by active inflammatory lesions, and transbronchial biopsy is characterized by a prominent peribronchiolar infiltrate of mononuclear cells (macrophages and lymphocytes), while BAL often presents excess neutrophilia. This phenotype is important to recognize as it is treatable with azithromycin: after 3–6 months of azithromycin therapy, the forced expiratory volume in 1 second (FEV$_1$) decline may be reversible (defined as an FEV$_1$ and/or FVC increase to >90% of the best posttransplant values). HRCT typically shows air trapping, tree-in-bud opacities and peribronchiolar infiltrates, of which the last two features may improve after azithromycin therapy [32, 59, 60]. Apart from treating ARAD, azithromycin may also prevent it [61]. On the other hand, some patients do not respond to azithromycin therapy, with persistent shortness of breath and BAL neutrophilia. This azithromycin resistant neutrophilia compromises survival and is a risk factor for later CLAD [62].

Other causes of ALAD can be capillary leak syndrome, anastomotic problems (e.g., dehiscence of bronchial anastomoses) and pulmonary embolism, among others. Infection and allograft rejection remain, however, the leading cause of rehospitalization after lung transplant (Fig. 22.5).

Fig. 22.5 Rehospitalisation post lung transplant. This figure shows the hospitalizations reported on the 1-year, 3-year, and 5-year follow-up. All follow-ups between January 2009 and June 2017 were included. (Based on data from the International Society of Heart and Lung Transplantation)

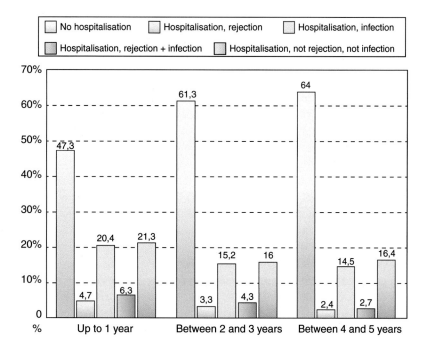

Chronic Lung Allograft Dysfunction

This part will mainly focus on the causes of long-term deterioration of pulmonary function, but one has to keep in mind that due to the chronic use of immunosuppressive drugs, lung transplant patients have an increased risk to develop malignant conditions (e.g., lymphoproliferative disorder), infections, or other complications (e.g., increased cardiovascular risk, kidney failure, among others).

CLAD is a term that encompasses chronic lung dysfunction after transplantation that is not explained by other conditions. CLAD is defined as a persistent (at least 3 weeks), often progressive, decline in pulmonary function (FEV$_1$ with/without FVC) $\geq 20\%$ from baseline (baseline defined as the average of the two best posttransplant values for FEV$_1$ and FVC obtained at least 3 weeks apart) [32, 63]. Potential CLAD is defined as a persistent (at least 3 weeks), otherwise unexplained decline in pulmonary function $\geq 10\%$ from baseline. Potential CLAD should always trigger an in-depth investigation of possible causes of pulmonary function decline, including blood sampling (HLA-antibodies, infection parameters), full pulmonary function testing (measurement of total lung capacity (TLC) and residual volume (RV), in addition to spirometry), transbronchial biopsy specimen analysis, BAL with total and differential cell count, and chest HRCT with inspiratory and expiratory imaging. If no cause is found, trial therapy with azithromycin should be started to differentiate between CLAD and ARAD (see Fig. 22.6) [32, 63]. Definite CLAD is a term used when all other causes are treated or excluded, azithromycin trial therapy was not or only partially successful, and lung allograft dysfunction continues for at least 3 months [63]. CLAD is a common long-term complication, its prevalence increasing over post lung transplantation time (Fig. 22.7) [11].

There are several different terms in the literature: CLAD, BOS, chronic rejection, and obliterative bronchiolitis (OB) are used interchangeably, which needs clarification. OB is a histopathologic term that was the main finding

initially described in autopsies from patients who were believed to have died of chronic rejection. Because of the clinical need for a clinical definition instead of a histological one, the term bronchiolitis obliterans syndrome (BOS) was proposed, which was defined by spirometry by Cooper et al. [64]. A few years ago, more and more patients with an FEV$_1$-decline associated with a restrictive pulmonary defect were reported, which led to the introduction of restrictive allograft syndrome (RAS) [65]. CLAD should not be used as a synonym for BOS or RAS, but includes all cases of BOS and RAS and mixed phenotypes of RAS and BOS. CLAD encompasses multiple causes of chronic lung dysfunction and is therefore also no synonym for chronic rejection.

Thus, CLAD is an umbrella term, not a final diagnosis. Furthermore, before the use of the term CLAD, other causes of a decreased pulmonary function must be excluded, and reversibility after azithromycin must be assessed. Therefore, potential CLAD patients should be thoroughly investigated to find a specific cause of persistent decreased pulmonary function. There are several non-CLAD causes of pulmonary function decline (previously referred to as non-BOS, non-RAS CLAD) [32]. These can be either allograft-related (persistent infection, persistent acute rejection, anastomotic strictures, disease recurrence) or non-allograft-related (pleural disorders, diaphragmatic dysfunction, obesity, ascites, and chronic kidney failure, among others), or a combination of both. Despite the possibility of specific treatment, patients with identifiable causes of chronic pulmonary function decline show equally decreased survival compared to BOS or RAS [32, 66].

When no specific cause is found, and the FEV$_1$ decline is not only persistent but also purely obstructive (FEV$_1$/FVC < 0.70, with no drop in TLC) the term BOS should be used to describe this clinical phenotype (Fig. 22.8a). BOS accounts for approximately 70% of CLAD patients [65, 67]. Histopathological reports from transbronchial biopsies and autopsy specimens show fibrotic lesions of the bronchioles, known as OB lesions, with sur-

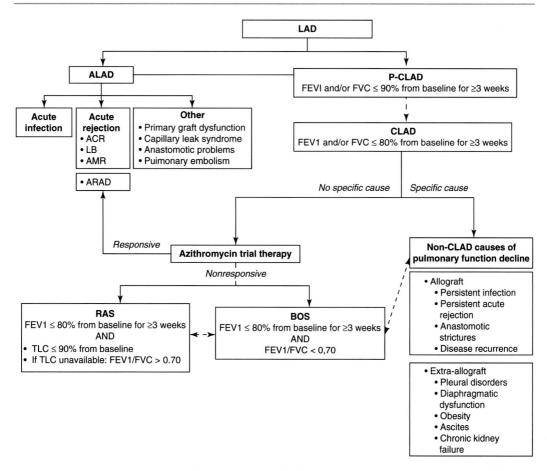

Fig. 22.6 Diagnosis of chronic lung allograft dysfunction [32]. In the case of suspected CLAD, all other causes of a decrease in FEV1 should be excluded. If no cause is found, a trial therapy with azithromycin should be started. If a patient is responsive (defined as an improvement in FEV1 with ≥10% after 3–6 months azithromycin), this phenotype is referred to as ARAD. If a patient is nonresponsive, further investigations should differentiate between BOS and RAS. LAD lung allograft dysfunction, FEV_1 forced expiratory volume in 1 second, FVC forced vital capacity, TLC total lung capacity, ALAD acute lung allograft dysfunction, CLAD chronic lung allograft dysfunction, P-CLAD potential chronic lung allograft dysfunction, ACR acute cellular rejection, LB lymphocytic bronchiolitis, AMR antibody-mediated rejection, ARAD azithromycin responsive allograft dysfunction, RAS restrictive allograft syndrome, BOS bronchiolitis obliterans syndrome

rounding normal parenchyma, as well as collapse lesions [68, 69]. HRCT changes, like air trapping with or without bronchiectasis, can be observed (Fig. 22.8b). There should be no persistent infiltrates on HRCT. In contrast to ARAD, BOS is not fully responsive to azithromycin therapy [32].

A persistent FEV_1 decline with no specific cause, accompanied by a persistent decline in TLC (>10% compared to baseline) is defined as restrictive allograft syndrome (RAS) (Fig. 22.8c), also referred to as restrictive CLAD (r-CLAD).

RAS accounts for approximately 30% of CLAD [65, 67]. When TLC is not available, FEV_1/FVC can be used as a surrogate marker ($FEV_1/FVC > 0.70$). RAS has a lower survival rate compared to BOS, and the cause of this poor prognosis is unclear [32, 70]. Histopathology obtained from explanted lungs shows pleural and septal thickening and parenchymal fibrosis in the lung periphery [65]. HRCT demonstrates changes such as interstitial opacities, ground-glass opacities, upper lobe dominant fibrosis, and honeycombing (Fig. 22.8d) [32]. The RAS phenotype is still a very heterogeneous entity, and there are no clear-cut guidelines for diagnosis. As a result, there is some overlap with other (histological) phenotypes, such as acute fibrinous and organizing pneumonia (AFOP), pleuroparenchymal fibroelastosis (PPFE) and diffuse alveolar damage (DAD). There is still debate whether these phenotypes are pathological subtypes of RAS or represent separate clinical entities [71].

These CLAD subtypes are not permanent, and there may be some overlap: some patients initially display a typical FEV_1 decline compatible with BOS, but may subsequently develop the RAS phenotype. The frequency of each subtype

Fig. 22.7 Kaplan Meier CLAD curve after lung transplantation. Lung transplantations performed from January 2004 till December 2015 in UZ Leuven, Belgium were included. CLAD chronic lung allograft dysfunction, LTx lung transplantation

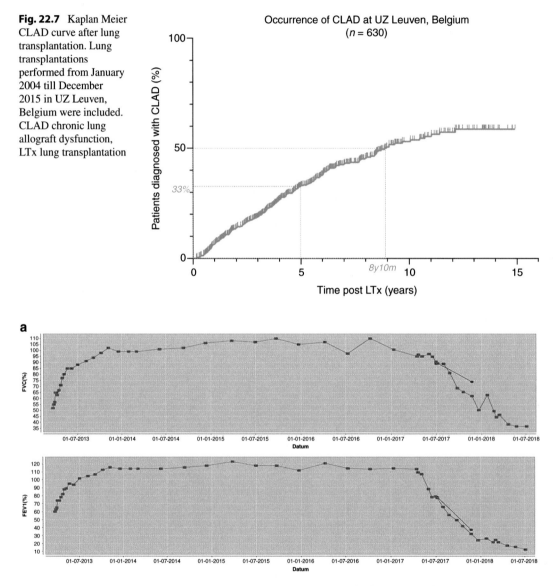

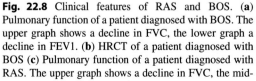

Fig. 22.8 Clinical features of RAS and BOS. (**a**) Pulmonary function of a patient diagnosed with BOS. The upper graph shows a decline in FVC, the lower graph a decline in FEV1. (**b**) HRCT of a patient diagnosed with BOS (**c**) Pulmonary function of a patient diagnosed with RAS. The upper graph shows a decline in FVC, the middle graph a decline in FEV1 and the lower graph a decline in TLC. (**d**) HRCT of a patient diagnosed with RAS. BOS bronchiolitis obliterans syndrome, FVC forced vital capacity, FEV1 forced expiratory volume in 1 second, HRCT high resolution computed tomography, RAS restrictive allograft syndrome, TLC total lung capacity

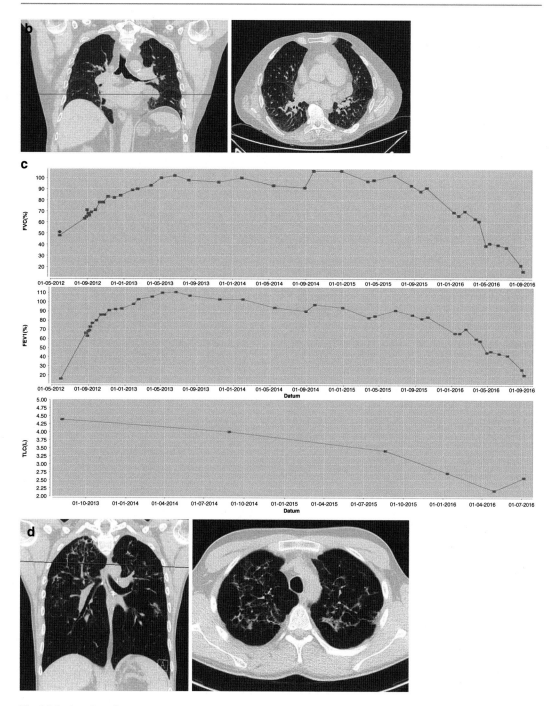

Fig. 22.8 (continued)

can be found in Fig. 22.9. Development of persistent parenchymal infiltrates on HRCT seems predictive of the conversion from BOS to RAS, even when initially the pulmonary function status is not consistent with a restrictive pattern. Likewise, some patients may first develop RAS, but end up with the classical BOS phenotype after the resolution of their infiltrates. Table 22.5 shows an overview of the key features of the phenotypes of CLAD [32]. Many factors may contribute to the development of CLAD. Reported risk factors for RAS and BOS seem fairly similar and are summed up in Table 22.6 [72–74].

As mentioned before, every lung transplant patient receives life-long treatment with immunosuppressive drugs in order to avoid graft rejection [31]. Treatment of CLAD by increasing or shifting immunosuppression (cyclosporin to tacrolimus, azathioprine to mycophenolate) and/ or steroids results at best in a temporary slowing the decline of pulmonary function [75, 76]. The

addition of azithromycin may improve lung function in a subset of CLAD patients (mainly the BOS phenotype), even if they were not fully responsive to azithromycin therapy before, due to various anti-inflammatory and immunomodulatory properties, mainly targeting neutrophils [77–79]. There is also evidence that prophylactic azithromycin initiated at discharge post lung transplantation can reduce CLAD prevalence and improve CLAD-free survival and pulmonary function [79, 80]. Also, several new therapies have been introduced, which may attenuate CLAD progression: total lymphoid irradiation (TLI), extracorporeal photophoresis (ECP), fundoplication, mTOR inhibitors, montelukast (a leukotriene receptor antagonist), and pirfenidone [81–88]. Whether it may be beneficial to lower immunosuppressive therapy, a therapeutic approach already practiced in other solid organ transplantation patients, e.g., kidney transplantation patients, remains elusive [89–92].

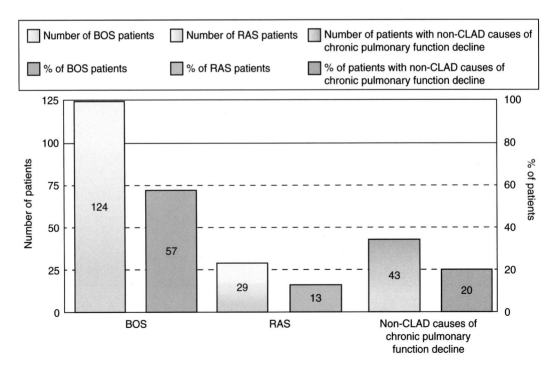

Fig. 22.9 Prevalence of causes of chronic pulmonary function decline [66]. CLAD chronic lung allograft dysfunction, RAS restrictive allograft syndrome, BOS bronchiolitis obliterans syndrome

Table 22.5 Key features of the main phenotypes of chronic lung allograft dysfunction [32]

Entity	Classic BOS	RAS
Pulmonary function	Obstructive (FEV$_1$/FVC < 0.70)	Restrictive (TLC ≤ 90% of stable baseline value) and/or FEV$_1$/FVC > 0.70
	FEV$_1$ ≤ 80% of stable baseline value	FEV$_1$ decline ≤80% of stable baseline value
HRCT thoracic imaging	No/minimal infiltrates	Infiltrates usually present
	Air trapping usually present	With/without air trapping
	With/without bronchiectasis	With/without bronchiectasis
Histopathology	OB (difficult to diagnose by transbronchial biopsy specimen)	Parenchymal/pleural fibrosis with/without OB
Clinical course	Typically progressive but may stabilize	Tends to be relentlessly progressive
	May evolve to RAS	May start as or coincide with BOS
	Recipients may have coexistent chronic bacterial infection	
Other	Usually responds poorly to pharmacologic therapies	Correlates with the presence of early diffuse alveolar damage posttransplant

BOS bronchiolitis obliterans syndrome, *RAS* restrictive allograft syndrome, *FEV$_1$* forced expiratory volume in 1 second, *FVC* forced vital capacity, *TLC* total lung capacity, *OB* obliterative bronchiolitis

Table 22.6 Risk factors for RAS and BOS [72–74]

Allo-immune dependent risk factors
Acute allograft rejection
Acute cellular rejection –A-grade
Acute antibody mediated rejection
Lymphocytic bronchiolitis
Azithromycin responsive allograft dysfunction
HLA mismatch
Allo-immune independent risk factors
Primary graft dysfunction
Gastroesophageal reflux and microaspiration
Infection and colonization
Viral
Bacterial
Fungal
Persistent neutrophil influx and sequestration (elevated BAL neutrophilia)
Airway eosinophilia (elevated BAL eosinophilia)
Recipient age
Donor age
Autoimmunity (e.g., collagen V sensitization)
Ischemic time
Air pollution
Genetic factors

BOS bronchiolitis obliterans syndrome, *RAS* restrictive allograft syndrome, *BAL* bronchoalveolar lavage

Conclusion

Lung transplantation is a life-saving intervention in patients with advanced lung disease. Although the technical aspects of the procedure have evolved significantly since the earlier days of the technique, the main challenge to precision and long-term survival after lung transplantation is the recognition and management of CLAD. Prevention of CLAD is an important approach as therapeutic strategies have been largely unsuccessful. CLAD, however, covers different phenotypes, with different pathophysiological mechanisms and different clinical characteristics. Specifically tailored therapeutic regimes have yet to be developed. Nevertheless, lung transplantation is moving forward: with more and more experience in all centers, survival is improving (Fig. 22.10) and will hopefully soon reach the level of other solid organ transplantations.

Fig. 22.10 Kaplan Meier Survival curve after lung transplantation. Lung transplantations performed in UZ Leuven, Belgium from July 1991 till December 2018 in the KU Leuven Lung Transplant Unit were included

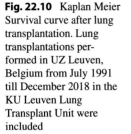
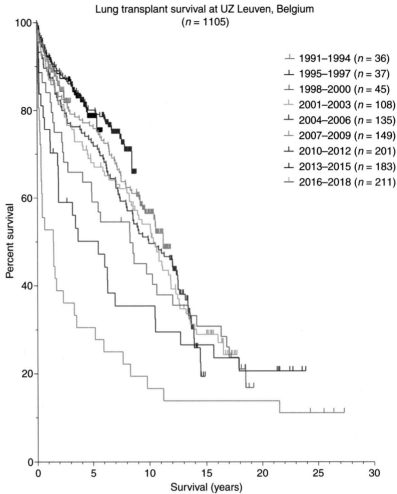

Lung transplant survival at UZ Leuven, Belgium
(n = 1105)

⊥ 1991–1994 (n = 36)
⊥ 1995–1997 (n = 37)
⊥ 1998–2000 (n = 45)
⊥ 2001–2003 (n = 108)
⊥ 2004–2006 (n = 135)
⊥ 2007–2009 (n = 149)
⊥ 2010–2012 (n = 201)
⊥ 2013–2015 (n = 183)
⊥ 2016–2018 (n = 211)

References

1. Benfield JR, Wain JC. The history of lung transplantation. Chest Surg Clin N Am. 2000;10:189–99, xi.
2. Steen S, Sjöberg T, Pierre L, et al. Transplantation of lungs from a non-heart-beating donor. Lancet. 2001;357:825–9.
3. Burke CM, Theodore J, Baldwin JC, et al. Twenty-eight cases of human heart-lung transplantation. Lancet. 1986;1:517–9.
4. Theodore J, Jamieson SW, Burke CM, et al. Physiologic aspects of human heart-lung transplantation. Pulmonary function status of the post-transplanted lung. Chest. 1984;86:349–57.
5. Yusen RD, Edwards LB, Kucheryavaya AY, et al. The registry of the International Society for Heart and Lung Transplantation: thirty-first adult lung and heart-lung transplant report--2014; focus theme: retransplantation. J Heart Lung Transplant. 2014;33:1009–24.
6. Frost AE. Donor criteria and evaluation. Clin Chest Med. 1997;18:231–7.
7. Wille KM, Harrington KF, deAndrade JA, et al. Disparities in lung transplantation before and after introduction of the lung allocation score. J Heart Lung Transplant. 2013;32:684–92.
8. Van Raemdonck D, Neyrinck A, Verleden GM, et al. Lung donor selection and management. Proc Am Thorac Soc. 2009;6:28–38.
9. Ceulemans LJ, Monbaliu D, Verslype C, et al. Combined liver and lung transplantation with extended normothermic lung preservation in a patient with end-stage emphysema complicated by drug-induced acute liver failure. Am J Transplant. 2014;14:2412–6.
10. Cypel M, Yeung JC, Hirayama S, et al. Technique for prolonged normothermic ex vivo lung perfusion. J Heart Lung Transplant. 2008;27:1319–25.
11. Chambers DC, Yusen RD, Cherikh WS, et al. The registry of the International Society for Heart and

Lung Transplantation: thirty-fourth adult lung and heart-lung transplantation report-2017; focus theme: allograft ischemic time. J Heart Lung Transplant. 2017;36:1047–59.

12. Hart A, Smith JM, Skeans MA, et al. OPTN/SRTR 2016 annual data report: kidney. Am J Transplant. 2018;18(Suppl 1):18–113.

13. Weill D, Benden C, Corris PA, et al. A consensus document for the selection of lung transplant candidates: 2014--an update from the Pulmonary Transplantation Council of the International Society for Heart and Lung Transplantation. J Heart Lung Transplant. 2015;34:1–15.

14. Nathan SD. Lung transplantation: disease-specific considerations for referral. Chest. 2005;127:1006–16.

15. Kotloff RM, Thabut G. Lung transplantation. Am J Respir Crit Care Med. 2011;184:159–71.

16. Somers J, Ruttens D, Verleden SE, et al. A decade of extended-criteria lung donors in a single center: was it justified? Transpl Int. 2015;28:170–9.

17. Smits JM, van der Bij W, Van Raemdonck D, et al. Defining an extended criteria donor lung: an empirical approach based on the Eurotransplant experience. Transpl Int. 2011;24:393–400.

18. Schiavon M, Falcoz P-E, Santelmo N, et al. Does the use of extended criteria donors influence early and long-term results of lung transplantation? Interact Cardiovasc Thorac Surg. 2012;14:183–7.

19. Bittle GJ, Sanchez PG, Kon ZN, et al. The use of lung donors older than 55 years: a review of the United Network of Organ sharing database. J Heart Lung Transplant. 2013;32:760–8.

20. Carrier M, Lizé J-F. Québec-Transplant Programs. Impact of expanded-criteria donors on patient survival after heart, lung, liver and combined organ transplantation. Transplant Proc. 2012;44:2231–4.

21. Ingemansson R, Eyjolfsson A, Mared L, et al. Clinical transplantation of initially rejected donor lungs after reconditioning ex vivo. Ann Thorac Surg. 2009;87:255–60.

22. Fildes JE, Archer LD, Blaikley J, et al. Clinical outcome of patients transplanted with marginal donor lungs via ex vivo lung perfusion compared to standard lung transplantation. Transplantation. 2015;99:1078–83.

23. Cypel M, Keshavjee S. Extending the donor pool: rehabilitation of poor organs. Thorac Surg Clin. 2015;25:27–33.

24. Cypel M, Rubacha M, Yeung J, et al. Normothermic ex vivo perfusion prevents lung injury compared to extended cold preservation for transplantation. Am J Transplant. 2009;9:2262–9.

25. Cypel M, Yeung JC, Liu M, et al. Normothermic ex vivo lung perfusion in clinical lung transplantation. N Engl J Med. 2011;364:1431–40.

26. De Vleeschauwer SI, Wauters S, Dupont LJ, et al. Medium-term outcome after lung transplantation is comparable between brain-dead and cardiac-dead donors. J Heart Lung Transplant. 2011;30:975–81.

27. Bartosik W, Egan JJ, Wood AE. The Novalung interventional lung assist as bridge to lung transplantation for self-ventilating patients - initial experience. Interact Cardiovasc Thorac Surg. 2011;13:198–200.

28. Hoetzenecker K, Donahoe L, Yeung JC, et al. Extracorporeal life support as a bridge to lung transplantation-experience of a high-volume transplant center. J Thorac Cardiovasc Surg. 2018;155:1316–1328.e1.

29. Vasanthan V, Garg M, Maruyama M, et al. Extended bridge to heart and lung transplantation using pumpless extracorporeal lung assist. Can J Cardiol. 2017;33:950.e11–3.

30. Mayes J, Niranjan G, Dark J, et al. Bridging to lung transplantation for severe pulmonary hypertension using dual central Novalung lung assist devices. Interact Cardiovasc Thorac Surg. 2016;22:677–8.

31. Scheffert JL, Raza K. Immunosuppression in lung transplantation. J Thorac Dis. 2014;6:1039–53.

32. Verleden GM, Raghu G, Meyer KC, et al. A new classification system for chronic lung allograft dysfunction. J Heart Lung Transplant. 2014;33:127–33.

33. Sato M, Hwang DM, Ohmori-Matsuda K, et al. Revisiting the pathologic finding of diffuse alveolar damage after lung transplantation. J Heart Lung Transplant. 2012;31:354–63.

34. Castro CY. ARDS and diffuse alveolar damage: a pathologist's perspective. Semin Thorac Cardiovasc Surg. 2006;18:13–9.

35. Snell GI, Yusen RD, Weill D, et al. Report of the ISHLT Working Group on Primary Lung Graft Dysfunction, part I: definition and grading-A 2016 Consensus Group statement of the International Society for Heart and Lung Transplantation. J Heart Lung Transplant. 2017;36:1097–103.

36. Christie J, Keshavjee S, Orens J, et al. Potential refinements of the International Society for Heart and Lung Transplantation primary graft dysfunction grading system. J Heart Lung Transplant. 2008;27:138.

37. Christie JD, Van Raemdonck D, de Perrot M, et al. Report of the ISHLT Working Group on Primary Lung Graft Dysfunction part I: introduction and methods. J Heart Lung Transplant. 2005;24:1451–3.

38. Suzuki Y, Cantu E, Christie JD. Primary graft dysfunction. Semin Respir Crit Care Med. 2013;34:305–19.

39. Shah RJ, Diamond JM, Cantu E, et al. Objective estimates improve risk stratification for primary graft dysfunction after lung transplantation. Am J Transplant. 2015;15:2188–96.

40. Diamond JM, Lee JC, Kawut SM, et al. Clinical risk factors for primary graft dysfunction after lung transplantation. Am J Respir Crit Care Med. 2013;187:527–34.

41. Christie JD, Kotloff RM, Ahya VN, et al. The effect of primary graft dysfunction on survival after lung transplantation. Am J Respir Crit Care Med. 2005;171:1312–6.

42. Lee JC, Christie JD. Primary graft dysfunction. Clin Chest Med. 2011;32:279–93.

43. Whitson BA, Prekker ME, Herrington CS, et al. Primary graft dysfunction and long-term pulmonary function after lung transplantation. J Heart Lung Transplant. 2007;26:1004–11.

44. Daud SA, Yusen RD, Meyers BF, et al. Impact of immediate primary lung allograft dysfunction on bronchiolitis obliterans syndrome. Am J Respir Crit Care Med. 2007;175:507–13.

45. Fiser SM, Tribble CG, Long SM, et al. Ischemia-reperfusion injury after lung transplantation increases risk of late bronchiolitis obliterans syndrome. Ann Thorac Surg. 2002;73:1041–7; discussion 1047–8.

46. Lee JC, Christie JD. Primary graft dysfunction. Proc Am Thorac Soc. 2009;6:39–46.

47. Bermudez CA, Adusumilli PS, McCurry KR, et al. Extracorporeal membrane oxygenation for primary graft dysfunction after lung transplantation: long-term survival. Ann Thorac Surg. 2009;87:854–60.

48. Vlasselaers D, Verleden GM, Meyns B, et al. Femoral venoarterial extracorporeal membrane oxygenation for severe reimplantation response after lung transplantation. Chest. 2000;118:559–61.

49. Novick RJ, Stitt LW, Al-Kattan K, et al. Pulmonary retransplantation: predictors of graft function and survival in 230 patients. Pulmonary retransplant registry. Ann Thorac Surg. 1998;65:227–34.

50. Nosotti M, Tarsia P, Morlacchi LC. Infections after lung transplantation. J Thorac Dis. 2018;10:3849–68.

51. Roden AC, Aisner DL, Allen TC, et al. Diagnosis of acute cellular rejection and antibody-mediated rejection on lung transplant biopsies: a perspective from members of the pulmonary pathology society. Arch Pathol Lab Med. 2017;141:437–44.

52. Fishman JA. Infection in solid-organ transplant recipients. N Engl J Med. 2007;357:2601–14.

53. Yusen RD, Edwards LB, Kucheryavaya AY, et al. The registry of the International Society for Heart and Lung Transplantation: thirty-second official adult lung and heart-lung transplantation report--2015; focus theme: early graft failure. J Heart Lung Transplant. 2015;34:1264–77.

54. De Vito Dabbs A, Hoffman LA, Iacono AT, et al. Are symptom reports useful for differentiating between acute rejection and pulmonary infection after lung transplantation? Heart Lung. 2004;33:372–80.

55. Stewart S, Fishbein MC, Snell GI, et al. Revision of the 1996 working formulation for the standardization of nomenclature in the diagnosis of lung rejection. J Heart Lung Transplant. 2007;26:1229–42.

56. Loupy A, Lefaucheur C. Antibody-mediated rejection of solid-organ allografts. N Engl J Med. 2018;379:1150–60.

57. Levine DJ, Glanville AR, Aboyoun C, et al. Antibody-mediated rejection of the lung: a consensus report of the International Society for Heart and Lung Transplantation. J Heart Lung Transplant. 2016;35:397–406.

58. Benzimra M, Calligaro GL, Glanville AR. Acute rejection. J Thorac Dis. 2017;9:5440–57.

59. Vanaudenaerde BM, Meyts I, Vos R, et al. A dichotomy in bronchiolitis obliterans syndrome after lung transplantation revealed by azithromycin therapy. Eur Respir J. 2008;32:832–43.

60. Verleden GM, Vos R, De Vleeschauwer SI, et al. Obliterative bronchiolitis following lung transplantation: from old to new concepts? Transpl Int. 2009;22:771–9.

61. Vos R, Vanaudenaerde BM, Ottevaere A, et al. Long-term azithromycin therapy for bronchiolitis obliterans syndrome: divide and conquer? J Heart Lung Transplant. 2010;29:1358–68.

62. Vandermeulen E, Verleden SE, Ruttens D, et al. BAL neutrophilia in azithromycin-treated lung transplant recipients: clinical significance. Transpl Immunol. 2015;33:37–44.

63. Verleden GM, Glanville AR, Lease ED, et al. Chronic lung allograft dysfunction: definition, diagnostic criteria and approaches to treatment. A consensus report from the pulmonary council of the ISHLT. J Heart Lung Transplant. 2019;38(5):493–503.

64. Cooper JD, Billingham M, Egan T, et al. A working formulation for the standardization of nomenclature and for clinical staging of chronic dysfunction in lung allografts. International Society for Heart and Lung Transplantation. J Heart Lung Transplant. 1993;12:713–6.

65. Sato M, Waddell TK, Wagnetz U, et al. Restrictive allograft syndrome (RAS): a novel form of chronic lung allograft dysfunction. J Heart Lung Transplant. 2011;30:735–42.

66. Van Herck A, Verleden SE, Sacreas A, et al. Validation of a post-transplant chronic lung allograft dysfunction classification system. J Heart Lung Transplant. 2019;38(2):166–73. https://doi.org/10.1016/j.healun.2018.09.020.

67. Verleden SE, Vandermeulen E, Ruttens D, et al. Neutrophilic reversible allograft dysfunction (NRAD) and restrictive allograft syndrome (RAS). Semin Respir Crit Care Med. 2013;34:352–60.

68. Verleden SE, Vasilescu DM, McDonough JE, et al. Linking clinical phenotypes of chronic lung allograft dysfunction to changes in lung structure. Eur Respir J. 2015;46:1430–9.

69. Verleden SE, Vasilescu DM, Willems S, et al. The site and nature of airway obstruction after lung transplantation. Am J Respir Crit Care Med. 2014;189:292–300.

70. Verleden SE, Todd JL, Sato M, et al. Impact of CLAD phenotype on survival after lung retransplantation: a multicentre study. Am J Transplant. 2015;15:2223–30.

71. von der Thüsen JH. Pleuroparenchymal fibroelastosis: its pathological characteristics. Curr Respir Med Rev. 2013;9:238–47.

72. Verleden SE, Ruttens D, Vandermeulen E, et al. Bronchiolitis obliterans syndrome and restrictive allograft syndrome: do risk factors differ? Transplantation. 2013;95:1167–72.

73. Verleden GM, Vos R, Vanaudenaerde B, et al. Current views on chronic rejection after lung transplantation. Transpl Int. 2015;28:1131–9.

74. Meyer KC, Raghu G, Verleden GM, et al. An international ISHLT/ATS/ERS clinical practice guideline: diagnosis and management of bronchiolitis obliterans syndrome. Eur Respir J. 2014;44:1479–503.

75. Glanville AR, Aboyoun CL, Morton JM, et al. Cyclosporine C2 target levels and acute cellular rejection after lung transplantation. J Heart Lung Transplant. 2006;25:928–34.

76. Cairn J, Yek T, Banner NR, et al. Time-related changes in pulmonary function after conversion to tacrolimus in bronchiolitis obliterans syndrome. J Heart Lung Transplant. 2003;22:50–7.

77. Verleden GM, Vanaudenaerde BM, Dupont LJ, et al. Azithromycin reduces airway neutrophilia and interleukin-8 in patients with bronchiolitis obliterans syndrome. Am J Respir Crit Care Med. 2006;174:566–70.

78. Gerhardt SG, McDyer JF, Girgis RE, et al. Maintenance azithromycin therapy for bronchiolitis obliterans syndrome: results of a pilot study. Am J Respir Crit Care Med. 2003;168:121–5.

79. Vos R, Vanaudenaerde BM, Verleden SE, et al. A randomised controlled trial of azithromycin to prevent chronic rejection after lung transplantation. Eur Respir J. 2011;37:164–72.

80. Ruttens D, Verleden SE, Vandermeulen E, et al. Prophylactic azithromycin therapy after lung transplantation: post hoc analysis of a randomized controlled trial. Am J Transplant. 2016;16:254–61.

81. Fisher AJ, Rutherford RM, Bozzino J, et al. The safety and efficacy of total lymphoid irradiation in progressive bronchiolitis obliterans syndrome after lung transplantation. Am J Transplant. 2005;5:537–43.

82. Benden C, Speich R, Hofbauer GF, et al. Extracorporeal photopheresis after lung transplantation: a 10-year single-center experience. Transplantation. 2008;86:1625–7.

83. Meloni F, Cascina A, Miserere S, et al. Peripheral CD4(+)CD25(+) TREG cell counts and the response to extracorporeal photopheresis in lung transplant recipients. Transplant Proc. 2007;39:213–7.

84. Davis RD, Lau CL, Eubanks S, et al. Improved lung allograft function after fundoplication in patients with gastroesophageal reflux disease undergoing lung transplantation. J Thorac Cardiovasc Surg. 2003;125:533–42.

85. Gullestad L, Iversen M, Mortensen S-A, et al. Everolimus with reduced calcineurin inhibitor in thoracic transplant recipients with renal dysfunction: a multicenter, randomized trial. Transplantation. 2010;89:864–72.

86. Snell GI, Valentine VG, Vitulo P, et al. Everolimus versus azathioprine in maintenance lung transplant recipients: an international, randomized, double-blind clinical trial. Am J Transplant. 2006;6:169–77.

87. Verleden GM, Verleden SE, Vos R, et al. Montelukast for bronchiolitis obliterans syndrome after lung transplantation: a pilot study. Transpl Int. 2011;24:651–6.

88. Vos R, Verleden SE, Ruttens D, et al. Pirfenidone: a potential new therapy for restrictive allograft syndrome? Am J Transplant. 2013;13:3035–40.

89. Rajab A, Pelletier RP, Henry ML, et al. Excellent clinical outcomes in primary kidney transplant recipients treated with steroid-free maintenance immunosuppression. Clin Transpl. 2006;20:537–46.

90. Cantarovich D, Vistoli F, Soulillou J-P. Immunosuppression minimization in kidney transplantation. Front Biosci. 2008;13:1413–32.

91. Steiner RW. Steroid-free chronic immunosuppression in renal transplantation. Curr Opin Nephrol Hypertens. 2012;21:567–73.

92. Weaver DJ, Selewski D, Janjua H, et al. Improved cardiovascular risk factors in pediatric renal transplant recipients on steroid avoidance immunosuppression: a study of the Midwest Pediatric Nephrology Consortium. Pediatr Transplant. 2016;20:59–67.

Karen C. Dugan and Bhakti K. Patel

The first positive-pressure mechanical ventilators became available in the 1950s during the poliomyelitis epidemic and showed a significant mortality benefit. At that time, the goal of mechanical ventilation was to restore ventilation [1]. Now, mechanical ventilation is one of the most common interventions implemented in the intensive care unit, and its indications have been expanded [2]. However, the main goals have remained the same: to improve gas exchange and relieve respiratory distress while allowing the patient and their lungs to heal.

Ventilator-Induced Lung Injury

There is growing evidence that mechanical ventilation can cause worsening injury in previously damaged lung and initiation of damage in normal lungs, termed ventilator-induced lung injury (VILI). Accordingly, the goal of mechanical ventilation is to not only provide adequate oxygenation and ventilation but to mitigate damage caused by the ventilator itself. Alveolar overdis-

tension, atelectrauma, and biotrauma are considered the principal mechanisms behind VILI. Pathologically, it is characterized by diffuse alveolar damage, which consists of inflammatory cell-infiltrates, hyaline membranes, increased vascular permeability, and pulmonary edema [3].

Alveolar Overdistension

Alveolar overdistension is the over distension of lung units caused by an increased transpulmonary pressure either in the setting of excessive pressure (barotrauma) or volume (volutrauma) [4]. When airflow is zero at end inspiration, the transpulmonary pressure (Ptp) is the alveolar pressure (Palv) minus the intrapleural pressure (Pip) [5] (Fig. 23.1).

$$Ptp = Palv - Pip$$

There is no well-accepted clinical method for measuring the transpulmonary pressure, and therefore identifying alveolar overdistension is challenging. There are, nevertheless, many surrogate measures to estimate the transpulmonary pressure and help limit overdistension along with atelectasis, which will be detailed below.

K. C. Dugan
Kaiser Permanente, Pulmonary and Critical Care,
Portland, OR, USA
e-mail: karen.dugan@uchospitals.edu

B. K. Patel (✉)
University of Chicago, Department of Medicine,
Section of Pulmonary and Critical Care,
Chicago, IL, USA
e-mail: bpatel@medicine.bsd.uchicago.edu

© Springer Nature Switzerland AG 2020
J. L. Gomez et al. (eds.), *Precision in Pulmonary, Critical Care, and Sleep Medicine*,
Respiratory Medicine, https://doi.org/10.1007/978-3-030-31507-8_23

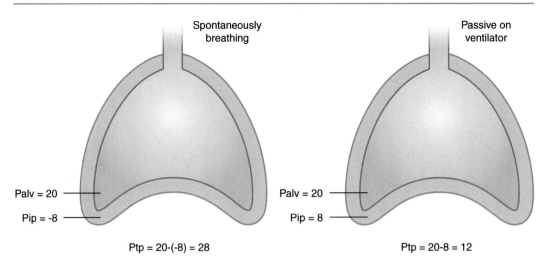

Spontaneously breathing

Passive on ventilator

Palv = 20

Pip = -8

Ptp = 20-(-8) = 28

Palv = 20

Pip = 8

Ptp = 20-8 = 12

Fig. 23.1 Transpulmonary pressure differences between spontaneously breathing and passive patients

Atelectrauma

Atelectrauma is the repetitive opening and closing of terminal lung units causing lung injury [6]. It is caused by a small or negative transpulmonary pressure at the end of exhalation [7]. Similar to alveolar overdistension, prevention of atelectrauma depends on optimizing the transpulmonary pressure.

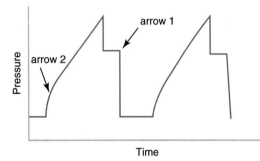

Fig. 23.2 Evidence of restrictive lung disease on the ventilator. Elevation of plateau pressure (arrow 1) and low shoulder on the pressure curves (arrow 2)

Biotrauma

Biotrauma is characterized by ventilator-induced release of inflammatory mediators that can exacerbate lung injury [8].

Because mechanical ventilation can cause VILI, the goal is to support the patient's oxygenation and ventilation, while reducing and ultimately preventing damage caused by the ventilator. The strategies to reduce VILI, based on the pathophysiology of the lung disease, will be outlined below.

Restrictive Disorders of the Lung

In restrictive lung diseases, the compliance of the lung is reduced, and thus, a greater pressure is required to generate a defined tidal volume. Common causes of decreased lung compliance are interstitial lung disease, cardiogenic pulmonary edema, and acute respiratory distress syndrome (ARDS). Most often, identification of a restrictive

disorder of the lung is through a patient's medical history and imaging. However, clues on the ventilator that a patient has a restrictive disorder include decreased compliance, increased plateau pressure, and a low shoulder on the early portion of the pressure versus time tracing [9] (Fig. 23.2). Most research in mechanical ventilation has been performed in patients with ARDS and can be extrapolated to patients with interstitial lung disease. In order to reduce VILI in patients with restrictive lung disorders, strategies to optimize the transpulmonary pressure and decrease both alveolar overdistension and atelectasis will be outlined below.

Low Tidal Volume Ventilation in ARDS

Patients with acute respiratory distress syndrome (ARDS) have areas of nonaerated lung units interspersed with relatively normal aerated lung units [10]. Because of this, there is a smaller volume of lung available for ventilation, and a smaller tidal volume should be used to prevent regional overdistension of the normal, aerated lung. The 2000 ARDSNet trial (also referred to as the ARMA trial) intended to prove this. Patients with ARDS were randomized to a lung-protective strategy with low tidal volume (6 mL/kg ideal body weight) versus high tidal volume (12 mL/kg ideal body weight). The trial was stopped early given a significant decrease in mortality in the low tidal volume group (31% vs. 40%) when compared to the high tidal volume group. The number needed to treat was 11 to prevent one death with an absolute risk reduction of 9% [11]. A more recent Cochrane meta-analysis confirmed these results, and low tidal volume has become the standard of care [12].

Low Tidal Volume Ventilation in Non-ARDS

Low tidal volume ventilation (LTVV) in critically ill and surgical patients without ARDS is also associated with better clinical outcomes, although the data are limited and based on small randomized, controlled trials (RCT) and observational studies [13, 14]. Recently, the PReVENT study randomized critically ill patients without ARDS to either LTVV versus intermediate tidal volume ventilation (10 mL/kg ideal body weight) [15]. However, a majority of the patients in both groups did not achieve their target volumes, and thus, it is difficult to come to a conclusion regarding the potential benefit of LTVV versus intermediate tidal volume ventilation in non-ARDS patients [16].

Prone Positioning

Prone positioning has been used since the 1970s to treat refractory hypoxemia in patients with ARDS. It is thought that placing a patient prone allows for a more even distribution of transpulmonary pressure, resulting in more homogenous lung aeration [17]. In 2013, Guerin et al. published a randomized, controlled trial comparing prone positioning to supine positioning in patients with severe ARDS. There was a significant mortality benefit when compared to the supine position [18]. Proning patients with severe ARDS has become the standard of care.

Plateau Pressure

A surrogate measure of alveolar pressure, the plateau pressure (Pplat) is the pressure applied to the alveoli at end inspiration. It is measured in a passive patient on the ventilator as the pressure during an inspiratory hold maneuver (Fig. 23.3). It can also be calculated in a spontaneously breathing patient by a method using the expiratory time constant (Υ_E).

$$\text{Pplat} = \left[\left(Vt \times PIP \right) - \left(Vt \times PEEP \right) \right] / \left[Vt + \left(\Upsilon_E + Vi \right) \right]$$

where Vi is the inspiratory flow, PIP is the peak inspiratory pressure, Vt is the tidal volume, PEEP is the positive end-expiratory pressure, and Υ_E is estimated from the slope of the passive expiratory flow curve between 0.1 and 0.5 seconds [19].

The plateau pressure is often taken as an approximation of end-inspiratory lung-distending pressure, or transpulmonary pressure. During full ventilator support, the plateau pressure is determined by the tidal volume (Vt), compliance of the respiratory system (Crs), and positive end-expiratory pressure (PEEP) [20]. Therefore, changes in tidal volume and PEEP can alter the plateau pressure.

$$\text{Pplat} = Palv = Vt / Crs + PEEP$$

In the ARMA trial, comparing LTVV versus high tidal volume ventilation, patients randomized to low tidal volumes had a goal plateau pressure less than 30 mmHg, whereas those patients randomized to high tidal volumes had a goal plateau pressure less than 50 cmH2O. Because of these goals and the mortality improvement in the LTVV arm, current guidelines recommend a plateau pressure less than 30 cmH2O when titrating PEEP and tidal volume [21].

However, using the plateau pressure does not take into consideration the intrapleural pressure, and is oftentimes a poor approximation of the transpulmonary pressure. In spontaneously breathing patients, the intrapleural pressure is oftentimes negative. In these patients, the plateau pressure will commonly underestimate the transpulmonary pressure, potentially leading to alveolar overdistension (Fig. 23.1). In passive patients with poor chest compliance, such as obesity, abdominal compartment syndrome, or ascites, the intrapleural pressure is oftentimes excessively positive, leading to overestimation of the transpulmonary pressure and causing atelectasis [22].

Protocolized PEEP

PEEP is the pressure applied by the ventilator at end expiration. It is used to increase the functional residual capacity, recruit collapsed lung, and improve oxygenation [23]. However, deter-

mining the optimal level of PEEP is difficult, as too much PEEP may lead to alveolar overdistension and too little PEEP may lead to atelectasis.

The ALVEOLI trial set out to determine if an "open lung" model with higher levels of PEEP improved mortality; 549 patients were enrolled in which 273 patients were assigned to a low PEEP strategy and 276 patients were randomly assigned to a high PEEP strategy [24] (Table 23.1). In both groups, a goal plateau pressure of less than 30 cmH2O was recommended.

There was improvement in oxygenation and compliance in the higher PEEP group, but no clinically significant difference in outcomes was seen. A meta-analysis confirmed these findings, but did show an improved mortality with higher PEEP in patients with moderate-to-severe ARDS [25].

Interestingly, in a post hoc analysis, Calfee et al. performed latent class modeling to identify subphenotypes within ARDS patients using clinical and biological data from the ALVEOLI trial, along with the ARMA trial. They found two subphenotypes, with one phenotype (Phenotype 2) identified as hyperinflammatory with a higher incidence of acidosis, shock, and plasma concentrations of inflammatory biomarkers when compared to the other phenotype (Phenotype 1). They used data from the ALVEOLI trial to determine if there were differences in response to the high PEEP strategy versus the low PEEP strategy based on phenotype. They found that patients with phenotype 1 had improved mortality when treated with a low PEEP strategy in contrast to phenotype 2 which had improved mortality and more ventilator-free days when treated with a high PEEP strategy [26]. Given these findings, tailoring a PEEP strategy based on phenotype

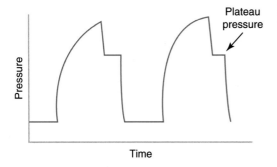

Fig. 23.3 Plateau pressure assessed during an inspiratory hold

Table 23.1 High versus low PEEP strategies employed in the ALVEOLI trial

Lower PEEP/higher FiO2													
FiO2	0.3	0.4	0.4	0.5	0.5	0.6	0.7	0.7	0.7	0.8	0.9	0.9	0.9	1
PEEP	5	5	8	8	10	10	10	12	14	14	14	16	18	18–24

Higher PEEP/lower FiO2													
FiO2	0.3	0.3	0.3	0.3	0.3	0.4	0.4	0.5	0.5	0.5–0.8	0.8	0.9	1	1
PEEP	5	8	10	8	12	14	16	16	18	20	22	22	22	24

may lead to better outcomes and should be studied in a randomized controlled study.

Driving Pressure

Even in the era of LTVV, target tidal volumes do not necessarily take into account the varying proportion of lung that is available for ventilation. Because respiratory system compliance is strongly related to the volume of functional, aerated lung, it is thought that optimizing the driving pressure ($\Delta P = Vt/Crs$, where Crs is the compliance of the respiratory system) by titrating tidal volume normalized to aerated lung size can improve lung protection, decrease VILI, and improve mortality [27]. The driving pressure can be easily measured at the bedside as the plateau pressure (measured during an inspiratory pause) minus PEEP.

Although no prospective study has been conducted assessing titration of the driving pressure and clinically relevant endpoints, Amato et al. performed a retrospective analysis including eight randomized, controlled trials and found that ΔP was a better predictor of mortality than plateau pressure or tidal volume. They also found that decreases in tidal volume or increases in PEEP driven by random treatment group assignments were beneficial only if associated with a decrease in ΔP [28]. Physiologically, this is logical since application of PEEP that recruits lung will improve compliance and reduce ΔP, whereas application of PEEP that causes over distension of the lung will reduce compliance and increase ΔP. This was a retrospective study and it is difficult to conclude that modifying driving pressure will improve outcomes. Rather, it may be a marker of ARDS severity. Prospective studies are needed.

Case Study A 35-year-old female admitted to the hospital with pancreatitis is urgently transferred to the intensive care unit with worsening hypoxemia. She is immediately intubated following transfer. Her current ventilator settings are as follows: a mode of assist control, tidal volume of 350 mL (6 mL/kg ideal body weight), respiratory rate of 28 breaths/minute, PEEP of 5 cmH2O and fraction of oxygen 100%. Her oxygen saturation is 89% and her ABG is pH 7.25, PaO2 60 mmHg, and PaCO2 50 mmHg. Her plateau is measured while she remains paralyzed after intubation and is 35 cmH2O. Her calculated driving pressure is 30 cmH2O. What ventilator changes would you make?

To improve both the plateau and the driving pressure, there are a few changes you can make. First, you decrease the tidal volume. However, both the driving pressure and plateau pressure remain elevated. This means that the drop in tidal volume likely led to worsening atelectasis. Next, you decide to increase the PEEP. If lung is recruited with increasing the PEEP, the plateau should decrease or increase less than the increase in applied PEEP. The driving pressure should then decrease. With a PEEP titration up to 15 cmH2O, the plateau decreases to 30 cmH2O and the driving pressure improves to 15 cmH2O. In this case, the high plateau and driving pressure was likely a consequence of atelectasis and poor chest wall compliance secondary to the patient's pancreatitis.

Recruitment Maneuvers, Best Respiratory System Compliance

Recruitment maneuvers are designed to recruit more alveoli using incremental increases in PEEP. Previous trials have shown improvements in oxygenation and respiratory system compliance, but have failed to show improvements in clinically relevant outcomes [29]. The ARDS Trial investigators performed a multicenter, randomized controlled trial comparing the ARDSNet LTVV, low PEEP strategy in the control arm to a lung recruitment strategy with recruitment maneuvers, and PEEP titrated to best respiratory system compliance in patients [30]. In the intervention group, patients were initially given neuromuscular blockade, and then PEEP was increased to 25 cmH2O for 1 minute, then 35 cmH2O for 1 minute, and then 45 cmH2O for 2 minutes. The PEEP was then reduced to

23 cmH2O and down titrated by 3 cmH2O every 4 minutes until a PEEP of 11 cmH2O. The respiratory system compliance was calculated at each stage (Crs = Vt/ΔP). The optimal PEEP was identified as 2 plus the PEEP at which the highest respiratory compliance was achieved. There was a statistically increased risk of death in the intervention group, and therefore, recruitment maneuvers and titrated PEEP based on measured respiratory system compliance should not be undertaken.

Esophageal Pressure

As discussed previously, the plateau pressure does not take into account the intrapleural pressure and consequently, in many cases of mechanically ventilated patients, is a poor surrogate marker for transpulmonary pressure and assessment of lung overdistension or atelectasis. Measuring the intrapleural pressure, however, is invasive and fraught with significant complications. Therefore, the most commonly used surrogate measure to estimate intrapleural pressure is esophageal manometry [31].

To measure the esophageal pressure, an air-filled catheter with a balloon near its distal end, also known as the esophageal balloon, is inserted through the nose or mouth and advanced to the stomach at 60 cm. The balloon is inflated with the minimum volume recommended by the manufacturer, and confirmation of intragastric placement is done by gentle epigastric compression with a transient change in pressure. The catheter is then withdrawn slowly into the esophagus to 40 cm until the appearance of cardiac oscillations. The validity of the esophageal measurement can be done at end-expiratory occlusion, both in spontaneously breathing and passive patients. In spontaneous breathing patients, the patient's inspiratory effort generates a similar change in airway pressure at end-expiratory occlusion. In contrast, in a passive patient, a clinician must manually compress the chest wall or abdomen to increase the esophageal pressure (Pes). The positive change in esophageal pressure should be the same as the airway pressure. Once placement and validity are confirmed, the transpulmonary pressure can be calculated [32, 33] (Fig. 23.4).

$$\text{Transpulmonary pressure} = \text{Palv} - \text{Pip}$$

$$\text{Estimated transpulmonary pressure} = \text{Pplat} - \text{PEEP} - \text{change in Pes}$$

Although some studies show physiologic improvement in patients when esophageal balloons are used, uncertainties exist concerning the reliability in estimating the intrapleural pressure. Pleural pressure varies within the pleural space because of both gravitational gradients and regional heterogeneity. Therefore, esophageal manometry measured at one location oftentimes cannot identify alveolar overdistension or atelectasis in patients with heterogeneous lung disease, such as ARDS [34].

In the EPVent study, 61 patients with ARDS were randomized to optimal PEEP as determined by esophageal balloon manometry and transpulmonary pressure estimates both at end-expiratory (Ptpe) and at end-inspiratory (Ptp) as compared

to standard of care with a low PEEP titration strategy (see Table 23.1). In the esophageal balloon manometry group, PEEP was titrated to a goal Ptpe while keeping the Ptp less than 25 cmH2O (Table 23.2). Average PEEP was 17 cmH2O in the intervention group versus 10 cmH2O in the control group. The study was stopped early given improved oxygenation and compliance in the esophageal balloon group, but no statistically significant changes were found in clinical outcomes [35]. A multicentered trial was recently completed, comparing esophageal balloon manometry to a high PEEP titration strategy (see Table 23.1). It showed no difference in a composite outcome of ventilator-free days and death, but did show a statistically significant decrease in rescue therapies. In contrast to the EpVent study, which used a low PEEP strategy, mean PEEP between the intervention and control groups were not different, possibly leading to a lack of separation between the groups and a negative result [36].

Stress Index

The stress index is a measure of the linearity of the pressure-time waveform under constant inspiratory flow during control ventilation [9]. Assessment of the stress index may only be performed in passive patients. A linear increase of the waveform (stress index = 1) indicates ideal compliance and alveolar recruitment [20]. When

the stress index is >1, the waveform becomes concave. This indicates that the alveoli are overdistended and tidal volume, PEEP, or both should be decreased. In contrast, when the stress index is <1, the waveform becomes convex. This indicates atelectasis, and PEEP should be increased in order to recruit more lung (Fig. 23.5).

Pressure-Volume Curves

Pressure-volume Curves are displayed on the ventilator with volume as a function of pressure. The slope of the curve is Crs [20]. To optimize PEEP and Vt from pressure-volume curves, the physician applies either different tidal volumes or PEEP in sequence with constant inspiratory flow. The plateau pressure is performed at end-inspiration after each breath and the pressure-volume curve is constructed from the different plateau pressures that correspond to the administered volumes or PEEP [37]. The curve is then examined for both an upper and lower inflection point. The upper inflection point is thought to indicate alveolar overdistension, and therefore the volume or PEEP should be reduced below this point. In contrast, the lower inflection point is thought to indicate atelectasis and the PEEP (or volume) should be increased above this point [9] (Fig. 23.6).

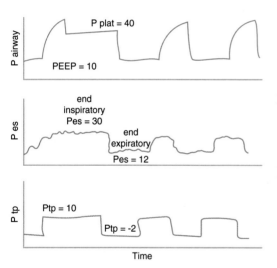

Fig. 23.4 Example of esophageal balloon manometry. Top waveform: airway pressure with an inspiratory pause demonstrating plateau pressure (Pplat). Middle waveform: esophageal pressure (Pes), measured both at end inspiration and expiration. Bottom waveform: calculated transpulmonary pressure (Ptp)

Electrical Impedance Tomography

Several studies have assessed lung heterogeneity, alveolar recruitment, and overdistension in patients with ARDS using computed tomography (CT) [38]. In one study, CT images performed at end expiration in patients with ARDS at a PEEP

Table 23.2 Transpulmonary pressure goals in the intervention group versus PEEP goals in the control group

Esophageal pressure guided group											
FiO2	0.4	0.5	0.5	0.6	0.6	0.7	0.7	0.8	0.8	0.9	0.9	1.0
Ptp	0	0	2	2	4	4	6	6	8	8	10	10

Control group											
FiO2	0.3	0.4	0.4	0.5	0.5	0.6	0.7	0.7	0.7	0.8	0.9	0.9	0.9	1
PEEP	5	5	8	8	10	10	10	12	14	14	14	16	18	20–24

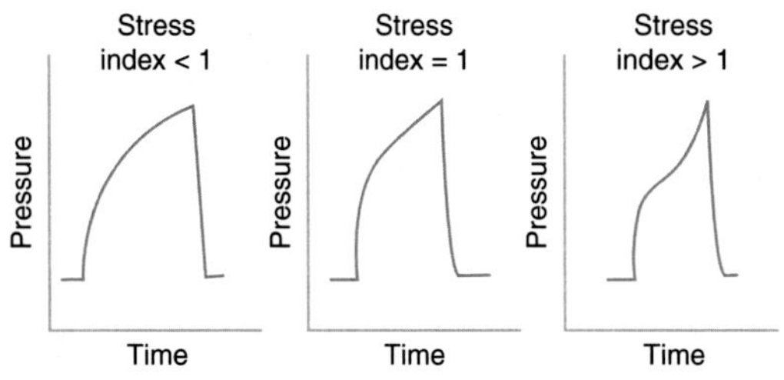

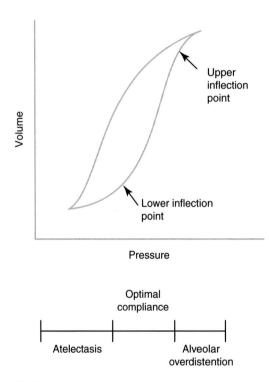

Fig. 23.5 Stress index assessed on the pressure-time curves

Fig. 23.6 Pressure-volume curve

of 5 cmH2O and a PEEP of 15 cmH2O were able to identify collapsed alveoli that regain inflation [39, 40]. However, CT imaging is not performed at the bedside and is therefore unavailable for continual measurement and mechanical ventilator titration in critically patients. In contrast, electrical impedance tomography (EIT) is a noninvasive, nonradiologic, portable imaging modality of ventilation that can be used in the titration of mechanical ventilation [41]. Electrodes are placed on the chest, each of which send and receive small, alternating electrical impulses with each other [42]. Impedance is measured between and among the electrode array. Data are acquired

and processed into two-dimensional slices. These two-dimensional images have been shown to correlate with radiographic changes in assessing regional heterogeneity [43]. EIT's application is still primarily in the research setting, but it may prove to be a beneficial tool in the future.

Spontaneous Breathing

There is significant controversy regarding the benefits and harms of spontaneous breathing in patients with ARDS. Spontaneous breathing can improve alveolar recruitment and reduce the risk of ventilator-induced diaphragm dysfunction while also avoiding the risks of heavy sedation and neuromuscular blockade [44]. However, spontaneous breathing can also produce alveolar overdistension from increased transpulmonary pressure and high tidal volumes in the setting of a high drive to breathe (also known as patient-self-inflicted lung injury, or P-SILI) [45]. In one study, neuromuscular blockade was associated with reduced mortality. However, a multicentered, randomized controlled trial, the ROSE trial conducted by the PETAL network, was completed comparing neuromuscular blockade to placebo. It was stopped at the second interim analysis for futility [46].

Noninvasive Ventilation

Noninvasive ventilation is the use of ventilator support without an invasive airway, but delivered via a facial or nasal mask or helmet. Its use in patients with acute hypoxemic respiratory failure rose initially after observational trials reported substantial improvements in mortality and intubation rates [47, 48]. However, a recent randomized, controlled trial comparing nasal cannula oxygen with noninvasive ventilation with a facemask in patients with acute hypoxemic failure showed harm in patients assigned to noninvasive ventilation [49]. A single-centered trial comparing noninvasive ventilation delivered via helmet compared to face mask resulted in a reduction in intubation rates and mortality [50]. The most recent ERS/ATS clinical practice guidelines, therefore, do not offer any recommendations about the use of noninvasive ventilation in acute hypoxemic respiratory failure [51].

Obstructive Disorders of the Lung

In contrast to restrictive disorders, compliance is often normal or high in obstructive disorders of the lung. However, airway narrowing results in increased airways resistance in obstructive disorders. Therefore, greater peak pressures may be required to deliver a tidal volume. Common causes of obstructive lung disease include asthma, chronic obstructive pulmonary disease (COPD), and bronchiectasis. Similar to restrictive disorders of the lungs, obstructive lung disease is commonly identified by a patient's history or imaging. Clues on the ventilator that a patient may have an obstructive disorder include elevated peak inspiratory pressure without concomitant increase in the plateau pressure, prolonged expiratory flow, and a high shoulder on the early portion of the pressure versus time tracing [9] (Fig. 23.7). In order to reduce VILI in patients with obstructive lung disease, strategies to limit the transpulmonary pressure via reduction in dynamic overinflation will be outlined below.

Auto-PEEP and Dynamic Overinflation

Auto-PEEP occurs when there is insufficient time for exhalation prior to inspiration, leading to air trapping [52]. It is commonly seen in obstructive lung diseases when the increased expiratory resistance leads to prolonged expiration or patients with high minute volumes and short expiratory times. On the ventilator, it can be identified when the expiratory flow tracing shows persistent end-expiratory flow [9]. It can be quantitated with an end-expiratory hold as the pressure at end expiration minus extrinsic PEEP (Fig. 23.8). Auto-PEEP leads to dynamic hyperinflation and elevated transpulmonary pressures, increasing the risk of VILI via alveolar overdistension. Reduction of auto-PEEP can be achieved by increasing expiration time either by decreasing the respiratory rate, decreasing the tidal volume, or increasing inspira-

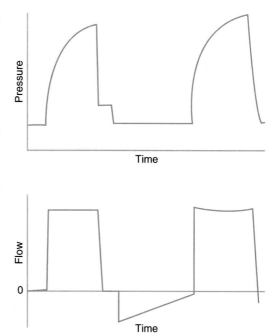

Fig. 23.7 Evidence of obstructive lung disease on the ventilator. Elevation of peak airway pressure without elevation of the plateau pressure and prolonged expiratory flow

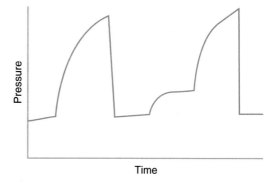

Fig. 23.8 Auto-PEEP as evidenced by an elevation in pressure during an end-expiratory hold

tory flow (thus decreasing time of inhalation and increasing time of expiration).

Ventilator Asynchrony

Patients, depending on their underlying pathophysiology, differ extraordinarily in their breathing patterns and desire for tidal volume, respiratory rate, flow, and inspiratory and expiratory times [9]. The initial ventilator settings do not align with a patient's needs often and may result in abnormal ventilator interactions, termed ventilator asynchrony. Identifying the type of ventilator asynchrony will allow the intensivist to adjust ventilator parameters to improve patient comfort and potentially impact clinical outcomes.

Breath Stacking

Breath stacking, also known as double triggering, occurs when a patient's inspiratory effort continues into the set ventilator exhalation and results in larger delivered tidal volumes (Fig. 23.9). It is seen in patients with high respiratory drives on volume-controlled ventilation, oftentimes when set to low tidal volumes [53]. Once breath stacking is observed, there are two changes that can be made to the ventilator in order reduce its occurrence: switching to pressure-assisted ventilation or adding a T-pause to inspiration. It has been

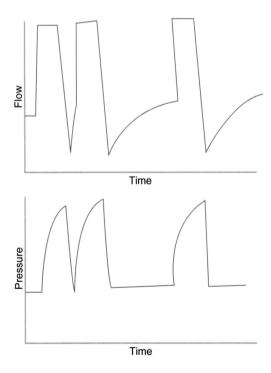

Fig. 23.9 Breath stacking

shown that increasing sedation or analgesia does not improve breath stacking [54].

Reverse Triggering

Identifiable only with esophageal balloon placement, reverse triggering is the initiation of inspiratory effort and diaphragmatic contraction after passive insufflation of the lungs with a ventilator-induced breath [55]. Similar to breath stacking, it can result in a larger tidal volume if the inspiratory effort is strong enough to initiate a ventilator-assisted breath prior to completion of exhalation. There are no known effective strategies to reduce reverse triggering.

Ineffective Triggering

The ventilator is triggered to deliver a breath when it perceives a drop in airway pressure or flow [56]. Ineffective triggering occurs when an inspiratory effort is not detected by the ventilator, and therefore, a ventilator-initiated breath does not occur [57]. This can be detected as a decrease in airway pressure with a simultaneous increase in inspiratory flow that is not followed by a breath (Fig. 23.10). Ineffective triggering is most commonly seen in two circumstances: the trigger sensitivity is set too low or in the setting of auto-PEEP. If the trigger sensitivity is too low, this can be changed easily on the ventilator. In the setting of auto-PEEP, the patient must overcome the level of auto-PEEP before the pressure or flow change can trigger a ventilator-assisted breath. Therefore, if auto-PEEP is the cause of ineffective triggering, one can employ methods to reduce auto-PEEP discussed previously. In addition, increasing the external PEEP will reduce the pressure or flow change needed to initiate a breath.

Auto-Cycling

In contrast to ineffective triggering, auto-cycling is the inappropriate delivery of a breath in the absence of an inspiratory effort by the patient.

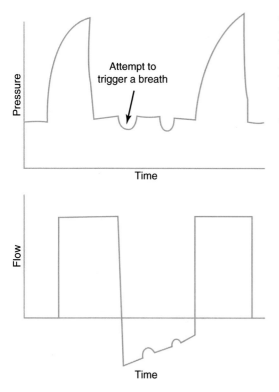

Fig. 23.10 Ineffective triggering

This occurs when the trigger sensitivity is too low and external factors trigger the breath, such as cardiac oscillations or in the setting of circuit leaks or condensation in the tubing [58]. Auto-cycling should be suspected in patients with a high respiratory rate, especially if the breaths match cardiac oscillations or in the presence of a cuff leak or significant condensation in the tubing. The trigger sensitivity should be increased and the underlying cause fixed.

Inspiratory Flow Mismatching

Inspiratory flow mismatching occurs when the patient's flow demand is higher than what is set by the ventilator. Typically, this can be fixed easily with increasing the inspiratory flow delivery [57].

Conclusion

Mechanical ventilation is lifesaving, with the goals of improving gas exchange and reducing the work of breathing in patients with underlying lung disease. However, personalizing mechanical ventilation according to the underlying patho-physiologic disease allows for reduction in VILI and improvement in outcomes.

References

1. Slutsky AS. History of mechanical ventilation. From vesalius to ventilator-induced lung injury. Am J Respir Crit Care Med. 2015;101(10):1106–15.
2. Tobin MJ. Physiologic basis of mechanical ventilation. Ann Am Thorac Soc. 2018;15(1):S49–52.
3. Slutsky AS, Ranieri VM. Ventilator-induced lung injury. N Engl J Med. 2013;369:2126–36.
4. Grieco DL, Chen L, Bouchard L. Transpulmonary pressure: importance and limits. Ann Transl Med. 2017;5(14):285.
5. Loring SH, Topulos GP, Hubmayr RD. Transpulmonary pressure: the importance of precise definitions and limiting assumptions. Am J Respir Crit Care Med. 2016;194(12):1452–7.
6. De Prost N, Ricard JD, Saumon G, Dreyfss D. Ventilator-induced lung injury: historical perspectives and clinical implications. Ann Intensive Care. 2011;1(1):28.
7. Lee WL, Slutsky AS. Acute hypoxemic respiratory failure and ARDS. In: Broaddus VC, Mason RJ, Ernst JD, King TE, Lazarus SC, Murray JF, et al., editors. Murray and Nadel's textbook of respiratory medicine. Philadelphia: Elsevier Saunders; 2016. p. 1740–60. Print.
8. Curley GF, Laffey JG, Zhang H, Slutsky AS. Biotrauma and ventilator induced lung injury: clinical implications. Chest. 2016;150(5):1109–17.
9. Schmidt G. Ventilator waveforms: clinical interpretation. In: Hall JB, Schmidt GA, Kress JP, editors. Principles of critical care medicine. New York: McGraw Hill; 2015. p. 411–24. Print.
10. Gattinoni L, Caironi P, Pelosi P, Goodman LR. What has computed tomography taught us about the acute respiratory distress syndrome? Am J Respir Crit Care Med. 2001;17:1701–11.
11. The Acute Respiratory Distress Syndrome Network. Ventilation with lower tidal volumes as compared with traditional tidal volumes for acute lung injury and the acute respiratory distress syndrome. N Engl J Med. 2000;342(18):1301–8.
12. Petrucci N, Iacovelli I. Ventilation with lower tidal volumes versus traditional tidal volumes in adults for acute lung injury and acute respiratory distress syndrome. Cochrane Database Syst Rev. 2003;(3):CD003844.
13. Neto AS, et al. Association between use of lung-protective ventilation with lower tidal volumes and clinical outcomes among patients without acute respiratory distress syndrome: a meta-analysis. JAMA. 2012;308(16):1651–9.

14. Futier E, Constant JM, Paugam-Burtz C, et al. Trial of intraoperative low-tidal-volume ventilation in abdominal surgery. N Engl J Med. 2013;369(5):428–37.
15. Writing Group for the PReVENT Investigators. Effect of a low vs intermediate tidal volume strategy on ventilator-free days in intensive care unit patients without ARDSA randomized clinical trial. JAMA. 2018;320(18):1872–80.
16. Rubenfeld GD, Shankar-Hari M. Lessons from ARDS for non-ARDS research remembrance of trials past. JAMA. 2018;320(18):1863–5.
17. Pelosi P, Brazzi L, Gattinoni L. Prone position in acute respiratory distress syndrome. Eur Respir J. 2002;20(4):1017–28.
18. Guerin C, Reignier J, Richard JC, Beuret P, Gacouin A, Boulain T, et al. Prone positioning in severe acute respiratory distress syndrome. N Engl J Med. 2013;268(23):2159–68.
19. Hess DR. Respiratory mechanics in mechanically ventilated patients. Respir Care. 2014;59(11):1773–94; Macintyre NR. Mechanical ventilation. In: Broaddus VC, Mason RJ, Ernst JD, King TE, Lazarus SC, Murray JF, et al., editors. Murray and Nadel's textbook of respiratory medicine. Philadelphia: Elsevier Saunders; 2016. p. 1761–77. Print.
20. Hess DR. Respiratory mechanics in mechanically ventilated patients. Respir Care. 2014;59(11):1773–94.
21. Fan E, Del Sorbo L, Goligher EW, Hodgson CL, Nunshi L, Walkey AJ, et al. An Official American Thoracic Society/European Society of Intensive Care Medicine/Society of Critical Care Medicine Clinical Practice Guideline: mechanical ventilation in adult patients with acute respiratory distress syndrome. Am J Respir Crit Care Med. 2017;195(9):1253–63.
22. Macintyre NR. Mechanical ventilation. In: Broaddus VC, Mason RJ, Ernst JD, King TE, Lazarus SC, Murray JF, et al., editors. Murray and Nadel's textbook of respiratory medicine. Philadelphia: Elsevier Saunders; 2016. p. 1761–77. Print.
23. Villar J. The use of P.E.E.P. in the treatment of A.R.D.S. In: Matalon S, Sznajder JL, editors. Acute respiratory distress syndrome. NATO ASI series (advanced science institutes series), vol. 297. Boston: Springer; 1998.
24. Brower RG, Lanken PN, MacIntyre N, National Heart, Lung, and Blood Institute ARDS Clinical Trials Network, et al. Higher versus lower positive end-expiratory pressures in patients with the acute respiratory distress syndrome. N Engl J Med. 2004;351(4):327–36.
25. Briel M, Meade M, Mercat A, Brower RG, Talmor D, Walter SD, et al. Higher vs lower positive end-expiratory pressure in patients with acute lung injury and acute respiratory distress syndrome: systematic review and meta-analysis. JAMA. 2010;303(9):865–73.
26. Calfee CS, Delucchi K, Parsons PE, Thompson BT, Ware LB, Matthay MA, et al. Latent class analysis of ARDS subphenotypes: analysis of data from two randomized controlled trials. Lancet Respir Med. 2014;2(8):611–20.
27. Tonetti T, Vasques F, Rapetti F, Maiolo G, Collino F, Romitti F, et al. Driving pressure and mechanical power: new targets for VILI prevention. Ann Transl Med. 2017;5(14):286.
28. Amato MAP, Meade MO, Slutsky AS, Brochard L, Costa EL, Schoenfeld DA, et al. Driving pressure and survival in the acute respiratory distress syndrome. N Engl J Med. 2015;372(8):747–55.
29. Meade MO, Cook DJ, Guyatt GH, Slutsky AS, Arabi YM, Cooper DJ, et al. Ventilation strategy using low tidal volumes, recruitment maneuvers, and high positive end-expiratory pressure for acute lung injury and acute respiratory distress syndrome. JAMA. 2008;299(6):637–45.
30. ART Investigators. Effect of lung recruitment and titrated positive end-expiratory pressure (PEEP) vs low PEEP on mortality in patients with acute respiratory distress syndrome. JAMA. 2017;318(14):1335–45.
31. Sahetya S, Brower R. The promises and problems of transpulmonary pressure measurements in ARDS. Curr Opin Crit Care. 2016;22(1):7–13.
32. Piraino T, Cook DJ. Optimal PEEP guided by esophageal balloon Manometry. Respir Care. 2011;56(4):510–3.
33. Soroksky A, Esquinas A. Goal-directed mechanical ventilation: are we aiming at the right goals? A proposal for an alternative approach aiming at optimal lung compliance, guided by esophageal pressure in acute respiratory failure. Crit Care Res Prac. 2012;2012:597932.
34. Akoumianaki E, Maggiore SM, Valenza F, Bellani G, Jubran A, Loring SH, et al. The application of esophageal pressure measurement in patients with respiratory failure. Am J Respir Crit Care Med. 2014;189(5):520–31.
35. Talmor D, Sarge T, Malhotra A, O'Donnell CR, Ritz R, Lisbon A, et al. Mechanical ventilation guided by esophageal pressure in acute lung injury. N Engl J Med. 2008;359(20):2095–104.
36. Beitler JR, Sarge T, Banner-Goodspeed VM, Gong MN, Cook D, Novack V, et al. Effect of titrating positive end-expiratory pressure (PEEP) with an esophageal pressure-guided strategy vs. an empirical high PEEP-FiO2 strategy on death and days free from mechanical ventilation among patients with acute respiratory distress syndrome. JAMA. 2019;321(9):846–57.
37. Lu Q, Rouby J-J. Measurement of pressure volume curves in patients on mechanical ventilation: methods and significance. Crit Care. 2000;4(2):91–100.
38. Caironi P, Langer T, Gattinoni L. Acute lung injury/acute respiratory distress syndrome pathophysiology: what we have learned from computed tomography scanning. Curr Opin Crit Care. 2008;14(1):64–9.
39. McKown AC, Ware LB. Quantification of lung recruitment by respiratory mechanics and CT imaging: what are the clinical implications? Ann Transl Med. 2016;4(7):145.

40. Gattinoni L, Caironi P, Cressoni M, Chiumello D, Ranieri VM, Quintel M, et al. Lung recruitment in patients with the acute respiratory distress syndrome. N Engl J Med. 2006;354(17):1775–86.
41. Lobo B, Hermosa C, Abella L, Gordo F. Electrical impedance tomography. Ann Transl Med. 2018;6(2):26.
42. Walsh BK, Smallwood CD. Electrical impedance tomography during Mechanical Ventilation. Respir Care. 2016;61(1):1417–24.
43. Frerichs I, Amato MBP, van Kaam AH, Tingay DG, Zhao Z, Grychtol B, et al. Chest electrical impedance tomography examination, data analysis, terminology, clinical use and recommendations: consensus statement of the TRanslational EIT developmeNt stuDy group. Thorax. 2017;72(1):83–93.
44. Mauri T, Cambiaghi B, Spinelli E, Langer T, Grasselli G. Spontaneous breathing: a double-edged sword to handle with care. Ann Transl Med. 2017;5(14):292.
45. Brochard L, Slutsky A, Pesenti A. Mechanical Ventilation to minimize progression of lung injury and acute respiratory failure. Am J Respir Crit Care Med. 2017;195(4):438–42.
46. The National Heart, Lung, and Blood Institute PETAL Clinical Trials Network. Early neuromuscular blockade in the acute respiratory distress syndrome. N Engl J Med. 2019;380(21):1997–2008.
47. Hilbert G, Gruson D, Vargas F, et al. Noninvasive ventilation in immunosuppressed patients with pulmonary infiltrates, fever, and acute respiratory failure. N Engl J Med. 2001;344(7):481–7.
48. Antonelli M, Conti G, Bufi M, Costa MG, Lappa A, Rocco M, et al. Noninvasive ventilation for treatment of acute respiratory failure in patients undergoing solid organ transplantation: a randomized trial. JAMA. 2000;283(2):235–41.
49. Frat JP, Thille B, Mercat A, Girault C, Ragot S, Pervet S, et al. High flow oxygen through nasal cannula in acute hypoxemic respiratory failure. N Engl J Med. 2015;372(23):2185–96.
50. Patel BK, Wolfe KS, Pohlman AS, Hall JB, Kress JP. Effect of noninvasive Ventilation delivery by helmet vs face mask on the rate of endotracheal intubation in patients with acute respiratory distress syndrome. JAMA. 2016;315(22):2435–41.
51. Scala R, Pisani L. Noninvasive ventilation in acute respiratory failure: which recipe for success? Eur Respir Rev. 2018;27(149):1–15.
52. Marini JJ. Ventilator-associated problems related to obstructive lung disease. Respir Care. 2013;58(6):938–49.
53. Pohlman MC, McCallister KE, Schweikert WD, Pohlman AS, Nigos CP, Krishnan JA, et al. Excessive tidal voiume from breath stacking during lung-protective Ventilation for acute lung injury. Crit Care Med. 2008;36(11):3019–22.
54. Changues G, Kress JP, Pohlman A, Patel S, Poston J, Jabir S, et al. Impact of ventilator adjustment and sedation-analgesia practices on severe asynchrony in patients ventilated in assist-control mode. Crit Care Med. 2013;41(9):2177–87.
55. Akoumianaki E, Lyazidi A, Rey N, Matamis D, Perez-Martinez N, Giraud R, et al. Mechanical ventilation-induced reverse-triggered breaths. Chest. 2013;143(4):927–38.
56. Murias G, Lucangelo U, Blanch L. Patient-ventilator asynchrony. Curr Opin Crit Care. 2016;22(1):53–9.
57. Subira C, de Haro C, Magrans R, Fernandez R, Blanch L. Minimizing asynchronies in mechanical ventilation: current and future trends. Respir Care. 2018;63(4):464–78.
58. Noujeim C, BouAkl I, El-Khatib M, Bou-Khalil P. Ventilator auto-cycling from cardiogenic oscillations: case report and review of literature. Nurs Crit Care. 2013;18(5):222–8.

Precision Medicine for Cigarette Smoking Addiction

Stephen R. Baldassarri

Key Point Summary

- *Cigarette smoking addiction is a chronic condition* that requires long-term care.
- *Combination behavioral and pharmacotherapy* is the gold standard treatment for cigarette smoking addiction.
- *Precision medicine* for cigarette smoking addiction holds great promise to develop novel treatment concepts that can improve long-term abstinence rates among people who smoke.
- The precision medicine *approaches* for smoking addiction to date include targeting of: (1) *sex differences*; (2) *genetic differences* in brain nicotine receptors; (3) *pharmacogenetic differences* in nicotine metabolism; and (4) host differences with respect to *comorbid conditions*.
- *Harm reduction* is precision medicine for individuals who are unable or unwilling to abstain from drug use. Common tobacco harm reduction strategies include use of snus or other smokeless tobacco, electronic cigarettes, and heat-not-burn tobacco.

S. R. Baldassarri (✉)
Department of Internal Medicine, Section of Pulmonary, Critical Care, and Sleep Medicine, Yale School of Medicine, New Haven, CT, USA
e-mail: stephen.baldassarri@yale.edu

General Considerations for Prevention, Diagnosis, and Treatment of Cigarette Smoking Addiction

Case #1

A 55-year-old woman presented to the emergency department with acute shortness of breath that occurred at home. A family member reported the patient had a productive cough with yellow sputum and subjective fevers for 10 days. The patient smoked approximately 1 pack of tobacco cigarettes daily since the age of 13. She had made several attempts to stop smoking, but was unsuccessful. On exam, she was hypoxemic, confused, unable to speak in full sentences, and in severe respiratory distress. She was intubated and mechanically ventilated. Chest imaging revealed a large right hilar mass and multiple large, discrete pulmonary nodules consistent with metastatic disease. A brain MRI demonstrated metastases and cerebral edema. Lung biopsy ultimately confirmed a diagnosis of extensive stage small cell lung adenocarcinoma. The patient recovered from her initial acute illness and initiated chemotherapy. Eight months later, she again became ill and died.

© Springer Nature Switzerland AG 2020
J. L. Gomez et al. (eds.), *Precision in Pulmonary, Critical Care, and Sleep Medicine*, Respiratory Medicine, https://doi.org/10.1007/978-3-030-31507-8_24

Physicians care for individuals suffering the consequences of long-term cigarette smoking every day. *Tobacco cigarette smoking* is currently the leading cause of preventable death in the United States and has been attributed to more than 20 million premature deaths since 1965 [1]. Chronic smoking is widely recognized as a major cause of pulmonary diseases including chronic obstructive pulmonary disease and lung cancer [1]. Clinically, smoking is a symptom and outward manifestation of a deeper problem: tobacco cigarette addiction. Drug addiction is best understood as a combination of two key elements: First, an acquired disease of the brain that is characterized by compulsive drug taking despite the desire to stop taking the drug and is consistent with severe substance use disorder [2]; second, a maladaptive pattern of learned behavior influenced by environmental, social, psychologic, and physiologic mechanisms [3]. Addiction is a chronic disease, characterized by periods of relapse and remission. Since cigarette smoking is not associated with the destructive behavior that commonly characterizes addictions to alcohol and other psychoactive drugs of abuse, smoking is frequently overlooked as an addiction. Nonetheless, cigarette smoking is at least as addictive in nature as heroin use [4].

Nicotine is the primary (though not sole) addictive and psychoactive substance in tobacco smoke [5]. However, it is worth noting that cigarette smoke is a complex mixture of more than 7000 chemicals, and other smoke constituents are likely psychoactive and may play a role in maintaining addiction to cigarettes [5]. Smoke inhalation is a rapid and highly efficient mechanism to deliver drugs to the brain [6]. It has been well established that large tobacco companies spent many years carefully engineering cigarettes to be highly addictive to users through manipulation of nicotine chemistry and various additives that facilitated smoke inhalation [7].

Tobacco use disorder is characterized by tobacco use patterns that lead to clinically significant impairment or distress [8]. In the context of individuals who suffer from pulmonary diseases,

combustible cigarette smoking is the most consequential form of tobacco consumption. Smoking cessation and maintenance of abstinence are thus critical central elements of optimal patient care.

Cigarette smoking typically occurs as part of a complex interplay between addiction, medical illness, psychiatric illness, and social stress. While nearly half of the US population smoked during the peak of the tobacco epidemic, control efforts and education have helped reduce this to just under 15% at present [9]. However, this means that current smoking is now concentrated more heavily among people of low socioeconomic status and individuals with mental illness. Consequently, treatment efforts are more complicated and challenging in this patient population (see section on "Comorbid Conditions Complicating Smoking").

Prevention

It is critical to prevent young people from initiating cigarette smoking. Data strongly suggest that an earlier age of onset of smoking predicts chronic smoking and failure to quit permanently [10–12]. Early age use of nicotine fundamentally alters the developing brain in a way that is more likely to create and sustain addiction [13, 14]. Prevention efforts in the United States have been largely successful to date, with teen and adult smoking rates currently at an all-time low [9]. Tobacco control policies in the United States have included public education about the dangers of smoking, taxation of cigarettes, banning of flavored cigarettes, clean-air laws that prohibit smoking indoors, and in some states, increasing the legal smoking age to 21 years [15]. In 2009, the Family Smoking Prevention and Tobacco Control Act was signed into law, which gave the Food and Drug Administration (FDA) the authority to regulate tobacco products to protect public health. One controversial proposal that is currently under review is the possibility of requiring tobacco companies to reduce the nicotine content in cigarettes to very low (i.e., nonaddictive) levels to prevent initiation of smoking and subsequent addiction to cigarettes among youth and nonsmokers who try smoking [16].

Table 24.1 Essential history-taking for clinicians

Topic	Question	Significance
Smoking history		
Age of initiation	"When did you start smoking?"	Earlier age → increased difficulty to stop
Time-to-first-cigarette (TTFC)	"How many minutes after waking do you smoke?"	Determine level of nicotine dependence. TTFC within 5 minutes signifies high level of nicotine dependence
Smoking intensity	"How many cigarettes do you smoke each day?"	Establish "pack-years" smoking *Note*: This metric may *not* accurately quantify exposure
Motivation	"How do you feel about your smoking?" "Do you feel your smoking causes you any problems?"	Nonjudgmental, open-ended question. Allows patient to explore reasons for cessation Establish patient's insight and motivation to stop smoking
Readiness to stop smoking	"Would you like to stop smoking?"	Understand motivation to stop smoking
Prior quit attempts	"Were there any other prior methods that helped you stop smoking in the past?"	Tailor treatment plan to patient's preference and prior experience
Past medical history		
Medical	"Do you have any past or current medical problems or concerns?"	Identify smoking-related illness Presence of smoking-related illness indicates a high level of smoking addiction
Psychiatric	"Do you have any past or current mental health problems or concerns?"	Identify conditions that may complicate tobacco treatment
Social history		
Drug use disorders	"Do you use alcohol, drugs, or any other substances?"	Identify conditions that may complicate tobacco treatment
Social stress	"Do you have stress in your life?"	Identify conditions that may complicate tobacco treatment Involve social work when needed
Smoking contacts	"Do you live with anyone else who smokes?"	More difficult to stop smoking if partner smokes Target partner for treatment if applicable

Diagnosis

Asking individuals about smoking behavior is the most important way to diagnose smoking addiction. In some cases, individuals smelling of smoke are identified by physicians and other clinic or hospital staff. It is highly recommended to screen all individuals entering any medical facility for current or past cigarette smoking. Daily cigarette use is typical for smoking addiction. Nondaily cigarette smokers tend to differ somewhat from daily smokers and may have different reasons for smoking (i.e., weight control or cue exposure) [17]. The diagnostic and treatment approaches described further from this point are aimed primarily at daily cigarette smokers who have cigarette addiction.

History-taking is critical for identifying the duration and intensity of smoking, degree of drug dependence, and other comorbid conditions that may complicate treatment efforts. The essential elements of the history are summarized in Table 24.1. In general, it is important to establish the age of onset of smoking and the number of packs smoked per day at the peak. "Pack-years" the product of number of packs per day multiplied by the number of years smoked provides an estimate of cumulative smoke exposure that has demonstrated a dose-response relationship to adverse events such the development of chronic lung disease and lung cancer [1]. Based on these data, current lung cancer screening guidelines in the United States recommend screening individuals aged 55–80 years who have a 30 pack-year smoking history and currently smoke or have stopped smoking within the past 15 years [18]. Pack-years are an imperfect exposure measure because they fail to account for individual differences in smoking intensity. For example, one person might smoke one-fourth of a cigarette each time, while another might smoke seven-eighth of a cigarette. These exposures, over time, are vastly different. Furthermore, data indicate that *any* cigarette smoke exposure (i.e., one cigarette smoked daily) increases the risk of smoking-related diseases [19]. Nonetheless, studies linking validated smoking exposure biomarkers, such as cotinine or carbon monoxide to health outcomes, have not been done.

Assessing the degree of nicotine dependence is one important metric for understanding the severity of cigarette addiction and can be assessed using a validated scoring system such as the Fagerström Test for Nicotine Dependence [20]. Prior smoking quit attempts, medications used, and severity of past withdrawal and cravings are important to determine.

Physical examination provides additional clues both to current and past cigarette smoking. The smell of smoke may be noted on the patients' clothing upon presentation to the clinic and should not be ignored or dismissed. Signs of chronic lung and heart disease such as wheezing, diminished breath sounds, coughing during exam, sputum production, hoarseness, elevated jugular venous pressure, leg swelling, or cyanosis may indicate medical consequences of chronic smoking. It is critical to take note of patients who wear supplemental oxygen, since concomitant smoking while on oxygen therapy poses a significant fire hazard [21].

Finally, when in doubt, biomarkers of smoking exposure can be easily assessed. While the gold standard for diagnosis is measurement of serum cotinine [22], a portable exhaled breath carbon monoxide (CO) monitor is a convenient device used to rapidly assess current smoking status [23]. A level of greater than six parts per billion (ppb) of CO indicates likely smoking within, in the past several hours [23, 24], which is typical for individuals with smoking addiction.

Treatment

Treatment for smoking addiction may have the single biggest positive impact on a patient's health. Unfortunately, management is frequently complex and time-consuming, and response to treatment is frequently limited (despite being cost-effective) [25]. As a result, many providers view treatment efforts as low-yield, which can reduce physician engagement in fully addressing the problem [26]. Other challenges include a fragmented health system that may not integrate medical and psychiatric treatment, inadequate resources and low reimbursement for preventive care, and high workload likely limit treatment of smoking addiction [27].

Combination of behavioral and pharmacologic therapies provides optimal treatment for smoking addiction, though either of the modality also significantly increases the odds of successful treatment [28].

Behavioral treatment is tailored to the needs of each individual and is an important precision medicine modality for smoking addiction. This is the more difficult treatment to provide because it is much more time-consuming than prescribing pharmacotherapy and typically requires specialized training to deliver the optimal dose for patients. The most important initial step prior to delivering behavioral treatment is to determine the patient's level of motivation and insight. Do they want to stop smoking and do they think their smoking is a problem? If the answer to either of these questions is "No," the provider must direct effort to changing the answers to "Yes." *Motivational interviewing (MI)* is the method commonly used to achieve this goal and typically requires specialized training to optimize the intervention [29]. MI is a patient-centered technique that allows patients to explore and discover their own reasons to change their behavior. The interviewer's use of open-ended questions, empathy, and nonjudgmental disposition are the key elements. The role of the interviewer is to support the patient's efforts to resolve ambivalence and find compelling reasons to take action for positive change.

Table 24.2 Pharmacotherapy[a]

Controller medications	On-demand/as-need medications
Nicotine transdermal patch	Nicotine lozenge
Varenicline (Chantix)	Nicotine gum
Bupropion SR (Wellbutrin, Zyban)[b]	Nicotine nasal spray
	Nicotine inhaler

[a]All medications can be used safely in combination. Monitor for development of neuropsychiatric symptoms (which could reflect severe withdrawal) in all patients regardless of methods used
[b]Caution needed in patients with seizure or eating disorders

Pharmacologic treatment is a critical element of treating smoking addiction and significantly increases the odds of achieving abstinence (Table 24.2) [28]. Treatments are usefully categorized as controller medications (i.e., long-acting drugs) and on-demand medications (i.e., short-acting drugs). Controller and on-demand therapeutics should be combined for optimal results. There are a total of seven FDA-approved treatments. Among these, there are three FDA-approved controller medications: (1) nicotine patch; (2) varenicline (Chantix); and (3) bupropion (Wellbutrin/Zyban). The four FDA-approved on-demand medications are as follows: (1) nicotine gum; (2) nicotine lozenge; (3) nicotine inhaler; and (4) nicotine nasal spray. Medications can be safely used in combination and for a prolonged period of time. Precision medicine approaches to treatment described below are emerging and might help optimize the initial choice of treatment.

Follow Up

It is critical to assess the patient's response to treatment. Since cigarette addiction is a chronic condition, patients require frequent and longitudinal follow-up. Treatment failure and relapses are common [30] and must be expected as part of the normal treatment course. Consequently, adjustments to treatment regimens are frequently required. There are three typical scenarios that occur in clinical practice: (1) failure to achieve any initial period of abstinence; (2) achieving short-term abstinence, followed by relapse into smoking; and (3) long-term abstinence with a sustained remission.

Failure to achieve abstinence may indicate one or more problems. First, there may be inadequate motivation or desire to stop smoking on the part of the patient. This is a critical pre-requisite that should be assessed at every visit. If motivation or insight are lacking, an exploration of the patient's views and understanding using MI is the best approach. As previously noted, MI skills are specialized and typically best provided by an individual who has been formally trained in the techniques [29].

Second, the prescribed medication regimen may fail to adequately control *withdrawal* symptoms (Table 24.3). The presence and severity of withdrawal symptoms should be assessed at the initial visit and at every follow-up visit. The presence of withdrawal symptoms indicates that the initial treatment regimen was insufficient and requires greater intensity. Options include the

Table 24.3 Common smoking withdrawal symptoms

Withdrawal symptoms
Neurologic/psychiatric symptoms
Depression
Anxiety
Irritability
Anger
Restlessness
Difficulty concentrating
Fatigue
Cravings to smoke
Sleep disturbances
Insomnia
Nightmares/vivid dreams
Frequent awakenings
Sleepiness
Respiratory symptoms
Cough (rebound in cough sensitivity)
Sore throat (withdrawal from smoking additives such as menthol)
Gastrointestinal symptoms
Increased appetite/weight gain
Constipation
Nausea

following: (1) increasing the dose of nicotine replacement; (2) adding an additional controller medication; and (3) adding an additional on-demand medication.

Third, cigarette craving may not be adequately suppressed. While withdrawal symptoms characterize physical symptoms and typically abate within several days to a few weeks of abstinence, [31] cravings may persist for much longer. Finally, comorbid psychiatric and substance use disorders may require treatment (see section on "Comorbid Conditions Complicating Smoking").

General Principles of Novel Concepts with Relevance for Precision Medicine

Precision medicine for treatment of smoking addiction is extremely promising and still in the early stages of development. Since smoking addiction, like many diseases, involves the interplay between environmental and genetic factors that influence predisposition, precision medicine has great potential to revolutionize treatment approaches. Novel treatment concepts that have been investigated to date include targeting of: (1) sex differences; (2) genetic differences in brain nicotine receptors; (3) pharmacogenetic differences in nicotine metabolism; and (4) host differences with respect to comorbid conditions. We will explore these treatment concepts below.

Sex Differences in Smoking Addiction

Case #2

Mr. and Mrs. Smith are in their mid-50s. They met at a bar 30 years ago, at which time they shared a cigarette. They have smoked cigarettes daily since that time. When Mr. Smith was diagnosed with coronary artery disease earlier this year, the couple decided to seek professional help to stop smoking. They are each evaluated separately by an advanced practitioner registered nurse (APRN). Mr. Smith reports that he smokes his first cigarette within 5 minutes of waking. He notes strong cravings to smoke during his work day and must take frequent breaks to go outside. He enjoys the "uplifting" effect but does not particularly enjoy the taste or ritual of smoking. Mrs. Smith, on the other hand, reports smoking her first cigarette in the mid-morning after she arrives at work. She feels that smoking gives her relief from work-related stress, and she enjoys going outside as an "escape." She has frequently contemplated quitting smoking and is quite confident in her ability to do so. However, she is significantly concerned about weight gain, which occurred many years ago when she had stopped smoking for 6 months.

Sex differences in disease states and response to therapy are critical to examine and have traditionally been overlooked due to the historical exclusion of women from research studies. In more recent decades, this topic has garnered significant attention and has been studied extensively. There is a large amount of evidence to suggest a differential response to smoking cessation treatments between men and women. Much of the literature has focused on the response to nicotine itself [32]. Meta-analyses of nicotine patch trials have found that women had lower odds of achieving smoking cessation by this method as compared with men [33]. Additional meta-analysis evidence emerged that women appeared to respond relatively more favorably to varenicline as compared with the nicotine patch [34]. These observations led to a hypothesis that non-nicotine factors of smoking might be more important for women as compared with men.

However, the recent large randomized controlled trial (EAGLES) of over 8000 participants examining neuropsychiatric safety in various FDA-approved tobacco treatments, including varenicline, bupropion, and nicotine replacement therapy, did not observe significant sex differences in either primary smoking cessation quit rate outcomes or with respect to which treatment was administered [35].

Taken in totality, the data suggest that there may be sex differences in response to treatment *on average*. Future precision medicine approaches would be wise to consider sex effects in the context of many other individual characteristics at play (such as level of nicotine dependence and comorbidities) that influence treatment outcomes.

Genetic Differences in Brain Nicotine Receptors

The effects of genetics on smoking behavior and outcome have been difficult to tease out because of the complex and chronic nature of smoking addiction. Simply measuring cumulative smoking dose exposure is impossible, since users vary in the degree and frequency to which they puff a cigarette. As noted, pack-years is a highly imprecise but commonly used estimate of smoke exposure. Furthermore, our understanding of smoking addiction as a chronic disease has made identification of a meaningful endpoint difficult. A famous author once noted: "To cease smoking is the easiest thing I ever did. I ought to know because I've done it a thousand times" [36]. Thus, understanding the outcome among people with smoking addiction is difficult since relapse is common.

The *CHRNA5* gene encodes the alpha 5 nicotinic receptor structure and function [37]. Polymorphism in this gene alters receptor channel permeability and has been implicated in the development of nicotine dependence and adverse health outcomes including COPD [38, 39]. However, full understanding of the genetic mechanisms underlying smoking behavior is incomplete, and additional studies are required. Further development of genetic predictors of susceptibility to addiction and addiction-related illnesses will be critical developments with implications for prevention efforts, diagnosis, and treatment.

Pharmacogenetic Differences in Nicotine Metabolism

Case #3

Mrs. Johnson is a 47-year-old woman who has smoked one half pack of cigarettes daily since the age of 17. Last year, she developed a persistent cough productive of yellow sputum and dyspnea on exertion. Pulmonary function testing was normal. A chest computed tomography (CT) scan showed evidence of air trapping and mild emphysematous changes. As a result of her ongoing symptoms and a diagnosis of COPD, she decided to seek assistance to stop smoking. She was assessed with the nicotine metabolite ratio (NMR) blood biomarker, a surrogate for *CYP2A6* activity. She was found to be a slow metabolizer of nicotine. Based on the available evidence [40], she was prescribed the combination of a daily nicotine patch along with nicotine lozenges to use as needed. At her first follow-up visit 2 weeks later, she reported complete smoking abstinence with minimal side effects. She was maintained on dual NRT and monitored in follow-up every 3 months.

Biomarkers that identify individual differences in the metabolism of the key drugs of interest have the potential to customize initial therapeutic approaches. Nicotine metabolism occurs primarily through the liver enzyme cytochrome P450 2A6 [41]. The primary metabolism product is cotinine (COT), which itself is metabolized by the liver to trans-3′-hydroxycotinine (3HC) [42]. The ratio between 3HC and COT measured in human plasma or saliva was noted to be highly correlated with the oral clearance of nicotine, indicating that 3HC:COT might be useful as a surrogate marker of *CYP2A6* activity and nicotine clearance [43]. Given that multiple genetic variants in the gene coding *CYP2A6* [44], metabolism of nicotine varies significantly among individuals.

Data supporting the hypothesis that slower nicotine metabolism might affect smoking quit rates are mixed. A few early studies found an association between slow metabolism and higher quit rates in different populations who were enrolled in smoking cessation trials [45, 46]. Furthermore, normal nicotine metabolizers had better response to varenicline compared with slow nicotine metabolizers [40]. Similarly to the impact of genetic variation in nicotine receptors in smoking behaviors, pharmacogenetics of nicotine metabolism are only partially understood, but represent an important advance in our understanding of nicotine addiction and management.

Comorbid Conditions Complicating Smoking

Case #4

Mr. Jones is a 36-year-old male combat Veteran who was seen by his primary care physician for a routine physical examination. He reported no current or past health problems aside from a 7-year history of chronic back pain. He had begun smoking cigarettes daily at the age of 14 and enlisted in the military at age 18. He completed several tours of duty in Iraq and Afghanistan and suffered a serious back injury during his service that required surgery. Upon return to civilian life, he struggled briefly with heroin addiction and eventually enrolled himself into a methadone maintenance program. He currently takes methadone each day and has not suffered a relapse into injection drug use. From a psychiatric standpoint, he has had intermittent symptoms of depressed mood, nightmares, and hypersensitivity to environmental stimuli. He has not had suicidal thoughts or actions, but notes that living with chronic back pain is a daily struggle. He has never contemplated smoking cessation.

Comorbid psychiatric and medical conditions are extremely common among people with cigarette addiction, particularly those who present for treatment in medical settings [47]. It is critical to realize that many of these comorbidities may be *undiagnosed* conditions that require significant attention. Cigarette addiction bridges the intersection between mental and physical health. As a result, a multidisciplinary approach to care that addresses the comorbid conditions is critical to providing precision medicine and adequately treating smoking addiction (Table 24.4).

It is essential to understand *why* people smoke, what "benefit" they might derive from smoking, and how this perceived benefit fits with their specific comorbidities. Like all drugs, cigarettes provide a therapeutic effect for users despite their significant toxicity and health risks (Table 24.5). If we understand the underlying reasons for drug use, our treatments have a better chance of succeeding if we precisely address the underlying problems specific to the patient.

Psychiatric illness is particularly common among people who smoke, and cessation rates in this population are substantially lower compared

Table 24.4 Comorbidities requiring attention

Comorbid condition	Actions
Depression	Specialty referral; antidepressant prescription; cognitive behavioral therapy
Anxiety	Specialty referral; antidepressant prescription; cognitive behavioral therapy
Attention-deficit hyperactivity disorder (ADHD)	Specialty referral; stimulant prescription
Substance use disorders	
Opioids	Ensure access and adherence to buprenorphine or methadone
Alcohol	Naltrexone, counseling programs
Other drug use	Specialty referral
Pain	Specialty referral; nonopioid pain management strategies whenever possible
Stress	Psychosocial support; behavioral counseling, social work consultation

Table 24.5 Effects of cigarette smoking in people with comorbid conditions

Comorbidity/symptom	Smoking effect
Depression	Mood elevation
Anxiety	Relaxation
Attention-deficit hyperactivity disorder (ADHD)	Improved focus, attention
Chronic pain	Analgesia
Alcohol use disorder	Synergistic euphoric effect with alcohol
Opioid use disorder	Synergistic euphoric effect with opioids; reduced sedation, less constipation
Obesity	Weight loss, appetite suppression
Fatigue/sleepiness	Stimulant, increased alertness; synergistic with caffeine
Constipation	Gastrointestinal stimulant

Note: In cases of prolonged addiction, ongoing cigarette use may act to prevent withdrawal symptoms (as opposed to providing pleasurable effects)

with those without these conditions [48]. The common conditions encountered in clinical settings include mood disorders such as depression or bipolar disorder, attention disorders (i.e., ADHD), and cognitive disorders (i.e., schizophrenia). As noted above, the antidepressant bupropion has been demonstrated to be effective for smoking cessation (though in practice, most people with depression who smoke require multiple treatment modalities). For smokers who present in medical settings, it is wise to screen for mental illness if there is not one reported in the history. Questioning patients about mood, anxiety state, and cognitive function may uncover new diagnoses that require specialized care. It is also critical to note that smoking cessation may unmask an underlying mood disorder if severe withdrawal occurs. All patients, but particularly those with underlying mood disorders, need to be monitored carefully for the development of severe neuropsychiatric effects during a cessation attempt.

Other drug use disorders commonly coexist with psychiatric illness, either as contributors to these conditions or as a means to self-medicate for symptoms. Alcohol and/or opioid use in particular are drugs that work synergistically with cigarettes in a manner that reinforces smoking [49]. Smoking is nearly universal in people with opioid use disorder, and the commonly used treatments for smoking addiction appear to be much less effective in this population. The optimal timing for promoting smoking abstinence in people with other drug use disorders is unclear.

Psychosocial stress is a second factor that is closely linked with smoking and frequently coexists with psychiatric illness. People who smoke frequently more commonly have lower socioeconomic status and less access to care, which creates both barriers to treatment and prevention of relapse [50]. Stress is known to result in hormonal changes and increases in systemic inflammation [51]. The precise neurobiological mechanisms by which stress impacts behavior continues to be an area of active investigation, but it is clear that people with smoking addiction are prone to its adverse effects. Studies have consistently shown that stress increases cravings to smoke and also increases the rewarding effects from smoking [52].

Medical illnesses commonly result from chronic smoking and likely have a bidirectional relationship with mental illness [53]. Clinicians encounter patients at various stages of chronic diseases, including COPD, asthma-COPD overlap, ILD, lung cancer, and coronary disease, among others. It is important to note that patients who continue to smoke despite awareness of medical diagnoses likely represent a more highly addicted subpopulation compared with smokers more generally. However, frank discussions about the impact of smoking on the underlying disease process and acute illnesses related to chronic diseases may serve as teachable moments that can increase motivation to achieve smoking abstinence [54, 55]. Finally, as described in the example case, chronic pain syndromes may significantly complicate treatment efforts for smoking abstinence, particularly given that cigarettes have known analgesic effects [56, 57].

Future Directions

Smoking addiction is much more difficult to treat today compared with half a century ago when nearly half the US population smoked. The remaining individuals who smoke are more highly addicted, complex medically and psychiatrically, and have more social and economic stressors that impede abstinence. Novel approaches that address both the addiction to nicotine and the psychological stressors that perpetuate smoking are critical to continued efforts to promote public health.

Tobacco Harm Reduction

Harm reduction is an approach to treatment that involves minimizing the risks of drug use to the individual without discontinuing the drug completely. It typically refers to interventions that occur outside of traditional physician prescribing practices. Harm reduction is precision medicine for individuals who are either unable or unwilling to stop using a drug. The idea is to replace the drug or modify its administration such that it is less likely to harm the individual. This might include substituting with a drug that has a similar mechanism of action but a different route of administration and/or lower addictive potential. The administration of methadone maintenance for people with opioid injection drug use is the classic example. The use of clean needles for injection drug users is a second example.

Among people who smoke cigarettes, there are three potential options for harm reduction, all of which remain controversial among public health experts: (1) snus or other forms of oral tobacco; (2) electronic cigarettes; and (3) heat-not-burn tobacco.

Snus is smokeless tobacco that delivers nicotine and other chemical constituents via absorption through the buccal mucosa. One of the most interesting lines of evidence supporting use of snus as harm reduction comes from Sweden, where the product is commonly used. The use of snus in Sweden is linked to lower rates of tobacco smoking, and Sweden experienced the largest reduction in smoking-related diseases from 1976 to 2002 [58–60]. Though snus has not been definitively linked to oral cancer and other health problems, concerns remain given that the products contain tobacco-specific nitrosamines and other carcinogens. Nonetheless, snus is dramatically less toxic than cigarette smoking. Despite the Swedish experience, skepticism remains in the United States regarding promotion of snus as a harm reduction strategy [61, 62].

Electronic cigarettes (ECs) are battery-operated devices that heat and aerosolize a liquid solution that may contain nicotine [63]. They do not contain tobacco. ECs carry toxicants to the body but are significantly less toxic than conventional cigarettes [64]. Multiple lines of evidence suggest that a complete switch from conventional smoking to exclusive EC use reduces toxic exposure and probably reduces harm [65, 66]. However, there is evidence that EC aerosol has harmful pulmonary and cardiovascular effects [67, 68]. The harms of chronic EC use remain unknown.

ECs were shown to be more effective for smoking cessation compared with traditional nicotine replacement in a randomized controlled trial performed in the United Kingdom [69]. Epidemiologically, the rise of EC use has coincided with a decline in conventional cigarette smoking in the United States between 2007 and 2018 [70, 71]. Nevertheless, recommending EC use for patients who smoke remains controversial among healthcare providers [72, 73]. From a harm-reduction standpoint, exclusive EC use might benefit patients if they can completely eliminate combustible cigarette smoking. However, concerns about potential additive toxicities from dual use of ECs and combustible products remain.

Heat-not-burn tobacco (HNBT) products operate similarly to ECs, but actually contain tobacco. HNBT does not involve combustion and delivers fewer toxicants per puff to users as compared with cigarettes [74]. The products have developed a market in Japan, but to date are not commonly used in the United States. One study that examined nicotine delivery from various products found that HNBT delivered nicotine less efficiently than cigarettes and high-power ECs and more efficiently than low-power ECs

[75]. Studies to assess long-term health effects of HNBT will be important to determine if use of these products reduces harm compared with combustible cigarettes.

Summary

Cigarette smoking addiction is the most common preventable cause of death in the United States. Prevention efforts are critical because once the addiction takes hold it is very difficult to treat and is marked by frequent abstinence attempts, relapse, and low sustained abstinence over time. As a result, harm reduction strategies may become increasingly important as the smoking population becomes more highly concentrated with people who have other comorbidities complicating treatment efforts.

Thus, smoking addiction is a chronic disease that must be managed longitudinally. Periods of relapse and remission are the norm. The combination of behavioral and pharmacotherapy remains the gold standard for treatment. Precision medicine approaches to treatment are promising and will continue to develop to reduce the burden of this critical health problem.

References

1. National Center for Chronic Disease Prevention and Health Promotion (US) Office on Smoking and Health. The health consequences of smoking-50 years of progress: a report of the surgeon general. Atlanta: Centers for Disease Control and Prevention (US); 2014.
2. Volkow ND, Koob GF, McLellan AT. Neurobiologic advances from the brain disease model of addiction. N Engl J Med. 2016;374(4):363–71.
3. Lewis M. Brain change in addiction as learning, not disease. N Engl J Med. 2018;379(16):1551–60.
4. Stolerman IP, Jarvis MJ. The scientific case that nicotine is addictive. Psychopharmacology. 1995;117(1):2–10.
5. Benowitz NL. Nicotine addiction. N Engl J Med. 2010;362(24):2295–303.
6. Tiwari G, Tiwari R, Sriwastawa B, Bhati L, Pandey S, Pandey P, et al. Drug delivery systems: an updated review. Int J Pharm Investig. 2012;2(1):2.
7. Proctor RN, Proctor R. Golden holocaust: origins of the cigarette catastrophe and the case for abolition. Berkeley: University of California Press; 2011.
8. Substance-Related and Addictive Disorders. Diagnostic and statistical manual of mental disorders. DSM library. Arlington: American Psychiatric Association; 2013.
9. Wang TW, Asman K, Gentzke AS, Cullen KA, Holder-Hayes E, Reyes-Guzman C, et al. Tobacco product use among adults—United States, 2017. Morb Mortal Wkly Rep. 2018;67(44):1225.
10. Breslau N, Peterson EL. Smoking cessation in young adults: age at initiation of cigarette smoking and other suspected influences. Am J Public Health. 1996;86(2):214–20.
11. Khuder SA, Dayal HH, Mutgi AB. Age at smoking onset and its effect on smoking cessation. Addict Behav. 1999;24(5):673–7.
12. Chassin L, Presson CC, Sherman SJ, Edwards DA. The natural history of cigarette smoking: predicting young-adult smoking outcomes from adolescent smoking patterns. Health Psychol. 1990;9(6):701.
13. Dwyer JB, McQuown SC, Leslie FM. The dynamic effects of nicotine on the developing brain. Pharmacol Ther. 2009;122(2):125–39.
14. Slotkin TA. Cholinergic systems in brain development and disruption by neurotoxicants: nicotine, environmental tobacco smoke, organophosphates. Toxicol Appl Pharmacol. 2004;198(2):132–51.
15. Levy DT, Chaloupka F, Gitchell J. The effects of tobacco control policies on smoking rates: a tobacco control scorecard. J Public Health Manag Pract. 2004;10(4):338–53.
16. Apelberg BJ, Feirman SP, Salazar E, Corey CG, Ambrose BK, Paredes A, et al. Potential public health effects of reducing nicotine levels in cigarettes in the United States. N Engl J Med. 2018;378:1725.
17. Shiffman S, Dunbar MS, Scholl SM, Tindle HA. Smoking motives of daily and non-daily smokers: a profile analysis. Drug Alcohol Depend. 2012;126(3):362–8.
18. Moyer VA. Screening for lung cancer: US Preventive Services Task Force recommendation statement. Ann Intern Med. 2014;160(5):330–8.
19. Bjartveit K, Tverdal A. Health consequences of smoking 1–4 cigarettes per day. Tob Control. 2005;14(5):315–20.
20. Heatherton TF, Kozlowski LT, Frecker RC, Fagerstrom KO. The Fagerstrom test for nicotine dependence: a revision of the Fagerstrom tolerance questionnaire. Br J Addict. 1991;86(9):1119–27.
21. Lacasse Y, LaForge J, Maltais F. Got a match? Home oxygen therapy in current smokers. London: BMJ Publishing Group Ltd; 2006.
22. Vartiainen E, Seppälä T, Lillsunde P, Puska P. Validation of self reported smoking by serum cotinine measurement in a community-based study. J Epidemiol Community Health. 2002;56(3):167–70.
23. Deveci SE, Deveci F, Açik Y, Ozan AT. The measurement of exhaled carbon monoxide in healthy smokers and non-smokers. Respir Med. 2004;98(6):551–6.
24. Middleton ET, Morice AH. Breath carbon monoxide as an indication of smoking habit. Chest. 2000;117(3):758–63.

25. Hoogendoorn M, Feenstra TL, Hoogenveen RT, Rutten-van Mölken MPMH. Long-term effectiveness and cost-effectiveness of smoking cessation interventions in patients with COPD. Thorax. 2010;65(8):711–8.

26. Leone FT, Evers-Casey S, Graden S, Schnoll R. Behavioral economic insights into physician tobacco treatment decision-making. Ann Am Thorac Soc. 2015;12(3):364–9.

27. Blumenthal DS. Barriers to the provision of smoking cessation services reported by clinicians in underserved communities. J Am Board Fam Med. 2007;20(3):272–9.

28. 2008 PHS Guideline Update Panel, Liaisons, and Staff. Treating tobacco use and dependence: 2008 update U.S. Public Health Service Clinical Practice Guideline executive summary. Respir Care. 2008;53(9):1217–22.

29. Rollnick S, Miller WR. What is motivational interviewing? Behav Cogn Psychother. 1995;23(4):325–34.

30. Shiffman S. A cluster-analytic classification of smoking relapse episodes. Addict Behav. 1986;11(3):295–307.

31. Shiffman SM, Jarvik ME. Smoking withdrawal symptoms in two weeks of abstinence. Psychopharmacology. 1976;50(1):35–9.

32. Perkins KA. Sex differences in nicotine versus nonnicotine reinforcement as determinants of tobacco smoking. Exp Clin Psychopharmacol. 1996;4(2):166–77.

33. Perkins KA, Scott J. Sex differences in long-term smoking cessation rates due to nicotine patch. Nicotine Tob Res. 2008;10(7):1245–51.

34. Smith PH, Mazure CM, McKee SA, Weinberger AH, Emme E, Zhang J. Sex differences in smoking cessation pharmacotherapy comparative efficacy: a network meta-analysis. Nicotine Tob Res. 2016;19(3):273–81.

35. Anthenelli RM, Benowitz NL, West R, St Aubin L, McRae T, Lawrence D, et al. Neuropsychiatric safety and efficacy of varenicline, bupropion, and nicotine patch in smokers with and without psychiatric disorders (EAGLES): a double-blind, randomised, placebo-controlled clinical trial. Lancet. 2016;387(10037):2507–20.

36. Kuehn BM. Could a novel vaccine help smokers quit? JAMA. 2005;294(8):891–2.

37. Saccone NL, Wang JC, Breslau N, Johnson EO, Hatsukami D, Saccone SF, et al. The CHRNA5-CHRNA3-CHRNB4 nicotinic receptor subunit gene cluster affects risk for nicotine dependence in African-Americans and in European-Americans. Cancer Res. 2009;69(17):6848–56.

38. Liu JZ, Tozzi F, Waterworth DM, Pillai SG, Muglia P, Middleton L, et al. Meta-analysis and imputation refines the association of 15q25 with smoking quantity. Nat Genet. 2010;42:436.

39. Cho MH, McDonald M-LN, Zhou X, Mattheisen M, Castaldi PJ, Hersh CP, et al. Risk loci for chronic obstructive pulmonary disease: a genome-wide association study and meta-analysis. Lancet Respir Med. 2014;2(3):214–25.

40. Lerman C, Schnoll RA, Hawk LW Jr, Cinciripini P, George TP, Wileyto EP, et al. Use of the nicotine metabolite ratio as a genetically informed biomarker of response to nicotine patch or varenicline for smoking cessation: a randomised, double-blind placebo-controlled trial. Lancet Respir Med. 2015;3(2):131–8.

41. Nakajima M, Yamamoto T, Nunoya KI, Yokoi T, Nagashima K, Inoue K, et al. Role of human cytochrome P4502A6 in C-oxidation of nicotine. Drug Metab Dispos. 1996;24(11):1212–7.

42. Nakajima M, Yamamoto T, Nunoya K, Yokoi T, Nagashima K, Inoue K, et al. Characterization of CYP2A6 involved in 3′-hydroxylation of cotinine in human liver microsomes. J Pharmacol Exp Ther. 1996;277(2):1010–5.

43. Dempsey D, Tutka P, Jacob P, Allen F, Schoedel K, Tyndale RF, et al. Nicotine metabolite ratio as an index of cytochrome P450 2A6 metabolic activity. Clin Pharmacol Ther. 2004;76(1):64–72.

44. Haberl M, Anwald B, Klein K, Weil R, Fu C, Gepdiremen A, et al. Three haplotypes associated with CYP2A6 phenotypes in Caucasians. Pharmacogenet Genomics. 2005;15(9):609–24.

45. Ho MK, Mwenifumbo JC, Al Koudsi N, Okuyemi KS, Ahluwalia JS, Benowitz NL, et al. Association of nicotine metabolite ratio and CYP2A6 genotype with smoking cessation treatment in African-American light smokers. Clin Pharmacol Ther. 2009;85(6):635–43.

46. Kaufmann A, Hitsman B, Goelz PM, Veluz-Wilkins A, Blazekovic S, Powers L, et al. Rate of nicotine metabolism and smoking cessation outcomes in a community-based sample of treatment-seeking smokers. Addict Behav. 2015;51:93–9.

47. Rojewski AM, Baldassarri S, Cooperman NA, Gritz ER, Leone FT, Piper ME, et al. Exploring issues of comorbid conditions in people who smoke. Nicotine Tob Res. 2016;18(8):1684–96.

48. McClave AK, McKnight-Eily LR, Davis SP, Dube SR. Smoking characteristics of adults with selected lifetime mental illnesses: results from the 2007 National Health Interview Survey. Am J Public Health. 2010;100(12):2464–72.

49. McKee SA, Krishnan-Sarin S, Shi J, Mase T, O'Malley SS. Modeling the effect of alcohol on smoking lapse behavior. Psychopharmacology. 2006;189(2):201–10.

50. Slopen N, Kontos EZ, Ryff CD, Ayanian JZ, Albert MA, Williams DR. Psychosocial stress and cigarette smoking persistence, cessation, and relapse over 9–10 years: a prospective study of middle-aged adults in the United States. Cancer Causes Control. 2013;24(10):1849–63.

51. Yudkin JS, Kumari M, Humphries SE, Mohamed-Ali V. Inflammation, obesity, stress and coronary heart disease: is interleukin-6 the link? Atherosclerosis. 2000;148(2):209–14.

52. Childs E, De Wit H. Effects of acute psychosocial stress on cigarette craving and smoking. Nicotine Tob Res. 2010;12(4):449–53.

53. Katon WJ. Clinical and health services relationships between major depression, depressive symptoms, and general medical illness. Biol Psychiatry. 2003;54(3):216–26.

54. Demers RY, Neale AV, Adams R, Trembath C, Herman SC. The impact of physicians' brief smoking cessation counseling: a MIRNET study. J Fam Pract. 1990;31(6):625–9.

55. Gritz ER, Fingeret MC, Vidrine DJ, Lazev AB, Mehta NV, Reece GP. Successes and failures of the teachable moment: smoking cessation in cancer patients. Cancer. 2006;106(1):17–27.

56. Volkman JE, DeRycke EC, Driscoll MA, Becker WC, Brandt CA, Mattocks KM, et al. Smoking status and pain intensity among OEF/OIF/OND veterans. Pain Med. 2015;16(9):1690–6.

57. Ditre JW, Heckman BW, Zale EL, Kosiba JD, Maisto SA. Acute analgesic effects of nicotine and tobacco in humans: a meta-analysis. Pain. 2016;157(7):1373.

58. Lund KE, Scheffels J, McNeill A. The association between use of snus and quit rates for smoking: results from seven Norwegian cross-sectional studies. Addiction. 2011;106(1):162–7.

59. Ramstrom LM, Foulds J. Role of snus in initiation and cessation of tobacco smoking in Sweden. Tob Control. 2006;15(3):210–4.

60. Foulds J, Ramstrom L, Burke M, Fagerström K. Effect of smokeless tobacco (snus) on smoking and public health in Sweden. Tob Control. 2003;12(4):349–59.

61. Mejia AB, Ling PM, Glantz SA. Quantifying the effects of promoting smokeless tobacco as a harm reduction strategy in the USA. Tob Control. 2010;19(4):297–305.

62. Benowitz NL. Smokeless tobacco as a nicotine delivery device: harm or harm reduction? Clin Pharmacol Ther. 2011;90(4):491–3.

63. Baldassarri SR, Bernstein SL, Chupp GL, Slade MD, Fucito LM, Toll BA. Electronic cigarettes for adults with tobacco dependence enrolled in a tobacco treatment program: a pilot study. Addict Behav. 2018;80:1–5.

64. Goniewicz ML, Knysak J, Gawron M, Kosmider L, Sobczak A, Kurek J, et al. Levels of selected carcinogens and toxicants in vapour from electronic cigarettes. Tob Control. 2014;23(2):133–9.

65. National Academies of Sciences, Engineering, and Medicine (U.S.). Committee on the Review of the Health Effects of Electronic Nicotine Delivery Systems. In: Stratton K, Kwan LY, Eaton DL, editors. Public health consequences of E-cigarettes. Washington, DC: The National Academies Press; 2018. 774 p.

66. Shahab L, Goniewicz ML, Blount BC, et al. Nicotine, carcinogen, and toxin exposure in long-term e-cigarette and nicotine replacement therapy users: a cross-sectional study. Ann Intern Med. 2017;166:390.

67. Chun LF, Moazed F, Calfee CS, Matthay MA, Gotts JE. Pulmonary toxicity of e-cigarettes. Am J Phys Lung Cell Mol Phys. 2017;313(2):L193–206.

68. Benowitz NL, Fraiman JB. Cardiovascular effects of electronic cigarettes. Nat Rev Cardiol. 2017;14(8):447.

69. Hajek P, Phillips-Waller A, Przulj D, Pesola F, Myers Smith K, Bisal N, et al. A randomized trial of E-cigarettes versus nicotine-replacement therapy. N Engl J Med. 2019;380:629.

70. Jamal A, Homa DM, O'Connor E, Babb SD, Caraballo RS, Singh T, et al. Current cigarette smoking among adults – United States, 2005–2014. MMWR Morb Mortal Wkly Rep. 2015;64(44):1233–40.

71. Babb S, Malarcher A, Schauer G, Asman K, Jamal A. Quitting smoking among adults – United States, 2000–2015. MMWR Morb Mortal Wkly Rep. 2017;65(52):1457–64.

72. Baldassarri SR, Chupp GL, Leone FT, Warren GW, Toll BA. Practise patterns and perceptions of chest health care providers on electronic cigarette use: an in-depth discussion and report of survey results. J Smok Cessat. 2018;13(2):72–7.

73. Steinberg MB, Giovenco DP, Delnevo CD. Patient–physician communication regarding electronic cigarettes. Prev Med Rep. 2015;2:96–8.

74. Haziza C, de La Bourdonnaye G, Skiada D, Ancerewicz J, Baker G, Picavet P, et al. Evaluation of the tobacco heating system 2.2. Part 8: 5-day randomized reduced exposure clinical study in Poland. Regul Toxicol Pharmacol. 2016;81:S139–S50.

75. Farsalinos KE, Yannovits N, Sarri T, Voudris V, Poulas K. Nicotine delivery to the aerosol of a heat-not-burn tobacco product: comparison with a tobacco cigarette and e-cigarettes. Nicotine Tob Res. 2018;20(8):1004–9.

Implementing COPD Precision Medicine in Clinical Practice

Don D. Sin

Key Point Summary

- Precision medicine in COPD is being enabled by advances in phenotyping and molecular techniques that have begun to clarify the heterogeneity of COPD endotypes.
- Blood eosinophil count is a promising predictive biomarker of clinical responses to inhaled corticosteroids (ICS) in COPD.
- Azithromycin therapy in COPD may be targeted to those with GOLD 2 disease severity, ex-smokers, and those 65 years of age and older.
- The combined genomics/biomarker-based approach to drug discovery and development is currently favored in COPD and may lead to novel therapeutics.

Introduction

Chronic obstructive pulmonary disease (COPD) is an inflammatory condition of the lung that afflicts 300 million people worldwide [1]. Approximately

D. D. Sin (✉)
University of British Columbia Centre for Heart Lung Innovation (HLI), Department of Medicine, St. Paul's Hospital, Vancouver, BC, Canada
e-mail: don.sin@hli.ubc.ca

3.2 million individuals die from COPD every year, and it is projected to become the fourth leading cause of death by 2040, responsible for 4.4 million deaths annually [1]. COPD is also a leading cause of hospitalizations in many countries around the world, and in the U.S., COPD is the second leading cause of disability-adjusted life years (DALYs) lost [2]. COPD is a progressive disease whose natural course is punctuated by periods of acute worsening of symptoms, which are called acute exacerbations of COPD [3]. Most of the COPD morbidity and mortality occur during these periods of exacerbations, which often lead to urgent visits to physicians' offices and emergency departments, and hospitalizations.

COPD as a Heterogeneous Disorder

COPD is defined based on a physiologic abnormality: a reduced forced expiratory volume in 1 second (FEV_1) to forced vital capacity (FVC) ratio, which can be detected reliably with spirometry [3]. COPD is thus characterized by persistent airflow limitation that is not fully reversible with bronchodilators [3]. However, as there are many different disease processes that lead to airflow limitation, COPD is pathophysiologically a heterogeneous disorder. Indeed, Vestbo and Lange have argued that a reduced FEV_1/FVC ratio is analogous to fever (for which there is a wide differential diagnosis), and as such, it does not provide any clues regarding the etiology or molecular drivers of its underlying cause [4].

© Springer Nature Switzerland AG 2020
J. L. Gomez et al. (eds.), *Precision in Pulmonary, Critical Care, and Sleep Medicine*,
Respiratory Medicine, https://doi.org/10.1007/978-3-030-31507-8_25

Pathologically, key features of COPD include airway remodeling and emphysema. Airway remodeling is characterized by narrowing of small airways, which are defined as airways less than 2 mm in diameter, and reduction in the total number of these airways [5]. Because resistance in the airways is inversely related to the fourth power of their radius, even small reductions in airway caliber can lead to significant airflow impairment. In mild COPD, however, airway caliber may be relatively normal [6]. Even in the absence of any significant airflow limitation, patients with mild COPD, defined by a reduced FEV_1/FVC and normal FEV_1 values, demonstrate significant loss in the number of small airways [7]. For example, Koo et al. recently showed using microimaging techniques that individuals with mild COPD had 40% fewer terminal bronchioles than smokers without any airflow limitation [7].

Emphysema is also present in most patients with COPD, though the extent of the disease is extremely variable across patients. On average, the alveolar surface area available for gas exchange, which is a surrogate for the severity of emphysema, decreases as emphysema burden increases. Compared to smokers without COPD, those with mild COPD, according to the Global initiative for Chronic Obstructive Lung Disease (GOLD) grade 1 definition, demonstrate an approximate 25% increase in emphysema burden, while those in GOLD grade 2 (i.e., with moderate COPD defined by FEV_1 between 50 and 79% of predicted) experience a 40% increase, and those in GOLD grade 4 (i.e., very severe COPD defined by FEV_1 less 30% of predicted) show an 80% increase in emphysema severity [7].

The distribution of emphysema is also variable. In cigarette smoke-related COPD, there is an upper lobe predominance of disease and emphysema is mostly located in the center of secondary lobules (termed centrilobular emphysema). In COPD related to alpha-1 antitrypsin deficiency (A1ATD), emphysema is predominantly found in the lower lobes and is characterized by complete destruction of secondary lobules (termed panlobular emphysema). In some COPD patients, however, the disease is predominantly located near the pleural surface (termed paraseptal emphysema). In many, there is a combination of paraseptal and

centrilobular emphysema. In biomass-related COPD, there is very little emphysema and most of the airflow limitation is attributed to small airway disease [8]. Other morphologic phenotypes in COPD include bronchiectasis and pulmonary arterial hypertension. In general, the pulmonary arterial hypertension of COPD is relatively mild and does not require specific pulmonary vasodilators [9]. Interestingly, however, the diameter of pulmonary artery has been shown to relate to risk of exacerbations [10]. The mechanism for this observed epidemiological relationship is unknown.

Clinically, patients most often complain of dyspnea on exertion and reduced health status. However, in a subset of patients, symptoms of cough and sputum production are the predominant feature. Traditionally, these patients have been labelled as having "chronic bronchitis." Another 10–30% of patients have features of asthma including prior history of childhood or adolescent asthma, atopy, and chronic rhinitis [11]. Over 60% of patients with mild COPD demonstrate positive reaction to methacholine challenge, consistent with airway hyperresponsiveness [12], and are referred to as having "asthma-COPD overlap syndrome" (ACOS) or "asthma-COPD overlap" (ACO) [13]. These ACO patients have greater symptom burden, more exacerbations and faster disease progression of disease than COPD without asthma features. Nevertheless, these patients have been largely excluded from trials of COPD and asthma drugs, leading to a scarcity of high quality data to guide therapeutic choices in ACO patients, although there is a general consensus that inhaled corticosteroids with long-acting bronchodilators should be first-line therapies [14].

Molecular characterization of COPD has been challenging, and the exact pathophysiology of COPD is unknown. In animal models of COPD (e.g., smoke-exposed mice, rats or guinea pigs for 3–6 months), many molecular pathways have been shown to be important players in COPD. These include pathways involving matrix metallopeptidases 9 and 12 (MMP9 and MMP12), C-C chemokine receptor type 5 and 6 (CCR5 and CCR6), tumor necrosis factor (TNF), interleukin 1 (IL-1), myeloperoxidase (MPO), club cell protein 16 (CC16), cathepsin S (CTSS), endothelial monocyte activating protein 2 (EMAPII), surfactant protein D

(SPD) [15], bone morphogenetic protein (BMP-6) [16], fibroblast growth factor-2 (FGF2) [17], ATP binding cassette A1 (ABCA1) [18], and ADAM Metallopepsidase Domain 9 (ADAM9) [19, 20], to name a few. However, only *SERPINA1*, the gene encoding alpha-1-antitrypsin protein, has been definitively implicated in COPD pathogenesis.

Precision Medicine in COPD

Traditionally, pharmaceutical companies have treated differences in phenotypes of COPD as "noise" and used large sample sizes to "drown out" this noise, especially in large phase III randomized controlled trials (RCTs). Accordingly, most of the evidence to support the current management of COPD have been generated from large RCTs, which have yield "average" data [21]. However, in clinical practice, there is no such thing as an average patient; physicians treat individual patients. Given the heterogeneity of COPD with respect to its phenotypes and endotypes (defined as molecular processes that lead to

the phenotype), clinical implementation of RCT results has been challenging.

Dissimilar to this traditional approach of "one-size-fits-all", precision medicine is defined as an *"approach for disease treatment and prevention that takes into account individual variability in genes, environment, and lifestyle for each person"* [22]. By considering a person's biology, exposures and lifestyle, precision medicine determines tailored approaches to prevent and treat disease [23, 24]. Precision medicine in COPD is being enabled by advances in phenotyping and molecular techniques that have begun to clarify the heterogeneity of COPD endotypes [25, 26]. Although clinicians have been practicing some form of precision medicine for decades, the launch of the Precision Medicine Initiative in 2015 by the National Institutes of Health (NIH) and other organizations has led to advances in discovery and implementation [24], with promises of a better future for patients. In this chapter, we provide examples of successful COPD precision medicine implementations (Table 25.1), and discuss how precision medicine will shape new therapeutic approaches in COPD.

Table 25.1 Examples of precision therapies in COPD

Interventions	Biomarker(s) or clinical trait(s)	Clinical context
Inhaled Corticosteroids	Blood eosinophil count (≥300 cells/uL)	Frequent exacerbator[a] on long-acting bronchodilator(s)
Supplemental home oxygen	PaO2 < 55 mm Hg (room air) OR PaO2 < 60 mm Hg (room air) + right sided heart failure or polycythemia	No role in exercise or intermittent oxygen desaturation
LVRS	Upper lobe predominant emphysema + low exercise capacity[b]	Very symptomatic despite maximal inhaler therapy and pulmonary rehabilitation Not a candidate for lung transplantation
Alpha-1-antitrypsin replacement	Blood alpha-1-antitrypin level (≤ 11 umol/L) or *SERPINA1* genotyping or electrophoresis	Rapid loss in lung function Symptomatic
Low-dose prophylaxis with azithromycin	Non or ex-smokers or GOLD 2 disease or Age ≥ 65 years	Frequent exacerbator despite maximal inhaler therapy
IgG replacement therapy	Serum IgG (<7 g/L)	Repeated hospitalizations for AECOPD despite maximal inhaler therapy and azithromycin Exacerbations are mostly related to recurrent respiratory tract infections
LAMA over LABA	BMI <20 kg/m² or GOLD 4 disease severity	LABA and LAMA have similar effectiveness except in those these traits (low BMI and high GOLD grade)

Abbreviations: *AECOPD* acute exacerbations of COPD, *BMI* body mass index, *GOLD* Global initiative for chronic Obstructive Lung Disease, *LABA* long-acting beta-2 adrenergic agonist, *LAMA* long-acting muscarinic antagonist, *LVRS* lung volume reduction surgery, *PaO₂* arterial partial pressure of oxygen
[a]Frequent exacerbator is defined as a patient who has two or more exacerbations per year or at least one hospitalization per year
[b]defined as <25 Watts for females and < 40 Watts for males on standard cardiopulmonary exercise test

Precision Medicine in the Use of Inhaled Corticosteroids

The most commonly used maintenance therapy in COPD is inhaled corticosteroids (ICS). ICS were first developed for asthma therapy, but with the realization that COPD airways were also inflamed, ICS have been used to control the inflammatory component of the disease [27]. However, unlike in asthma, where steroid-responsive Th2 cytokines and eosinophils are the major molecular drivers, the inflammatory process of COPD, which is characterized by neutrophils, is relatively resistant to corticosteroids [28]. Moreover, ICS use has been associated with adverse effects, including increased risk of bone demineralization, osteoporosis, vertebral and long-bone fractures, skin bruising, and cataracts [29]. In COPD, but not in asthma, ICS use has also been associated with increased risk of pneumonia (more on this later). Nonetheless, the two bestselling COPD drugs in the world contain ICS. In COPD, ICS are used in conjunction with a long-acting ß$_2$-agonist (LABA) typically in a fixed dose formulation (ICS/LABA combination).

GOLD and other COPD expert committees recommend against the use of ICS monotherapy and suggest that ICS be used only in combination with a LABA and/or a long-acting muscarinic antagonist (LAMA) for COPD patients who have a history of recurrent exacerbations (defined as having two or more exacerbations per year or one or more hospitalizations per year) [3]. In this setting, compared with LABA alone, ICS/LABA combination reduces exacerbations by approximately 10–20%, which translates to a number-needed-to-treat (NNT) of 34 patients to prevent one patient from experiencing an exacerbation per year [30]. The NNT to prevent one patient from experiencing a hospitalization is approximately 50–100 per year [30]. There is another method of calculating NNT based on the number of exacerbations rather than individuals. The method based on exacerbation as the unit of analysis is called event-based NNT, while that based on patients as the unit of analysis is called a person-based NNT. In general, person-based NNTs are preferred over event-based NNTs

because they are clinically easier to understand, as physicians treat patients not exacerbations [31], and because the original NNT calculations were based on dichotomous, not recurring, events. Since patients can have more than one exacerbation, event-based NNTs are generally smaller than person-based NNTs. In the case of ICS/LABA therapy compared with placebo, the event-based NNT is 4 per year, while the person-based NNT is 15–20 per year [32, 33].

More recently, ICS/LABA combinations have been mixed together with a LAMA in a fixed dose combination, leading to ICS/LABA/LAMA inhalers. A meta-analysis by Cazzola et al. suggested that compared with a LABA/LAMA fixed dose combination, ICS/LABA/LAMA was associated with a significant reduction in the rate of exacerbations [33]. The NNT, however, was high at 39 patients per year. Compared to LABA or LAMA alone (rather than dual bronchodilators), the NNT was slightly smaller at 22 [33].

Although eosinophils are not thought to be important players in the pathogenesis of COPD, blood eosinophil count may be predictive of clinical responses to ICS in COPD. Siddiqui et al. showed in the Foster 48 week Trial to Reduce Exacerbations in COPD (FORWARD) trial that ICS/LABA combination (beclomethasone/formoterol) therapy resulted in a 46% reduction in the risk of exacerbations over 1 year compared with formoterol alone in COPD patients with a blood eosinophil count of 280 cells/uL or more [34]. In contrast, among those with blood eosinophil count less than 110 cells/uL, the relative risk reduction was a non-significant 22%. Similar findings have been noted by others [35, 36]. Interestingly, in the Indacaterol-Glycopyrronium versus Salmeterol-Fluticasone for COPD Exacerbations (FLAME) study, the use of a LABA/LAMA (indacaterol/glycopyrronium) significantly reduced exacerbation rates compared to ICS/LABA (fluticasone/salmeterol) therapy in COPD patients whose blood eosinophil count was less than 150 cells/uL [37]. Above this threshold, the rates of exacerbation were similar between ICS/LABA and LABA/LAMA groups. In the most recent InforMing the PAthway of *COPD* Treatment (IMPACT) study, the beneficial effects of ICS/LABA/LAMA (fluticasone/

vilanterol/umeclidinium) combination compared with LABA/LAMA (vilanterol/umeclidinium) therapy were larger in patients with a blood eosinophil count of 150 cells/uL or greater compared to those who had counts lower than this level (32% relative reduction vs. 12%) [38]. Based on these studies, blood eosinophil count could play a role in predicting ICS response among COPD patients, although it should be noted that the relationship between blood and sputum eosinophil counts is relatively weak and blood eosinophil counts do not predict future risk of exacerbations [39].

In Cazzola et al.'s meta-analysis, the addition of ICS to LABA/LAMA combination was associated with an NNT of 9 patients per year when only patients with blood eosinophil count 300 cells/uL or more were considered (compared with an NNT of 47 for those whose eosinophil counts were less than 300 cells/uL) [33]. Interestingly, the risk of pneumonia related to ICS does not appear to be related to blood eosinophil count [40]. The risk is mostly related to potency of ICS, prior history of tuberculosis or pneumonia, and GOLD grade of severity with the risk rapidly rising when FEV_1 is <50% of predicted [41]. Thus, in COPD, the use of an ICS-containing regimen should be guided by a history of recurrent or frequent exacerbations (two or more per year) and blood eosinophil count 300 cells/uL or more. Although there is no firm evidence, experts recommend the use of ICS in COPD patients with features of asthma, including a prior or current history of asthma, significant airway hyperresponsiveness, and atopy [42]. ICS should be used very cautiously or avoided entirely in patients without these "traits" or in those with a prior history of pneumonia or tuberculosis. In those with the latter trait or those with GOLD 3 or 4 disease, lower potency formulations should be considered.

Precision Medicine in the Use of Bronchodilators

Bronchodilators are the first-line therapy for most symptomatic patients with COPD [3]. They reduce breathlessness, improve exercise perfor-mance, and prevent exacerbations. The most commonly used bronchodilators for COPD are LABAs, which predominantly target ß2-adrenergic receptors in airway smooth muscle, and LAMAs, which predominantly target the M3 muscarinic acetylcholine receptors in airway smooth muscle. Although there is some variation in reported results, on average, these bronchodilators reduce the risk of exacerbations by ~15–30% compared to placebo over 12 months [43–46], which translates to a person-based NNT of approximately 10–15 patients per year to prevent one or more exacerbations. Although the NNT is higher than most "precise" therapies, given the relatively low-cost of bronchodilators, a paucity of adverse side effects, and symptomatic benefit for patients, they remain the preferred first-line therapies for most symptomatic patients.

Although LABAs and LAMAs have similar effects, the Prevention of Exacerbations in Tiotropium (POET) study showed a slight advantage of tiotropium over salmeterol for exacerbation prevention [47]. On average, those who were assigned to tiotropium had a 17% lower risk of exacerbation over 1 year compared with those who used salmeterol. Intriguingly, the largest relative risk difference in exacerbation between tiotropium and salmeterol arms of the study was observed in patients with GOLD grade 4 disease severity and those with a body mass index (BMI) less than 20 kg/m^2. While the overall person-based NNT was 25 patients per year in favor of tiotropium, the NNT was eight for these two subgroups of patients. In those with GOLD grade 4 disease or BMI < 20 kg/m^2, tiotropium is clearly the preferred choice.

Precision Medicine in the Use of Antibiotic Prophylaxis

It is now a common practice to use daily or thrice-weekly regimen of azithromycin (250 mg/d) therapy for exacerbation prevention in patients with repeated exacerbations despite maximal bronchodilator treatment (generally, ICS/LABA/LAMA combination therapy). Overall, in such patients, low-dose azithromycin therapy reduces the risk of exacerbations by approximately 25%, with a person-based NNT of nine over 12 months [48]. However, long-term azithromycin therapy is associated with anti-microbial resistance and reduced hearing acuity, among other side effects. The number needed to harm (NNH; the number of patients needed to treat before one patient experiences an adverse effect from the drug) is approximately 18 patients per year [48]. As such, more targeted therapy for subgroups who are most likely to benefit from antibiotic therapies is desired. The Azithromycin for Prevention of Exacerbations study showed that the salutary effects of azithromycin were most pronounced in patients with GOLD 2 disease severity (hazard ratio (HR), 0.55; 95% CI, 0.40–0.75), ex-smokers (HR, 0.65; 95% CI, 0.55–0.77), and those 65 years of age and older (HR, 0.59; 95% CI, 0.47–0.74) [49]. Thus, azithromycin therapy may be targeted to patients in these subgroups and avoided in other patients.

Precision Medicine in the Use of Non-Pharmacologic Therapies

Non-pharmacologic therapies, including supplemental oxygen and lung volume reduction surgery, should be considered in patients with COPD. Supplemental oxygen therapy should be prescribed for patients with resting hypoxemia on room air. The Medical Research Council study showed that in patients with resting hypoxemia ($PaO_2 \leq 55$ mmHg on room air, or $PaO_2 < 60$ mmHg with evidence of right-sided heart failure or raised hematocrit), the use of continuous home oxygen therapy reduced mortality by ~50% with a person-based NNT of 5 over 5 years [50]. Similarly, the U.S. based Nocturnal Oxygen Treatment Trial (NOTT) showed a 50% relative risk reduction in mortality with continuous vs. nocturnal oxygen supplementation, with an NNT of 5 over 2 years [51]. In contrast, in the recently completed Long-Term Oxygen Treatment Trial (LOTT), supplemental oxygen therapy did not significantly modify mortality or risk of hospitalization among patients with moderate resting desaturation (89–93% oxyhemoglobin saturation on pulse oximetry) or those with

moderate exercise-related oxygen desaturation [52]. Thus, pulse oximetry or arterial blood gases may be used as biomarkers to identify subgroups of patients who are likely to benefit from supplemental oxygen therapy.

Lung volume reduction surgery (LVRS) has been evaluated for treatment of COPD. The National Emphysema Treatment Trial (NETT) showed that overall, there was no survival difference between those treated with LVRS (plus standard therapy) vs. those treated with standard non-surgical therapy alone [53]. However, in patients whose emphysema predominantly affected the upper lobes (as judged on thoracic computed tomography (CT)), and in those who demonstrated low exercise capacity (defined as less than 25 Watts for female and 40 Watts for male patients on standard cardiopulmonary exercise test), LVRS was effective in reducing mortality with a person-based NNT of 7 over 5 years. However, given the cost and the potential perioperative morbidity and mortality associated with LVRS, this procedure has not been widely adopted in clinical practice, even in this favorable subgroup of patients.

More recently, endoscopic lung volume reduction (EVLR) therapy using valves or coils has been evaluated. In general, EVLR methods have produced disappointing results and indeed, in one study, the use of an endobronchial valve was associated with increased risk of COPD hospitalization and hemoptysis [54], and an NNH for COPD exacerbation of 13 per year. However, investigators found in a post hoc analysis that the benefits of EVLR were observed largely in patients who did not demonstrate any significant collateral ventilation. Targeting of endobronchial valves to those who did not show collateral ventilation of the ipsilateral airway segment (using the Chartis System) was associated with a significantly reduced exacerbation risk, at an NNT of 13 per year [55]. The Zephyr Endobronchial Valve System has now received approval from the U.S. Food and Drug Administration (FDA). The current NNT is likely too high for widespread adoption and additional studies are needed to identify subgroups of patients in whom EVLR therapy will produce even greater efficacy.

It is well established that respiratory viral pathogens are the most common triggers of acute exacerbations of COPD. Immunoglobulins, which can be pathogen-specific or broadly neutralizing, are important first-line defenses against respiratory pathogens, and their deficiency has been associated with frequent pneumonias and bronchiectasis. Leitao Filho et al. showed in the MACRO and Simvastatin for the Prevention of Exacerbations in Moderate-to-Severe COPD (STATCOPE) cohorts that approximately one in four to one in five patients with COPD have reduced serum total immunoglobulin levels (IgG), consistent with immunodeficiency [56, 57]. Most importantly, those who had IgG deficiency, especially IgG1 and IgG2 deficiencies, demonstrated a 50–100% increase in the risk of exacerbations leading to hospitalization. A case series indicates that treatment of these individuals with immunoglobulin replacement therapy significantly reduces the risk of exacerbations [58]. Thus, in patients with IgG immunodeficiency who experience recurrent hospitalizations despite maximal inhaler therapy and chronic prophylactic azithromycin therapy, intravenous immunoglobulin replacement therapy may be considered.

Application of Precision Medicine in Drug Discovery

Overall, the pace of new drug development in respiratory diseases has been extremely slow. Although the world market for asthma and COPD therapeutics is 35 billion USD/yr., only one new class of medications has been introduced for COPD patients over the past 30 years [59]. The cumulative probability of respiratory drugs reaching the clinic is only 3% (from phase I to approval), whereas it is 14% for HIV/AIDS drugs and 7% for cancer therapeutics [59]. The greatest attrition occurs during phase II and III studies, mostly owing to lack of efficacy, which accounts for approximately 60% of the failures [60]. Traditionally, pharmaceutical companies have relied on preclinical animal models to assess potential therapeutic targets and compounds.

However, because they are poorly predictive of the human condition, they have been largely abandoned in favor of genomics-based approaches to drug discovery and development in COPD [60, 61].

The genomics-based approach has two major components: (1) genetic linkage to the drug target and (2) availability of 'response biomarkers' to gauge drug efficacy or 'predictive biomarkers' to determine groups of patients who are likely to respond to the drug [60]. Support from human genetics studies for drug targets improves the success rate of drugs in phase II studies by 50–100%, while the availability of response or predictive biomarkers increases the success rate by two- to threefold [60]. By implementing a combined genomics/biomarker approach, one major therapeutic company in respiratory sciences has increased the success rate from drug nomination across all therapeutic areas to completion of phase III studies by fivefold, from 4% to 19% [62]. Pharmacogenomics, which combines pharmacology and genetics to study how genes affect patient responses to particular drugs, is still in its infancy in COPD.

Precision Medicine to Prevent Rapid Loss of Lung Function in COPD?

Another major challenge in COPD precision medicine is developing prognostic biomarkers of "disease activity". In COPD, disease activity is generally defined as rapid decline in lung function over time. In general, there are three distinct patterns of lung function trajectory in COPD patients: (1) accelerated decline, especially after age 40 years; (2) reduced lung growth during childhood but normal decline as an adult; and (3) a mix of the previous two trajectories, which leads to severe disease at a younger age [63]. Although at the population-level these patterns are distinct, at an individual level there is tremendous heterogeneity and overlap of patterns over time. To date, there is no single blood- or lung-based biomarker that can predict the trajectory of lung function decline in a single individual. In the absence of such tools, it is not surprising that there are no current therapies, aside from smoking cessation, that can modify disease progression or mortality in COPD. As noted previously, while there are many genes that have been reproducibly associated with COPD risk, there are no genes (apart from the alpha 1 anti-trypsin gene) that are associated with disease progression and FEV_1 decline.

In a recent study by Zafari et al., clinical variables associated with rapid decline in lung function were used to develop a "calculator" to predict progression of disease at an individual level for patients with mild to moderate COPD [64]. They showed that five clinical features (i.e., smoking status, baseline FEV_1, BMI, sex, and airway hyperresponsiveness) were responsible for 1/3 of the variation in FEV_1 values over time within a single individual. They exploited this knowledge to create a tool where clinicians can input these parameters and obtain the probability that their patient will progress to higher grades of COPD over 10 years (available at: http://resp.med.ubc.ca/software/ipress/epic/fev1pred/). Data from this tool can be used by clinicians to target high-risk patients (i.e., those who are likely to progress) with intense smoking cessation programs or pharmacologic (e.g., LAMA) and non-pharmacologic therapies (e.g., pulmonary rehabilitation) for disease modification. The effects of these interventions can be serially and dynamically assessed using this online tool to determine whether the interventions have made any material difference to the patients' overall risk over time. Formal evaluation of the utility of tools such as this to improve health outcomes is not yet available.

Conclusion

COPD is now in the era of precision medicine. The traditional "one-size-fits-all" approach is no longer acceptable to patients, physicians and payers. To fully implement precision medicine, however, better therapeutics and biomarkers are needed to predict therapeutic responses and gauge disease activity. Biomarkers can be blood or sputum tests, or more broadly, precision imaging [65] or other phenotyping tools [66]. This will enable application of current and novel therapeutics beyond the "average" patient to the "individual" patient in clinical practice.

References

1. Foreman KJ, Marquez N, Dolgert A, et al. Forecasting life expectancy, years of life lost, and all-cause and cause-specific mortality for 250 causes of death: reference and alternative scenarios for 2016–40 for 195 countries and territories. Lancet. 2018;392(10159):2052–90.
2. Collaborators USBoD, Mokdad AH, Ballestros K, et al. The state of US health, 1990–2016: burden of diseases, injuries, and risk factors among US states. JAMA. 2018;319(14):1444–72.
3. Vogelmeier CF, Criner GJ, Martinez FJ, et al. Global strategy for the diagnosis, management, and prevention of chronic obstructive lung disease 2017 report: GOLD executive summary. Eur Respir J. 2017;49(3):pii: 1700214.
4. Vestbo J, Lange P. COPD drugs: the urgent need for innovation. Lancet Respir Med. 2014;2(1):14–5.
5. Hogg JC. Pathophysiology of airflow limitation in chronic obstructive pulmonary disease. Lancet. 2004;364(9435):709–21.
6. Hogg JC, Pare PD, Hackett TL. The contribution of small airway obstruction to the pathogenesis of chronic obstructive pulmonary disease. Physiol Rev. 2017;97(2):529–52.
7. Koo HK, Vasilescu DM, Booth S, et al. Small airways disease in mild and moderate chronic obstructive pulmonary disease: a cross-sectional study. Lancet Respir Med. 2018;6(8):591–602.
8. Camp PG, Ramirez-Venegas A, Sansores RH, et al. COPD phenotypes in biomass smoke- versus tobacco smoke-exposed Mexican women. Eur Respir J. 2014;43(3):725–34.
9. Kovacs G, Agusti A, Barbera JA, et al. Pulmonary vascular involvement in chronic obstructive pulmonary disease. Is there a pulmonary vascular phenotype? Am J Respir Crit Care Med. 2018;198(8):1000–11.
10. Wells JM, Washko GR, Han MK, et al. Pulmonary arterial enlargement and acute exacerbations of COPD. N Engl J Med. 2012;367(10):913–21.
11. Leung JM, Sin DD. Asthma-COPD overlap syndrome: pathogenesis, clinical features, and therapeutic targets. BMJ. 2017;358:j3772.
12. Tkacova R, Dai DL, Vonk JM, et al. Airway hyperresponsiveness in chronic obstructive pulmonary disease: a marker of asthma-chronic obstructive pulmonary disease overlap syndrome? J Allergy Clin Immunol. 2016;138(6):1571–9 e10.
13. Sin DD, Miravitlles M, Mannino DM, et al. What is asthma-COPD overlap syndrome? Towards a con-

sensus definition from a round table discussion. Eur Respir J. 2016;48(3):664–73.

14. Woodruff PG, van den Berge M, Boucher RC, et al. American thoracic society/national heart, lung, and blood institute asthma-chronic obstructive pulmonary disease overlap workshop report. Am J Respir Crit Care Med. 2017;196(3):375–81.

15. Pilecki B, Wulf-Johansson H, Stottrup C, et al. Surfactant protein D deficiency aggravates cigarette smoke-induced lung inflammation by upregulation of ceramide synthesis. Front Immunol. 2018;9:3013.

16. Verhamme FM, De Smet EG, Van Hooste W, et al. Bone morphogenetic protein 6 (BMP-6) modulates lung function, pulmonary iron levels and cigarette smoke-induced inflammation. Mucosal Immunol. 2019;12(2):340.

17. Kim YS, Hong G, Kim DH, et al. The role of FGF-2 in smoke-induced emphysema and the therapeutic potential of recombinant FGF-2 in patients with COPD. Exp Mol Med. 2018;50(11):150.

18. Sonett J, Goldklang M, Sklepkiewicz P, et al. A critical role for ABC transporters in persistent lung inflammation in the development of emphysema after smoke exposure. FASEB J. 2018;32(12):6724–36. fj201701381.

19. Wang X, Polverino F, Rojas-Quintero J, et al. A disintegrin and a metalloproteinase-9 (ADAM9): a novel proteinase culprit with multifarious contributions to COPD. Am J Respir Crit Care Med. 2018;198(12):1500–18.

20. Polverino F, Rojas-Quintero J, Wang X, et al. A disintegrin and metalloproteinase domain-8: a novel protective proteinase in chronic obstructive pulmonary disease. Am J Respir Crit Care Med. 2018;198(10):1254–67.

21. Schork NJ. Personalized medicine: time for one-person trials. Nature. 2015;520(7549):609–11.

22. National Institutes of Health. What is precision medicine? Your guide to understanding genetic conditions. Available at https://ghr.nlm.nih.gov/primer/precision-medicine/definition. Accessed 23 June 2018.

23. Nimmesgern E, Benediktsson I, Norstedt I. Personalized medicine in Europe. Clin Transl Sci. 2017;10(2):61–3.

24. Collins FS, Varmus H. A new initiative on precision medicine. N Engl J Med. 2015;372(9):793–5.

25. Aronson SJ, Rehm HL. Building the foundation for genomics in precision medicine. Nature. 2015;526(7573):336–42.

26. McCarthy JJ, McLeod HL, Ginsburg GS. Genomic medicine: a decade of successes, challenges, and opportunities. Sci Transl Med. 2013;5(189):189sr4.

27. Hogg JC, Chu F, Utokaparch S, et al. The nature of small-airway obstruction in chronic obstructive pulmonary disease. N Engl J Med. 2004;350(26):2645–53.

28. Barnes PJ. Corticosteroid resistance in patients with asthma and chronic obstructive pulmonary disease. J Allergy Clin Immunol. 2013;131(3):636–45.

29. Park HY, Man SF, Sin DD. Inhaled corticosteroids for chronic obstructive pulmonary disease. BMJ. 2012;345:e6843.

30. Suissa S. Number needed to treat in COPD: exacerbations versus pneumonias. Thorax. 2013;68(6):540–3.

31. Aaron SD, Fergusson DA. Exaggeration of treatment benefits using the "event-based" number needed to treat. Can Med Assoc J. 2008;179(7):669–71.

32. Suissa S. Number needed to treat: enigmatic results for exacerbations in COPD. Eur Respir J. 2015;45(4):875–8.

33. Cazzola M, Rogliani P, Calzetta L, Matera MG. Triple therapy versus single and dual long-acting bronchodilator therapy in COPD: a systematic review and meta-analysis. Eur Respir J. 2018;52(6):1801586.

34. Siddiqui SH, Guasconi A, Vestbo J, et al. Blood eosinophils: a biomarker of response to extrafine beclomethasone/formoterol in chronic obstructive pulmonary disease. Am J Respir Crit Care Med. 2015;192(4):523–5.

35. Pavord ID, Lettis S, Locantore N, et al. Blood eosinophils and inhaled corticosteroid/long-acting beta-2 agonist efficacy in COPD. Thorax. 2016;71(2):118–25.

36. Pascoe S, Locantore N, Dransfield MT, Barnes NC, Pavord ID. Blood eosinophil counts, exacerbations, and response to the addition of inhaled fluticasone furoate to vilanterol in patients with chronic obstructive pulmonary disease: a secondary analysis of data from two parallel randomised controlled trials. Lancet Respir Med. 2015;3(6):435–42.

37. Wedzicha JA, Banerji D, Chapman KR, et al. Indacaterol-glycopyrronium versus salmeterol-fluticasone for COPD. N Engl J Med. 2016;374(23):2222–34.

38. Lipson DA, Barnhart F, Brealey N, et al. Once-daily single-inhaler triple versus dual therapy in patients with COPD. N Engl J Med. 2018;378(18):1671–80.

39. Hastie AT, Martinez FJ, Curtis JL, et al. Association of sputum and blood eosinophil concentrations with clinical measures of COPD severity: an analysis of the SPIROMICS cohort. Lancet Respir Med. 2017;5(12):956–67.

40. Pavord ID, Lettis S, Anzueto A, Barnes N. Blood eosinophil count and pneumonia risk in patients with chronic obstructive pulmonary disease: a patient-level meta-analysis. Lancet Respir Med. 2016;4(9):731–41.

41. Sin DD, Tashkin D, Zhang X, et al. Budesonide and the risk of pneumonia: a meta-analysis of individual patient data. Lancet. 2009;374(9691):712–9.

42. Leung JM, Sin DD. Inhaled corticosteroids in COPD: the final verdict is. Eur Respir J. 2018;52(6):pii: 1801940.

43. Calverley PM, Anderson JA, Celli B, et al. Salmeterol and fluticasone propionate and survival in chronic obstructive pulmonary disease. N Engl J Med. 2007;356(8):775–89.

44. Sin DD, Man J, Sharpe H, Gan WQ, Man SF. Pharmacological management to reduce exacer-

bations in adults with asthma: a systematic review and meta-analysis. JAMA. 2004;292(3):367–76.

45. Tashkin DP, Celli B, Senn S, et al. A 4-year trial of tiotropium in chronic obstructive pulmonary disease. N Engl J Med. 2008;359(15):1543–54.

46. Zhou Y, Zhong NS, Li X, et al. Tiotropium in early-stage chronic obstructive pulmonary disease. N Engl J Med. 2017;377(10):923–35.

47. Vogelmeier C, Hederer B, Glaab T, et al. Tiotropium versus salmeterol for the prevention of exacerbations of COPD. N Engl J Med. 2011;364(12):1093–103.

48. Albert RK, Connett J, Bailey WC, et al. Azithromycin for prevention of exacerbations of COPD. N Engl J Med. 2011;365(8):689–98.

49. Han MK, Tayob N, Murray S, et al. Predictors of chronic obstructive pulmonary disease exacerbation reduction in response to daily azithromycin therapy. Am J Respir Crit Care Med. 2014;189(12):1503–8.

50. Report of the Medical Research Council Working Party. Long term domiciliary oxygen therapy in chronic hypoxic cor pulmonale complicating chronic bronchitis and emphysema. Lancet. 1981;1(8222):681–6.

51. Nocturnal Oxygen Therapy Trial Group. Continuous or nocturnal oxygen therapy in hypoxemic chronic obstructive lung disease: a clinical trial. Ann Intern Med. 1980;93(3):391–8.

52. Long-Term Oxygen Treatment Trial Research G, Albert RK, Au DH, et al. A randomized trial of long-term oxygen for COPD with moderate desaturation. N Engl J Med. 2016;375(17):1617–27.

53. Fishman A, Martinez F, Naunheim K, et al. A randomized trial comparing lung-volume-reduction surgery with medical therapy for severe emphysema. N Engl J Med. 2003;348(21):2059–73.

54. Sciurba FC, Ernst A, Herth FJ, et al. A randomized study of endobronchial valves for advanced emphysema. N Engl J Med. 2010;363(13):1233–44.

55. Criner GJ, Sue R, Wright S, et al. A multicenter randomized controlled trial of zephyr endobronchial valve treatment in heterogeneous emphysema (LIBERATE). Am J Respir Crit Care Med. 2018;198(9):1151–64.

56. Leitao Filho FS, Ra SW, Mattman A, et al. Serum IgG subclass levels and risk of exacerbations and hospitalizations in patients with COPD. Respir Res. 2018;19(1):30.

57. Leitao Filho FS, Won Ra S, Mattman A, et al. Serum IgG and risk of exacerbations and hospitalizations in chronic obstructive pulmonary disease. J Allergy Clin Immunol. 2017;140(4):1164–7.

58. Cowan J, Gaudet L, Mulpuru S, et al. A retrospective longitudinal within-subject risk interval analysis of immunoglobulin treatment for recurrent acute exacerbation of chronic obstructive pulmonary disease. PLoS One. 2015;10(11):e0142205.

59. Barnes PJ, Bonini S, Seeger W, Belvisi MG, Ward B, Holmes A. Barriers to new drug development in respiratory disease. Eur Respir J. 2015;45(5):1197–207.

60. Cook D, Brown D, Alexander R, et al. Lessons learned from the fate of AstraZeneca's drug pipeline: a five-dimensional framework. Nat Rev Drug Discov. 2014;13(6):419–31.

61. Churg A, Sin DD, Wright JL. Everything prevents emphysema: are animal models of cigarette smoke-induced chronic obstructive pulmonary disease any use? Am J Respir Cell Mol Biol. 2011;45(6):1111–5.

62. Morgan P, Brown DG, Lennard S, et al. Impact of a five-dimensional framework on R&D productivity at AstraZeneca. Nat Rev Drug Discov. 2018;17(3):167–81.

63. Lange P, Celli B, Agusti A, et al. Lung-function trajectories leading to chronic obstructive pulmonary disease. N Engl J Med. 2015;373(2):111–22.

64. Zafari Z, Sin DD, Postma DS, et al. Individualized prediction of lung-function decline in chronic obstructive pulmonary disease. Can Med Assoc J. 2016;188(14):1004–11.

65. Washko GR, Parraga G. COPD biomarkers and phenotypes: opportunities for better outcomes with precision imaging. Eur Respir J. 2018;52(5):1801570.

66. Leung JM, Obeidat M, Sadatsafavi M, Sin DD. Introduction to precision medicine in COPD. Eur Respir J. 2019;53(4):1802460.

Part VII

Enabling Widespread Adoption of Precision Medicine

Precision Medicine for All: Minority Health

26

Victor E. Ortega and Juan C. Celedón

Introduction

Racial and ethnic disparities in respiratory health can be broadly defined as significant differences in the prevalence, morbidity, or mortality from respiratory diseases that are linked to racial ancestry or ethnicity. Such disparities cannot be solely explained by race- or ethnic-specific genetic variants, as race and ethnicity are strongly correlated with socioeconomic status and, ultimately, environmental or lifestyle factors that affect respiratory health [1, 2]. Current evidence suggests that: (1) racial or ethnic minorities of African descent have worse outcomes for many respiratory diseases than non-Hispanic whites, and (2) individuals from different racial and ethnic groups respond differently to certain drugs [3–6].

According to the US Census Bureau, the US population will be more racially and ethnically diverse over the next 50 years, as Hispanics increase from one in six US residents to one in

V. E. Ortega (✉)
Department of Internal Medicine, Center for Precision Medicine, Wake Forest School of Medicine, Medical Center Boulevard, Winston-Salem, NC, USA
e-mail: vortega@wakehealth.edu

J. C. Celedón
Medicine, Epidemiology and Human Genetics, University of Pittsburgh, Pittsburgh, PA, USA

Pediatric Pulmonary Medicine, Children's Hospital of Pittsburgh of UPMC, Pittsburgh, PA, USA
e-mail: juan.celedon@chp.edu

three during this period [7]. The increased diversity of the US population has resulted in an unprecedented need for genomic (and other omics) studies for the development of precision approaches that can be applied to members of different racial and ethnic groups. Race and ethnicity are nominal terms that imply a particular ancestral background while also encompassing a lifelong social experience (Table 26.1) [8]. Genomic studies stratified according to these terms have been challenged because these categories do not apply similarly to individuals with different ancestral backgrounds [8, 9].

Over the past two decades, high-throughput genomic technologies have added an unprecedented level of complexity to the analysis and interpretation of data from different racial or ethnic groups with varying interindividual ancestral backgrounds [2, 10]. The vast majority of genomic studies have been performed in subjects of European descent, but there has been a recent increase in genomic studies including different racial and ethnic groups [11]. The advent of next-generation whole-genome sequencing has allowed for a more rapid expansion of diverse catalogues of human genome variation, which facilitate genetic studies of racial and ethnic minorities [12].

In this chapter, we review the basis for the variability in genomic diversity in commonly used ethnic and racial categories and the challenges involved in multiethnic genomic studies. We discuss specific examples of genomic studies in health (lung function) and respiratory disease (chronic obstructive pulmonary disease (COPD) and asthma) where clear racial or ethnic differences have been demonstrated in disease risk or severity and drug response (pharmacogenetics). Finally, we review findings from recent epigenome-wide association studies and discuss new approaches to study genetic and environmental factors related to complex respiratory diseases.

The US Population Is Increasingly Diverse and Multiethnic

Over the past 500 years, the admixture of Native American, African, and European populations has resulted in the varying ancestral backgrounds of contemporary US racial and ethnic groups, including Puerto Ricans, Mexican Americans, and African Americans (Table 26.1). Within Hispanic subgroups, Puerto Ricans have, on average, a higher proportion of African ancestry but a lower proportion of Native American ancestry than Mexican Americans. Compared to non-Hispanic whites or members of most Hispanic groups, African Americans and Afro-Caribbeans have, on average, a greater proportion of African ancestry but a lower proportion of European ancestry [13, 14].

The remarkable variability in ancestral background among individuals within a specific self-identified ethnic group is thus not adequately captured by current ethnic and racial designations employed by the US Census Bureau and biomedical researchers [1]. The identification and use of ancestry-informative genetic markers throughout the genome has demonstrated that the distribution of African, Native American, and European ancestry in individuals from a specific ethnic group varies according to multiple factors, including (1) self-reported ethnicity, as the racial ancestry of Hispanics varies across different Hispanic subgroups (e.g., Puerto Ricans vs. Mexican Americans); (2) area of residence, as, for example, the average proportion of African ancestry is higher in African Americans living in the Eastern United States than in other areas; and (3) familial generation, as, for example, the average proportion of African ancestry in African Americans can change in each subsequent generation due to racial admixture [14–16].

Table 26.1 Commonly used terms related to race and ethnicity

Term	Definition	Examples
Race	Historical and commonly used term for a group of people based on physical features (including hair or skin color) which reflect a common ancestral and geographical origin	White, black, Asian, African American, American Indian, Native Hawaiian
Ethnicity	Social group resulting from shared cultural factors, ancestry, language, diet, and physical features traditionally associated with race	Hispanic, non-Hispanic
Ancestry	Term to define a person's genetic, family, and geographic origins which can be quantified categorically or as a proportion based on ancestry-informative genetic markers	European, African, Asian, Amerindian
European	Inhabitant of Europe or an individual with ancestral origins from Europe, but is also used as synonym for white	European, white, European white
White	People of European ancestral origins, which can indicate race but also ethnicity	European, Caucasian, Caucasoid
Caucasian	Popular racial term for white race based on Blumenbach's eighteenth-century term for people who lived in Caucasus	European, white, Caucasoid
Black	Racial category for people of African ancestral origins	African, Afro-Caribbean
African	Racial category for people who self-identify as African while excluding European and other ancestries	Black, African American
Hispanic	Ethnic category used interchangeably with Latino that signifies people of Spanish ancestral origins, irrespective of race	Puerto Ricans, Mexicans, Colombians, Costa Ricans, Cubans

Sub-Saharan African ancestry is the most ancient of ancestries, resulting in more recombination events and fewer co-inherited DNA variants over a shorter genomic region. In contrast, European ancestry is the result of a more recent bottleneck event that resulted in a loss of genetic diversity, as the first modern humans are thought to have migrated to Europe from Africa approximately 40,000 years ago [17]. Thus, subjects of European descent have DNA variants that are co-inherited over longer distances across DNA (i.e., are in linkage disequilibrium (LD)). Based on LD patterns, individual DNA variants are less likely to tag the same groups of variants in subjects of African descent than those of European descent. Further, more extensive genotyping is required to characterize the genetic diversity in subjects of African descent than those of European descent. Differences in genetic ancestry also result in varying allelic frequencies throughout the genome, particularly for rare variants, which are more frequent in genomes of African descent [17, 18]. Genomic studies must thus consider ancestral background as a major determinant of genomic variation, which influences disease risk, disease severity, and responsiveness to drugs [3].

Lung Function: A Heritable Trait that Varies According to Genetic Ancestry

Lung function measures help characterize respiratory health, and reduced lung function is associated with increased morbidity and mortality from respiratory diseases. Large population-based studies in the United States and elsewhere have shown differences in lung function across racial or ethnic groups [19–21], leading the American Thoracic Society and the European Respiratory Society to recommend using racial- or ethnic-specific reference values for lung function measures [19, 22].

Ancestry-based genetic studies have shown that African ancestry impacts lung function in admixed ethnic groups in the same direction predicted by current, nominal race-based predictive equations [14, 16, 23]. In three independent studies of African American adults, Brazilians, and Puerto Rican children, the proportion of global African ancestry was inversely associated with the forced expiratory volume in 1 second (FEV_1) and forced vital capacity (FVC) [14, 16, 24]. In Mexicans and Mexican Americans from two studies, the east-to-west variation in regional Native American ancestry in Mexico was inversely associated with lung function [25]. Moreover, the percentage of global Native American ancestry has been associated with higher FEV_1 and FVC, as well as with reduced risk of airflow obstruction and COPD among Hispanics in Costa Rica and New Mexico [26, 27]. Thus, whereas Native American ancestry is positively associated with increased lung function in Hispanics, African ancestry is negatively associated with lung function in Hispanics and African Americans. This relationship between continental ancestry and lung function in racially admixed populations could provide insights into causal mechanisms underlying racial or ethnic disparities in respiratory health.

Genome-wide association studies (GWAS) in large cohorts, primarily of European descent, have identified numerous lung function susceptibility variants [28–30]. Among the largest of these was a GWAS of 144,318 subjects of European descent, which identified 97 susceptibility genes for lung function. In that study, a genetic risk score (GRS) based on 95 single nucleotide polymorphisms (SNPs) was shown to be associated with COPD [29]. Of note, some of the lung function genes identified in subjects of European descent (including *HHIP, FAM13A,* and *PTCH1*) were subsequently associated with lung function in a study of African Americans with asthma [31].

Recent studies have focused on the genetics of lung function in US minority populations. A GWAS of 11,822 Hispanics from the Hispanic Community Health Study/Study of Latinos (HCHS/SOL) identified eight novel loci for lung function, of which three replicated in non-Hispanic whites. Whole-genome admixture mapping identified a novel locus on *AGMO,* which was replicated in subjects of European descent [32]. A subsequent meta-analysis of GWAS in 90,715 subjects, including 8429 subjects of

African descent and 11,775 Hispanics, confirmed prior findings in subjects of European descent (e.g., for *HHIP*), while discovering 60 novel loci, 43 of which were unique to Hispanics and subjects of African descent [33]. This illustrates how studying diverse cohorts provides insight into racial- or ethnic-specific (Table 26.2) and "cosmopolitan" genetic determinants of lung function, which have variable allelic frequencies across racial/ethnic groups (Fig. 26.1). In the next section, we discuss ancestry-based studies and GWAS performed in diverse cohorts of smokers, which have identified novel loci for COPD risk (Fig. 26.2).

Precision Medicine Approaches May Improve COPD Inequalities

COPD, a genetically complex respiratory disease, affects an estimated 64 million individuals worldwide and is the third leading specific cause of death in the United States [46]. Cigarette smoking may interact with racial ancestry in determining COPD progression. Compared to non-Hispanic whites, African Americans have greater smoking-related decline in lung function and COPD mortality [47, 48], as well as increased risk of, and impairment from, COPD exacerbations [49]. Such findings may be partly due to

Table 26.2 Novel loci identified in diverse, multiethnic genome-wide studies

Gene symbol	Variant	Trait	Race/ethnic group	Reference
KIF25	rs76656601	FEV1/FVC	Hispanics	Burkart et al. [32]
ZSWIM7	rs4791658	FEV1	Hispanics	Burkart et al. [32]
HAL	rs145174011	FEV1/FVC	Hispanics	Burkart et al. [32]
KCNE2	rs28593428	FEV1/FVC	Hispanics	Burkart et al. [32]
GPR126	rs262113	FEV1/FVC	Hispanics	Burkart et al. [32]
AGMO	rs4133185	FEV1	Hispanics	Burkart et al. [32]
RYR2	rs3766889	FEV1	African ancestry	Wyss et al. [33]
EN1/MARCO	rs114962105	FVC	African ancestry	Wyss et al. [33]
CADPS	rs111793843	FEV1/FVC	African ancestry	Wyss et al. [33]
HDC	rs180930492	FEV1/FVC	African ancestry	Wyss et al. [33]
CPT1C	rs147472287	FEV1/FVC	African ancestry	Wyss et al. [33]
FAM19A2	rs348644	COPD	African Americans	Parker et al. [34]
KLHL7/ NUPL2	rs858249	COPD	Hispanics	Chen et al. [35]
DLG2	rs286499	COPD	Hispanics	Chen et al. [35]
DBH	rs1108581	FEV1 in at-risk current/ ex-smokers	Whites, African Americans	Lutz et al. [36]
PDZD2	rs7709630	COPD	Hispanics	Burkart et al. [32]
SERPINA1	rs2402444	Severe COPD	African Americans	Prokopenko et al. [37]
ADRA1B	rs10515807	Asthma	African ancestry	Mathias et al. [38]
PRNP	rs6052761	Asthma	African ancestry	Mathias et al. [38]
PYHIN1	rs1102000	Asthma	African Americans	Torgerson et al. [39]
PTCHD3	rs660498	Asthma	African Americans	White et al. [40]
PTGES	rs11788591	EMR-based asthma	African ancestry	Almoguera et al. [41]
SLC24A4	rs77441273	BDR in asthma	Hispanics	Drake et al. [42]
SLC22A15	rs1281748	BDR in asthma	Mexicans	Drake et al. [42]
PAPPA2	rs77977790	BDR in asthma	Puerto Ricans	Drake et al. [42]
NCOA3	rs115501901	BDR in asthma	Puerto Ricans	Drake et al. [42]
PRKG1	rs7903366	BDR in asthma	African Americans, Hispanics	Spear et al. [43]
NFKB1	rs28450894	BDR in asthma	Hispanics	Mak et al. [44]

Table highlights novel variant by reference sequence number (rs) identified by whole-genome association studies (GWAS) or admixture mapping in diverse multiethnic meta-analyses or studies focused on specific ethnic or racial groups. *BDR* bronchodilator response

genetic ancestry, as the proportion of global African ancestry determined by genetic markers was inversely associated with FEV_1/FVC [34] and modified the estimated effects of cigarette smoking on lung function decline among African Americans [23]. In contrast to findings in African Americans, a study of former and current smokers in New Mexico showed that Hispanics had lower risk of COPD and reduced decline in lung function than non-Hispanic whites that was not explained by differences in smoking habits [26]. One hypothesis to explain these findings is that there is a protective effect conferred by Native American ancestry against the detrimental effects of tobacco use on lung function among Hispanics.

To date, GWAS of COPD among former and current smokers of predominantly European descent have identified 43 susceptibility loci [50]. The first such GWAS identified the region containing the α-nicotinic acetylcholine receptor genes (*CHRNA3/5*) and *IREB2* (an adjacent antioxidant pathway gene) as COPD susceptibility loci [51]. Subsequent GWAS implicated loci associated with lung function in general populations (*HHIP* and *FAM13A*) on COPD risk while also identifying a novel locus for COPD (*CYP2A6*, a nicotine addiction pathway gene) [52, 53].

GWAS in multiethnic cohorts including former/current smokers and affected subjects have identified novel loci for COPD risk. In the COPDGene study, a meta-analysis of GWAS of COPD in non-Hispanic whites and African Americans confirmed known susceptibility loci (*CHRNA3, FAM13A, HHIP*) and identified *RIN3* as a novel susceptibility locus [54]; a follow-up admixture mapping analysis identified a novel locus for airflow obstruction (*FAM19A2*) in African Americans [34]. A subsequent GWAS of lung function in 9919 former and current smokers (including 3260 African Americans) confirmed multiple susceptibility loci for lung function and COPD, which were related to nicotine addiction (*CHRNA3/5, CYP2A6*) and other pathways (*HHIP, TGFB2, FAM13A, RIN3, AGPHD1, IREB2, MMP12*) while identifying a novel locus for COPD in *DBH* [36]. The first whole-genome sequencing study of severe COPD, which included 1794 subjects (of whom

844 were African Americans) from the Boston Early-Onset COPD and COPDGene studies, confirmed known loci for COPD (*HHIP, TNS1, CHRNA3/5, SERPINA6/1*) and identified a novel low-frequency *SERPINA1* variant as associated with severe COPD in African Americans [37].

Among Hispanics, a COPD GWAS meta-analysis in studies of Costa Ricans, Hispanics from New Mexico, and Hispanics in the US Multi-Ethnic Study of Atherosclerosis (MESA) provided suggestive evidence for two novel loci while confirming *FAM13A* as a susceptibility locus for COPD [35]. More recently, a GWAS in a subgroup of Hispanic ever smokers from HCHS/SOL identified a novel locus for COPD on *PDZD2* [32].

To date, genetic variants known to confer susceptibility to COPD have been primarily located in noncoding regulatory regions of the genome and cumulatively account for only a small proportion of disease heritability. This "missing heritability" of COPD could be explained by nongenetic mechanisms such as epigenetic regulation. Indeed, a few studies have linked cigarette smoking to DNA methylation signals that regulate the expression of genes related to nicotine addiction and COPD pathogenesis, but such studies have been limited by small sample size and lack of racial diversity [55].

Multiethnic epigenetic studies may increase our understanding of health disparities in COPD, since smoking habits vary across racial and ethnic groups [23, 26]. In a study of sputum samples from former and current smokers in New Mexico, methylation of the promoter region of 12 genes was higher in Hispanics than in non-Hispanic whites, and Native American ancestry was inversely associated with DNA methylation among Hispanics. Lung function and COPD risk loci identified by GWAS are highly represented among differentially methylated loci associated with COPD, further emphasizing the need for future studies of COPD epigenetics in racial and ethnic minorities [56].

While many genetic determinants of lung function and COPD overlap between racial and ethnic groups despite having variable allelic frequencies (Fig. 26.2), studies in increasingly

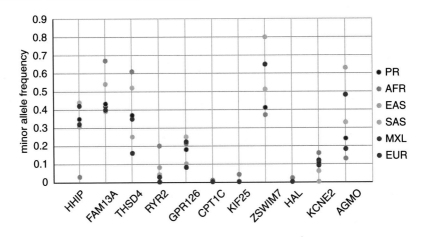

Fig. 26.1 Allele frequencies of different lung function loci by race or ethnic group. Lung function loci were among the first identified in general populations or loci subsequently discovered in minority ethnic groups denoted by reference sequence number (rs). Minor or less common, variant allele frequencies are based on data from the 1000 Genomes Project Phase 3. Abbreviations from each group are as follows: *CEU* Utah residents with ancestry from northern and western Europe; *PR* Puerto Ricans; *AFR* African descent populations, including African Americans, African Caribbeans, and Africans from Nigeria; *EAS* East Asians; *SAS* South Asians; *MXL* Mexican Americans from Los Angeles; and *EUR* European descent populations from the United States and Europe [45]

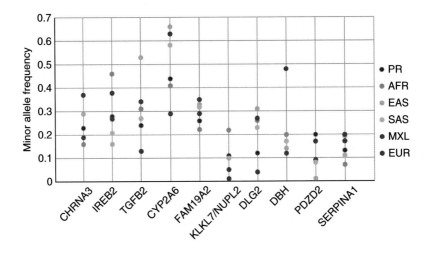

Fig. 26.2 Allele frequencies of different COPD risk loci by race or ethnic group. COPD loci were among the first identified in general populations or subsequently discovered in minority ethnic groups denoted by reference sequence number (rs). Minor or less common, variant allele frequencies are based on data from the 1000 Genomes Project Phase 3. Abbreviations from each group are as follows: *CEU* Utah residents with ancestry from northern and western Europe; *PR* Puerto Ricans; *AFR* African descent populations, including African Americans, African Caribbeans, and Africans from Nigeria; *EAS* East Asians; *SAS* South Asians; *MXL* Mexican Americans from Los Angeles; and *EUR* European descent populations from the United States and Europe [45]

diverse cohorts demonstrate that there are complex genetic architectures in/near ancestry-specific risk loci (Table 26.2). Future large-scale studies should improve our understanding of the relationship among ancestry-specific and "cosmopolitan" genetic determinants of lung function and COPD, gene-by-tobacco smoke or biomass smoke interactions, and epigenetic regulation on the pathogenesis of COPD in racial and ethnic minorities.

Precision Medicine Approaches May Improve Asthma Disparities

Asthma affects an estimated 300 million individuals worldwide and is the most common chronic respiratory disease of childhood in the United States [57]. Racial/ethnic asthma disparities are well recognized in the United States, where disease prevalence is highest in Puerto Ricans and African Americans, intermediate in non-Hispanic whites, and lowest in Mexican Americans [4, 5, 58, 59]. Puerto Ricans and African Americans also have greater morbidity and mortality from asthma than non-Hispanic whites or Mexican Americans [4, 5, 58, 59]. Despite such disparities, more genetic studies of asthma have been conducted in non-Hispanic whites than in Puerto Ricans or African Americans.

To date, GWAS of asthma have identified approximately 76 susceptibility loci, albeit with varying degrees of subsequent replication [50]. A GWAS of physician-diagnosed asthma in 10,365 cases and 16,110 control subjects of European descent first identified the chromosome 17q21 locus as conferring susceptibility to asthma [60]. The first GWAS of asthma in African Americans and Afro-Caribbeans identified the α-1B-adrenergic receptor (ADRA1B) and prion-related protein (PRNP) genes as novel susceptibility loci, while replicating a locus previously identified in family-based linkage studies (DPP10) [38, 61]. The first multiethnic GWAS meta-analysis of asthma, including subjects of African descent, Hispanics, and non-Hispanic whites, confirmed some of the prior findings in subjects of European descent while identifying an ethnic-specific locus (PYHIN1) in subjects of African descent [39]. This meta-analysis, together with the one in subjects of European descent and a subsequent admixture mapping analysis in Puerto Ricans and Mexican Americans, confirmed as "cosmopolitan" susceptibility loci for asthma the 17q21 locus, IL1RL1, TSLP, and IL33 [39, 60, 62].

Because asthma prevalence differs between Puerto Ricans and Mexican Americans, GWAS of combined Hispanic subgroups could obscure ethnic-specific associations in Hispanic subgroups. The first meta-analysis of asthma GWAS in Puerto Ricans, which included 2144 cases and 2893 control subjects, found genome-wide significant associations between multiple SNPs within the 17q21 locus [39, 60, 62, 63] while confirming findings for SNPs in IL1Rl, TSLP, and GSDMB from GWAS in other racial and ethnic groups [63]. In a GWAS of 1227 African American children, the 17q21 locus was not associated with asthma, consistent with prior weak associations found in studies of subjects of African descent. Although only 3 of 53 prior asthma risk loci from studies of non-Hispanic whites were replicated and a novel locus was identified in PTCHD3, these results must be cautiously interpreted due to the relatively small sample size of the study [40].

A GWAS of 21,644 subjects with and without asthma defined according to the presence of International Classification of Diseases (ICD) codes analyzed data from two ancestral groups identified on the basis of genetic markers [41]. This study confirmed the 17q21 locus as an asthma-susceptibility locus in subjects of European descent but not in those of African descent. Two novel loci were identified in subjects of European descent (TEK and HMGA1) and one unique to subjects of African descent (PTGES) [41]. More recently, a large multi-ancestry meta-analysis of 23,948 cases and 118,538 control subjects identified 878 SNPs in 18 genetic loci as significantly associated with asthma in a multi-ancestry meta-analysis and an European ancestry meta-analysis [64]. In that study, there were no statistically significant results in the African ancestry, Japanese ancestry, or Latino ancestry meta-analyses, which could be explained by having insufficient statistical power in subgroups of non-European ancestry [64].

Current evidence shows that many asthma-susceptibility genetic variants are shared across racial or ethnic groups ("cosmopolitan"), while others may be unique to, or have greater effects in, specific racial or ethnic groups (Table 26.2). Because some alleles in cosmopolitan loci have variable allelic frequencies across racial/ethnic groups, they could contribute to health disparities observed in asthma (Fig. 26.3).

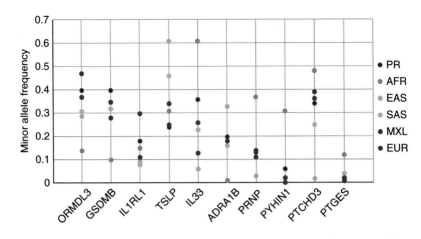

Fig. 26.3 Allelic frequencies of different asthma risk loci by race or ethnic group. Asthma loci first identified in subjects of European descent and/or subsequently discovered in minority groups are denoted by reference sequence number (rs). Allelic frequencies for minor or less common variants are based on data from the 1000 Genomes Project Phase 3. Abbreviations from each group are as follows: *CEU* Utah residents with ancestry from northern and western Europe; *PR* Puerto Ricans; *AFR* African descent populations, including African Americans, African Caribbeans, and Africans from Nigeria; *EAS* East Asians; *SAS* South Asians; *MXL* Mexican Americans from Los Angeles; and *EUR* European descent populations from the United States and Europe [45]

Racial or ethnic differences in response to therapies for asthma have been described across different drug classes and could underlie disparities in asthma morbidity. Findings from a large surveillance trial and retrospective analyses of clinical trials suggested that African Americans respond less favorably to long-acting β_2-adrenergic receptor agonist (LABA) drugs than non-Hispanic whites [65, 66]. Moreover, Puerto Ricans with asthma have been shown to be less responsive to short-acting β_2-agonists (SABA) than Mexican Americans, a finding that could be explained by ethnic-specific differences in the frequency of risk alleles and/or chronic psychosocial stress [67, 68].

The most studied locus for inhaled β_2-agonist response is that encoding the receptor target of the drug, the β_2-adrenergic receptor gene (*ADRB2*). *ADRB2* has a common coding SNP, Gly[16]Arg, which has been extensively studied in pharmacogenetic studies of asthma [68, 69]. Gly[16]Arg has in vitro effects on β_2-agonist-induced receptor downregulation [70]. Arg[16] homozygotes have been shown to have greater bronchodilator response to SABA than Gly[16] homozygotes in non-Hispanic whites and Puerto Ricans [71, 72].

Genotype-stratified studies found that Gly[16]Arg genotypes were associated with lung function and clinical response to regular albuterol therapy, but not with response to LABA [73–77].

Gly[16]Arg is common (allelic frequency of 40–60%) and thus unlikely to influence lack of response to LABA, because most individuals with asthma experience beneficial effects [65, 78]. A rare variant in *ADRB2* (Thr[164]Ile) has strong in vitro effects and could influence uncommon adverse or impaired responses to LABA [79, 80]. Sequencing of *ADRB2* identified rare variants associated with severe asthma exacerbations among LABA-treated non-Hispanic whites with the Thr[164]Ile variant and among African Americans with a promoter 25-base pair insertion variant [69]. A combined GWAS and admixture mapping study of SABA bronchodilator response in Hispanics also identified rare variants in solute carrier proteins (*SLC24A4* and *SLC22A15*) and β_2-adrenergic receptor pathway genes (*ADCY9, SPATS2L, THRB*) as pharmacogenetic loci [42, 81, 82]. Rare variants differ according to genetic ancestry and, thus, may contribute to disparities in asthma drug response [17, 18].

GWAS of response to short-acting bronchodilators have identified susceptibility loci for bronchodilator response in cohorts including predominantly non-Hispanic white subjects with asthma [42, 81, 83]. GWAS in diverse cohorts have identified potential susceptibility loci for bronchodilator response in Puerto Ricans [42] and African Americans [43, 84, 85]. The first study to use whole-genome sequencing to identify susceptibility loci for response to SABA included 1141 African American and Hispanic children with asthma and identified 32 novel regions containing rare and common variants in pathways for β$_2$-adrenergic receptor signaling (*ADAMTS3* and *COX18*), inflammation (*NFKB1* and *PLCB1*), and ciliopathy (*DNAH5*). The *NFKB1* variant (rs28450894) that was associated with reduced bronchodilator response was more frequent in African Americans [44]. Whole-genome sequencing was ideal to provide information on both rare and novel pharmacogenetic variants in this minority cohort (Table 26.2).

Most known susceptibility variants for asthma are in regulatory noncoding genomic regions and altogether account for less than 5% of the observed heritability [64]. This finding and the rise in asthma prevalence in industrialized countries from the 1960s to at least the 1990s strongly suggest a major role for environmental exposures in the "asthma epidemic." In this context, epigenetic studies are invaluable to better understand environmental influences on gene expression and identifying markers of disease development and progression [86–88]. A genome-wide study of DNA methylation in peripheral blood mononuclear cells from 97 African American and Hispanic children with asthma and 97 control subjects identified 73 differentially methylated genomic regions associated with asthma that were enriched for pathways related to mucus hypersecretion, inflammation, innate immunity, and nitric oxide synthesis [89]. Such findings await replication in other cohorts.

Considerable interest has arisen to study DNA methylation in nasal epithelium as a surrogate for DNA methylation in bronchial epithelium. In a study of 36 African American subjects with atopic asthma and 36 non-atopic African American controls, 186 genomic regions were differentially methylated by atopic asthma, encompassing pathways related to collagen and the extracellular matrix, immunity, and allergic inflammation [90]. More recently, a genome-wide study of DNA methylation in nasal epithelium from 477 Puerto Rican school-aged children identified 8664 CpG sites that were significantly associated with atopy and atopic asthma, with false discovery rate (FDR) corrected p-values ranging from 9.58×10^{-17} to 2.18×10^{-22} for the top 30 CpGs for atopy [91]. Several of these top CpGs were located near genes associated with immune response or epithelial barrier function, and a high proportion of significant CpGs were associated with changes in gene expression. Of the 30 top CpGs for atopy, 28 were replicated in two independent cohorts of subjects with African American and European ancestry, with similar results for atopic asthma. Moreover, a 30-CpG panel accurately classified children according to atopic asthma (area under the receiver operating characteristic curve of 0.95–0.99 in the Puerto Rican cohort and 0.85–0.88 in the replication cohorts). Taken together, these findings suggest a key role for epigenetic regulation of the airway epithelium in the pathogenesis of atopic asthma and support the feasibility of using the nasal methylome in future longitudinal studies. Such studies may identify methylation marks that precede disease development or predict treatment response in subjects with asthma, including in minority populations.

Conclusions

Racial and ethnic disparities in respiratory health are due to the interplay between non-modifiable (genetic) risk factors and modifiable (socioeconomic and environmental) risk factors occurring over an individual's lifetime [9]. GWAS in diverse cohorts have identified common susceptibility variants for lung function and respiratory diseases, but such variants explain only a small proportion of observed heritability. Future studies that focus on rare genetic variants and regulation of gene expression in racial and ethnic minorities may help account for some of the missing heritability. Indeed, efforts are underway to perform large whole-genome sequencing of studies in diverse cohorts, and recent epigenomic and transcriptomic studies of airway epithelium in asthma lend strong support to the advantage of conducting multi-omics studies in diverse cohorts to further our understanding of disparities in respiratory diseases according to race/ethnicity. Such knowledge, coupled with improved access to high-quality healthcare for all, will improve the prevention, diagnosis, and treatment of respiratory diseases in underrepresented minorities, ultimately leading to the elimination of unacceptable disparities in respiratory health.

Acknowledgments Dr. Ortega's contribution was supported by grant K08 HL118128 from the US National Institute of Health (NIH). Dr. Celedón's contribution was supported by grants HL117191, HL119952, and MD011764 from the US NIH.

Conflicts of Interest Dr. Victor E. Ortega has nothing to disclose. Dr. Juan C. Celedón has received research materials from GSK and Merck (inhaled steroids) and Pharmavite (vitamin D and placebo capsules), to provide medications free of cost to participants in NIH-funded studies.

References

1. Cooper RS, Nadkarni GN, Ogedegbe G. Race, ancestry, and reporting in medical journals. JAMA. 2018;320(15):1531–2.
2. Celedon JC, Burchard EG, Schraufnagel D, Castillo-Salgado C, Schenker M, Balmes J, et al. An American Thoracic Society/National Heart, Lung, and Blood Institute Workshop report: addressing respiratory health equality in the United States. Ann Am Thorac Soc. 2017;14(5):814–26.
3. Bonham VL, Callier SL, Royal CD. Will precision medicine move us beyond race? N Engl J Med. 2016;374(21):2003–5.
4. Moorman JE, Akinbami LJ, Bailey CM, Zahran HS, King ME, Johnson CA, et al. National surveillance of asthma: United States, 2001–2010. Vital Health Stat 3. 2012;(35):1–58.
5. Homa DM, Mannino DM, Lara M. Asthma mortality in U.S. Hispanics of Mexican, Puerto Rican, and Cuban heritage, 1990–1995. Am J Respir Crit Care Med. 2000;161(2 Pt 1):504–9.
6. Keet CA, McCormack MC, Pollack CE, Peng RD, McGowan E, Matsui EC. Neighborhood poverty, urban residence, race/ethnicity, and asthma: rethinking the inner-city asthma epidemic. J Allergy Clin Immunol. 2015;135(3):655–62.
7. Bureau USC. U.S. Census Bureau Projections Show a Slower Growing, Older, More Diverse Nation a Half Century from Now 2012 [updated December 12, 2012; cited 2014 December 4, 2014]. Available from: https://www.census.gov/newsroom/releases/archives/population/cb12-243.html.
8. Braun L, Fausto-Sterling A, Fullwiley D, Hammonds EM, Nelson A, Quivers W, et al. Racial categories in medical practice: how useful are they? PLoS Med. 2007;4(9):e271.
9. Ellison GT, Smart A, Tutton R, Outram SM, Ashcroft R, Martin P. Racial categories in medicine: a failure of evidence-based practice? PLoS Med. 2007;4(9):e287.
10. Ortega VE, Meyers DA. Implications of population structure and ancestry on asthma genetic studies. Curr Opin Allergy Clin Immunol. 2014;14(5):381–9.
11. Bustamante CD, Burchard EG, De la Vega FM. Genomics for the world. Nature. 2011;475(7355):163–5.
12. Johnston HR, Hu YJ, Gao J, O'Connor TD, Abecasis GR, Wojcik GL, et al. Identifying tagging SNPs for African specific genetic variation from the African Diaspora Genome. Sci Rep. 2017;7:46398.
13. Choudhry S, Burchard EG, Borrell LN, Tang H, Gomez I, Naqvi M, et al. Ancestry-environment interactions and asthma risk among Puerto Ricans. Am J Respir Crit Care Med. 2006;174(10):1088–93.
14. Kumar R, Seibold MA, Aldrich MC, Williams LK, Reiner AP, Colangelo L, et al. Genetic ancestry in lung-function predictions. N Engl J Med. 2010;363(4):321–30.
15. Bryc K, Durand EY, Macpherson JM, Reich D, Mountain JL. The genetic ancestry of African Americans, Latinos, and European Americans across the United States. Am J Hum Genet. 2015;96(1):37–53.
16. Pino-Yanes M, Thakur N, Gignoux CR, Galanter JM, Roth LA, Eng C, et al. Genetic ancestry influences asthma susceptibility and lung function among Latinos. J Allergy Clin Immunol. 2015;135(1):228–35.
17. Marth G, Schuler G, Yeh R, Davenport R, Agarwala R, Church D, et al. Sequence variations in the public human genome data reflect a bottlenecked population history. Proc Natl Acad Sci U S A. 2003;100(1):376–81.
18. The 1000 Genomes Project Consortium, Abecasis GR, Auton A, Brooks LD, DePristo MA, Durbin RM, et al. An integrated map of genetic variation from 1,092 human genomes. Nature. 2012;491(7422):56–65.
19. Quanjer PH, Stanojevic S, Cole TJ, Baur X, Hall GL, Culver BH, et al. Multi-ethnic reference values for spirometry for the 3-95-yr age range: the

global lung function 2012 equations. Eur Respir J. 2012;40(6):1324–43.

20. Hankinson JL, Odencrantz JR, Fedan KB. Spirometric reference values from a sample of the general U.S. population. Am J Respir Crit Care Med. 1999;159(1):179–87.

21. Duong M, Islam S, Rangarajan S, Teo K, O'Byrne PM, Schunemann HJ, et al. Global differences in lung function by region (PURE): an international, community-based prospective study. Lancet Respir Med. 2013;1(8):599–609.

22. Miller MR, Hankinson J, Brusasco V, Burgos F, Casaburi R, Coates A, et al. Standardisation of spirometry. Eur Respir J. 2005;26(2):319–38.

23. Aldrich MC, Kumar R, Colangelo LA, Williams LK, Sen S, Kritchevsky SB, et al. Genetic ancestry-smoking interactions and lung function in African Americans: a cohort study. PLoS One. 2012;7(6):e39541.

24. Menezes AM, Wehrmeister FC, Hartwig FP, Perez-Padilla R, Gigante DP, Barros FC, et al. African ancestry, lung function and the effect of genetics. Eur Respir J. 2015;45(6):1582–9.

25. Moreno-Estrada A, Gignoux CR, Fernandez-Lopez JC, Zakharia F, Sikora M, Contreras AV, et al. Human genetics. The genetics of Mexico recapitulates Native American substructure and affects biomedical traits. Science. 2014;344(6189):1280–5.

26. Bruse S, Sood A, Petersen H, Liu Y, Leng S, Celedon JC, et al. New Mexican Hispanic smokers have lower odds of chronic obstructive pulmonary disease and less decline in lung function than non-Hispanic whites. Am J Respir Crit Care Med. 2011;184(11):1254–60.

27. Chen W, Brehm JM, Boutaoui N, Soto-Quiros M, Avila L, Celli BR, et al. Native American ancestry, lung function, and COPD in Costa Ricans. Chest. 2014;145(4):704–10.

28. Soler Artigas M, Loth DW, Wain LV, Gharib SA, Obeidat M, Tang W, et al. Genome-wide association and large-scale follow up identifies 16 new loci influencing lung function. Nat Genet. 2011;43(11):1082–90.

29. Wain LV, Shrine N, Artigas MS, Erzurumluoglu AM, Noyvert B, Bossini-Castillo L, et al. Genome-wide association analyses for lung function and chronic obstructive pulmonary disease identify new loci and potential druggable targets. Nat Genet. 2017;49(3):416–25.

30. Repapi E, Sayers I, Wain LV, Burton PR, Johnson T, Obeidat M, et al. Genome-wide association study identifies five loci associated with lung function. Nat Genet. 2010;42(1):36–44.

31. Li X, Howard TD, Moore WC, Ampleford EJ, Li H, Busse WW, et al. Importance of hedgehog interacting protein and other lung function genes in asthma. J Allergy Clin Immunol. 2011;127(6):1457–65.

32. Burkart KM, Sofer T, London SJ, Manichaikul A, Hartwig FP, Yan Q, et al. A genome-wide association study in Hispanics/Latinos identifies novel signals for lung function. The Hispanic community health study/study of Latinos. Am J Respir Crit Care Med. 2018;198(2):208–19.

33. Wyss AB, Sofer T, Lee MK, Terzikhan N, Nguyen JN, Lahousse L, et al. Multiethnic meta-analysis identifies ancestry-specific and cross-ancestry loci for pulmonary function. Nat Commun. 2018;9(1):2976.

34. Parker MM, Foreman MG, Abel HJ, Mathias RA, Hetmanski JB, Crapo JD, et al. Admixture mapping identifies a quantitative trait locus associated with FEV1/FVC in the COPDGene Study. Genet Epidemiol. 2014;38(7):652–9.

35. Chen W, Brehm JM, Manichaikul A, Cho MH, Boutaoui N, Yan Q, et al. A genome-wide association study of chronic obstructive pulmonary disease in Hispanics. Ann Am Thorac Soc. 2015;12(3):340–8.

36. Lutz SM, Cho MH, Young K, Hersh CP, Castaldi PJ, McDonald ML, et al. A genome-wide association study identifies risk loci for spirometric measures among smokers of European and African ancestry. BMC Genet. 2015;16:138.

37. Prokopenko D, Sakornsakolpat P, Loehlein Fier H, Qiao D, Parker MM, McDonald MN, et al. Whole genome sequencing in severe chronic obstructive pulmonary disease. Am J Respir Cell Mol Biol. 2018;59(5):614–22.

38. Mathias RA, Grant AV, Rafaels N, Hand T, Gao L, Vergara C, et al. A genome-wide association study on African-ancestry populations for asthma. J Allergy Clin Immunol. 2010;125(2):336–46.e4.

39. Torgerson DG, Ampleford EJ, Chiu GY, Gauderman WJ, Gignoux CR, Graves PE, et al. Meta-analysis of genome-wide association studies of asthma in ethnically diverse North American populations. Nat Genet. 2011;43(9):887–92.

40. White MJ, Risse-Adams O, Goddard P, Contreras MG, Adams J, Hu D, et al. Novel genetic risk factors for asthma in African American children: Precision Medicine and the SAGE II Study. Immunogenetics. 2016;68(6–7):391–400.

41. Almoguera B, Vazquez L, Mentch F, Connolly J, Pacheco JA, Sundaresan AS, et al. Identification of four novel loci in asthma in European American and African American populations. Am J Respir Crit Care Med. 2017;195(4):456–63.

42. Drake KA, Torgerson DG, Gignoux CR, Galanter JM, Roth LA, Huntsman S, et al. A genome-wide association study of bronchodilator response in Latinos implicates rare variants. J Allergy Clin Immunol. 2014;133(2):370–8.

43. Spear ML, Hu D, Pino-Yanes M, Huntsman S, Eng C, Levin AM, et al. A genome-wide association and admixture mapping study of bronchodilator drug response in African Americans with asthma. Pharmacogenomics J. 2018;19(3):249–59.

44. Mak ACY, White MJ, Eckalbar WL, Szpiech ZA, Oh SS, Pino-Yanes M, et al. Whole-genome sequencing of Pharmacogenetic drug response in racially diverse children with asthma. Am J Respir Crit Care Med. 2018;197(12):1552–64.

45. Sudmant PH, Rausch T, Gardner EJ, Handsaker RE, Abyzov A, Huddleston J, et al. An integrated map of structural variation in 2,504 human genomes. Nature. 2015;526(7571):75–81.

46. Rabe KF, Hurd S, Anzueto A, Barnes PJ, Buist SA, Calverley P, et al. Global strategy for the diagnosis, management, and prevention of chronic obstructive pulmonary disease: GOLD executive summary. Am J Respir Crit Care Med. 2007;176(6):532–55.

47. Chatila WM, Wynkoop WA, Vance G, Criner GJ. Smoking patterns in African Americans and whites with advanced COPD. Chest. 2004;125(1):15–21.

48. Dransfield MT, Davis JJ, Gerald LB, Bailey WC. Racial and gender differences in susceptibility to tobacco smoke among patients with chronic obstructive pulmonary disease. Respir Med. 2006;100(6):1110–6.

49. Han MK, Curran-Everett D, Dransfield MT, Criner GJ, Zhang L, Murphy JR, et al. Racial differences in quality of life in patients with COPD. Chest. 2011;140(5):1169–76.

50. Institute NHGRIatEB. NHRGI-EBI catalog of published genome-wide association studies 2018. Available from: https://www.ebi.ac.uk/gwas/.

51. Pillai SG, Ge D, Zhu G, Kong X, Shianna KV, Need AC, et al. A genome-wide association study in chronic obstructive pulmonary disease (COPD): identification of two major susceptibility loci. PLoS Genet. 2009;5(3):e1000421.

52. Cho MH, Boutaoui N, Klanderman BJ, Sylvia JS, Ziniti JP, Hersh CP, et al. Variants in FAM13A are associated with chronic obstructive pulmonary disease. Nat Genet. 2010;42(3):200–2.

53. Cho MH, Castaldi PJ, Wan ES, Siedlinski M, Hersh CP, Demeo DL, et al. A genome-wide association study of COPD identifies a susceptibility locus on chromosome 19q13. Hum Mol Genet. 2012;21(4):947–57.

54. Cho MH, McDonald ML, Zhou X, Mattheisen M, Castaldi PJ, Hersh CP, et al. Risk loci for chronic obstructive pulmonary disease: a genome-wide association study and meta-analysis. Lancet Respir Med. 2014;2(3):214–25.

55. Vucic EA, Chari R, Thu KL, Wilson IM, Cotton AM, Kennett JY, et al. DNA methylation is globally disrupted and associated with expression changes in chronic obstructive pulmonary disease small airways. Am J Respir Cell Mol Biol. 2014;50(5):912–22.

56. Morrow JD, Glass K, Cho MH, Hersh CP, Pinto-Plata V, Celli B, et al. Human lung DNA methylation quantitative trait loci colocalize with chronic obstructive pulmonary disease genome-wide association loci. Am J Respir Crit Care Med. 2018;197(10):1275–84.

57. Masoli M, Fabian D, Holt S, Beasley R. The global burden of asthma: executive summary of the GINA Dissemination Committee report. Allergy. 2004;59(5):469–78.

58. Akinbami L, Moorman J, Bailey C, Zahran H, King M, Johnson C, et al. Trends in asthma prevalence, health care use, and mortality in the United States,

2001–2010. Hyattsville: National Center for Health Statistics; 2012.

59. Rose D, Mannino DM, Leaderer BP. Asthma prevalence among US adults, 1998–2000: role of Puerto Rican ethnicity and behavioral and geographic factors. Am J Public Health. 2006;96(5):880–8.

60. Moffatt MF, Gut IG, Demenais F, Strachan DP, Bouzigon E, Heath S, et al. A large-scale, consortium-based genomewide association study of asthma. N Engl J Med. 2010;363(13):1211–21.

61. Koppelman GH, Stine OC, Xu J, Howard TD, Zheng SL, Kauffman HF, et al. Genome-wide search for atopy susceptibility genes in Dutch families with asthma. J Allergy Clin Immunol. 2002;109(3):498–506.

62. Galanter JM, Gignoux CR, Torgerson DG, Roth LA, Eng C, Oh SS, et al. Genome-wide association study and admixture mapping identify different asthma-associated loci in Latinos: the Genes-environments & Admixture in Latino Americans study. J Allergy Clin Immunol. 2014;134(2):295–305.

63. Yan Q, Brehm J, Pino-Yanes M, Forno E, Lin J, Oh SS, et al. A meta-analysis of genome-wide association studies of asthma in Puerto Ricans. Eur Respir J. 2017;49(5):1601505. https://doi.org/10.1183/13993003.01505-2016.

64. Demenais F, Margaritte-Jeannin P, Barnes K, Cookson W, Altmuller J, Ang W, et al. Multiancestry association study identifies new asthma risk loci that colocalize with immune-cell enhancer marks. Nat Genet. 2018;50(1):42–53.

65. Nelson HS, Weiss ST, Bleecker ER, Yancey SW, Dorinsky PM, Group SS. The Salmeterol multicenter asthma research trial: a comparison of usual pharmacotherapy for asthma or usual pharmacotherapy plus salmeterol. Chest. 2006;129(1):15–26.

66. Wechsler ME, Castro M, Lehman E, Chinchilli VM, Sutherland ER, Denlinger L, et al. Impact of race on asthma treatment failures in the asthma clinical research network. Am J Respir Crit Care Med. 2011;184(11):1247–53.

67. Naqvi M, Thyne S, Choudhry S, Tsai HJ, Navarro D, Castro RA, et al. Ethnic-specific differences in bronchodilator responsiveness among African Americans, Puerto Ricans, and Mexicans with asthma. J Asthma. 2007;44(8):639–48.

68. Brehm J, Ramratnam S, Tse SM, Croteau-Chonka D, Pino-Yanes M, Rosas-Salazar C, et al. Stress and bronchodilator response in children with asthma. Am J Respir Crit Care Med. 2015;192(1):47–56.

69. Hawkins GA, Tantisira K, Meyers DA, Ampleford EJ, Moore WC, Klanderman B, et al. Sequence, haplotype, and association analysis of ADRbeta2 in a multiethnic asthma case-control study. Am J Respir Crit Care Med. 2006;174(10):1101–9.

70. Ortega VE, Hawkins GA, Moore WC, Hastie AT, Ampleford EJ, Busse WW, et al. Effect of rare variants in ADRB2 on risk of severe exacerbations and symptom control during longacting beta agonist treatment in a multiethnic asthma population: a genetic study. Lancet Respir Med. 2014;2(3):204–13.

71. Green SA, Turki J, Innis M, Liggett SB. Amino-terminal polymorphisms of the human beta 2-adrenergic receptor impart distinct agonist-promoted regulatory properties. Biochemistry. 1994;33(32):9414–9.

72. Choudhry S, Ung N, Avila PC, Ziv E, Nazario S, Casal J, et al. Pharmacogenetic differences in response to albuterol between Puerto Ricans and Mexicans with asthma. Am J Respir Crit Care Med. 2005;171(6):563–70.

73. Lima JJ, Thomason DB, Mohamed MH, Eberle LV, Self TH, Johnson JA. Impact of genetic polymorphisms of the beta2-adrenergic receptor on albuterol bronchodilator pharmacodynamics. Clin Pharmacol Ther. 1999;65(5):519–25.

74. Taylor DR, Drazen JM, Herbison GP, Yandava CN, Hancox RJ, Town GI. Asthma exacerbations during long term beta agonist use: influence of beta(2) adrenoceptor polymorphism. Thorax. 2000;55(9):762–7.

75. Israel E, Chinchilli VM, Ford JG, Boushey HA, Cherniack R, Craig TJ, et al. Use of regularly scheduled albuterol treatment in asthma: genotype-stratified, randomised, placebo-controlled cross-over trial. Lancet. 2004;364(9444):1505–12.

76. Wechsler ME, Kunselman SJ, Chinchilli VM, Bleecker E, Boushey HA, Calhoun WJ, et al. Effect of beta2-adrenergic receptor polymorphism on response to longacting beta2 agonist in asthma (LARGE trial): a genotype-stratified, randomised, placebo-controlled, crossover trial. Lancet. 2009;374(9703):1754–64.

77. Bleecker ER, Nelson HS, Kraft M, Corren J, Meyers DA, Yancey SW, et al. Beta2-receptor polymorphisms in patients receiving salmeterol with or without fluticasone propionate. Am J Respir Crit Care Med. 2010;181(7):676–87.

78. Bleecker ER, Postma DS, Lawrance RM, Meyers DA, Ambrose HJ, Goldman M. Effect of ADRB2 polymorphisms on response to longacting beta2-agonist therapy: a pharmacogenetic analysis of two randomised studies. Lancet. 2007;370(9605):2118–25.

79. Busse WW, Bateman ED, Caplan AL, Kelly HW, O'Byrne PM, Rabe KF, et al. Combined analysis of asthma safety trials of long-acting beta2-agonists. N Engl J Med. 2018;378(26):2497–505.

80. Green SA, Cole G, Jacinto M, Innis M, Liggett SB. A polymorphism of the human beta 2-adrenergic receptor within the fourth transmembrane domain alters ligand binding and functional properties of the receptor. J Biol Chem. 1993;268(31):23116–21.

81. Green SA, Rathz DA, Schuster AJ, Liggett SB. The Ile164 beta(2)-adrenoceptor polymorphism alters salmeterol exosite binding and conventional agonist coupling to G(s). Eur J Pharmacol. 2001;421(3):141–7.

82. Himes BE, Jiang X, Hu R, Wu AC, Lasky-Su JA, Klanderman BJ, et al. Genome-wide association analysis in asthma subjects identifies SPATS2L as a novel bronchodilator response gene. PLoS Genet. 2012;8(7):e1002824.

83. Duan QL, Lasky-Su J, Himes BE, Qiu W, Litonjua AA, Damask A, et al. A genome-wide association study of bronchodilator response in asthmatics. Pharmacogenomics J. 2014;14(1):41–7.

84. Israel E, Lasky-Su J, Markezich A, Damask A, Szefler SJ, Schuemann B, et al. Genome-wide association study of short-acting beta2-agonists. A novel genome-wide significant locus on chromosome 2 near ASB3. Am J Respir Crit Care Med. 2015;191(5):530–7.

85. Padhukasahasram B, Yang JJ, Levin AM, Yang M, Burchard EG, Kumar R, et al. Gene-based association identifies SPATA13-AS1 AS a pharmacogenomic predictor of inhaled short-acting beta-agonist response in multiple population groups. Pharmacogenomics J. 2014;14(4):365–71.

86. Gref A, Merid SK, Gruzieva O, Ballereau S, Becker A, Bellander T, et al. Genome-wide interaction analysis of air pollution exposure and childhood asthma with functional follow-up. Am J Respir Crit Care Med. 2017;195(10):1373–83.

87. Buro-Auriemma LJ, Salit J, Hackett NR, Walters MS, Strulovici-Barel Y, Staudt MR, et al. Cigarette smoking induces small airway epithelial epigenetic changes with corresponding modulation of gene expression. Hum Mol Genet. 2013;22(23):4726–38.

88. Baccarelli A, Wright RO, Bollati V, Tarantini L, Litonjua AA, Suh HH, et al. Rapid DNA methylation changes after exposure to traffic particles. Am J Respir Crit Care Med. 2009;179(7):572–8.

89. Yang IV, Pedersen BS, Liu A, O'Connor GT, Teach SJ, Kattan M, et al. DNA methylation and childhood asthma in the inner city. J Allergy Clin Immunol. 2015;136(1):69–80.

90. Yang IV, Pedersen BS, Liu AH, O'Connor GT, Pillai D, Kattan M, et al. The nasal methylome and childhood atopic asthma. J Allergy Clin Immunol. 2017;139(5):1478–88.

91. Forno E, Wang T, Qi C, Yan Q, Xu C, Boutaoui N, et al. A genome-wide study of DNA methylation in nasal epithelium and atopy and atopic asthma in children. Lancet Respir Med. 2019;7(4):336–46.

Education for the Practice of Precision Medicine in PCCSM: Creating Tomorrow's Workforce

27

Shyoko Honiden and Margaret Ann Pisani

Introduction

Rapid technological advances in the past decade allow data generation in a high-resolution, high-throughput fashion, often based on "-omics" platforms. Precision medicine is no longer a theoretical dream, but an attainable reality. Despite this, uptake has been slow and fragmented, in part due to a dearth of collaborative and well-organized education for the frontline physicians. Lack of familiarity has contributed to lack of confidence and, at times, overt provider skepticism.

Adding to the challenge is the need for a paradigm shift in the way we interpret evidence. Traditional evidence-based medicine is derived from data generated through studying large cohorts and populations. Physicians have been trained to temper enthusiasm, until sufficient high-quality and reproducible evidence is available. Precision medicine operates under new assumptions that counter this paradigm. While outliers are often discounted or overlooked in randomized trial design, data generated from a singular patient – who may have a particularly poor or high response to a given drug, for example – in fact forms the basis of precision medicine [1].

Integrated and wide adoption of precision medicine will require a deliberate investigation into the root cause of implementation challenges. Uncovered challenges need to be analyzed through the lens of education and curriculum development. Only then can we work on creating tomorrow's workforce, equipped with knowledge, behaviors, and skills necessary to weave together traditional evidence-based practice and precision medicine.

We employ a "5-why" approach, often utilized in root case analysis, in thinking about the challenges of developing robust curricula for precision medicine education [2]. The 5-why approach starts with a problem statement which is then examined in an iterative interrogative approach. This helps uncover the layers of interconnected problems that need to be addressed to craft a solution.

Problem Statement: *While exponential technological advances have occurred, precision medicine practice has not been widely adopted.*

Why: *Why are providers not embracing precision medicine?*

Explanation: *Adoption has been sluggish due to provider unease.*

Providers remain uneasy about integrating precision medicine into practice. Even in areas

S. Honiden · M. A. Pisani (✉)
Yale School of Medicine, New Haven, CT, USA
e-mail: Shyoko.Honiden@yale.edu; Margaret.Pisani@yale.edu

© Springer Nature Switzerland AG 2020
J. L. Gomez et al. (eds.), *Precision in Pulmonary, Critical Care, and Sleep Medicine*, Respiratory Medicine, https://doi.org/10.1007/978-3-030-31507-8_27

such as cancer testing where there is most consensus, recommendations vary when physicians are surveyed, often leading to inappropriate testing. In one study, practicing physicians in Texas were asked to participate in a case-based survey, where they were asked to make genetic testing and management recommendations for healthy at-risk relatives of patients with cancer. Whether the patient carried a *BRCA1* mutation or a variant of uncertain significance, the vast majority of physicians recommended screening of healthy family members, and typically testing ordered in these simulated scenarios was more comprehensive than guideline recommendations [3]. Similar variability and deviation from guideline recommendations were noted when physicians were surveyed about a healthy *BRCA1* mutation carrier management approach [4]. Indeed, a number of studies have shown that referral to trained genetic counselors led to anywhere from 8% to 26% revision of genetic testing orders, including many orders that were outright cancelled [5, 6]. Traditionally, genomics has been the subspecialty domain of a handful of geneticists. However, referral to these specialists cannot be relied upon as the solution, as there is a shortage of geneticists in the workforce [7]. Additionally, as the domain in which precision medicine is practiced expands from rare diseases and oncology to more common diseases such as COPD and asthma, improving genomic literacy across all subspecialties including pulmonary and critical care medicine has become critical.

Why: *Why are providers uneasy?*

Explanation: *Provider unease is in part fueled by skepticism toward precision medicine.*

Physicians remain ambivalent toward opportunities made available through precision medicine. Of physicians surveyed in Pennsylvania, only about half of respondents felt that precision medicine would help provide better medical care or that it was the future of medicine [8]. Age and gender had no significant influence upon physician attitudes in this survey, and acceptance of other technologies, such as electronic health records, was not associated with a more positive attitude toward precision medicine.

Providers who have practiced long enough can recite many examples of recommended practices that ultimately became refuted entirely or fell out of favor (e.g., the use of drotecogin alpha for sepsis, total parenteral nutrition, tight glucose control during critical illness) [9]. Early adopters of new treatment or technologies have sometimes been forced to take a jolting u-turn based on subsequent discrepant data. Physicians are expected to be careful and calculated until robust and generalizable data derived from multiple cohorts become available. The explosion of literature around evidence-based practice educational interventions supports this physician culture [10].

The cornerstone of evidence-based medicine (EBM) is that there is an accepted hierarchy for classifying evidence. Large, randomized controlled trials (RCTs) are given the most weight in this system [11]. Meticulous data analysis in RCTs ensures that confounders are accounted for, and central tendency (i.e., means, medians) are used to describe, for example, an expected treatment response to a given drug. Outliers are generally discounted. Precision medicine is ultimately an *n-of-one* enterprise. Vast amounts of data are generated not on a population level, but rather at a micro-individual level. The outlier responses are specifically what is analyzed in-depth in precision medicine. While there has been less cognitive dissonance in adopting precision medicine to better understand rare genetic diseases for which no large trials exist (and will likely never exist), how to factor in this new technology for more common scenarios has been unclear. At present, physicians are given little guidance about how to reconcile traditional clinical decision-making approaches anchored in EBM with the opportunities afforded by precision medicine.

The lack of consensus or guidelines which specify how and when -omics platforms should be integrated into practice additionally fuels concerns [12]. Availability of clear consensus will help increase physician buy-in, but will also enable uniform curriculum development from an educational perspective. While genomic medicine is clearing the first hurdle by accumulating bench to bedside translational (T1) research, T2 research that answers questions surrounding effectiveness and leads to guideline formation is still in its infancy [13]. For most conditions, the clinical utility of incorporating precision medicine into practice has not yet been outlined [14, 15].

Why: *Why are providers skeptical?*

Explanation: *Provider skepticism persists because there are insufficient structured, collaborative educational opportunities across the various stages of medical training.*

Physician skepticism, unease, and at best ambivalence cannot be countered without more robust and coordinated education for physicians. Thankfully, despite obvious challenges, significant progress has been made to enhance educational opportunities.

Undergraduate and Graduate Medical Education

At the undergraduate medical education level, most US and Canadian medical schools had not yet innovated their medical genetics curriculum in year 1 and/or 2 to include modern genomic medicine, according to a survey representing the academic year 2004–2005 [16]. To aid medical schools with curriculum development, in 2013 the Association for Professors of Human and Medical Genetics (APHMG) released a framework for a genetics curriculum. This included competencies and specific learning objectives in the topics of (a) genomic organization, (b) application of knowledge of genomic variation in normal populations and disease phenotypes, (c) basic concepts of emerging testing technologies (including expression, microarrays, and exome and whole-genome sequencing), (d) information technology (including websites and resources for the interpretation of genomic variation), and (e) the implications and limitations of direct-to-consumer (DTC) genetic testing. While not yet universal, very quickly after this release in 2013, nearly 50% of surveyed genetics course directors had started to access and use the APHMG curriculum as a guide for curriculum development or to evaluate their existing curriculum for the academic year 2013–2014 [17].

The looming question has been whether new curriculum development translates to durable changes in physician behavior and ultimately patient outcomes. In education research, Kirkpatrick's education outcome hierarchy is often used as a metric to define education success [18]. At the lowest Kirkpatrick level, success of an educational program is assessed through learner reactions to the content delivered. For example, a post-workshop survey might assess whether the learners found the material useful. In Kirkpatrick's level two, educators attempt to assess how much knowledge has increased after the training. This is often done in a pre-/post-workshop format. Sustained increase in knowledge (e.g., months later) is often hard to demonstrate. At level three, educators assess application of knowledge gained and determine whether learner behavior (in a real-world setting) has changed. And, finally, at the highest level, level four, education researchers analyze whether patient outcomes have improved.

Needless to say, higher levels of Kirkpatrick educational outcomes are hard to achieve and to ascertain with confidence. Even with concerted efforts at improving genomics curriculum at Icahn School of Medicine at Mount Sinai, for example, only 6% of students felt that the curriculum had adequately prepared them to practice precision medicine from a self-efficacy perspective [19].

At the Graduate Medical Education level, the Training Residents in Genomics (TRIG) working group was formed in 2010 through the Association of Pathology Chairs, Pathology Residency Director section. Through collaboration with multiple societies and aided by funding from an R25 grant, the TRIG working group successfully developed a genomics curriculum with tools for implementation [20]. The original curriculum included exercises that followed a breast cancer patient through different levels of genetic testing ranging from single gene testing all the way to whole-exome sequencing. These genomics workshops were expanded to include practicing physicians through a team-based learning approach and also led to the development of "train the trainer" handbook and toolkits to ease implementation at other institutions. The handbook includes workshop questions and answers, tips for implementation, as well as handouts and slide presentations that could be used. Most commendable has been the recent addition of a specialty-agnostic version of this genomics curriculum as of 2017, which would allow for adaptation in any disease or subspecialty, in a flexible and portable "plug and play" format. Given the success of the TRIG working group, an undergraduate medical education version was formed, named UTRIG, under the undergraduate medical education section of APHMG. While the APHMG genetics curriculum published in 2013 helped foster curricular innovation, surveys of US and Canadian medical schools suggested schools were still introducing genomics as a stand-alone topic. The goal of UTRIG was to help graduate genomic-literate future physicians across all specialties and to integrate genomics education across relevant topics in the preclinical years to highlight relevance and application that could be revisited in clinical years. This integration is likely vital to allow for learner application of knowledge attained in patient care scenarios (Kirkpatrick level three), without which patient outcome improvements (Kirkpatrick level four) could not be realized. As with TRIG, UTRIG has been committed to developing educational tools and faculty manuals in parallel to ensure successful implementation and to empower education leaders who themselves may be learning new material as modern genomics evolve rapidly.

Competency Assessment Through Entrustable Professional Activities

Assuming robust curriculum is designed and implemented, how else should educators examine education outcomes through the lens of graduate medical education assessment and evaluation?

The National Human Genome Research Institute convened the Inter-Society Coordinating Committee for Practitioner Education in Genomics (ISCC). The ISCC recently published a paper outlining a shared framework for developing genomics practice competencies that could be customized for various subspecialties. In the era of milestone assessments, the ISCC came up with five entrustable professional activities (EPAs) that could become the basis of competency assessment (a sample adapted version for interstitial pulmonary fibrosis shown in Table 27.1). EPAs are observable and measurable behaviors that allow for competency-based decisions about whether a trainee can be "entrusted" to assume responsibility in a defined domain. Under each of the EPAs are the newly expanded eight ACGME core competencies – patient care, knowledge for practice, practice-based learning and improvement, interpersonal and communication skills, professionalism, systems-based practice, interprofessional collaboration, and personal and professional development [21].

Ongoing Education for Practicing Providers

Reaching practicing providers out of training programs is undoubtedly a challenge. According to data from the Federation of State Medical Boards (FSMB) through the end of 2016, a little over half of the practicing physicians are over 50 years old, and three-quarters of the active workforce in the United States is over the age of 40 [22]. This means that even "relatively young" physicians were trained in an era before undergraduate and graduate medical education started to intensify modern genomics content. Much of what current practicing physicians learned formally, therefore, is now obsolete. Practicing physicians face competing demands. More is expected in terms of continuing education for maintaining professional certification and documentation in the context of daily patient care. Adding genomics literacy in the vast to-do list could be met with some resistance in this landscape, unless educational content is focused, relevant, digestible and bite-sized to fit

Table 27.1 Five core entrustable professional activities proposed by the Inter-Society Coordinating Committee for Physician Education in Genomics (ISCC) to assess physician competency in genomic medicine

Proposed EPA domains for genomic medicine competency assessment	
Family history	Elicit, document, and act on relevant family history pertinent to the patient's clinical status
Adaptation in pulmonary medicine	*Elicit, document, and act on relevant family history pertinent to a patient suspected of familial interstitial pulmonary fibrosis. Explain findings to patient, including implications for other family members*
Genomic testing	Use genomic testing to guide patient management
Adaptation in pulmonary medicine	*Use genomic testing to guide management of interstitial pulmonary fibrosis. Be able to explain how different genomic changes may result in different phenotypes and be prepared to order, interpret, and communicate results effectively*
Patient treatment based on genomic testing	Use genomic information to make treatment decisions
Adaptation in pulmonary medicine	*Recognize that genetic variants may predict responsiveness to anti-fibrotic therapies and utilize information to risk-stratify and individualize treatment*
Somatic genomics	Use genomic information to guide the diagnosis and management of cancer and other disorders involving somatic genetic changes
Adaptation in pulmonary medicine	*Explain benefits and limitations of somatic genomic testing to the patient such as those that affect fibroblast activation, oxidant stress, and senescence that may be relevant in lung fibrosis*
Microbial genomic information	Use genomic tests that identify microbial contributors to human health and disease, as well as genomic tests that guide therapeutics in infectious diseases
Adaptation in pulmonary medicine	*Explain the importance of the normal microbiome and be able to interpret genomics-based tests for diagnosis, monitoring, and treatment of infectious disease which may complicate or exacerbate underlying interstitial lung disease*

Adapted from Korf et al. [21]
Sample Adaptation for Interstitial Pulmonary Fibrosis

into a busy practitioner's schedule, and implemented in a flexible manner. The American College of Chest Physicians report on the effectiveness of continuing medical education (CME) activities was that, in general, the quality of evidence was low due to lack of standardization in CME approaches. Nevertheless, they outlined best practice recommendations when creating CME modules and encouraged the use of multimedia interventions, multiple exposures, as well as incorporation of multiple instructional techniques to ensure engagement and knowledge retention for providers [23].

Leveraging Characteristics of the Adult Learner

Adult learners do best when they see immediacy and relevance and feel engaged in the topic at hand [24]. To that end, some undergraduate and graduate medical education programs have offered trainees personal genotyping on a voluntary, confidential basis [25, 26]. There is, of course, nothing more relevant than your own personal genetic information to enhance engagement with the topic. Some educators have also wondered whether this experience will also enable better understanding of the complex implications from a patient perspective, by being a "consumer" themselves. Indeed, in the Stanford program, only about a third of the students who used personal genotyping data felt that they would have learned just as much had they used publicly available datasets. Despite some clear advantages, this approach has also raised a multitude of ethical concerns pertaining to lack of robust counseling infrastructure as well as implications for family members who may need to be screened themselves if a significant risk is uncovered [27].

At least in one institution, a pilot genomics curriculum was altered to exclude this personal testing component after much debate and was replaced by problem sets that included interpretation of anonymous genomes of individuals known to be at risk for diseases such as diabetes mellitus and cystic fibrosis [28].

A participatory approach to genetic education may be particularly palatable for the practicing physician. Direct-to-consumer genetic testing products are already available on the market, and physicians are encountering patients who have questions after completing self-testing. Offering personal genomic testing to physicians as a way to frame the educational content may thus increase relevance. At Cleveland Clinic, personal genomic testing was made available to staff at no cost as a way to increase physician familiarity [29]. Physicians who voluntarily signed up were asked to attend a 90-minute educational session prior to free personal testing. Optional pre- and posttest counseling was also made available to participants. 137 out of the 147 participants in this pilot project completed a survey. Only 39% of physicians reported that they were familiar with recent genomics research that may be impacting their patients. After completion, more than three quarters of the respondents felt that their personal genomic testing experience would benefit their patients directly.

What Are Specialty-Specific Genomic Opportunities in Pulmonary Medicine?

Recently, the joint National Heart and Lung Association-Cardiovascular Medical Research and Education Fund workshop released a report on how precision medicine might be used to manage patients with pulmonary vascular disease [30]. Specifically, the long-term vision would be to replace the current WHO pulmonary hypertension group designation with endophenotype mapping based on genomic signatures. The hope would be that such approaches would aid in earlier diagnosis, enhance precision of screening, and allow for personalized interventions or prevention of disease (long before the

disease actually manifests). In order for this to happen, better coordination of genomic data into large databases becomes necessary. Additional infrastructure development, such as a task force that will help define clinical trial protocols for pulmonary vascular disease that applies precision medicine principles, is much needed. Similarly, in chronic obstructive pulmonary disease (COPD), there is currently lack of well-organized large databases that will help uncover underlying molecular mechanisms that explain the wide-ranging clinical phenotypes of COPD observed. While alpha-1 antitrypsin deficiency is a definable known trait, those classically grouped as "asthma-COPD overlap," "eosinophilic COPD," and "frequent exacerbator" may also have molecular mechanisms that could be specifically targeted for therapy. For example, there are some preliminary studies that suggest that imbalances in microbial airway communities (i.e., dysbiosis rather than true new acquisition of bacteria) may be driving the latter "frequent exacerbator" clinical phenotype [31]. Changes in airway architecture and/or specific alterations in lung microbiome may be priming certain individuals to dysbiosis [32]. Among patients with interstitial pulmonary fibrosis (IPF), genome-wide association studies have identified several loci that interfere with host defense, cell-cell adhesion, and DNA repair that may help identify at-risk patients [33, 34]. A single-nucleotide polymorphism (SNP) variant that affects the mucin gene (*MUC5B*) is strongly associated with IPF [35]. Others are actively investigating how genetic variants may affect response to antifibrotic drugs, and the field of pharmacogenomics is in rapid evolution [36].

In severe asthma, biomarkers such as eosinophils and IgE levels, which are already being used, better define endotypes that help predict response to and utility of using one biologic agent over another [37]. Th-2-linked inflammation has been further linked to a measurable serum biomarker, periostin, and a favorable response to lebrikizumab (a Th-2, interleukin 13 targeted therapy) has been demonstrated [38]. Advances in asthma treatment have shown that precision approaches can be practically applied in polygenic diseases.

The above are just a few examples of the application of precision medicine and genomics to lung diseases but clearly many more opportunities exist.

Future of Pulmonary, Critical Care, and Sleep Medicine Training in Genomics and Personalized Medicine

There is currently no standard curriculum for training the next generation of PCCSM physicians in genomics and personalized medicine. In trying to develop educational tools at the postgraduate level that can educate trainees about the biology and clinical application of precision medicine, it seems best to develop a case-based learning approach. Developing a toolbox of demonstrative cases to illustrate the concepts of precision medicine including the importance of genotyping, when available, and understanding phenotypic responses in specific diseases appear to be the best approach to educating trainees. These cases should be paired with a structured reading curriculum to supply learners with the requisite background knowledge and an option for self-genotyping in a participatory model of genetic education. In addition, trainees should learn the importance of counseling patients regarding the benefits and the harms of genetic testing. Learning counseling skills should be through structured simulation training where learners have the opportunity to practice counseling and field questions from simulated patients. This piece is crucial as more genes that predict disease are discovered, but where treatments may not yet be available. The final piece of the curriculum development should include an understanding of the legislation and regulations surrounding genetic testing.

References

1. Beckmann JS, Lew D. Reconciling evidence-based medicine and precision medicine in the era of big data: challenges and opportunities. Genome Med. 2016;8(1):134.

2. CMS. The five whys tool for root cause analysis. https://www.cms.gov/Medicare/Provider-Enrollment-and-Certification/QAPI/downloads/FiveWhys.pdf. Cited 2018 September 24th, 2018.

3. Plon SE, Cooper HP, Parks B, Dhar SU, Kelly PA, Weinberg AD, et al. Genetic testing and cancer risk management recommendations by physicians for at-risk relatives. Genet Med. 2011;13(2):148–54.

4. Dhar SU, Cooper HP, Wang T, Parks B, Staggs SA, Hilsenbeck S, et al. Significant differences among physician specialties in management recommendations of BRCA1 mutation carriers. Breast Cancer Res Treat. 2011;129(1):221–7.

5. Miller CE, Krautscheid P, Baldwin EE, Tvrdik T, Openshaw AS, Hart K, et al. Genetic counselor review of genetic test orders in a reference laboratory reduces unnecessary testing. Am J Med Genet A. 2014;164A(5):1094–101.

6. Kotzer KE, Riley JD, Conta JH, Anderson CM, Schahl KA, Goodenberger ML. Genetic testing utilization and the role of the laboratory genetic counselor. Clin Chim Acta. 2014;427:193–5.

7. McGrath S, Ghersi D. Building towards precision medicine: empowering medical professionals for the next revolution. BMC Med Genet. 2016;9(1):23.

8. Kichko K, Marschall P, Flessa S. Personalized medicine in the U.S. and Germany: awareness, acceptance, use and preconditions for the wide implementation into the medical standard. J Pers Med. 2016;6(2):15.

9. Villar J, Perez-Mendez L, Aguirre-Jaime A, Kacmarek RM. Why are physicians so skeptical about positive randomized controlled clinical trials in critical care medicine? Intensive Care Med. 2005;31(2):196–204.

10. Albarqouni L, Hoffmann T, Glasziou P. Evidence-based practice educational intervention studies: a systematic review of what is taught and how it is measured. BMC Med Educ. 2018;18(1):177.

11. Guyatt G, Oxman AD, Akl EA, Kunz R, Vist G, Brozek J, et al. GRADE guidelines: 1. Introduction-GRADE evidence profiles and summary of findings tables. J Clin Epidemiol. 2011;64(4):383–94.

12. Feero WG, Green ED. Genomics education for health care professionals in the 21st century. JAMA. 2011;306(9):989–90.

13. Fort DG, Herr TM, Shaw PL, Gutzman KE, Starren JB. Mapping the evolving definitions of translational research. J Clin Transl Sci. 2017;1(1):60–6.

14. Evans JP, Khoury MJ. The arrival of genomic medicine to the clinic is only the beginning of the journey. Genet Med. 2013;15(4):268–9.

15. Manolio TA, Chisholm RL, Ozenberger B, Roden DM, Williams MS, Wilson R, et al. Implementing genomic medicine in the clinic: the future is here. Genet Med. 2013;15(4):258–67.

16. Thurston VC, Wales PS, Bell MA, Torbeck L, Brokaw JJ. The current status of medical genetics instruction in US and Canadian medical schools. Acad Med. 2007;82(5):441–5.

17. Plunkett-Rondeau J, Hyland K, Dasgupta S. Training future physicians in the era of genomic medicine:

trends in undergraduate medical genetics education. Genet Med. 2015;17(11):927–34.

18. Kirkpatrick D. Evaluation of training. In: Craig R, Mittel I, editors. Training and development handbook. New York: McGraw Hill; 1967. p. 87–112.

19. Eden C, Johnson KW, Gottesman O, Bottinger EP, Abul-Husn NS. Medical student preparedness for an era of personalized medicine: findings from one US medical school. Per Med. 2016;13(2):129–41.

20. Haspel RL, Atkinson JB, Barr FG, Kaul KL, Leonard DG, O'Daniel J, et al. TRIG on TRACK: educating pathology residents in genomic medicine. Per Med. 2012;9(3):287–93.

21. Korf BR, Berry AB, Limson M, Marian AJ, Murray MF, O'Rourke PP, et al. Framework for development of physician competencies in genomic medicine: report of the Competencies Working Group of the Inter-Society Coordinating Committee for Physician Education in Genomics. Genet Med. 2014;16(11):804–9.

22. Young A, Chaudhry HJ, Pei X, Arnhart K, Dugan M, et al. A census of actively licensed physicians. J Med Regul. 2016;103(2):7–21.

23. Moores LK, Dellert E, Baumann MH, Rosen MJ, American College of Chest Physicians Health and Science Policy Committee. Executive summary: effectiveness of continuing medical education: American College of Chest Physicians evidence-based educational guidelines. Chest. 2009;135(3 Suppl):1S–4S.

24. Knowles M. The adult learner: a neglected species. Houston: Golf Publishing Co.; 1984.

25. Salari K, Karczewski KJ, Hudgins L, Ormond KE. Evidence that personal genome testing enhances student learning in a course on genomics and personalized medicine. PLoS One. 2013;8(7):e68853.

26. Salari K, Pizzo PA, Prober CG. Commentary: to genotype or not to genotype? Addressing the debate through the development of a genomics and personalized medicine curriculum. Acad Med. 2011;86(8):925–7.

27. Garber KB, Hyland KM, Dasgupta S. Participatory genomic testing as an educational experience. Trends Genet. 2016;32(6):317–20.

28. Walt DR, Kuhlik A, Epstein SK, Demmer LA, Knight M, Chelmow D, et al. Lessons learned from the introduction of personalized genotyping into a medical school curriculum. Genet Med. 2011;13(1):63–6.

29. Sharp RR, Goldlust ME, Eng C. Addressing gaps in physician education using personal genomic testing. Genet Med. 2011;13(8):750–1.

30. Newman JH, Rich S, Abman SH, Alexander JH, Barnard J, Beck GJ, et al. Enhancing insights into pulmonary vascular disease through a precision medicine approach. A joint NHLBI-cardiovascular medical research and education fund workshop report. Am J Respir Crit Care Med. 2017;195(12):1661–70.

31. Dickson RP, Martinez FJ, Huffnagle GB. The role of the microbiome in exacerbations of chronic lung diseases. Lancet. 2014;384(9944):691–702.

32. Sidhaye VK, Nishida K, Martinez FJ. Precision medicine in COPD: where are we and where do we need to go? Eur Respir Rev. 2018;27(149):180022.

33. Fingerlin TE, Murphy E, Zhang W, Peljto AL, Brown KK, Steele MP, et al. Genome-wide association study identifies multiple susceptibility loci for pulmonary fibrosis. Nat Genet. 2013;45(6):613–20.

34. Thannickal VJ, Antony VB. Is personalized medicine a realistic goal in idiopathic pulmonary fibrosis? Expert Rev Respir Med. 2018;12(6):441–3.

35. Peljto AL, Zhang Y, Fingerlin TE, Ma SF, Garcia JG, Richards TJ, et al. Association between the MUC5B promoter polymorphism and survival in patients with idiopathic pulmonary fibrosis. JAMA. 2013;309(21):2232–9.

36. Oldham JM, Ma SF, Martinez FJ, Anstrom KJ, Raghu G, Schwartz DA, et al. TOLLIP, MUC5B, and the response to N-acetylcysteine among individuals with idiopathic pulmonary fibrosis. Am J Respir Crit Care Med. 2015;192(12):1475–82.

37. Canonica GW, Ferrando M, Baiardini I, Puggioni F, Racca F, Passalacqua G, et al. Asthma: personalized and precision medicine. Curr Opin Allergy Clin Immunol. 2018;18(1):51–8.

38. Corren J, Lemanske RF, Hanania NA, Korenblat PE, Parsey MV, Arron JR, et al. Lebrikizumab treatment in adults with asthma. N Engl J Med. 2011;365(12):1088–98.

Summary and Future Applications of Precision Medicine in Pulmonary, Critical Care, and Sleep Medicine

Jose L. Gomez, Naftali Kaminski, and Blanca E. Himes

Introduction

We are at the dawn of precision medicine, a transitional period fueled by technological advances in high-throughput assays for various types of biological data, imaging, sensors, data science, and computing. The application of these methods to large and deeply phenotyped cohorts coupled with our current understanding of disease pathogenesis are moving us closer to the widespread development and implementation of personalized therapies. The adoption of precision medicine across pulmonary, critical care, and sleep remains uneven, however, as can be gleaned by contrasting the reviews provided in preceding chapters.

J. L. Gomez
Pulmonary, Critical Care and Sleep Medicine Section, Department of Medicine, Yale University School of Medicine, New Haven, CT, USA

N. Kaminski
Pulmonary, Critical Care and Sleep Medicine, Department of Medicine, Yale University School of Medicine, New Haven, CT, USA

B. E. Himes (✉)
Department of Biostatistics, Epidemiology and Informatics, University of Pennsylvania, Philadelphia, PA, USA
e-mail: bhimes@pennmedicine.upenn.edu

Here, we summarize salient findings from each book section and major themes related to the future of precision medicine research and its implementation.

Genetics and Pharmacogenetics in Pulmonary, Critical Care, and Sleep Medicine

High-throughput genomic techniques have led to the discovery of loci linked to various pulmonary diseases and uncovered potential targets for drug development. In the case of rare diseases, where one or few loci confer a high proportion of disease susceptibility, substantial progress has been made in precision medicine. As discussed in the chapter on Diffuse Pulmonary Disorders, genotype-driven precision therapies are available or under study for patients with neonatal respiratory distress syndrome, cystic fibrosis, pulmonary alveolar proteinosis, pulmonary Langerhans cell histiocytosis, and alpha-1 antitrypsin deficiency (AATD) [1–6]. For these diseases and other rare ones of unknown origin, genetic evaluation can proceed in a relatively straightforward manner thanks to the availability of genome sequencing. A major barrier now is that ultra-rare, novel variants of uncertain significance are often identified via sequencing, and determining which of these may actually lead to observed traits is not straightforward [7]. Even when causal loci are identified, there may not be a treatment available. Identification of causal loci is nonetheless a helpful starting point that may lead to treatment identification as has been demonstrated successfully in some cases [8]. Genetic counselors play an important role in helping patients and their families navigate the process of searching for loci linked to disease and taking actions based on results.

For complex diseases, although most genomic findings have not yet changed clinical practice, some may soon lead to advances in precision medicine. For example, genetic studies of idiopathic pulmonary fibrosis (IPF) have begun to clarify why this disease occurs and identify new potential therapeutic targets. Because IPF is a diagnosis of exclusion, assigned only after various other conditions that present similarly have been ruled out, and IPF prognosis is poor, any clues regarding its origin are of great importance [9]. Further, distinguishing IPF from other interstitial lung diseases matters, as currently available anti-fibrotic therapies have been studied and approved for IPF patients but not those with other fibrosing idiopathic interstitial pneumonias [9]. Common and rare genetic factors conferring disease risk in IPF include variants in surfactant protein C (SFTPC), surfactant protein A2 (SFTPA), telomerase reverse transcriptase (TERT) and RNA component (TERC) [10–13], and Mucin 5B, Oligomeric Mucus/Gel-Forming (MUC5B) [14, 15]. Distinct genotypes found in these and other genes, which have implicated surfactants, mucociliary function, cell-cell adhesion and telomere maintenance as playing important roles in IPF pathobiology, may determine clinical phenotypes and novel therapies for IPF. The next stage is the conduct of prospective clinical trials to translate current IPF genetics observations into findings that may be implemented in clinical practice [16].

As demonstrated by genomics studies of COPD, genome-wide association studies (GWAS) with progressively larger sample sizes and increased coverage of genetic variants have been useful to identify reproducible disease risk loci. The largest COPD GWAS to date, consisting of 35,735 COPD cases defined by moderate to very severe airflow limitation and 222,076 controls with data on more than 6 million genetic variants, identified 82 genome-wide significant loci, at least 60 of which replicated in an independent cohort [17]. Effect sizes of these loci were relatively small (odds ratios 1.06–1.21) and together accounted for 7.0% of the COPD phenotypic variance, indicating that individual GWAS results are unlikely to serve as biomarkers. However, the identification of novel drug targets and pathways that may lead to the discovery of COPD endotypes is made possible by the study of these genes, as suggested by subsequent functional work of COPD-associated genes such as family with sequence similarity 13 member A (FAM13A), cholinergic receptor nicotinic alpha 3 subunit (CHRNA3), cholinergic receptor nicotinic alpha 5 subunit (CHRNA5), hedgehog interacting protein (HHIP), and matrix metallopeptidase 12 (MMP12). Beyond the many common variant associations identified for COPD, it is worth noting that the most validated genetic risk factor that accounts for 1–5% of COPD cases is the SERPINA1 variant that results in alpha-1 antitrypsin deficiency (AATD) [18]. Because this variant has not been identified via GWAS, further studies on the role of rare variants in subtypes of COPD may yield insights into other rare endotypes.

In the case of asthma, the most well-known and highly replicated genetic association signal is within the 17q21 locus, spanning genes ORMDL sphingolipid biosynthesis regulator 3 (ORMDL3) and gasdermin B (GSDMB) [19–21]. Although the exact mechanisms via which these genes are related to asthma is not yet known, functional studies are making progress in understanding their role in disease pathogenesis: overexpression of either ORMDL3 or GSDMB in mouse bronchial epithelium leads to increased airway remodeling and responsiveness [22, 23], and GSDMB protein induces pyroptosis of airway epithelia cells during inflammation [24]. Various immune pathway genes have also been associated with asthma, and contrasting association results obtained with specific asthma endotypes and other allergic diseases has helped clarify molecular processes that are unique versus shared across these conditions. Much work remains to yield novel therapies or identify novel genetics markers that are specific to asthma endotypes on the basis of GWAS findings.

In contrast to IPF, asthma and COPD, lung cancer is primarily caused by environmental exposures, such as tobacco smoke, that cause *non-inherited* somatic mutations [25]. While heritable genetic factors may influence individual response to environmental exposures and play a direct role in a minority of lung cancer cases, studies of somatic mutations have been the focus of much work and have advanced precision medicine for some types of lung cancer. Specifically, targeted treatments for various mutations involved in non-small cell lung cancer (NSCLC), which accounts for approximately 85% of all cases [26], have been identified. Notable examples include mutations of epidermal growth factor receptor (*EGFR*), anaplastic lymphoma kinase (*ALK*), and ROS Proto-Oncogene 1, Receptor Tyrosine Kinase (*ROS1*) [27, 28]. Testing of specific mutations that drive lung tumorigenesis where there is a chemotherapeutic drug available to target cells that harbor that mutation is currently recommended, and high-throughput sequencing has enabled the continued detection of additional driver mutations that contribute to lung cancer development and progression [29]. Many questions remain in lung cancer, including gaining traction on small cell lung cancer (SCLC), which is characterized by rapid growth, early metastasis, high molecular complexity, a large number of mutations in each tumor, and a very low 2-year survival rate [30, 31], as well as the identification of a broader range of mutations in NSCLC.

With the exception of lung cancer loci that have targeted drugs, few pharmacogenetic loci have been identified and widely replicated for most respiratory diseases. This is due in part to the limited number of large cohorts with appropriate and similarly captured drug response measures, which make studying these traits particularly challenging. Pharmacogenomics studies of bronchodilator and glucocorticoid response have been conducted for people with asthma and COPD, under the rationale that interindividual variability in the response to these drugs has a genetic component and that genetic variants may be useful to predict drug response or their side effects. Early reports from candidate gene studies of Adrenoceptor Beta 2 (*ADRB2*), the primary receptor target of β_2-agonists, found that variants of this gene were associated with bronchodilator response in people with asthma or COPD, but more recent meta-analysis have found few or no consistent associations between genotype and treatment response in COPD [32] and asthma [33]. Although some promising GWAS associations have been measured and are supported by functional data, such as spermatogenesis-associated serine-rich 2 like (*SPATS2L*) with bronchodilator response [34] and glucocorticoid-induced 1 (*GLCCI1*) with inhaled corticosteroid response [35], overall, pharmacogenetic studies over the past decade have failed to deliver medically actionable results, and it is unlikely that common genetic variants will serve as biomarkers of β_2-agonist or steroid responsiveness [36].

Biomarkers in Pulmonary, Critical Care, and Sleep Medicine

As described in several chapters, the search for, and discovery of, biomarkers has led to the evolution of syndrome definitions from symptom-centered diagnoses to more precise definitions based on genetics and other molecular changes. In pulmonary infections, the development of metagenomic testing has led to the identification of specific pathogens associated with illness in children without a previously identifiable pathogen [37]. The combination of metagenomics with novel sequencing platforms has also facilitated the analysis of sputum samples to identify bacterial pathogens with a turnaround time of 6 hours [38]. Additional expansion of these methods will enable rapid diagnosis and therapeutic changes in real time, rather than on culture-based methods, the current standard. Further, a deeper understanding of pathogens associated with infections is transforming how we prescribe and de-escalate therapy with antibiotics, which is of particular importance in the setting of increasing antibiotic resistance worldwide [39].

The search for biomarkers related to chronic airways obstruction has shown promise to discover endotypes of asthma, COPD and asthma-COPD overlap (ACO). Although COPD and asthma are considered distinct diseases, they share clinical manifestations, such as airway inflammation and obstruction. Consequently, the therapies used in their management overlap, as they are directed towards reducing airway inflammation and reversing bronchoconstriction. Some biomarkers have been developed for Type 2-driven asthma, while some for non-Type 2 asthma, COPD and ACO are only in the early stages of development. For example, eosinophils are used to predict therapeutic response and guide treatment in both asthma and COPD [40–42], including targeted treatments such as mepolizumab [43]. IgE, which correlates with the presence and severity of asthma, is another widely used biomarker that has driven the development of biologics like omalizumab [44]. With the exception of COPD related to AATD, no COPD-specific endotypes with clinically relevant treatments exist. Plasma fibrinogen qualified as the first FDA-approved biomarker for COPD, to be used for patient selection for enrollment into clinical trials to enrich for those who are at risk of disease worsening [45]. While identifying elevated plasma levels of fibrinogen as a biomarker is a step forward, fibrinogen lacks disease specificity and does not establish an endotype. Biomarker studies of asthma and COPD have made evident that no single gene or molecular biomarker will be sufficient to differentiate endotypes of these complex and multifactorial diseases. In fact, biomarker panels incorporating multiple markers in combination have shown increased efficacy over single biomarkers. Accurate and reproducible endotyping would be of great utility for the study and management of chronic airways obstructive diseases, enabling the development of treatments that target specific dysregulated pathways.

As is the case for obstructive airway disease, interstitial lung disease (ILD) refers to a large group of complex and highly heterogeneous diseases. Although shared characteristics of those with ILD include changes to the lung interstitium, distorted pulmonary architecture, and altered gas exchange ability of the lung, various molecular pathways underlie these traits. There are no molecular biomarkers in widespread clinical use for ILD, including IPF, although several exciting candidates are under study. For both IPF and non-IPF ILD, there is an urgent need to identify and validate biomarkers for early diagnosis, and monitor disease progression and outcomes [46]. Among the promising biomarkers for ILD and/or IPF are: 1) surfactant protein A (SFTPA) and surfactant protein D (SFTPD) [47], which are also supported by genetics studies [12, 48]; 2) telomere length, supported by the observations that a) telomere shortening is associated with cell death of airway epithelial cells and could explain the occurrence of disease in older individuals [49] and b) association of mutations in telomerase reverse transcriptase (encoded by the *TERT* gene) and telomerase RNA (encoded by *TERC*) that lead to abnormal telomere shortening have been observed in 8–15% of patients with familial pulmonary fibrosis [50, 51]; and 3) matrix metallopeptidase 7 (MMP7), the most studied and validated biomarker in IPF, whose elevated levels are associated with disease in multiple compartments (e.g., BAL, serum, lung tissue) and is related to extracellular matrix remodeling and fibroproliferation [52–56].

In addition to nucleic acid and protein biomarkers, imaging biomarkers have been adopted as diagnostic and therapeutic response tools, especially in lung cancer [57]. However, as illustrated in the chest imaging chapter, precision imaging is becoming an invaluable tool for the study and phenotyping of patients with chronic lung diseases such as COPD [58]. Therefore, the integration of biospecimen-derived and imaging biomarkers has the potential to transform disease classification and therapeutics. For IPF, detection of interstitial lung abnormalities via imaging are the best, albeit limited, approach for early detection of fibrosis [59, 60]. Another example of how imaging can be used for patient phenotyping is the use of machine learning to evaluate cardiac MRI changes of right ventricle (RV) failure in pulmonary hypertension, as work has demonstrated that patients with loss of effective contraction in the septum and free wall of the RV, along with reduced basal longitudinal motion, have worse RV failure. The combination of these cardiac MRI findings with traditional clinical characteristics and hemodynamics led to improved survival prediction and showed better separation of median survival between high- and low-risk groups [61]. Therefore, imaging integration with clinical characteristics improves patient identification and outcome prediction.

Phenotyping in Pulmonary, Critical Care, and Sleep Medicine

Phenotyping of pulmonary, critical care, and sleep-related conditions has become intertwined with the search for omics and imaging-based biomarkers. Although progress in phenotyping is made possible by the identification of biomarkers, the identification of biomarkers is made easier when distinct phenotypes of people are captured. Thus, phenotyping using clinical data and approaches besides high-throughput omics and imaging techniques remains relevant in precision medicine. The challenge of disease heterogeneity was salient for the complex conditions described, including IPF, COPD, sepsis, and acute respiratory distress syndrome (ARDS). The combination of deep phenotyping and identification of molecular profiles that characterize pathophysiologically heterogeneous conditions is currently the best approach to drug discovery. For example, the use of blood eosinophil count is a promising predictive biomarker of clinical response to inhaled corticosteroids in COPD [62–64]. Much work remains in the identification of more specific biomarkers and therapies for COPD and other diseases, as

can be gleaned from the chapters focused on complex respiratory conditions.

Sepsis and ARDS each cause substantial morbidity and mortality, and precision medicine approaches are sorely needed to improve outcomes related to them. Their study is challenged not only by disease heterogeneity but also by the fact that the entire course of disease is measured in days to weeks rather than months to years. Promising results from large-scale gene expression and targeted proteomics plasma studies suggest that biologically distinct patterns of expression may identify differential response to routine treatments applied in the intensive care unit (ICU). In sepsis, a gene expression signature with dysregulated adaptive immune signaling has evidence for a differential response to systemic steroid therapy [65, 66], whereas in ARDS, a hyperinflammatory pattern identified in plasma using targeted proteomics was favorably associated with randomized interventions including high positive end-expiratory pressure, volume conservative fluid therapy, and simvastatin therapy [67–70]. In the case of pulmonary arterial hypertension (PAH), a whole blood transcriptomic classifier led to the identification of a specific signature in vasodilator-responsive PAH that differentiates it from non-responsive PAH [71]. Replication of these critical care and PAH findings and the conduct of prospective studies evaluating expression signatures may lead to clinically useful results.

Sleep medicine is one of the most data-rich fields in medicine because of the increasing conduct of sleep studies that include remote collection of data from positive airway pressure (PAP) devices. The use of sophisticated analytical methods to identify distinct patterns of data captured during sleep has led to the characterization of distinct obstructive sleep apnea endotypes associated with adverse cardiovascular events [72]. Machine learning and computational tools [73, 74] are being further leveraged to develop better classification methods for various sleep disorders. These advances in phenotyping coupled to the discovery of biomarkers may yield striking changes in sleep precision medicine.

The Role of Sensors, Wearables and Health Information Technologies in Pulmonary, Critical Care, and Sleep Medicine

Along with efforts to capture molecular, imaging and phenotype data using traditional clinical and research approaches, precision medicine captures additional complementary data on the environment, behavior, patient-reported symptoms and outcomes, and medication use. The latter are made possible by advances in health information and sensor technologies, which have resulted in the creation of a wide range of mobile health (mHealth) platforms for disease self-management, research, and inclusion of novel data streams into provider-facing applications [75]. The use of these platforms has tremendous potential to benefit patients, providers, and the entire healthcare system although their documented clinical utility has not been established in most cases. While over 325,000 mobile applications (apps) are currently available, most are limited to providing information [76], and a relatively small proportion are dedicated to respiratory health. Functions provided by respiratory apps include medical education, messaging, diary logs, disease self-management, and educational games [77]. One of the largest mobile health tracking studies thus far was the Asthma Mobile Health Study. This project demonstrated the feasibility of using a mobile app to monitor asthma symptoms, but the lessons learned at study completion apply to most mobile health efforts: sustaining initial enthusiasm of an app is very difficult, there is selection bias in those enrolling and providing information, and data security concerns limit some subjects' willingness to share data [78]. Wearables, devices worn on the body to track bodily functions, have become a part of daily life. Most wearables are worn on a wrist or chest with functions that include tracking exercise, weight loss, sleep, and coping with stress [79]. Incorporating wearable data into respiratory studies may be an effective way to capture additional subject data to aid in phenotyping. Use of these technologies is still in the early stages, and despite some early progress, several barriers must

be overcome before mHealth is widely adopted and recommended by healthcare providers.

Concern for pollution's effect on health and broad demand for accessible environmental monitoring have led researchers and manufacturers to develop a number of low-cost, portable pollution sensors that are able to capture increasingly finer-scaled geographic differences in pollution. Such sensors broaden the scope of environmental studies that are possible: rather than rely on measures taken by regulatory monitors that are not able to account for the spatial and temporal heterogeneity of personal exposures, we are nearly able to measure individual exposure profiles. Although pollution measurements taken with low-cost sensors are less accurate and reliable than reference monitors, several studies have shown the feasibility and validity of using them to capture air pollution information across an area by deploying sensors in fixed-location networks, attaching them to vehicles, placing them in indoor spaces, and having people wear them to monitor personal exposures [80–82]. Ultimately, capturing personal exposure measures and integrating them into health monitoring tools will lead to improved precision medicine.

Precision Therapies in Pulmonary, Critical Care, and Sleep Medicine

In parallel to the advances in genomics, biomarkers, and phenotyping, therapeutics have improved by specific knowledge of underlying molecular changes associated with distinct diseases. Of pulmonary diseases, precision medicine advances are most notable in lung cancer, for which, as mentioned above, some so-called driver mutations can be targeted with specific chemotherapeutic agents. The demonstration that patients with NSCLC with activating mutations in EGFR could be successfully treated with the tyrosine kinase inhibitor gefitinib [83], led to the search for other specific mutations in NSCLC that could be drug targets. The subsequent identification of ALK and development of ALK inhibitors [84], as well as many other oncogenic drivers, has been associated with improved outcomes in lung cancer over the last 15 years [85]. Efforts to identify driver mutations in lung cancer continue, and greater personalized approaches to cancer therapy will result from an improved understanding of lung tumor evolution, by allowing physicians to anticipate which lung tumors will develop resistance to chemotherapeutic agents and which lung tumors have a propensity to recur or metastasize. Cystic fibrosis has also made significant advances in targeted therapies. The development of cystic fibrosis transmembrane conductance regulator (CFTR) modulators that correct for specific deficiencies in the CFTR channel [86–88] are a first generation of drugs that can potentially transform this devastating disease. Advances in lung cancer and cystic fibrosis offer hope that other domains of pulmonary, critical care, and sleep medicine may soon have precise therapeutics, based on knowledge of specific molecular changes that characterize diseases.

Lung transplantation, used as a rescue therapy for patients with advanced lung disease, requires close monitoring to identify allograft rejection. Identification of allograft rejection is currently based on clinical signs and invasive procedures, such as lung biopsy, and thus, novel methods to improve detection of allograft rejection would greatly improve care of patients after transplantation. A promising non-invasive approach to identify early rejection may be the quantification of donor-derived cell-free DNA, as a study demonstrated that subjects with average levels in the upper tertile had a 6.6-fold higher risk of developing allograft failure [89]. This and other biomarker studies may soon improve management of immunosuppression.

Mechanical ventilation is a life-saving intervention used to treat patients in the ICU that requires immediate attention to patient tolerance and real-time adjustments to minimize the risk of ventilator-induced injury and ventilator dyssynchrony [90]. Thus, mechanical ventilation is one of the most important practices in the ICU that is personalized to maximize the benefit of physiologic support while avoiding harm to patients. The sophisticated design of modern ventilators has enabled safer practice of telemedicine in the

ICU by allowing clinicians to evaluate patients remotely through video streams. Tele-ICU practices have also facilitated the redesign of care processes to improve outcomes in critical care [91], a demonstration of the power of thoughtful design of clinical interventions that use telemedicine.

Cigarette smoking is a key risk factor for multiple pulmonary diseases, particularly COPD and lung cancer. Consequently, smoking cessation is an essential intervention in clinical practice. Despite evidence of increased interest in quitting smoking over the past few decades (49.2% in 2000 versus 55.4% in 2015), successful quitting happens in less than 10% of smokers in the United States according to the Centers for Disease Control and Prevention [92]. Although these outcomes are multifactorial, pharmacogenetics of nicotine plays a role. Both GWAS and candidate gene studies have identified loci associated with response to smoking cessation agents. Specifically, there is evidence that polymorphisms in cytochrome genes (*CYP2A6*, *CYP2B6*), which are involved in nicotine metabolism, and cholinergic receptors (*CHRNA3*, *CHRNA4*, *CHRNA5*, *CHRNB4*) are associated with nicotine replacement therapy outcomes [93, 94]. Pharmacogenomic profiling may thus serve as an adjunctive measure in the selection of smoking cessation strategies [94].

Ongoing and Future Efforts in Pulmonary, Critical Care, and Sleep Precision Medicine

Several large studies are underway to identify endotypes for various pulmonary, critical care, and sleep conditions. A notable initiative aimed at driving precision medicine is the U.S. National Heart, Lung, and Blood Institute (NHLBI)'s Trans-Omics for Precision Medicine (TOPMed) Program. The early phase of this program included the generation of whole-genome sequencing data for patients with well-defined clinical phenotypes and outcomes from earlier NHLBI-funded studies [95]. As the program has continued, the subjects sequenced are increasingly diverse and various layers of omics data are being incorporated. Results from TOPMed are expected to lay a foundation for precision medicine to substantially improve in several complex respiratory diseases.

As noted in the chapter on Precision Medicine for All, an important limitation of precision medicine now is the lack of information on minority populations [96]. For example, despite significant advances in the understanding of the human genome and decreased sequencing costs, only 22% of GWAS participants are non-European [97]. Because some observed racial/ethnic and sex disparities in respiratory disease prevalence and severity may have a genetic basis, genetics and other omics studies must include diverse groups to inform precision medicine efforts. In addition to this issue being addressed by large studies such as TOPMed, individual researchers and healthcare providers need to be aware of the limitations of precision medicine approaches that result from studies based on non-diverse populations.

Translating genetic associations to disease understanding remains a major challenge, as the number of loci obtained via GWAS and next-generation sequencing studies outpaces the ability of functional studies to identify biological mechanisms. Factors that contribute to the slow translation include: 1) the time-consuming nature of functional studies given the need to tailor experiments to a particular complex disease phenotype and type of polymorphisms in a genomic region; 2) in order to test genes and variants for function, complex diseases have to be simplified into assays that may not capture the cell-specific, developmental, or environmental context necessary for functional elucidation of gene/variant function; and 3) several loci of interest are in gene deserts or genes with no annotated function, making the design of functional experiments even more difficult. Ongoing efforts to identify cell types using single-cell methods for expression, protein, and other molecular quantitative trait loci (e.g., splicing, histone modification) across various conditions and using high-throughput assays to annotate variant effects [98] will increase our understanding of genetic asso-

ciations. Some of these issues extend to other biomarkers even though they are "closer to phenotype" than genetic variants.

Beyond validating the accuracy of biomarkers, key issues related to their widespread use are establishing their practicality, availability, and cost-effectiveness [99]. Non-invasive biomarkers are more practical for clinical use than invasive ones [100], and thus, finding biomarkers in readily obtained bio-samples to represent more invasive ones may be a necessary step for some conditions such as fibrotic lung diseases. As stated in the chapter on Implementing COPD Precision Medicine in Clinical Practice, the fact that clinically valuable COPD genetic findings related to AATD are not yet readily adopted in clinical practice, raises an important consideration for implementation of genetic findings. Education and advances in regulatory processes are critical if we want to witness the full promise of precision medicine.

For precision medicine to thrive, current and future trainees in the specialty need to be aware of the principles of precision medicine, how these influence our current understanding of disease biology, diagnostics and therapeutics, and how they will transform pulmonary, critical care, and sleep medicine. Education in precision medicine cannot be overlooked and needs to be incorporated in fellowship training curricula, as well as educational conferences. The chapter on education for the practice of precision medicine expounds these ideas and provides guidance on a path forward.

Conclusion

Precision medicine is advancing with the availability and improvement of high-throughput assays for various types of biological data, imaging, sensors, data science and computing. Some rare pulmonary diseases and lung cancer already have personalized therapies available, while most complex respiratory, critical care, and sleep conditions are in the early stages of precision medicine. The study of highly heterogeneous diseases with large and deeply phenotyped cohorts is leading to the discovery of genetic and other molecular biomarkers that underlie distinct phenotypes. As early examples show, the identification of reproducible endotypes that leverage a broad range of data for each person leads to a better understanding of disease pathobiology, thereby enabling successful preventive strategies and novel drug discovery. The widespread implementation of precision medicine will require inclusion of diverse individuals in research and clinical studies, consideration of cost-effectiveness of novel interventions, and improved education of healthcare providers.

References

1. Nogee LM. Genetic causes of surfactant protein abnormalities. Curr Opin Pediatr. 2019;31(3):330–9.
2. Tsui JL, Estrada OA, Deng Z, et al. Analysis of pulmonary features and treatment approaches in the COPA syndrome. ERJ Open Res [Internet]. 2018;4(2). Available from: https://doi.org/10.1183/23120541.00017-2018.
3. Trapnell BC, Nakata K, Bonella F, et al. Pulmonary alveolar proteinosis. Nat Rev Dis Primers. 2019;5(1):16.
4. Gupta N, Vassallo R, Wikenheiser-Brokamp KA, McCormack FX. Diffuse cystic lung disease. Part I. Am J Respir Crit Care Med. 2015;191(12):1354–66.
5. Torres-Durán M, Lopez-Campos JL, Barrecheguren M, et al. Alpha-1 antitrypsin deficiency: outstanding questions and future directions. Orphanet J Rare Dis. 2018;13(1):114.
6. Schwentner R, Kolenová A, Jug G, et al. Longitudinal assessment of peripheral blood BRAFV600E levels in patients with Langerhans cell histiocytosis [Internet]. Pediatr Res. 2019;85(6):856–64. Available from: https://doi.org/10.1038/s41390-018-0238-y.
7. Richards S, Aziz N, Bale S, et al. Standards and guidelines for the interpretation of sequence variants: a joint consensus recommendation of the American College of Medical Genetics and Genomics and the Association for Molecular Pathology. Genet Med. 2015;17(5):405.
8. Might M, Wilsey M. The shifting model in clinical diagnostics: how next-generation sequencing and families are altering the way rare diseases are discovered, studied, and treated. Genet Med. 2014;16(10):736–7.
9. Raghu G, Remy-Jardin M, Myers JL, et al. Diagnosis of idiopathic pulmonary fibrosis. An official ATS/ERS/JRS/ALAT clinical practice guideline [Internet]. Am J Respir Crit Care Med. 2018;198(5):e44–68. Available from: https://doi.org/10.1164/rccm.201807-1255st.
10. Nogee LM, Dunbar AE, Wert SE, Askin F, Hamvas A, Whitsett JA. A mutation in the surfactant protein C gene associated with familial interstitial lung disease [Internet]. N Engl J Med. 2001;344(8):573–9. Available from: https://doi.org/10.1056/nejm200102223440805.
11. Kropski JA, Pritchett JM, Zoz DF, et al. Extensive phenotyping of individuals at risk for familial interstitial pneumonia reveals clues to the pathogenesis of interstitial lung disease. Am J Respir Crit Care Med. 2015;191(4):417–26.
12. Wang Y, Kuan PJ, Xing C, et al. Genetic defects in surfactant protein A2 are associated with pulmonary fibrosis and lung cancer. Am J Hum Genet. 2009;84(1):52–9.
13. Borie R, Tabèze L, Thabut G, et al. Prevalence and characteristics of TERT and TERC mutations in suspected genetic pulmonary fibrosis. Eur Respir J. 2016;48(6):1721–31.
14. Seibold MA, Wise AL, Speer MC, et al. A common MUC5B promoter polymorphism and pulmonary fibrosis. N Engl J Med. 2011;364(16):1503–12.
15. Roy MG, Livraghi-Butrico A, Fletcher AA, et al. Muc5b is required for airway defence. Nature. 2014;505(7483):412–6.
16. Mathai SK, Yang IV, Schwarz MI, Schwartz DA. Incorporating genetics into the identification and treatment of idiopathic pulmonary fibrosis. BMC Med. 2015;13:191.
17. Sakornsakolpat P, Prokopenko D, Lamontagne M, et al. Genetic landscape of chronic obstructive pulmonary disease identifies heterogeneous cell-type and phenotype associations. Nat Genet. 2019;51(3):494–505.
18. American Thoracic Society, European Respiratory Society. American Thoracic Society/European Respiratory Society statement: standards for the diagnosis and management of individuals with alpha-1 antitrypsin deficiency. Am J Respir Crit Care Med. 2003;168(7):818–900.
19. Moffatt MF, Gut IG, Demenais F, et al. A large-scale, consortium-based genomewide association study of asthma. N Engl J Med. 2010;363(13):1211–21.
20. Torgerson DG, Ampleford EJ, Chiu GY, et al. Meta-analysis of genome-wide association studies of asthma in ethnically diverse North American populations. Nat Genet. 2011;43(9):887–92.
21. Demenais F, Margaritte-Jeannin P, Barnes KC, et al. Multiancestry association study identifies new asthma risk loci that colocalize with immune-cell enhancer marks. Nat Genet. 2018;50(1):42–53.
22. Miller M, Rosenthal P, Beppu A, et al. ORMDL3 transgenic mice have increased airway remodeling and airway responsiveness characteristic of asthma. J Immunol. 2014;192(8):3475–87.
23. Das S, Miller M, Beppu AK, et al. GSDMB induces an asthma phenotype characterized by increased airway responsiveness and remodeling without lung inflammation. Proc Natl Acad Sci U S A. 2016;113(46):13132–7.

24. Panganiban RA, Sun M, Dahlin A, et al. A functional splice variant associated with decreased asthma risk abolishes the ability of gasdermin B to induce epithelial cell pyroptosis. J Allergy Clin Immunol. 2018;142(5):1469–78.e2.

25. Alberg AJ, Samet JM. Epidemiology of lung cancer. Chest. 2003;123(1 Suppl):21S–49S.

26. Molina JR, Yang P, Cassivi SD, Schild SE, Adjei AA. Non-small cell lung cancer: epidemiology, risk factors, treatment, and survivorship. Mayo Clin Proc. 2008;83(5):584–94.

27. Ai X, Guo X, Wang J, et al. Targeted therapies for advanced non-small cell lung cancer. Oncotarget. 2018;9(101):37589–607.

28. Mayekar MK, Bivona TG. Current landscape of targeted therapy in lung cancer. Clin Pharmacol Ther. 2017;102(5):757–64.

29. Meyerson M, Gabriel S, Getz G. Advances in understanding cancer genomes through second-generation sequencing. Nat Rev Genet. 2010;11(10):685–96.

30. Pleasance ED, Stephens PJ, O'Meara S, et al. A small-cell lung cancer genome with complex signatures of tobacco exposure. Nature. 2010;463(7278):184–90.

31. Byers LA, Rudin CM. Small cell lung cancer: where do we go from here? Cancer. 2015;121(5):664–72.

32. Nielsen AO, Jensen CS, Arredouani MS, Dahl R, Dahl M. Variants of the ADRB2 gene in COPD: systematic review and meta-analyses of disease risk and treatment response. COPD. 2017;14(4):451–60.

33. Slob EMA, Vijverberg SJH, Palmer CNA, et al. Pharmacogenetics of inhaled long-acting beta2-agonists in asthma: a systematic review. Pediatr Allergy Immunol. 2018;29(7):705–14.

34. Himes BE, Jiang X, Hu R, et al. Genome-wide association analysis in asthma subjects identifies SPATS2L as a novel bronchodilator response gene. PLoS Genet. 2012;8(7):e1002824.

35. Tantisira KG, Lasky-Su J, Harada M, et al. Genomewide association between GLCCI1 and response to glucocorticoid therapy in asthma [Internet]. N Engl J Med. 2011;365(13):1173–83. Available from: https://doi.org/10.1056/nejmoa0911353.

36. Mosteller M, Hosking L, Murphy K, et al. No evidence of large genetic effects on steroid response in asthma patients. J Allergy Clin Immunol. 2017;139(3):797–803.e7.

37. Schlaberg R, Queen K, Simmon K, et al. Viral pathogen detection by metagenomics and pan-viral group polymerase chain reaction in children with pneumonia lacking identifiable etiology. J Infect Dis. 2017;215(9):1407–15.

38. Charalampous T, Kay GL, Richardson H, et al. Nanopore metagenomics enables rapid clinical diagnosis of bacterial lower respiratory infection. Nat Biotechnol. 2019;37(7):783–92.

39. Blair JMA, Webber MA, Baylay AJ, Ogbolu DO, Piddock LJV. Molecular mechanisms of antibiotic resistance [Internet]. Nat Rev Microbiol. 2015;13(1):42–51. Available from: https://doi.org/10.1038/nrmicro3380.

40. Vedel-Krogh S, Nielsen SF, Lange P, Vestbo J, Nordestgaard BG. Blood eosinophils and exacerbations in chronic obstructive pulmonary disease. The Copenhagen general population study. Am J Respir Crit Care Med. 2016;193(9):965–74.

41. Bafadhel M, Greening NJ, Harvey-Dunstan TC, et al. Blood eosinophils and outcomes in severe hospitalized exacerbations of COPD [Internet]. Chest. 2016;150(2):320–8. Available from: https://doi.org/10.1016/j.chest.2016.01.026.

42. Pavord ID, Korn S, Howarth P, et al. Mepolizumab for severe eosinophilic asthma (DREAM): a multicentre, double-blind, placebo-controlled trial. Lancet. 2012;380(9842):651–9.

43. Guilleminault L, Ouksel H, Belleguic C, et al. Personalised medicine in asthma: from curative to preventive medicine. Eur Respir Rev [Internet]. 2017;26(143). Available from: https://doi.org/10.1183/16000617.0010-2016.

44. Berry A, Busse WW. Biomarkers in asthmatic patients: has their time come to direct treatment? J Allergy Clin Immunol. 2016;137(5):1317–24.

45. Miller BE, Tal-Singer R, Rennard SI, et al. Plasma fibrinogen qualification as a drug development tool in chronic obstructive pulmonary disease. Perspective of the chronic obstructive pulmonary disease biomarker qualification consortium [Internet]. Am J Respir Crit Care Med. 2016;193(6):607–13. Available from: https://doi.org/10.1164/rccm.201509-1722pp.

46. Ley B, Brown KK, Collard HR. Molecular biomarkers in idiopathic pulmonary fibrosis. Am J Physiol Lung Cell Mol Physiol. 2014;307(9):L681–91.

47. Takahashi H, Fujishima T, Koba H, et al. Serum surfactant proteins A and D as prognostic factors in idiopathic pulmonary fibrosis and their relationship to disease extent. Am J Respir Crit Care Med. 2000;162(3 Pt 1):1109–14.

48. Nathan N, Giraud V, Picard C, et al. Germline SFTPA1 mutation in familial idiopathic interstitial pneumonia and lung cancer. Hum Mol Genet. 2016;25(8):1457–67.

49. Naikawadi RP, Disayabutr S, Mallavia B, et al. Telomere dysfunction in alveolar epithelial cells causes lung remodeling and fibrosis. JCI Insight. 2016;1(14):e86704.

50. Armanios MY, Chen JJ-L, Cogan JD, et al. Telomerase mutations in families with idiopathic pulmonary fibrosis. N Engl J Med. 2007;356(13):1317–26.

51. Tsakiri KD, Cronkhite JT, Kuan PJ, et al. Adult-onset pulmonary fibrosis caused by mutations in telomerase. Proc Natl Acad Sci U S A. 2007;104(18):7552–7.

52. Rosas IO, Richards TJ, Konishi K, et al. MMP1 and MMP7 as potential peripheral blood biomarkers in idiopathic pulmonary fibrosis. PLoS Med. 2008;5(4):e93.

53. Bauer Y, White ES, de Bernard S, et al. MMP-7 is a predictive biomarker of disease progression in patients with idiopathic pulmonary fibrosis. ERJ Open Res [Internet]. 2017;3(1). Available from: https://doi.org/10.1183/23120541.00074-2016.

54. Tzouvelekis A, Herazo-Maya JD, Slade M, et al. Validation of the prognostic value of MMP-7 in idiopathic pulmonary fibrosis [Internet]. Respirology. 2017;22(3):486–93. Available from: https://doi.org/10.1111/resp.12920.

55. Richards TJ, Kaminski N, Baribaud F, et al. Peripheral blood proteins predict mortality in idiopathic pulmonary fibrosis. Am J Respir Crit Care Med. 2012;185(1):67–76.

56. White ES, Xia M, Murray S, et al. Plasma surfactant protein-D, matrix metalloproteinase-7, and osteopontin index distinguishes idiopathic pulmonary fibrosis from other idiopathic interstitial pneumonias [Internet]. Am J Respir Crit Care Med. 2016;194(10):1242–51. Available from: https://doi.org/10.1164/rccm.201505-0862oc.

57. O'Connor JPB, Aboagye EO, Adams JE, et al. Imaging biomarker roadmap for cancer studies. Nat Rev Clin Oncol. 2017;14(3):169–86.

58. Washko GR, Parraga G. COPD biomarkers and phenotypes: opportunities for better outcomes with precision imaging. Eur Respir J [Internet]. 2018;52(5). Available from: https://doi.org/10.1183/13993003.01570-2018.

59. Sack CS, Doney BC, Podolanczuk AJ, et al. Occupational exposures and subclinical interstitial lung disease. The MESA (multi-ethnic study of atherosclerosis) air and lung studies. Am J Respir Crit Care Med. 2017;196(8):1031–9.

60. Washko GR, Hunninghake GM, Fernandez IE, et al. Lung volumes and emphysema in smokers with interstitial lung abnormalities. N Engl J Med. 2011;364(10):897–906.

61. Dawes TJW, de Marvao A, Shi W, et al. Machine learning of three-dimensional right ventricular motion enables outcome prediction in pulmonary hypertension: a cardiac MR imaging study. Radiology. 2017;283(2):381–90.

62. Siddiqui SH, Guasconi A, Vestbo J, et al. Blood eosinophils: a biomarker of response to extrafine beclomethasone/formoterol in chronic obstructive pulmonary disease. Am J Respir Crit Care Med. 2015;192(4):523–5.

63. Pavord ID, Lettis S, Locantore N, et al. Blood eosinophils and inhaled corticosteroid/long-acting β-2 agonist efficacy in COPD. Thorax. 2016;71(2):118–25.

64. Pascoe S, Locantore N, Dransfield MT, Barnes NC, Pavord ID. Blood eosinophil counts, exacerbations, and response to the addition of inhaled fluticasone furoate to vilanterol in patients with chronic obstructive pulmonary disease: a secondary analysis of data from two parallel randomised controlled trials. Lancet Respir Med. 2015;3(6):435–42.

65. Scicluna BP, van Vught LA, Zwinderman AH, et al. Classification of patients with sepsis according to blood genomic endotype: a prospective cohort study. Lancet Respir Med. 2017;5(10):816–26.

66. Antcliffe DB, Burnham KL, Al-Beidh F, et al. Transcriptomic signatures in sepsis and a differential response to steroids. From the VANISH randomized trial. Am J Respir Crit Care Med. 2019;199(8):980–6.

67. Calfee CS, Delucchi K, Parsons PE, et al. Subphenotypes in acute respiratory distress syndrome: latent class analysis of data from two randomised controlled trials. Lancet Respir Med. 2014;2(8):611–20.

68. Famous KR, Delucchi K, Ware LB, et al. Acute respiratory distress syndrome subphenotypes respond differently to randomized fluid management strategy. Am J Respir Crit Care Med. 2017;195(3):331–8.

69. Calfee CS, Delucchi KL, Sinha P, et al. Acute respiratory distress syndrome subphenotypes and differential response to simvastatin: secondary analysis of a randomised controlled trial. Lancet Respir Med. 2018;6(9):691–8.

70. Sinha P, Delucchi KL, Thompson BT, et al. Latent class analysis of ARDS subphenotypes: a secondary analysis of the statins for acutely injured lungs from sepsis (SAILS) study. Intensive Care Med. 2018;44(11):1859–69.

71. Hemnes AR, Trammell AW, Archer SL, et al. Peripheral blood signature of vasodilator-responsive pulmonary arterial hypertension. Circulation. 2015;131(4):401–9; discussion 409.

72. Zinchuk AV, Jeon S, Koo BB, et al. Polysomnographic phenotypes and their cardiovascular implications in obstructive sleep apnoea. Thorax. 2018;73(5):472–80.

73. Malafeev A, Laptev D, Bauer S, et al. Automatic human sleep stage scoring using deep neural networks. Front Neurosci. 2018;12:781.

74. Willetts M, Hollowell S, Aslett L, Holmes C, Doherty A. Statistical machine learning of sleep and physical activity phenotypes from sensor data in 96,220 UK biobank participants. Sci Rep. 2018;8(1):7961.

75. Himes BE, Weitzman ER. Innovations in health information technologies for chronic pulmonary diseases. Respir Res. 2016;17:38.

76. research2guidance. mHealth economics 2017 report: status and trends in digital health | R2G [Internet]. [cited 2019 Jul 16]. Available from: https://research2guidance.com/product/mhealth-economics-2017-current-status-and-future-trends-in-mobile-health/.

77. Wu AC, Carpenter JF, Himes BE. Mobile health applications for asthma. J Allergy Clin Immunol Pract. 2015;3(3):446–8.e1–16.

78. Chan Y-FY, Wang P, Rogers L, et al. The asthma mobile health study, a large-scale clinical observational study using ResearchKit. Nat Biotechnol. 2017;35(4):354–62.

79. Rock Health. Healthcare consumers in a digital transition | Rock Health [Internet]. [cited 2019 Jul 8]. Available from: https://rockhealth.com/reports/healthcare-consumers-in-a-digital-transition/.

80. Alexeeff SE, Roy A, Shan J, et al. High-resolution mapping of traffic related air pollution with Google street view cars and incidence of cardiovascular events within neighborhoods in Oakland, CA. Environ Health. 2018;17(1):38.

81. Niedzwiecki MM, Walker DI, Vermeulen R, Chadeau-Hyam M, Jones DP, Miller GW. The exposome: molecules to populations. Annu Rev Pharmacol Toxicol. 2019;59:107–27.

82. Agache I, Miller R, Gern JE, et al. Emerging concepts and challenges in implementing the exposome paradigm in allergic diseases and asthma: a Practall document. Allergy. 2019;74(3):449–63.

83. Lynch TJ, Bell DW, Sordella R, et al. Activating mutations in the epidermal growth factor receptor underlying responsiveness of non–small-cell lung cancer to gefitinib. N Engl J Med. 2004;350(21):2129–39.

84. Kwak EL, Bang Y-J, Camidge DR, et al. Anaplastic lymphoma kinase inhibition in non–small-cell lung cancer. N Engl J Med. 2010;363(18):1693–703.

85. Politi K, Herbst RS. Lung cancer in the era of precision medicine. Clin Cancer Res. 2015;21(10):2213–20.

86. Ramsey BW, Davies J, McElvaney NG, et al. A CFTR potentiator in patients with cystic fibrosis and the G551D mutation. N Engl J Med. 2011;365(18):1663–72.

87. Taylor-Cousar JL, Munck A, McKone EF, et al. Tezacaftor-ivacaftor in patients with cystic fibrosis homozygous for Phe508del. N Engl J Med. 2017;377(21):2013–23.

88. Rowe SM, Daines C, Ringshausen FC, et al. Tezacaftor-ivacaftor in residual-function heterozygotes with cystic fibrosis. N Engl J Med. 2017;377(21):2024–35.

89. Agbor-Enoh S, Wang Y, Tunc I, et al. Donor-derived cell-free DNA predicts allograft failure and mortality after lung transplantation. EBioMedicine. 2019;40:541–53.

90. Subira C, de Haro C, Magrans R, Fernández R, Blanch L. Minimizing asynchronies in mechanical ventilation: current and future trends. Respir Care. 2018;63(4):464–78.

91. Lilly CM, Cody S, Zhao H, et al. Hospital mortality, length of stay, and preventable complications among critically ill patients before and after tele-ICU reengineering of critical care processes. JAMA. 2011;305(21):2175–83.

92. Babb S, Malarcher A, Schauer G, Asman K, Jamal A. Quitting smoking among adults - United States, 2000-2015. MMWR Morb Mortal Wkly Rep. 2017;65(52):1457–64.

93. Salloum NC, Buchalter ELF, Chanani S, et al. From genes to treatments: a systematic review of the pharmacogenetics in smoking cessation. Pharmacogenomics. 2018;19(10):861–71.

94. Chenoweth MJ, Tyndale RF. Pharmacogenetic optimization of smoking cessation treatment. Trends Pharmacol Sci. 2017;38(1):55–66.

95. National Heart, Lung, and Blood Institute (NHLBI). Trans-omics for precision medicine (TOPMed) Program [Internet]. [cited 2019 Jul 14]. Available from: https://www.nhlbi.nih.gov/science/trans-omics-precision-medicine-topmed-program.

96. Guglielmi G. Facing up to injustice in genome science [Internet]. Nature. 2019;568(7752):290–3. Available from: https://doi.org/10.1038/d41586-019-01166-x.

97. Gurdasani D, Barroso I, Zeggini E, Sandhu MS. Genomics of disease risk in globally diverse populations. Nat Rev Genet [Internet]. 2019. Available from: https://doi.org/10.1038/s41576-019-0144-0.

98. Starita LM, Ahituv N, Dunham MJ, et al. Variant interpretation: functional assays to the rescue. Am J Hum Genet. 2017;101(3):315–25.

99. Wu AC, Kiley JP, Noel PJ, et al. Current status and future opportunities in lung precision medicine research with a focus on biomarkers. An American thoracic society/national heart, lung, and blood institute research statement. Am J Respir Crit Care Med. 2018;198(12):e116–36.

100. Kim H, Ellis AK, Fischer D, et al. Asthma biomarkers in the age of biologics. Allergy Asthma Clin Immunol. 2017;13:48.

Index

A

Activated protein C therapy, 194
Active *Mycobacterium tuberculosis* (MTb) infection, 171, 172
Acute coronary syndromes, 185
acute exacerbation of COPD (AECOPD), 138, 141
Acute lung allograft dysfunction, 340–343
Acute lung allograft rejection, 342
Acute lung injury (ALI), 186
Acute Physiologic and Chronic Health Evaluation II (APACHE II), 323
Acute respiratory distress syndrome (ARDS), 267, 268, 340
    complex, non-Mendelian traits, genetic approaches, 269, 270
    critical care, precision medicine in, 272–274
    defining feature, 192
    definition, 186
    gene expression studies in, 279, 280
    genetics and search for causal intermediates, 275–277
    knowledge- and discovery-based genomics studies, 270–272
    P/F ratio, 187
    metabolomics studies in, 280, 281
    mortality, 191
    prognostic biomarkers
        critical illness, 192, 193
        estimation of extravascular lung water, 192
        heterogeneous treatment responses, 192
        hypothesis-based biomarkers, 191
        immunosuppression phenotype, 191
        metabolomics approaches, 192
        PERSEVERE and updated PERSEVERE XP platforms, 191
        proteomic approaches, 191
        pulmonary vascular permeability index, 192
        survival, 191
        transcriptomic profiling, 191
    targeted proteomics, 268–270
    theranostic biomarkers, 193, 194
Adrenoceptor Beta 2 (*ADRB2*), 419
African ancestry, 396
Air pollution, 305, 306

Air Quality Sensor Performance Evaluation Center (AQ-SPEC), 311
Airway clearance techniques, 59
Alcohol, 377
ALK gene's kinase domain, 93
Allele frequencies, of different COPD risk loci, 400, 402
Allergic diseases, 31
Allergic rhinitis, 31
Allergic-disease-associated loci, 31
Alpha-1 antitrypsin deficiency (A1AD), 18, 109, 137, 233–234, 414
Alveolar epithelial type II (AEC II) cells, 158
Alveolar overdistension, 355
Alveolar pentraxin 3 (PTX3), 176
Alveolar type II (AT2) cell homeostasis, 14
Alveolo-capillary barrier, 192
Anaplastic lymphoma kinase (*ALK*) fusion mutation, 93–94
Anaplastic lymphoma kinase (ALK) rearrangements, 208
Angiomyolipomas (AMLs), 16
Angiopoietin-2 (ANG2), 276
Annual direct contribution margin (ADCM), 327
Antibiotic prophylaxis, precision medicine in, 387, 388
Antimicrobial therapy, 186, 193
Anti-platelet therapy, 193
Anti-TNF-α monoclonal antibody therapy, 193
Apnea-hypopnea index (AHI), 258
Apoptosis, 158
Apparent heterogeneous response, 269
Aptamer-based assay, 250
Asthma
    asthma-associated loci, 27
    biologically informative endotype, 133
    biomarkers/therapeutic targets, 133
    blood eosinophil count heritability, 26
    bronchial constriction, 132
    bronchodilator and glucocorticoid medications, 25
    bronchodilator response heritability, 26
    characteristics, 26
    of childhood, 26
    clinical therapy, 26
    definition, 25
    endotypes, 26, 133